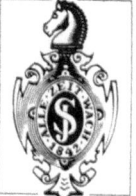

# ARTIFICIAL HEART 2

Proceedings of the 2nd International Symposium on Artificial Heart and Assist Device, August 13–14, 1987, Tokyo, Japan

Editor:
Tetsuzo Akutsu

Associate Editors:
Hitoshi Koyanagi, Setsuo Takatani, Kazunori Kataoka, Jack G. Copeland, Stuart L. Cooper, Peer M. Portner, David B. Geselowitz

Springer Japan KK

Tetsuzo Akutsu, M.D., Ph.D.
Vice-Director
National Cardiovascular Center
Research Institute
5-7-1 Fujishiro-dai
Suita, Osaka
565 Japan

ISBN 978-4-431-70544-4                    ISBN 978-4-431-65964-8 (eBook)
DOI 10.1007/978-4-431-65964-8

© Springer Japan 1988
Originally published by Springer-Verlag Tokyo Berlin Heidelberg New York London Paris in 1988
Softcover reprint of the hardcover 1st edition 1988

Publication of this proceedings was supported by the promotion fund of the Japan Keirin Association.

Typesetting: Asco Trade Typesetting Ltd., Hong Kong

## 2nd International Symposium on Artificial Heart & Assist Device
## August 13–14, 1987, Keidanren Kaikan, Tokyo, Japan

*Organized by*
Japan Research Promotion Society for Cardiovascular Diseases

*Sponsored by*
Ministry of Health and Welfare of Japan
Nihon Keizai Shimbun Inc.
Japanese Society for Artificial Organs
Japan Keirin Association

*Organizing Committee*
President: Hiroto Yoshioka
        (Japan Research Promotion Society for Cardiovascular Diseases)
Vice-President: Tetsuzo Akutsu
        (National Cardiovascular Center Research Institute)
Secretary General: Hitoshi Koyanagi
        (The Heart Institute of Japan, Tokyo Wemen's Medical College)

*Members*
Tetsuzo Akutsu (National Cardiovascular Center Research Institute)
Kenichi Asano (The Central Hospital Japanese National Railways)
Kazuhiko Atsumi (Institute for Medical Electronics, The University of Tokyo)
Koshichiro Hirosawa (The Heart Institute of Japan, Tokyo Wemen's Medical College)
Tadashi Inoue (Department of Surgery, Keio University)
Hitoshi Koyanagi (The Heart Institute of Japan, Tokyo Wemen's Medical College)
Hisao Manabe (National Cardiovascular Center)
Motoomi Nakamura (Research Institute of Angiocardiology, Kyushu University)
Yoshio Obunai (The Sakakibara Heart Institute)
Yasuhisa Sakurai (Institute of Biomedical Engineering, Tokyo Wemen's Medical College)
Atsuyoshi Takao (The Heart Institute of Japan, Tokyo Wemen's Medical College)
Kiichi Tsuchiya (School of Science and Engineering, Waseda University)

# Presidential Address

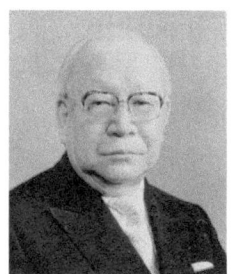

*President*
Hiroto Yoshioka

It is a great privilege for me to declare the 2nd International Symposium on Artificial Heart and Assist Devices open. As the president of the congress is at present incapacitated, in his stead I would like to deliver the opening address.

On behalf of the organizing committee and the Japan Research Promotion Society for Cardiovascular Diseases, I have the honor to extend a cordial welcome to each of the participants. First of all, I would like to thank them for their interest and efforts in helping to make this symposium possible; especial thanks go to the guests who have traveled here from the USA.

I would like to express my thanks to the Ministry of Health and Welfare of Japan, Nihon Keizai Shimbun (a newspaper company), and the Japanese Society for Artificial Organs for their kind assistance. Further, for financial support, we are greatly indebted to the Japan Keirin Association.

The Japan Research Promotion Society for Cardiovascular Diseases organized the Research Committee for the Development of Cardiac Assist Devices in 1982 and began equipping research facilities for the artificial heart in 1983. To promote progress in this field, we planned the 1st International Symposium on Artificial Heart and Assist Devices, which was held in August 1985. To this meeting, seven distinguished speakers from the USA and Europe were invited, who covered the areas of ventricular assist devices, total artificial hearts, and biomedical materials. About 200 participants from Japan contributed greatly to the academic sessions, which proved to be most informative and fruitful. The papers and discussions presented were reviewed repeatedly by the editorial board, and finally the proceedings of the first symposium, *Artificial Heart 1*, was published by Springer-Verlag Tokyo. This book achieved a worldwide distribution of 1000 copies and met with a positive critical reception.

I am certain that this second symposium will contribute greatly to the development of research in this field. I hope that the newest advances in this exciting and fast-moving area will lead to a third symposium with the assistance of the supporting organizations.

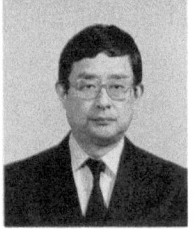

Hitoshi Koyanagi
Secretary General

# Greeting

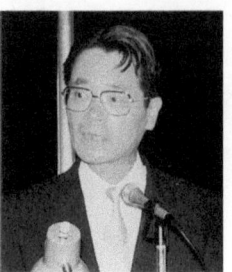

On behalf of the Ministry of Health and Welfare, it is a great honor to have been given this opportunity to say a few words at the opening of the 2nd International Symposium on Artificial Heart and Assist Devices.

As is widely known, the primary cause of death in Japan at present is cancer. In 1985, heart disease replaced cerebral apoplexy in the number two position. With the gradual aging of the population, I think that the importance of measures against cardiac diseases will become increasingly obvious.

Positive action has been taken in terms of primary care against heart disease including arteriosclerosis, and the results of this can now be seen. Following enormous efforts by doctors, the medical treatment of severe heart disease has improved remarkably. In Europe and the USA, in addition to transplantation, the clinical application of the artificial heart is showing rapid progress.

Japan has developed excellent techniques in the field of electronic devices and precision machines. We believe that the application and contribution of such techniques to the medical field, in other words, interdisciplinary research and development of an artificial heart can fulfil a very important role in the management of cardiovascular diseases, and thus we would like to give a positive support to all efforts made here.

It was against this background that the first international symposium was held 2 years ago, and its proceedings were published as *Artificial Heart 1*. This volume made a substantial contribution to worldwide research into the artificial heart. We are confident that with the present symposium research into the artificial heart will continue to make great strides and do much to increase health and welfare.

Kohji Takenaka
Director General of the
Health Policy Bureau,
the Ministry of
Health and Welfare

# Preface

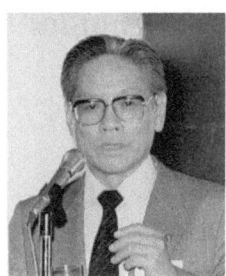

It is with great pleasure that we present here Artificial Heart 2 (Proceedings of the 2nd International Symposium on Artificial Heart and Assist Devices). The symposium was held in Tokyo on 13–14 August 1987 under the auspices of the Japan Research Promotion Society for Cardiovascular Diseases.

In the first symposium, also held in Tokyo, in 1985, seven distinguished investigators were invited from the USA and Europe. The symposium was divided into seven sessions according to the guest speakers' speciality. Following their presentations two designated researchers in Japan discussed the pertinent subject. This time, however, papers on the Japanese side were called for and selected by the program committee.

The subjects of the seven guest speakers, who were all from the USA, were as follows: 1) the second generation of ventricular assist devices (VAD) and total artificial hearts (TAH) under development, 2) clinical uses of VAD and TAH which include their applications as a bridge to heart transplantation and 3) biomaterials.

When considering the patients' quality of life with an implanted artificial heart, development of a totally implantable system including the energy source is essential. From the practical standpoint for clinical use, one way to solve the problems of heart replacement will be the cooperative use of artificial hearts and heart transplants. The concept of two-stage heart replacement introduced by Dr. D.A. Cooley in 1969 has now been widely accepted, and more than 100 clinical cases have been reported to date. Due to the shortage of donor hearts a strong demand for an artificial heart which can be used for years as a permanent system with guaranties in terms of safety and reliability has been increasing. To realise such a system, development of better materials is of prime importance.

The total number of VAD in clinical use in Japan is now over 100, and the results have been improving. To our regret, however, two-stage heart replacement is presently impossible in Japan since heart transplantation still may not be performed. In this respect we hope that a report by one group describing this topic as well as all the other exciting papers will be a good stimulant to us and will help us make further progress in this field in Japan.

Tetsuzo Akutsu

# Contributors

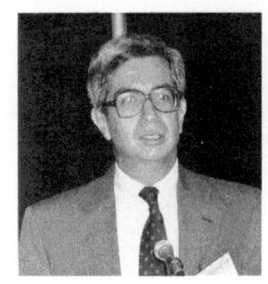
1. S.L. Cooper

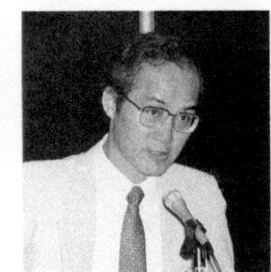
2. K. Hayashi

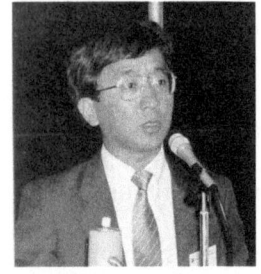
3. A. Takahara

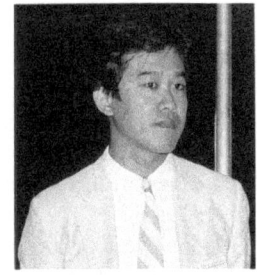
4. N. Yui

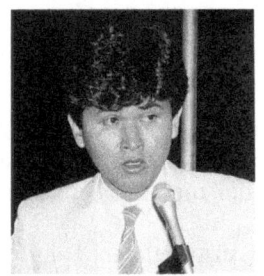
5. Y. Ito

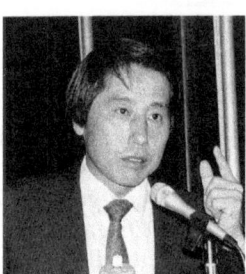
6. S.W. Kim

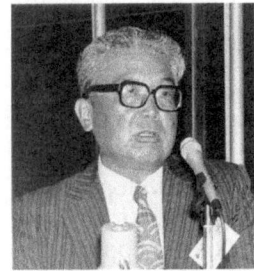
7. H. Miyama

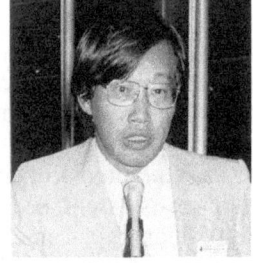
8. T. Matsuda

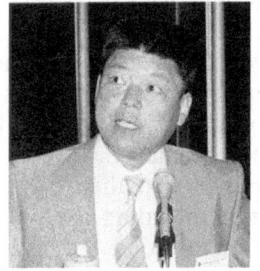
9. Y. Noishiki

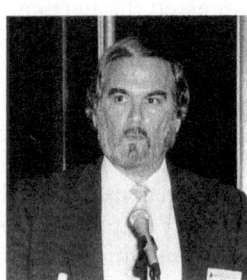
10. P.M. Portner

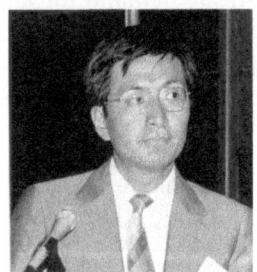
11. T. Nakamura

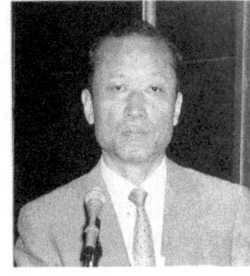
12. T. Akamatsu

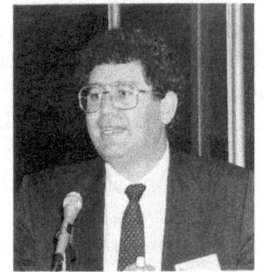
13. D.M. Lederman

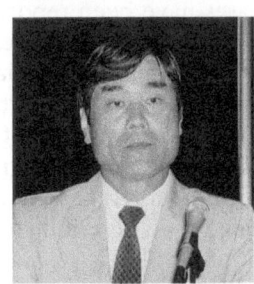
14. S. Nitta

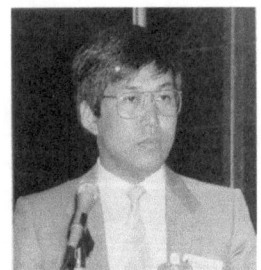
15. H. Irie

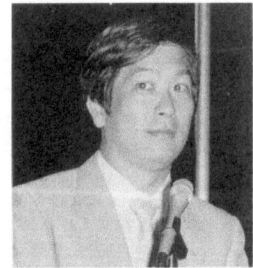
16. M. Umezu

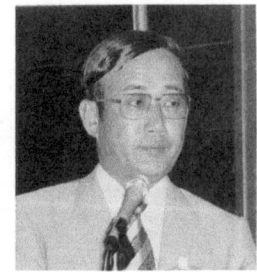
17. I. Yada

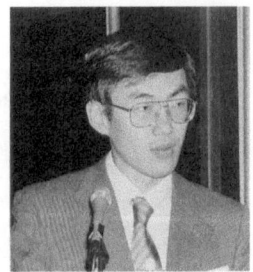
18. H. Adachi

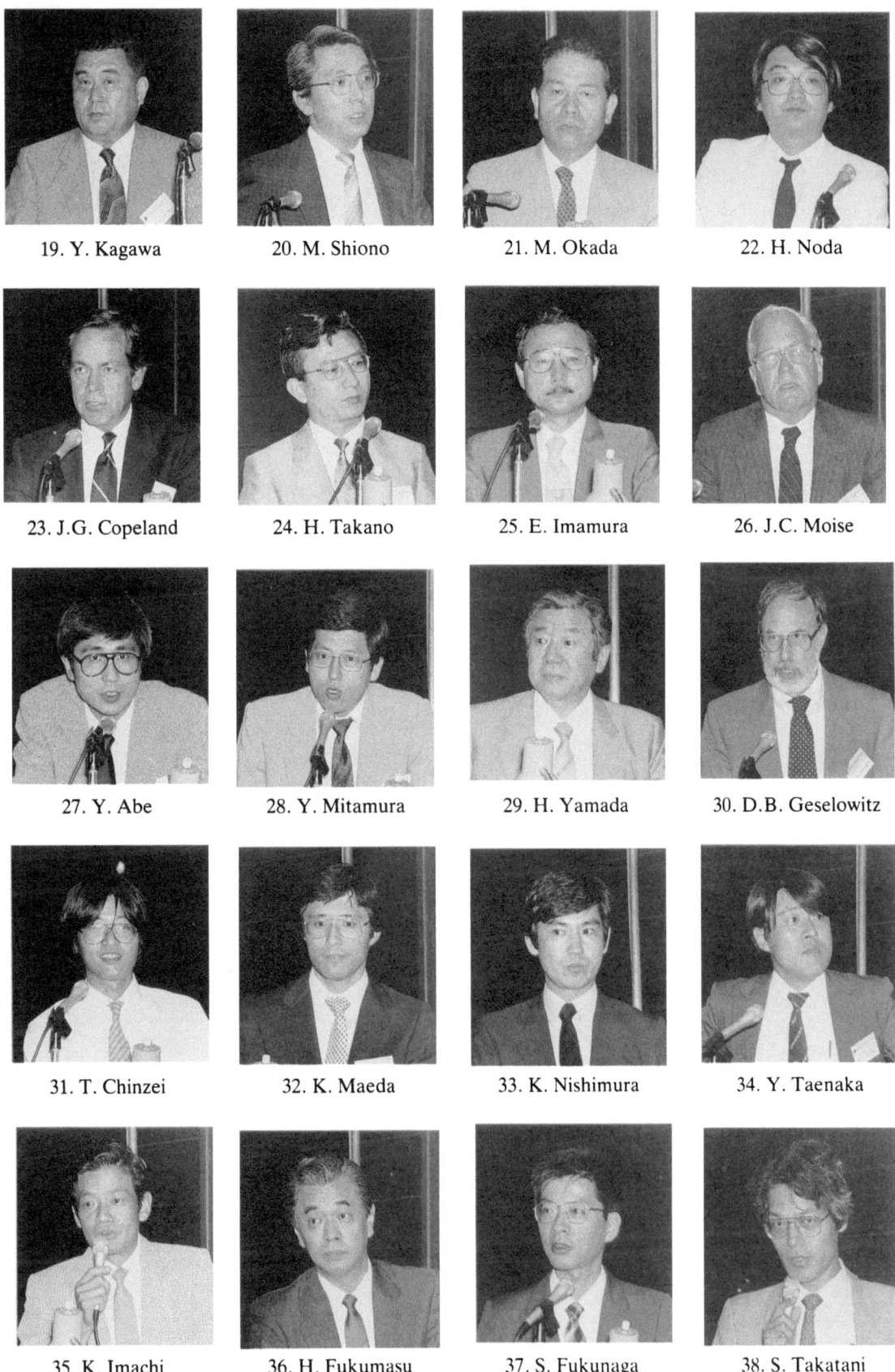

19. Y. Kagawa  20. M. Shiono  21. M. Okada  22. H. Noda

23. J.G. Copeland  24. H. Takano  25. E. Imamura  26. J.C. Moise

27. Y. Abe  28. Y. Mitamura  29. H. Yamada  30. D.B. Geselowitz

31. T. Chinzei  32. K. Maeda  33. K. Nishimura  34. Y. Taenaka

35. K. Imachi  36. H. Fukumasu  37. S. Fukunaga  38. S. Takatani

# Table of Contents

# Part I
# Biomaterials

# 1. Blood material interactions: Ex vivo investigations of polyurethanes

Stuart L. Cooper, Thomas A. Giroux, and Timothy G. Grasel[1]

**Summary.** A canine ex vivo series shunt was utilized to evaluate short-term blood compatibility of polyurethane block copolymers. The series shunt allows the evaluation of up to ten different materials simultaneously. Deposition of radiolabeled platelets and fibrinogen is quantified and used as a measure of thrombogenicity. The canine ex vivo experiment has been implemented in investigations of the roles of many aspects of polymer surface chemistry in platelet-surface and protein-surface interactions. This paper reviews some significant, recent results. The extent of microphase separation in polyurethane block copolymers has been found to affect surface properties and platelet-surface interactions. In addition, derivatization strategies for polyurethanes have been developed that enhance the specific adsorption of albumin, a surface passivating protein, and affect thrombogenicity as measured in the canine ex vivo model.

**Key words:** Polyurethane block copolymers—Thrombogenicity—Microphase separation—Alkyl derivatized polyurethanes

Recent advances leading to the implantation of artificial organs, and in particular, the successes and failures of artificial heart implants, have directed more attention to the development of blood-compatible materials. It is desirable to have a material which can withstand the rigors of a blood-contacting environment without the assistance of anticoagulants. Blood clot formation on the surface and in the vicinity of the valves of artificial hearts indicates that there is an incomplete understanding and control of artificial surface-induced thrombosis [1].

## Polyurethane block copolymers in blood-contacting applications

Polyurethane block copolymers are a diverse family of polymers that have a promising future as biomaterials [2, 3]. They have excellent physical properties, such as good fatigue and tensile strength, and surface properties that may be readily modified to alter their blood compatibility. Block copolymers are synthesized by the polymerization of alternating hard (high glass transition) and soft (low glass transition) segments, which, due to a thermodynamic incompatibility, tend to separate into two phases. The hard-segment phase consists of a diisocyanate, such as 4,4′-diphenylmethane diisocyanate [methylene bis(p-phenyldiisocyanate) MDI], polymerized with a chain extender, such as 1,4-butanediol (BD) or ethylene diamine (ED; Fig. 1.1). This phase is below its glass transition temperature, $T_g$, at service temperatures and tends to be glassy or semicrystalline. The soft-segment phase is based on an oligomeric macroglycol such as poly(tetramethylene oxide) (PTMO), poly(propylene oxide) (PPO), or poly(ethylene oxide) (PEO). This phase is above its $T_g$ at room temperature and tends to be amorphous and rubbery.

Copolymerization of the hard- and soft-segment components results in a material with a two-phase microstructure. In certain polyurethanes, phase separation has been linked to improved blood compatibility and has been shown to depend on the hard-segment/soft-segment ratio [2, 4]. At low hard- to soft-segment ratios, aggregates of hard segments act as crosslinks dissolved in a rubbery soft segment matrix and impart the good physical properties important to the practical applications of polyurethanes. Phase separation and bulk composition also strongly affect the surface properties of polyurethane block copolymers [2]. The surface composition of a polyurethane may not be the same as the bulk composition [2, 5, 6]. Polymers are dynamic materials and under a number of circumstances, it is possible for the surface to rearrange itself depending upon its environment. In an air or vacuum environment, the phase with the lower surface-air interfacial energy is expected to be dominant at the surface [7–9], while underwater it is anticipated that the phase with the lower surface-water interfacial energy would be present in excess at the surface. Thus, in air or a vacuum, it is possible for the apolar soft-segment phase to dominate at the surface, while underwater the polymer surface may have polar hard segments exposed, though the limited mobility of the hard segment may reduce the extent of underwater hard-segment enrichment. The ability of poly-

[1] Department of Chemical Engineering, University of Wisconsin, 1415 Johnson Drive, Madison, WI 53706, USA

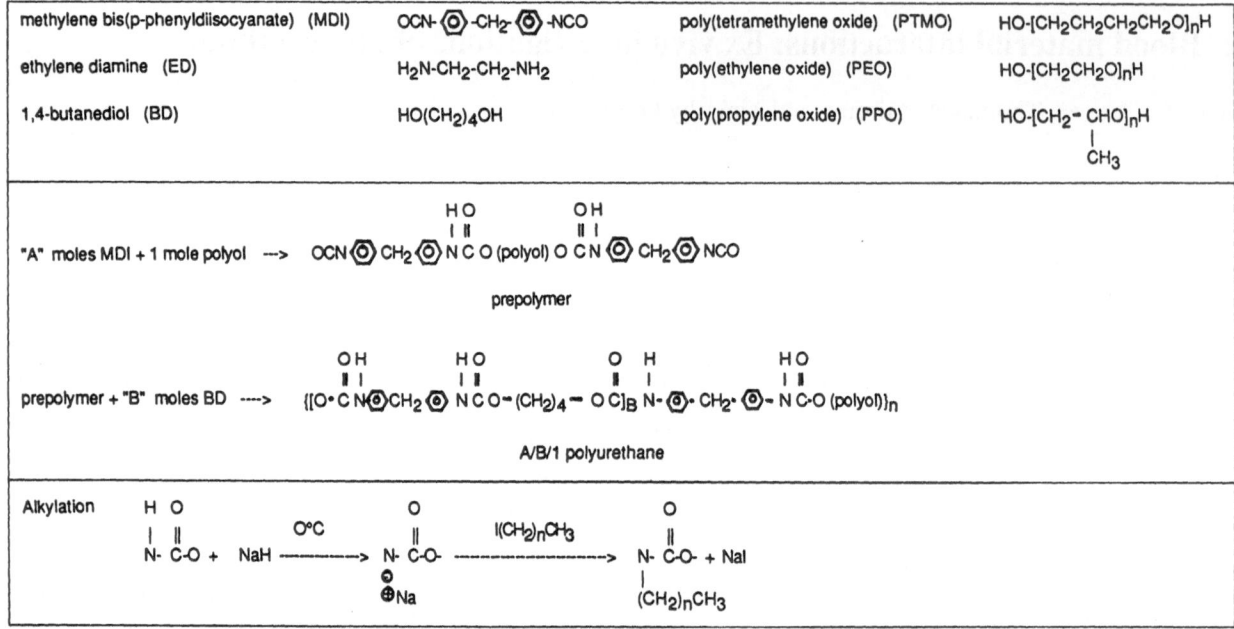

**Fig. 1.1.** Chemicals used in the synthesis of polyurethanes shown with simplified representations of polymerization and alkyl derivatization schemes

mers to change and adapt to their environment is an indication of the complexities of structure-property relationships in polyurethanes. It is thus of great interest to determine which polymer properties are directly related to blood compatibility [10, 11].

### Study of the blood compatibility of biomaterials

The evaluation of the blood compatibility of materials is complicated by the fact that the physiological response to the introduction of a synthetic material to the biological environment is very complex. In blood-contacting situations, protein adsorption, followed by platelet adhesion and activation, thrombus formation, and subsequent embolization are just some of the aspects of the physiological response that must be studied and understood.

Protein adsorption is envisioned as the first phenomenon to occur when blood contacts a foreign, synthetic surface [12]. Proteins adsorb, interact with the surface and with each other, and then possibly desorb or adsorb strongly and irreversibly. The surface of the foreign material tends to be coated entirely by proteins so that subsequent blood component interactions are influenced by an adsorbed protein layer. The effect of the polymer surface on the composition and structure of the adsorbed protein layer may affect further events in the coagulation cascade. Many researchers have investigated protein adsorption using in vitro experiments. A variety of techniques such as Fourier transform infrared spectroscopy (FTIR),

total internal reflectance fluorescence spectroscopy (TIRF), and radiolabeling have been utilized to compile many protein adsorption isotherms [13]. These data are indicative of protein affinity for the various materials examined. There are many plasma proteins that have significant roles in the physiological response to artificial surfaces. Albumin, fibrinogen, fibronectin, the gamma globulins, high molecular-weight kininogen, thrombin, and $\alpha_2$-macroglobulin are just some of the plasma proteins that have been studied by researchers [14–16]. The use of radiolabeled proteins in ex vivo experiments is common and the level of deposition is sometimes used as an indicator of blood compatibility [17, 18].

Platelet adhesion is another common parameter measured in ex vivo blood compatibility evaluations [19]. Adherent platelets are visualized utilizing scanning electron microscopy (SEM), photomicroscopy, or are measured by using radiolabeled platelets. In high-shear flow conditions, thrombi are composed of mostly platelets (white thrombi), while in low-shear flow thrombi with red blood cells (red thrombi) dominate [10]. The number of adherent platelets may be indicative of the material's thrombogenicity. Platelet morphology is used also as an indication of blood compatibility. After adhering, round platelets begin to spread, form pseudopodia, fully extend their pseudopodia, and become fully spread as they release their granular contents [20, 21]. Many of the released proteins assist the adhesion of additional platelets and are an important step in thrombus growth and development [22]. Examination of platelets using SEM allows their morphology to be visualized and thus gives a qualitative indication of the degree of platelet shape change.

The processes of thrombus growth and embolization are closely related to platelet adhesion and activation. Thus, they are examined using similar methods, especially visualization with microscopy, videodensitometry [23], or light scattering [24, 25].

The study of platelet adhesion, activation, and subsequent events at the blood-biomaterial interface involves complex phenomena. A canine ex vivo arteriovenous series shunt experiment has been developed to investigate protein adsorption and platelet adhesion onto several different materials simultaneously (Fig. 1.2) [26]. SEM is used to examine platelet activation and shape change on the polymeric test materials. The degree to which protein adsorption and platelet adhesion occur is used as a measure of short-term thrombogenicity. A material which has many adherent platelets and high fibrinogen deposition is considered to be thrombogenic. The canine ex vivo model has been used to investigate many different aspects of polymeric biomaterial blood compatibility [26–28], including the importance of polyurethane microphase separation [4] and the effect of derivatizing a base polyurethane with an alkyl chain to bind specifically albumin [5]. This paper reviews some significant results of these studies.

## Materials and methods

The polyurethanes used in the investigation of phase separation upon blood compatibility were laboratory-synthesized polymers with MDI and ED, comprising the hard segment and PTMO MW(1000), and PPO MW(1000) as the soft segments (Fig. 1.1). Hard- to soft-segment ratios were varied in the syntheses of these polyurethaneureas as 1.3/0.3/1 and 3/2/1 molar ratios of diisocyanate/chain extender/polyol were used. These materials were dissolved in $N,N$-dimethylacetamide (DMA) and cast onto polyethylene (PE) tubing before being subjected to the ex vivo evaluation.

A derivatized polyurethane was synthesized to take advantage of the potential interaction of albumin with the alkyl chains of fatty acids in the blood. First, a polyetherurethane with a 3/2/1 molar ratio of MDI, BD, and PTMO MW(1000) was synthesized. This polymer is referred to as the base polyurethane (PEU). An 18-carbon chain was attached to 10% of the urethane hydrogens of the base polymer using iodo-octadecane (Fig. 1.1). This material is designated PEU-C18-0.1 to represent the polyetherurethane (PEU) base, the 18-carbon chain (C18), and

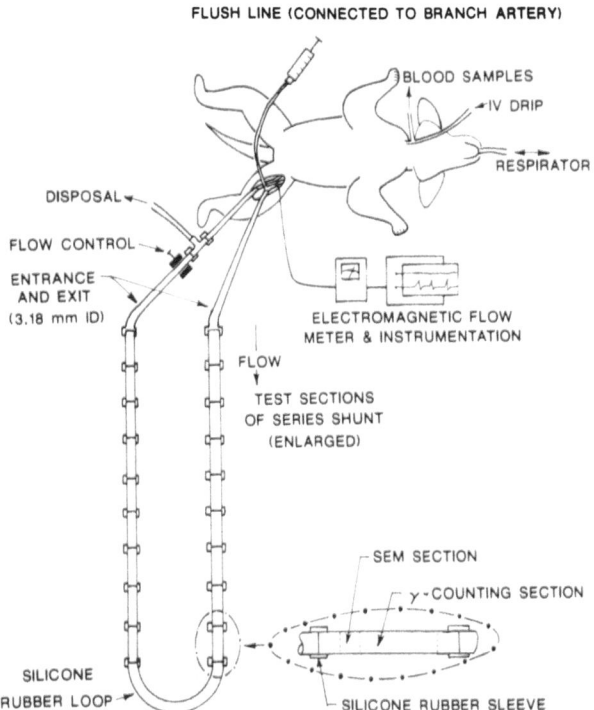

**Fig. 1.2.** Schema of ex vivo experiment showing an enlarged view of the series shunt. After Grasel and Cooper [4] by permission

the 10% level of urethane hydrogen substitution. The polymers were cast from DMA onto PE tubing and subjected to ex vivo evaluation. The details of the syntheses of these polymers have been published previously [4, 5, 29, 30].

The details of the canine ex vivo series shunt experiment have been published previously [4, 5, 26]. A brief summary of the methodology is presented here (Fig. 1.2). Adult mongrel dogs are screened with several hematological tests before and during experimentation. Fibrinogen radiolabeled with [125]I and [51]Cr-labeled platelets are introduced into the canine subject before the surgery begins. The polymers to be tested may be extruded into tubing form or cast on the inner surface of 3-mm ID polyethylene tubing segments. A series of tubing segments is connected together, filled with phosphate buffer, and then cannulated into the femoral artery and vein of the canine subject. Blood flow is allowed to begin, displacing the buffer. After a given amount of time (1–60 min), the artery is clamped, flow is stopped, and the blood is flushed out with buffer. The shunt is then fixed with 2% glutaraldehyde. The polymer segments are separated and made ready for gamma counting and SEM examination. A new series of test segments is inserted and the blood-contacting experiment begins again. This procedure is repeated for each time point of interest.

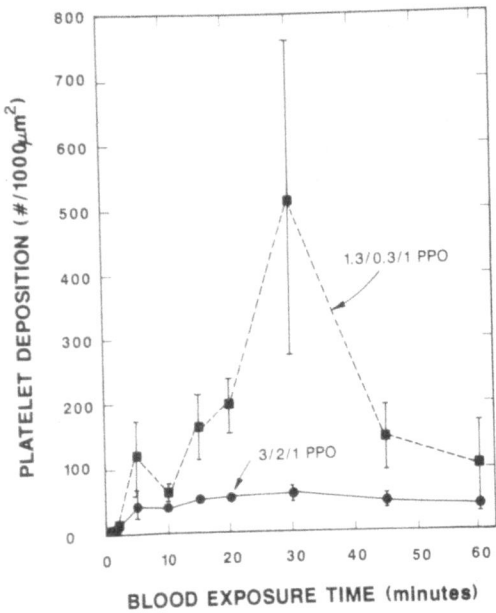

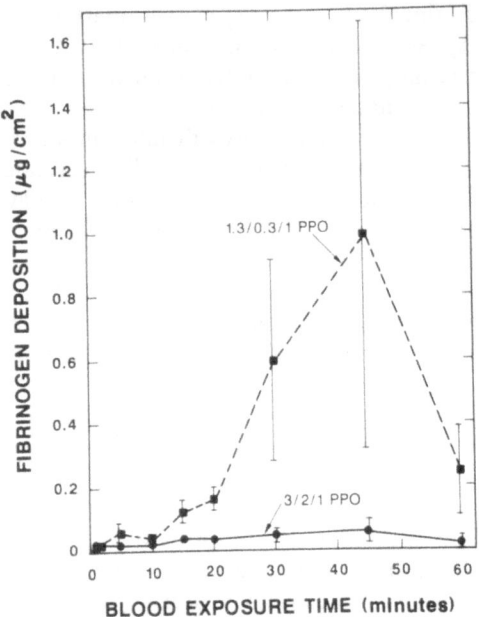

**Fig. 1.3.** Platelet deposition curves as determined in the ex vivo evaluation of 1.3/0.3/1 and 3/2/1 PPO based polyurethaneureas. After Grasel and Cooper [4] by permission

**Fig. 1.4.** Fibrinogen deposition curves for the 1.3/0.3/1 and 3/2/1 PPO-based polyurethaneureas. After Grasel and Cooper [4] by permission

## Results

The results of the ex vivo evaluation of the polymers based on PPO soft segments are shown in Figs. 1.3 and 1.4. Platelet and fibrinogen deposition profiles for the polyurethaneureas with PTMO soft segment are presented in Figs. 1.5 and 1.6. The PPO-based material with the 3/2/1 molar ratio of diisocyanate/chain extender/soft segment has a much lower level of adherent platelets than the 1.3/0.3/1 PTMO-based material. The results of fibrinogen deposition follow a similar pattern with deposition increasing in the order 3/2/1 PPO, 3/2/1 PTMO, 1.3/0.3/1 PPO, and 1.3/0.3/1 PTMO. The ordinates of Figs. 1.5 and 1.6 differ by an order of magnitude over those of Figs. 1.3 and 1.4. Platelet deposition peaks with 2500 platelets per 1000 $\mu m^2$ at 40 min for the 1.3/0.3/1 PTMO material. At 30 min of blood exposure, the 1.3/0.3/1 PPO material has 515 adherent platelets per $\mu m^2$. No large peaks in deposition are noted for the 3/2/1 PTMO- and PPO-based polymers. Peaks in fibrinogen adsorption closely follow the peaks in platelet adhesion. The maximum and sudden drop in the amount of adherent platelets and adsorbed protein is due to the competing processes of thrombus growth and embolization [26]. Protein and platelets adhere to the surface, and thrombi grow until they are large enough to be sheared off the surface. The thrombi consist mostly of platelets and attached fibrin or fibrinogen molecules. It is reasonable that sudden drops in the number of adherent platelets and adsorbed proteins would occur at similar time points. The fact that there are no large peaks in the platelet adhesion curves for the 3/2/1 PTMO- and PPO-based materials suggests that little thrombus formation and embolization is occurring or that the emboli are too small to detect. The possibility that the surface continuously induces and releases large numbers of tiny emboli cannot be discounted.

The results of the canine ex vivo evaluation of the polyetherurethane base polymer and its C18-derivatized counterpart are presented in Figs. 1.7 and 1.8. Error bars represent the standard errors of the mean for the three experiments performed. From Fig. 1.8, it can be seen that the PEU-C18-0.1 material adsorbs less fibrinogen and has fewer adherent platelets than the 3/2/1 PTMO material (PEU) from which it was synthesized. Platelet and fibrinogen deposition on the PEU-C18-0.1 polymer is consistently lower than on the base PEU and no large peaks in deposition are present. This is in direct contrast to another shorter-chain alkyl-grafted polymer shown in Figs. 1.7 and 1.8. The PEU-C2-0.1 polymer is briefly mentioned below and the blood-contacting experimental results are rationalized in terms of the potential for enhanced albumin adsorption on the C18-grafted polymer.

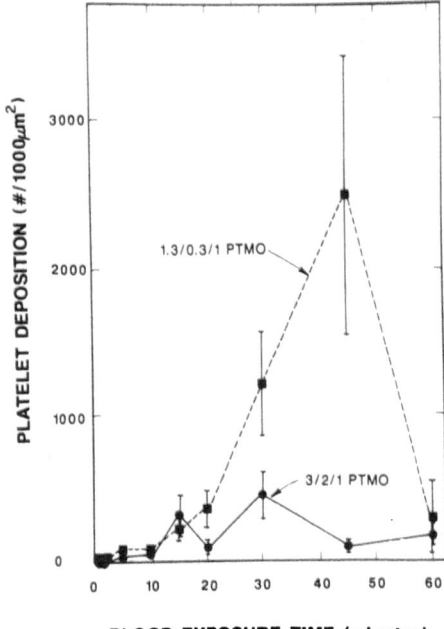

**Fig. 1.5.** Platelet deposition curves for the 1.3/0.3/1 and 3/2/1 PTMO-based polyurethaneureas. After Grasel and Cooper [4] by permission

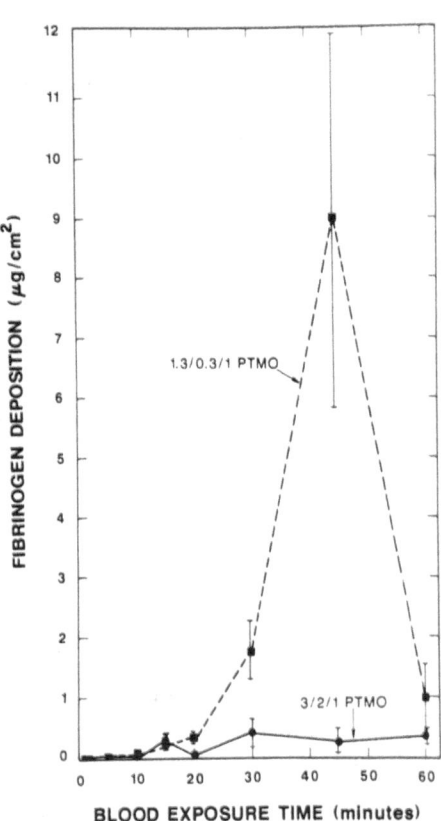

**Fig. 1.6.** Fibrinogen deposition curves for the 1.3/0.3/1 and 3/2/1 PTMO-based polyurethaneureas. After Grasel and Cooper [4] by permission

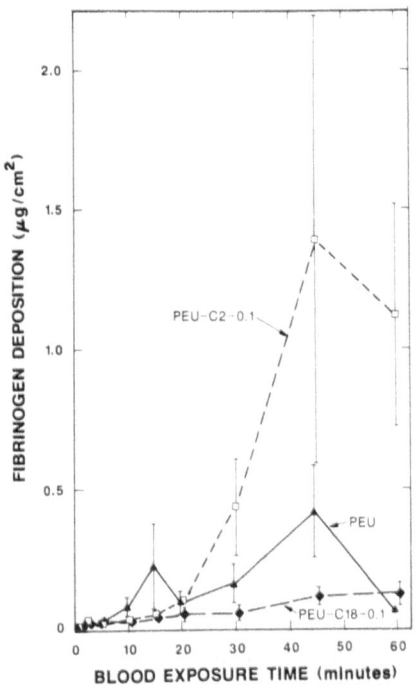

**Fig. 1.7.** Platelet deposition curves for the PEU, PEU-C2-0.1, and PEU-C18-0.1 materials. After Grasel et al. [5] by permission

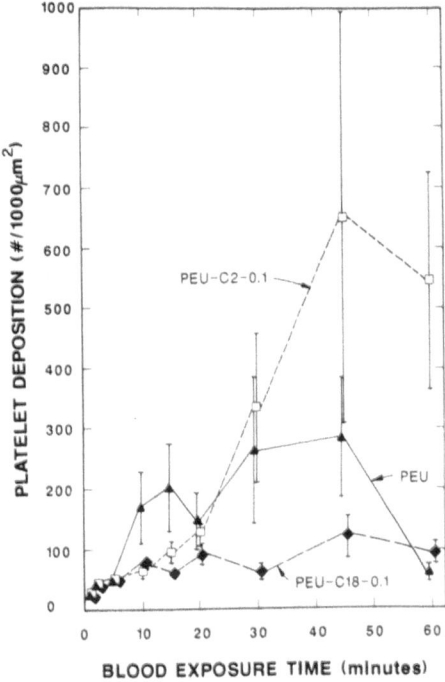

**Fig. 1.8.** Fibrinogen deposition curves for the PEU, PEU-C2-0.1, and PEU-C18-0.1 materials. After Grasel et al. [5] by permission

## Discussion

Polyurethaneureas with differing soft segments and different hard- to soft-segment ratios have been subjected to ex vivo evaluation in an attempt to determine the importance of various chemical characteristics upon blood compatibility [4]. Differential scanning calorimetry and dynamic mechanical testing were performed upon these materials and showed that the degree of phase separation increased as the hard- to soft-segment ratio increased. The polymers with a 3/2/1 diisocyanate/chain extender/soft-segment molar ratio were more highly phase-separated than the 1.3/0.3/1 materials. Combining the ex vivo results of Figs. 1.3–1.6 with this information suggests that blood compatibility is improved with the improved phase separation gained from higher hard- to soft-segment ratios. The authors conclude that phase separation and hard- to soft-segment ratios are primary determinants for the blood compatibility of the PPO- and PTMO-based polyurethaneureas.

The phase separation that has been discussed was determined utilizing bulk characterization methods and represents bulk microphase separation. The mediating parameter in the blood-contacting experiment would be expected to be the surface microphase separation, which is difficult to measure directly. Nevertheless, different compositions and bulk morphologies would be expected to yield different surface compositions and surface morphologies. Grasel and Cooper found evidence that two phases are present in significant amounts at the surface [4]. A controversial subject of continuing research is whether the surface is dominated by a soft-phase matrix with hard segment dispersed within it, or whether the surface consists of two relatively distinct phases.

In addition to phase separation, it was noted that the soft-segment composition has an effect on blood compatibility [4]. There is a significant difference between the blood-contacting behavior of the PTMO- and the PPO-based polyurethaneureas. The PPO-based polyurethaneureas examined were less thrombogenic in the canine ex vivo experiment. A surface's interfacial energy has been considered an important factor in biomaterial development. A low-energy surface is expected to initiate less adsorption than a higher-energy surface. Perhaps the PPO soft segment has a lower surface-water interfacial tension than PTMO. Contact angle data for these polyurethaneureas show that the PPO-based polymer was more hydrophilic. This could explain the difference in the blood response to these two polyurethaneureas.

In the study of the PPO- and PTMO-based polyurethaneureas, phase separation was affected by the various hard- to soft-segment ratios used. The effect of phase separation upon blood compatibility is convoluted with the effect of changing the hard- to soft-segment ratio. In further investigations, a polyetherurethane was derivatized in such a way as to vary the phase separation while holding the hard- to soft-segment ratio constant. The grafting of a short C2 side chain in varying percentages to the urethane hydrogen allows the disruption of the hydrogen bonding that greatly affects hard-segment aggregation. With a constant hard-segment content, increasing levels of derivatization decrease the phase separation. Additionally, there are other reasons for derivatizing a polyurethane to affect blood compatibility.

The derivatization of a material to enhance specific adsorption of nonthrombogenic proteins is a popular idea in biomaterial development. In blood, albumin is a fatty acid transport protein. On a biomaterial surface in contact with blood, albumin can be passivating, reducing the thrombogenicity of a material. The idea of grafting an alkyl chain to a polymer backbone to facilitate the specific adsorption of albumin has been proposed by Munro and co-workers [31, 32]. The ex vivo evaluation of the C18 grafted polyurethane has shown it to be less thrombogenic than its underivatized counterpart. However, it was found that the grafting of the C18 alkyl chain decreased phase separation [5]. To distinguish between the effect of decreased phase separation and the anticipated specific interaction between albumin and C18 chains, the same base polymer was grafted with a two-carbon chain (PEU-C2-0.1). Physical testing showed that the C2-grafted polymer was as poorly phase-separated as the C18-grafted material. The C2-grafted material was much more thrombogenic than the C18-grafted polymer and the PEU base material. Phase separation does not seem to be the dominant parameter in the blood compatibility of these materials. The C2-grafted material lacks the biospecific interaction with albumin that the C18-grafted polymer has. The results suggest that the C18-grafted polymer is specifically binding albumin and the thrombogenic nature of the base material is being suppressed.

The limited number of studies presented are a small sampling of the work performed on polyurethane biomaterials using the ex vivo method of evaluation. The flexibility of the technique has been demonstrated, and an example of the useful information derived from the experiment has been presented. In addition to the in vitro biomaterial evaluations that are commonly carried out in the laboratory, the canine ex vivo series shunt experiment has proven most useful and informative in determining the effects of polymer surface chemistry upon short-term blood compatibility. Research is continuing in our laboratory to determine the effectiveness of additional derivatized polyurethanes to further investigate the mechanisms of blood compatibility and to evaluate the interactions of polymer materials in a blood-contacting chronic shunt configuration.

**Acknowledgments.** This work was supported in part by the National Institutes of Health through grants HL-21001 and HL-24046.

# References

1. Coleman DL, Meuzelaar HLC, Kessler TR, McClennen WH, Richards JM, Gregonis DE (1986) Retrieval and analysis of a clinical total artificial heart. J Biomed Mater Res 20: 417–431
2. Lelah MD, Cooper SL (1986) Polyurethanes in medicine. CRC Press, Boca Raton
3. Boretos JW (1980) Past, present and future role of polyurethanes for surgical implants. Pure App Chem 52: 1851–1855
4. Grasel TG, Cooper SL (1986) Surface properties and blood compatibility of polyurethaneureas. Biomaterials 7: 315–328
5. Grasel TG, Pierce JA, Cooper SL (1987) Effects of alkyl grafting on surface properties and blood compatibility of polyurethane block copolymers. J Biomed Mater Res 21: 815–842
6. Yoon SC, Ratner BD (1986) Surface structure of segmented poly(etherurethanes) and poly(ether urethane ureas) with various perfluoro chain extenders. An x-ray photoelectron spectroscopic investigation. Macromolecules 19: 1068–1079
7. Lelah MD, Lambrecht LK, Young BR, Cooper SL (1983) Physicochemical characterization and *in vivo* blood tolerability of cast and extruded Biomer. J Biomed Mater Res 17: 1–22
8. Ratner BD, Paynter RW (1984) Polyurethane surfaces: the importance of molecular weight distribution, bulk chemistry, and casting conditions. In: Planck H, Egbers G, Syre I (eds) Polyurethanes in biomedical engineering. Elsevier, Amsterdam, pp 41–68
9. Paynter RW, Ratner BD, Thomas HR (1983) Polyurethane surfaces: an XPS study. Am Chem Soc Div Polym Chem Polym Prepr 24: 13–14
10. Hoffman AS (1982) Blood-biomaterials interactions: an overview. In: Cooper SL, Peppas NA (eds) Biomaterials: interfacial phenomena and applications. ACS Adv Chem Series 199: 3–8
11. Andrade JD, Nagaoka S, Cooper SL, Okano T, Kim SW (1987) Surfaces and blood compatibility: current hypotheses. ASAIO Trans 33: 75–84
12. Baier RE, Dutton RC (1969) Initial events in interactions of blood with a foreign surface. J Biomed Mater Res 3: 191–206
13. Andrade JD (1985) Surface and interfacial aspects of biomedical polymers' Vol 2. Protein adsorption. Plenum, New York
14. Young BR, Pitt WG, Cooper SL (1988) Protein adsorption on polymeric biomaterials. I. Adsorption isotherms. J Colloid Interfa Sci 124: 28–43
15. Vroman L, Adams AL (1986) Adsorption of proteins out of plasma and solutions in narrow spaces. J Colloid Interfa Sci 111: 391–402
16. Andrade JD, Hlady V (1987) Plasma protein adsorption—the big twelve. Ann NY Acad Sci 516: 158–172
17. Horbett TA, Cheng CM, Ratner BD, Hoffman AS, Hanson SR (1986) The kinetics of baboon fibrinogen adsorption to polymers: *in vitro* and *in vivo* studies. J Biomed Mater Res 20: 739–772
18. Schultz JS, Goddard JD, Ciarkowski A, Penner JA, Lindenauer SM (1977) An *ev vivo* method for the evaluation of biomaterials in contact with blood. Ann NY Acad Sci 283: 494–521
19. Cooper SL, Fabrizius DJ, Grasel TG (1986) Methods of assessment of thrombosis *ex vivo*. Ann NY Acad Sci 516: 572–585
20. Goodman SL, Lelah MD, Lambrecht LK, Cooper SL, Ablrecht RM (1984) *In vitro* vs. *ex vivo* platelet deposition on polymer surfaces. Scan Electron Microsc 1984: 279–290
21. Goodman SL, Grasel TG, Cooper SL, Albrecht RM (1988) Platelet shape-change and cytoskeletal reorganization on polyurethaneureas. J Biomed Mater Res (in press)
22. Anderson JM, Kottke-Marchant K (1985) Platelet interactions with biomaterials and artificial devices. CRC Crit Rev Biocompat 1: 111–204
23. Grabowski EF, Herther KK, Didisheim P (1974) Platelet aggregation quantified in an *ex vivo* chamber by means of videodensitometry. Thromb Diath Haemorrh [Suppl] 60: 127–134
24. Harker LA, Hanson SR, Hoffman AS (1977) Platelet kinetic evaluation of prosthetic material *in vivo*. Ann NY Acad Sci 283: 317–331
25. Hoffman AS, Hanson SR, Harker LA, Horbett TA, Ratner BD, Reynolds LO (1982) Thrombotic events on grafted polyacrylamide-Silastic surfaces as studied in a baboon. In: Cooper SL, Peppas NA (eds) Biomaterials: interfacial phenomena and applications. ACS Adv Chem Ser 199: 59–80
26. Lelah MD, Lambrecht LK, Cooper SL (1984) A canine *ex vivo* series shunt for evaluating thrombus deposition on polymer surfaces. J Biomed Mater Res 18: 475–496
27. Lelah MD, Grasel TG, Pierce JA, Cooper SL (1986) *Ex vivo* interactions and surface property relationships for polyetherurethanes. J Biomed Mater Res 20: 433–468
28. Lelah MD, Pierce JA, Lambrecht LK, Cooper SL (1985) Polyether-urethane ionomers: surface property/ *ex vivo* blood compatibility relationships. J Colloid Interfa Sci 104: 422–439
29. Saunders JH, Frisch KC (1962) Polyurethane chemistry and technology: Chemistry. Interscience, New York
30. Adibi K, George MH, Barrie JA (1979) Anionic synthesis of poly(urethane-g-acrylonitrile). Polymer 20: 483–487
31. Munro MS, Quattrone AJ, Ellsworth SR, Kulkarni P, Eberhart RC (1981) Alkyl substituted polymers with enhanced albumin affinity. ASAIO Trans 27: 499–501
32. Munro MS, Eberhart RC, Maki NJ, Brtink BE, Fry WJ (1983) Thromboresistant alkyl-derivitized polyurethanes. ASAIO J 6: 65–75

## Discussion

*Kataoka* (Tokyo Women's Medical College): Have you ever analyzed the protein composition of the passivated surface? Is the passivated surface stable over a long period of time?

*Cooper* (University of Wisconsin): We are at present working on the analysis of the passivated surface. It could be composed of proteins like albumin or it could be composed of membrane fragments from the platelet thrombi that have been removed from the surface and those lipid-like materials may be very biocompatible. So far, we have no definite evidence to present.

With regard to stability, we have been carrying out a chronic shunt experiment similar to the one Prof. Sefton uses at the University of Toronto. In this iliac artery to vein shunt, we have evidence of passivation in the dog for at least 24 h. I still do not think that this will be a permanent solution because of protein turnover and eventual occlusion. What also happens in the dog is that whereas the shunt can be kept open for months, platelet function slowly becomes degraded and the biomaterial begins to affect other hematological parameters and eventual failure is the result. It may not be that thromboembolism and passivation occurs repeatedly, but rather a more subtle degradation of platelet function occurs in the animal in the long term when its blood is exposed to synthetic materials.

*Portner* (Novacor Medical Corporation): How sensitive are the results or time-course of the chain of events to the flow?

*Cooper:* The results presented today are significant only for high arterial flows where white thrombus is the primary evidence of the incompatibility. We have done some studies using lower flows and in those cases we could obtain occlusion of the shunt. However, at low flows in the series shunt all materials begin to look alike. Thus, we need to go to high flows to prevent chemical contamination of the downstream surfaces. Certainly for venous flows and the like, we have no good predictive evidence from these animal experiments.

*Takahara* (Kyushu University): You mentioned the introduction of an alkyl group on the surface of a seg-

mented polyurethane. Are these reactions uniform or not? Does the microphase separated structure exist after the introduction of the alkyl group?

*Cooper:* We have studied this at some length. Our method of alkylation is different from that of Prof. Eberhart, which is a surface treatment. With the alkylation I described, the polymer chains are dissolved in solution and thus the whole polymer is alkylated. A solution cast surface is used in the animal experiments. From viscoelastic studies, such as dynamic mechanical testing, physical property measurements, and thermal analysis, we show that as we alkylate the NH group the material becomes more and more phase-mixed. Certainly, for ethyl group incorporation, increased phase mixing correlates with poor blood compatibility. These observations support the hypothesis that a fluctuating potential of hard and soft domains is required on the surface to give good biocompatibility.

*Kim* (University of Utah): Is the alkyl group exposed on the surface, causing some surface dynamics or mobility?

*Cooper:* We do not have very good evidence here. From the contact angle, which shows the surface to be very hydrophobic, there do appear to be alkyl groups on the surface. When a protein molecule comes down it can change the environment, so if the alkyl group is flattened out and the protein covers it, it may diffuse to a binding site on the protein. On studies we have done on albumin adsorption to these surfaces, there has been very little enhancement of protein adsorption except that the initial rate of albumin adsorption on the alkylated surfaces was higher than on the control material.

*Kim:* You used sulfonated polyurethanes. Have you measured any heparin activity on the surface?

*Cooper:* The material has some anticoagulant character. I made one material at 30% substitution. This material is water soluble and it does prolong clotting times. These sulfonate groups are placed every 1000 molecular weight along the chain because of the segmented nature of the polymer.

# 2. Mechanical properties of segmented polyether polyurethanes for blood pump applications

Kozaburo Hayashi[1]

**Summary.** The effects of test environment (cholesterol-lipid solution, saline solution, and room air), temperature (24°, 37°, and 50°C), and cyclic rate (0.8, 2, and 5 Hz) on the fatigue properties of Biomer and Toyobo TM5 polyurethanes were studied to obtain basic data for the design of artificial heart pumps and for the development of accelerated endurance test methods.

The mechanical properties of these materials deteriorated more significantly following immersion in plasma-analogous cholesterol-lipid solution than by exposure to saline solution or room atmosphere; this environmental effect was enhanced by cyclic deformation. Static and dynamic stress relaxation were greater at the higher ambient temperature. Although there was no significant difference in the stress relaxation behavior between the fatigue tests at 2 and 5 Hz at the same number of cycles, the stress reduction was much greater in the case of 0.8-Hz testing. These property changes were significantly less in Biomer than in Toyobo TM5 polyurethane. The material elasticity or flexibility did not significantly depend upon the ambient temperature or cyclic rate of fatigue testing.

The changes in the tensile properties of Toyobo TM5 polyurethane caused by the in vitro fatigue testing at the cyclic rate of 2 Hz in the cholesterol-lipid solution kept at 37°C were similar to the in vivo changes observed in the diaphragms of blood pumps implanted into animals.

**Key words:** Blood pump—Durability—Fatigue—Segmented polyurethane—Stress relaxation

Segmented polyether polyurethanes are believed to be one of the most favorable materials for cardiovascular applications owing to their excellent mechanical properties and blood compatibility. Since the materials used in blood pumps undergo cyclic deformation while in contact with blood, their fatigue properties and surface characteristics are very important for the long-term reliability and safety of implants. Although there are several reports on the interaction of polyurethanes with blood, their mechanical characteristics, particularly their fatigue properties, have not been documented well.

For blood pump diaphragms, we have been using Toyobo TM5 polyurethane (Toyobo Co., Osaka, Japan) since our preliminary evaluation tests have indicated that this material has relatively good mechanical properties and blood compatibility [1–5]. The effects of test environment, temperature, and cyclic rate have recently been studied in detail in an attempt to obtain basic data on the design of blood pumps as well as on the development of an accelerated endurance test and evaluation method. In this paper, these data are presented and compared with the results obtained from Biomer (Ethicon, Somerville, NJ, USA). The changes in the tensile properties of Toyobo TM5 polyurethane caused by the in vitro fatigue testing in the cholesterol-lipid solution are also compared with those observed in the diaphragms of blood pumps implanted into animals.

## Materials and method

The materials studied are Toyobo TM5 and Biomer polyurethanes. The soft segment of Toyobo TM5 is composed of polytetramethylene glycol and 4,4′-diphenylmethane diisocyanate (MDI), and the hard segment contains propylene diamine and MDI. The molecular weight of the soft segment of this material is 2000. The results obtained were compared with those of Biomer. This material is a similar segmented polyether polyurethane to Toyobo TM5, and its soft segment molecular weight is estimated to be around 1800. The procedures for fabricating test specimens of these materials have been reported elsewhere [2, 3, 5].

A miniature servohydraulic testing machine was used for uniaxial tensile as well as for static and dynamic fatigue testing in combination with a vidicon displacement analyzer for the noncontact measurement of specimen length [6]. Dynamic fatigue tests were carried out under conditions of 50% of mean strain ($\varepsilon_m$) and 10% of strain amplitude ($\varepsilon_a$) in strain-control, sine-waveform mode, usually at 2 Hz cyclic rate (f) in a plasma-analogous cholesterol-lipid solution kept at 37°C. For the study of environmental

[1]Department of Biomedical Control, Research Institute of Applied Electricity, Hokkaido University, Kita 12, Nishi 6, Kita-ku, Sapporo, 060 Japan

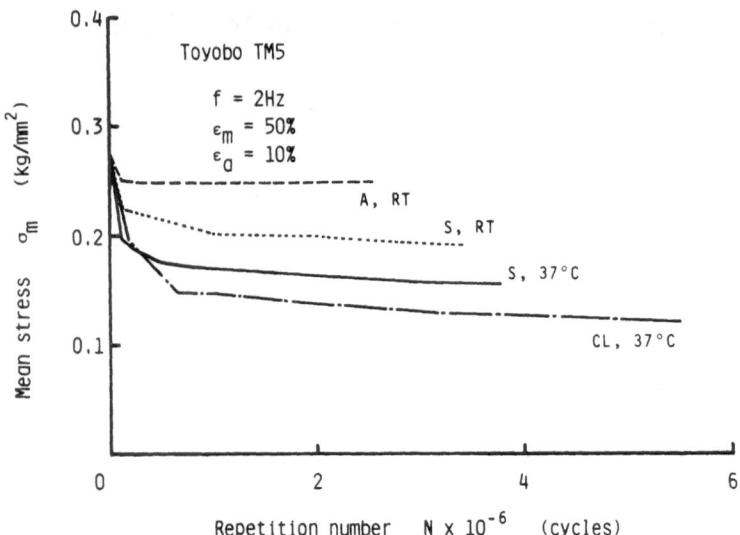

**Fig. 2.1.** Effect of test environment on the mean stress of TM5 polyurethane during fatigue testing. *A* air, *S* saline solution, *CL* cholesterol-lipid solution, *RT* room temperature. After Hayashi et al. [1]

effects, specimens were exposed to room atmosphere or immersed in a saline solution of 37°C during fatigue testing instead of being soaked in the cholesterol-lipid solution. Fatigue tests at the cyclic rates of 0.8 and 5 Hz were additionally carried out to study the effects of cyclic rate. Static fatigue tests, i.e., static stress relaxation tests, were performed applying 50% strain to the specimens immersed in the cholesterol-lipid solution at 37°C.

Tensile properties of the Toyobo TM5-made diaphragm assembled in a pusher plate-type left ventricular assist pump [7] were studied after implanting in a goat for 10 days and compared with the results obtained from the in vitro fatigue testing.

## Results and discussion

### Environmental effects

Blood pump diaphragms in contact with blood undergo cyclic deformation at a fairly large strain for a long duration. It would be ideal if we could carry out in vitro fatigue testing in blood maintained at the body temperature. However, this kind of testing is very difficult because of infection and contamination [8]. As a substitute for blood, we have been using a synthetic cholesterol-lipid solution, the composition of which is analogous to that of plasma [1]. This solution is similar to that used by Carmen and Mutha for the in vitro testing of silicone rubber heart-valve poppets [9].

As an example of the results obtained on the environmental effects on the fatigue behavior of polyurethanes, Fig. 2.1 shows the changes in the mean stress of TM5 polyurethane during fatigue tests in air at room temperature, in a saline solution, and in the

cholesterol-lipid solution of 37°C [1]. A significant decrease in the mean stress was observed in the very early stage of fatigue testing, which was more remarkable in the cholesterol-lipid solution than in the saline solution and in air. In all environments, the stress relaxation continued to proceed gradually even after several million cycles of deformation. Similar phenomena were observed on Biomer although the initial drop in the mean stress was significantly smaller than in Toyobo TM5.

Figure 2.2 summarizes the mean stress and stress/strain ratio of the two materials at the start of fatigue testing and those obtained after around 2 million cycles of deformation in various environments [5]. The stress/strain ratio is the ratio of stress amplitude, $\sigma_a$, to strain amplitude, $\varepsilon_a$, and represents the flexibility of a material under dynamic loading condition. This ratio also decreased significantly in TM5 polyurethane by the long-term cyclic deformation; the decrease was again greater in the cholesterol-lipid solution than in the saline solution. These results suggest that both water and lipid absorption occur in Toyobo TM5 polyurethane and they might change its mechanical properties.

In the case of Biomer, the effect of the immersion in the cholesterol-lipid solution on the dynamic stress relaxation was not much different from that in the saline solution, as shown in Fig. 2.2. The stress/strain ratio was very stable during fatigue testing and was not influenced by cyclic deformation or by environment. These results indicate that there is little effect of the constituents of the cholesterol-lipid solution on the mechanical properties of Biomer although humidity has some influence on the fatigue properties. There may be no lipid absorption into this material [10].

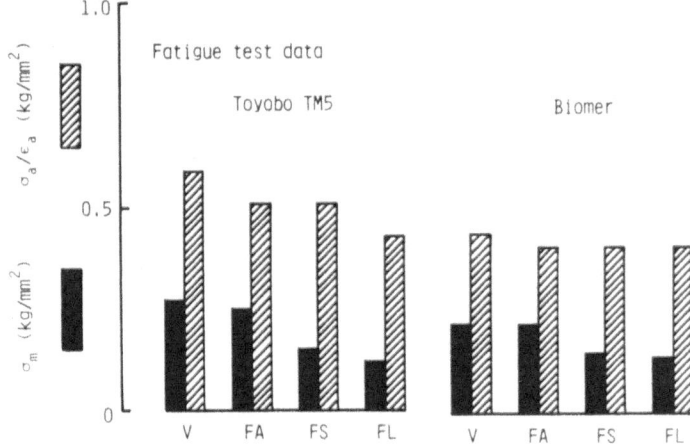

**Fig. 2.2.** Mean stresses $\sigma_m$ and stress/strain ratios $\sigma_a/\varepsilon_a$ of two materials measured at the start of fatigue tests and after around $2 \times 10^6$ cycles of fatigue testing in various environments under conditions of 50% mean strain, 10% strain amplitude, and 2Hz cyclic rate. *V* nonfatigued virgin, *FA* fatigued in air at room temperature, *FS* fatigued in saline solution at 37°C, *FL* fatigued in cholesterol-lipid solution at 37°C. After Hayashi [5]

## Effects of implantation

Tensile tests were performed on specimens cut out from the TM5-made diaphragm of a blood pump, which was implanted between the left atrium and descending thoracic aorta in a goat for 10 days [3]. In Fig. 2.3, the in vivo change in the tensile characteristics is compared with the in vitro change induced in the test specimens of the same material by 1-month fatigue testing ($5 \times 10^6$ cycles) in the cholesterol-lipid solution at 37°C or by 1-month immersion in the same solution under nonloading conditions. The tensile strength decreased to about 75% of that of the non-implanted, virgin diaphragm after only 10 days of implantation, which may be due to microcracks caused by lipids and/or some other blood constituents absorbed into the diaphragm material, although this observation has not been confirmed. The secant modulus at 30% elongation and the ultimate elongation at break were slightly decreased by the implantation.

The in vitro cyclic deformation in the cholesterol-lipid solution significantly decreased the secant modulus and ultimate elongation, which was greater than the change caused by the implantation. However, the reduction in the tensile strength by in vitro fatigue testing was less than the in vivo change. The large difference in the change in the elastic modulus and elongation between the in vivo implantation and in vitro testing might be attributed to the difference in the magnitude of the strains applied to the pump diaphragm and the sample specimens. In addition, the difference in the fabricating process used for the diaphragm and the sample sheet could result in a large variation in their mechanical properties. However, the in vivo change in the tensile properties of the diaphragm was similar to the in vitro change developed in the test specimens by the cyclic deformation in the cholesterol-lipid solution.

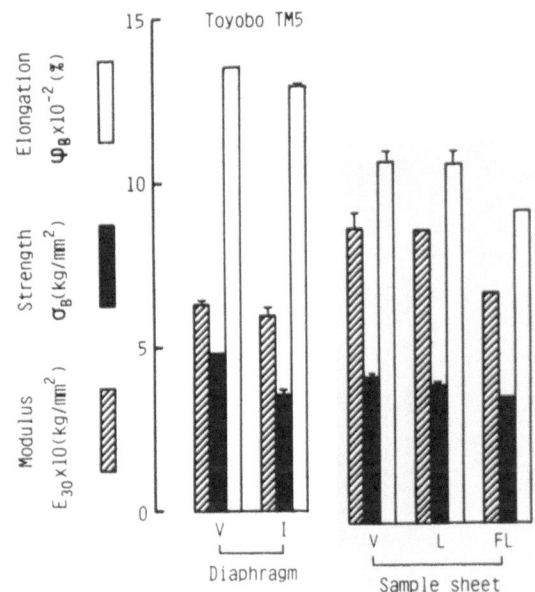

**Fig. 2.3.** Effects of 10-day implantation (I) on the secant modulus at 30% elongation $E_{30}$, tensile strength $\sigma_B$, and elongation at break $\phi_B$ of TM5 polyurethane-made blood pump diaphragm. The in vivo change in diaphragm characteristics is compared with the in vitro change observed in sample sheets by 1-month fatigue testing under conditions of 50% mean strain, 10% strain amplitude, 2-Hz cyclic rate, and 37°C temperature. L immersed in cholesterol lipid solution at 37°C. For other *abbreviations* see Fig. 2.2

## Effects of test temperature

The temperature dependence of the change in the mean stress during fatigue testing of TM5 polyurethane is shown in Fig. 2.4 [5]. With the increase in the ambient temperature, the dynamic stress relaxation became larger. At 50°C, the mean stress after $5 \times 10^6$ cycles was less than 30% of that measured at the beginning of the fatigue test. At this

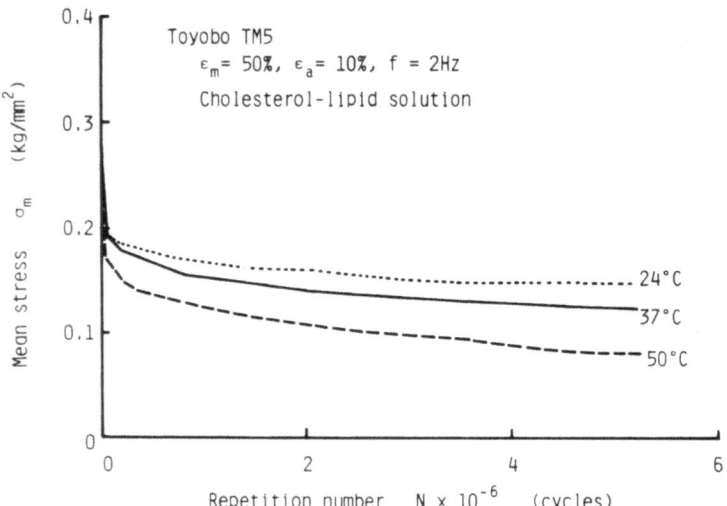

**Fig. 2.4.** Effect of ambient temperature on the change in the mean stress of TM5 polyurethane during fatigue testing. After Hayashi [5]

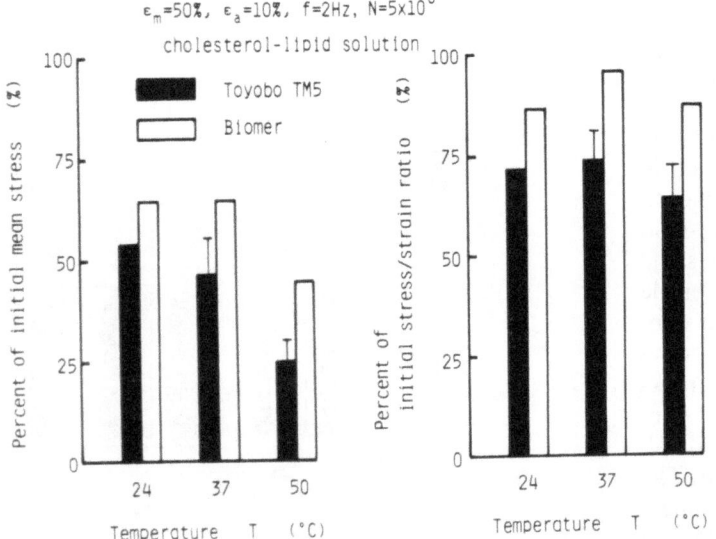

**Fig. 2.5.** Effect of test temperature on the change in the mean stress and stress/strain ratio developed by $5 \times 10^6$ cycles of fatigue testing

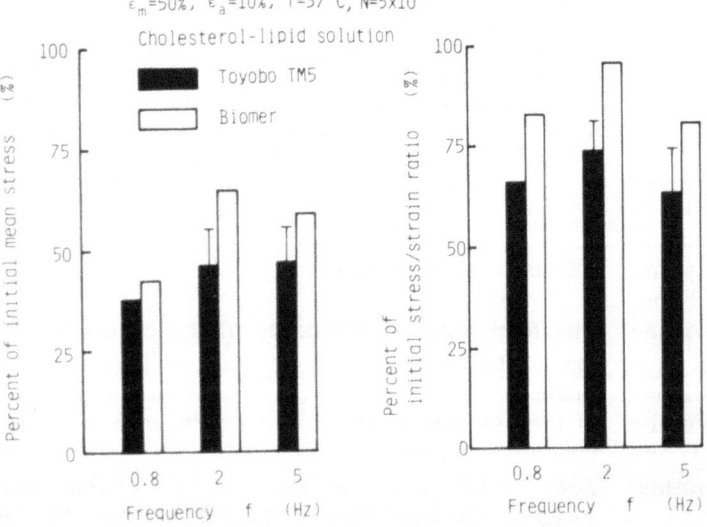

**Fig. 2.6.** Effect of cyclic rate on the change in the mean stress and stress/strain ratio developed by $5 \times 10^6$ cycles of fatigue testing

**Fig. 2.7.** Change in the stress measured during the static relaxation tests and that in the mean stress during the fatigue tests carried out in the cholesterol-lipid solution at various temperatures. *a* 1 h, *b* 10 h, *c* 100 h, *d* 500 h

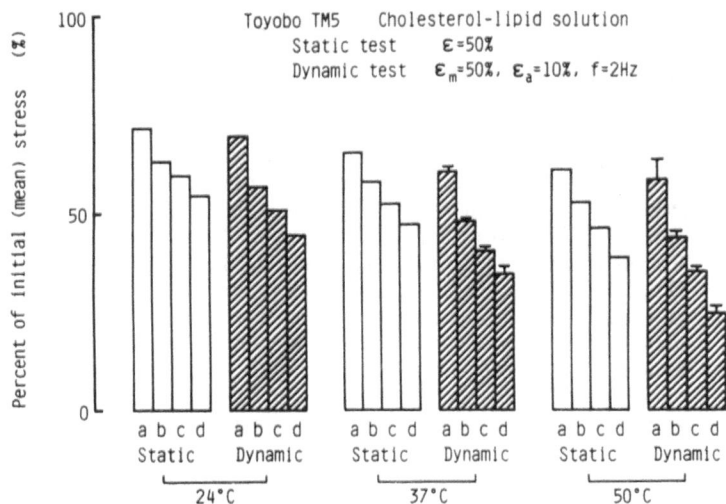

temperature, the stress relaxation continued to proceed quite rapidly even after $5 \times 10^6$ cycles of deformation.

Figure 2.5 summarizes the change in the mean stress and stress/strain ratio of the two materials caused by $5 \times 10^6$ cycles of deformation at different temperatures. Biomer also exhibited a large decrease in the mean stress regardless of the ambient temperature, although the degree of the stress relaxation was less than that with Toyobo TM5. The difference of temperature between 24° and 37°C had no significant influence on the dynamic stress relaxation. However, the elevation of test temperature to 50°C enhanced the stress relaxation remarkably in these materials. On the other hand, no significant temperature dependence was observed with the change in the dynamic flexibility, although the decrease in the stress/strain ratio was again larger in the TM5 polyurethane than in Biomer.

### Effects of cyclic rate

If the fatigue properties of a material are independent of strain rate, durability can be evaluated from accelerated testing at increased cyclic rates. Figure 2.6 summarizes the change in the mean stress and stress/strain ratio caused by fatigue tests carried out at different cyclic rates. The repetition number of $5 \times 10^6$ is equivalent to around 1740, 700, and 280 h for the cyclic rates of 0.8, 2, and 5 Hz, respectively. A time dependency or rate effect on the mean stress was observed in the case of 0.8 Hz testing, while there was no significant difference in the mean stress and stress/strain ratio between the fatigue tests at 2 and 5 Hz. As reported previously, the change in each parameter can be represented by a single curve regardless of the cyclic rate if plotted against the testing time [5]. These

data imply that the stress/strain ratio does not change much over long periods although the stress relaxation continues to proceed with time. Firure 2.6, suggests that the stress relaxation behavior might be different between static and dynamic loading conditions.

### Static and dynamic stress relaxation

To study the above-mentioned speculation in detail, stress relaxation tests were carried out under a constant strain ($\varepsilon = 50\%$), and the results were compared with the changes in the mean stress observed during fatigue testing. Firue 2.7 shows an example of the results obtained. A large difference is observed in the stress relaxation characteristics between the static and dynamic conditions irrespective of the ambient temperature. These results indicate that the long-term material behavior could not be predicted from the static stress relaxation test.

**Acknowledgments.** This research work was supported financially in part by a Research Grant for Cardiovascular Diseases (1982–1984, 1985–1987) from the Ministry of Health and Welfare and a Grant-in-Aid for Scientific Research (No. 60480323) from the Ministry of Education (all with Kozaburo Hayashi as the principal investigator).

### References

1. Hayashi K, Matsuda, T, Takano, H, Umezu, M (1984) Effects of immersion in cholesterol-lipid solution on the tensile and fatigue properties of elastomeric polymers for blood pump applications. J Biomed Mat Res 18: 939–951
2. Hayashi K, Takano H, Matsuda T, Umezu M (1985) Mechanical stability of elastomeric polymers for blood pump applications. J Biomed Mat Res 19: 179–193
3. Hayashi K, Matsuda T, Takano H, Umezu M, Taenaka

Y, Nakamura T (1985) Effects of implantation on the mechanical properties of the polyurethane diaphragm of left ventricular assist devices. Biomaterials 6: 82–88

4.  Hayashi K, Matsuda T, Nakamura T, Umezu M, Takano H (1985) Mechanical and ESCA studies of segmented polyether polyurethanes with various molecular weights for blood pump application. In: Nose Y, Kjellstrand C, Ivanovich P (eds) Progress in artificial organs—1985. Proceedings of 5th World Congress of International Society Artificial Organs, Chicago, 5–8 October, 1985. ISAO Press, Cleveland, pp 989–993

5.  Hayashi K (1987) Tensile and fatigue properties of segmented polyether polyurethanes. In: Planck H, Syre I, Dauner M, Egbers G (eds) Polyurethanes in biomedical engineering II. Elsevier, Amsterdam, pp 129–149

6.  Hayashi K, Nakamura T (1985) Material test system for the evaluation of mechanical properties of biomaterials. J Biomed Mat Res 19: 133–144

7.  Hayashi K, Nakamura T, Takano H, Umezu M, Taenaka Y, Matsuda T (1984) Design of pusher-plate-type left ventricular assist device based on mechanical analyses. Art Org 8: 204–214

8.  McMillin CR (1983) Physical testing of elastomers for cardiovascular applications. Art Org 7: 78–91

9.  Carmen R, Mutha SC (1972) Lipid absorption by silicone rubber heart valve poppets—In vivo and in vitro results. J Biomed Mat Res 6: 327–345

10. Boretos JW, Pierce WS, Baier RE, Leroy AF, Donachy HJ (1975) Surface and bulk characteristics of a polyether urethane for artificial hearts. J Biomed Mat Res 9: 327–340

# 3. Effect of segment structure on fatigue behavior of segmented polyurethaneureas in pseudobiological environments

Atsushi Takahara, Katsuya Takamori, and Tisato Kajiyama[1]

**Summary.** Segmented polyurethaneureas (SPUU) with various hard- and soft-segment components were prepared. The state of microphase separation was investigated by means of differential scanning calorimetry. After immersing in a lipid solution, the specimen showed a weight increase due to sorption of lipids. Acceleration of lipid sorption was observed under cyclic straining. Dynamic viscoelastic measurements revealed that the disordered hard segment lost its aggregation strength after lipid sorption. Where the aggregation strength of the hard-segment domain dropped due to lipid sorption, the SPUU showed reduced fatigue strength. However, the SPUU with an ordered hard-segment domain preserved its fatigue strength even after lipid sorption. The SPUU with a hydrophilic soft segment showed a decrease in molecular weight and a reduction in fatigue strength after immersion in an aqueous solution of hydrolytic enzyme.

**Key words:** Segmented polyurethaneureas—Fatigue—Lipid—Enzyme—Degradation—Microphase separated structure

When polymeric materials are in contact with body fluids, the surface of the materials becomes covered with components of body fluids, such as lipids, proteins, and blood cells. Since segmented polyurethaneureas (SPUUs) have excellent mechanical properties and blood compatibility, they have been used as blood-contacting blood components, such as diaphragms of blood pumps [1], vascular grafts [2], and other devices [3]. However, there have been several reports on the degradation of SPUU in vivo due to lipid adsorption or calcification [4, 5].

In this study, the effect of lipid sorption on the aggregation structure of SPUUs containing various hard and soft segments was investigated. The fatigue behavior of SPUUs after immersion in a lipid solution was also studied.

## Materials and method

The SPUUs were prepared by a prepolymer method. The soft segment consisted of polyethers or polyester diol and 4,4'-diphenylmethanediisocyanate (MDI). The polyethers used were polyethylene glycol (PEG), polytetramethylene glycol (PTMG), and polyester polycaprolactone diol (PCL). The hard segment was composed of diamine and MDI. The diamines were ethylenediamine (EDA), 1,2-propylenediamine (PDA), trimethylenediamine (TriMDA), and 4,4'-diaminodiphenylmethane (DAM). The molar ratio of MDI : polyether (polyester) : diamine is $2:1:1$. The structure is as follows:

Table 3.1 summarizes the chemical composition of SPUUs. These SPUUs are designated as "polyether-$(\overline{Mn})Y$" or "polyester$(\overline{Mn})Y$", where $\overline{Mn}$ is the average molecular weight of the polyether or polyester and Y represents the kind of diamine. The hard segment in PTMG$(\overline{Mn})$EDA/DAM is a random copolymer of MDI-EDA and MDI-DAM. Film specimens were prepared by casting each polymer from a solution of dimethylformamide (DMF) or dimethylacetamide (DMA) onto a clean glass plate. Biomer, a commercial SPUU, was also used in this study. The soft and hard segments of Biomer are reported to consist of MDI-PTMG with Mn of 1800 and MDI-EDA [6, 7].

[1]Department of Applied Chemistry, Faculty of Engineering, Kyushu University, 6-10-1 Hakozaki Higashi-ku, Fukuoka, 812 Japan

**Table 3.1.** Chemical compositions of segmented polyurethaneureas and their glass transition temperature and melting temperature of soft segment

| Sample name | Soft segment (Mn) | Hard segment | $T_g$/K[a] | $T_m$/K[b] |
|---|---|---|---|---|
| PTMG (856) EDA/DAM | MDI-PTMG (856) | MDI-EDA/DAM (3/2) | 223.9 | — |
| PTMG (1350) EDA/DAM | MDI-PTMG (1350) | MDI-EDA/DAM (3/2) | 205.7 | 221.2 |
| PTMG (2000) EDA/DAM | MDI-PTMG (2000) | MDI-EDA/DAM (3/2) | 196.6 | 275.0 |
| PTMG (856) PDA | MDI-PTMG (856) | MDI-PDA | 209.2 | — |
| PTMG (1350) PDA | MDI-PTMG (1350) | MDI-PDA | 193.1 | 260.5 |
| PTMG (2000) PDA | MDI-PTMG (2000) | MDI-PDA | 190.5 | 281.2 |
| Biomer | MDI-PTMG (1800) | MDI-EDA? | 199.5 | 273.0 |
| PEG (1000) EDA | MDI-PEG (1000) | MDI-EDA | 225.5 | 261.8 |
| PEG (1000) TriMDA | MDI-PEG (1000) | MDI-TriMDA | 234.8 | — |
| PCL (2000) EDA | MDI-PCL (2000) | MDI-EDA | | |
| PCL (2000) TriMDA | MDI-PCL (2000) | MDI-TriMDA | | |

[a] $T_g$ of soft segment
[b] $T_m$ of soft segment

The aggregation states of SPUUs were investigated by means of differential scanning calorimetry.

The film specimens of SPUUs were immersed in aqueous solutions of pepsin (2 mg/ml, pH 2.0) and lipid (lecithin 0.32 wt%; cholesterol 0.16 wt%; amino acids 0.5 wt%; NaCl 0.9 wt%) [7] at 310K. The lipid sorption experiment was carried out under both static and dynamic straining conditions. In the case of the dynamic condition, a sinusoidal deformation of the minimum and maximum strain amplitudes of ca. 5% and 205% was applied to the specimen immersed in the lipid solution. The amount of lipid sorbed by SPUU was evaluated from the weight difference of the specimen before and after exposure to the lipid solution. The state of sorbed lipid was investigated based on the dynamic viscoelastic measurements of the SPUU after immersing in the lipid solution.

The fatigue tests of SPUUs before and after immersion in each solution were carried out by a tensile fatigue tester with a constant imposed strain amplitude under a frequency of 9.26 Hz. The fatigue tester enables continuous measurement of modulus and mechanical loss tangent during the cyclic fatigue process [8]. Also, the fatigue tests were carried out in lipid or hydrolytic enzyme solutions at an ambient temperature of 310K.

## Results and discussion

### Aggregation states of SPUUs

The aggregation state of the hard segment and the state of microphase separation are closely related to the mechanical properties and to the degree of interaction with biological components. The glass transition temperature, $T_g$ of the soft segment of SPUUs is summarized in Table 3.1. The $T_g$ decreased with an increase in $\overline{Mn}$ of polyether. On the other hand, the melting temperature, $T_m$, of the soft segment of SPUU increased with $\overline{Mn}$ of polyether. These results indicate that the microphase separated structure of SPUU becomes more distinct with an increase in $\overline{Mn}$ of polyether in the soft segment.

The hard-segment structure also influences the state of microphase separation. The soft segment in PTMG($\overline{Mn}$)EDA/DAM showed higher $T_g$ and lower $T_m$ than in PTMG($\overline{Mn}$)PDA. PTMG($\overline{Mn}$)PDA gives a distinct X-ray diffraction pattern from the hard-segment crystallite compared with that of PTMG-($\overline{Mn}$)EDA/DAM. This indicates that the crystallite composed of the MDI-EDA/DAM hard segment is not as good as that of MDI-PDA [9]. Since the aggregation strength of hard segments in PTMG($\overline{Mn}$)-EDA/DAM is weaker than in PTMG($\overline{Mn}$)PDA, extensive phase mixing between the hard and soft segments occurred in PTMG($\overline{Mn}$)EDA/DAM. The $T_g$ of PEG(1000)EDA is lower than that of PEG(1000)-TriMDA. This indicates that the microphase separation of PEG(1000)EDA is more distinct than in PEG(1000)TriMDA. X-ray diffraction study and infrared measurements of these samples revealed that the hard-segment structure and the state of hydrogen bonding in MDI-TriMDA differ from those in MDI-EDA [10].

### Lipid sorption behavior of SPUU

It has been reported that silicone rubber heart valves degraded due to absorption of lipid from the blood [11]. Thus, the degree of interaction of lipid with SPUU surfaces is important with respect to the mechanical strength of SPUU. After immersing in a lipid solution at 310K, the specimen exhibited weight increases of 2%–5%. The relation between the state of microphase separation and the amount of lipid

**Fig. 3.1.** Temperature dependence of E' and E" for original PTMG (856) EDA/DAM (*1*) and PTMG (856) EDA/DAM after exposure to a lipid solution for 96 days (*2*)

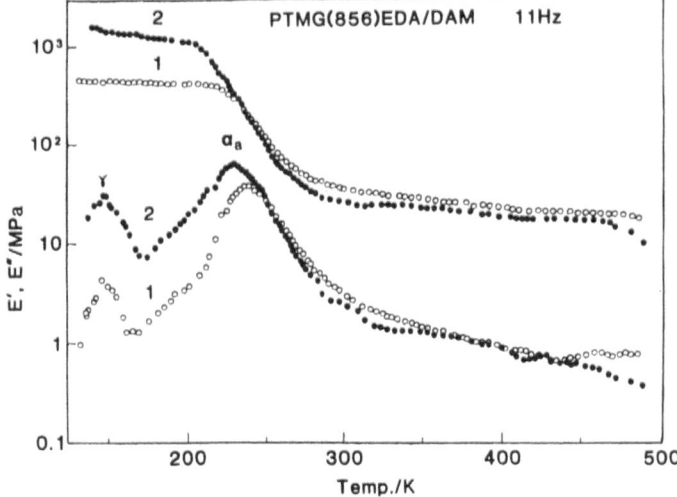

sorption is not clear. Figure 3.1 shows the variation in weight of PCL(2000)EDA with immersion time in a lipid solution at 310K under static and dynamic conditions. The specimen showed initially a sharp increase in weight. The amount of lipid sorbed under dynamic conditions is greater than under static condition. As yet, systematic estimation of lipid sorption has not been done for SPUU. The measurement of lipid absorption under cyclic deformation may be important from the viewpoint of evaluation of the performance of biomedical polymers.

Whether lipid molecules are absorbed into or adsorbed to SPUU is an important problem with respect to the degradation induced by interaction with lipids. Figure 3.2 shows the temperature dependence of the dynamic storage modulus, E', and dynamic loss modulus, E", for the original PTMG(856)EDA/DAM and that after immersing in a lipid solution for 96 days at 310K. The $\gamma$- and $\alpha_a$-absorptions are observed at around 150 and 255K, respectively. After immersing in the lipid solution, the $\alpha_a$-absorption temperature shifts to a lower temperature due to the plasticizing effect of the absorbed lipid. E' in the rubbery state decreased and dissociation of the hard-segment domain occurred at a lower temperature than in the original specimen. These results indicate that the aggregation strength of the hard-segment domain decreased due to lipid absorption. This behavior was observed only for the PTMG($\overline{Mn}$)EDA/DAM, in which the aggregation strength of the hard segment is weak.

**Influence of lipid sorption on fatigue strength of SPUU**

The fatigue behavior of SPUU was studied in the control specimens and specimens after immersion in a

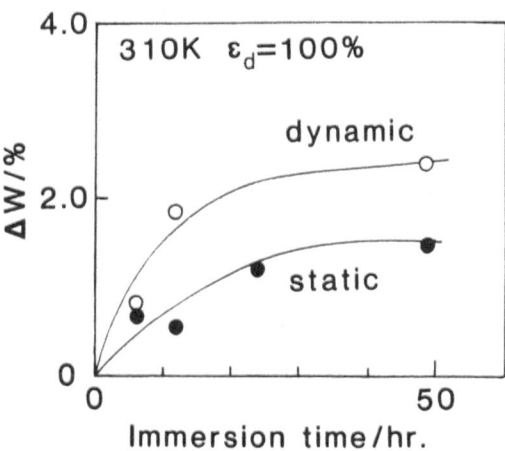

**Fig. 3.2.** Variation in weight increase of PCL (2000) EDA with time immersed in a lipid solution under static and dynamic conditions at 310K

lipid solution. Figure 3.3 shows the relations between fatigue lifetime and imposed strain amplitude for SPUU after immersing the specimen in a lipid solution for 96 days. The strain amplitude-fatigue lifetime behavior of the control samples of PTMG($\overline{Mn}$)-EDA/DAM and Biomer was similar to the curve 5 in Fig. 3.3. The fatigue strength for the original SPUU except for PEG(1000)TriMDA is sufficient for its application as a blood pump for an artificial heart system. The fatigue lifetimes of PTMG($\overline{Mn}$)EDA/DAM, PCL(2000)EDA, and PCL(2000)TriMDA after immersion in a lipid solution for 96 days were strikingly reduced at the same imposed strain amplitude. This may be caused by the absorbed lipids. Biomer, PTMG($\overline{Mn}$)PDA, and PEG(1000)EDA, where the

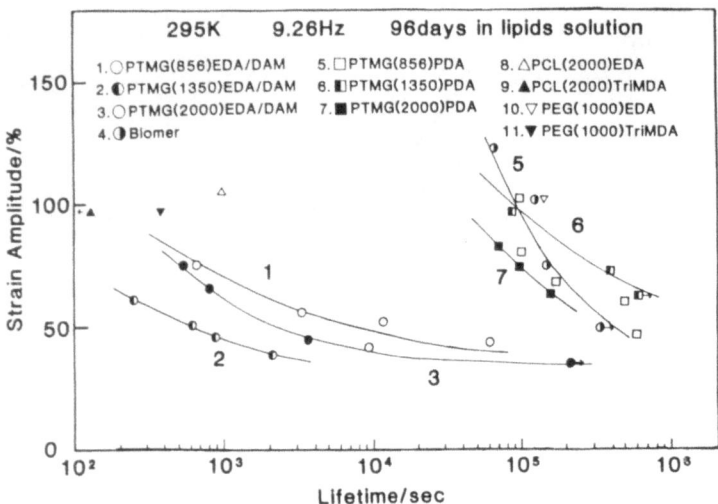

**Fig. 3.3.** Relation between fatigue lifetime and imposed strain amplitude for SPUU's after immersion in a lipids-solution for 96 days

hard segments have strong aggregation strength, did not show any reduction in fatigue strength. Even though PCL(2000)EDA has an MDI-EDA hard segment, this specimen showed reduction in fatigue strength; this is due to the phase mixing between the hard and soft segments caused by the interaction between ester group in the soft segment and urea group in the hard segment. The original SPUU containing the MDI-TriMDA hard segment showed a shorter fatigue lifetime than the SPUU containing the MDI-EDA hard segment. This is attributed to the weak aggregation of the hard segment. The SPUU with the MDI-TriMDA hard segment shows extensive reduction in fatigue strength after immersion in the lipid solution. This is due to the decrease in aggregation strength of the hard segment after lipid sorption.

Figure 3.4 shows the scanning electron micrograph of PTMG(1350)EDA/DAM, which was fatigue-fractured after immersing in a lipid solution for 96 days at 310 K under an imposed strain amplitude of 38%. The direction of cyclic straining is perpendicular to the fracture surface. This specimen showed a number of microcracks, which were propagated perpendicular to the direction of cyclic straining. In addition to the microcracks, a "mirror zone" was observed on the fatigue-fractured surface after lipid absorption: This is the slow growth area containing the origin of the fracture that is smooth and of high specular reflectivity. Since the original specimen did not show either "microcracks" or a "mirror zone" after fatigue fracture, these may be attributed to adsorbed lipids in the specimen. These results suggest that lipids absorbed by the specimen promote the formation and propagation of cracks. This behavior was only observed for the SPUU containing hard segments with weak aggregation strength. These microcracks may also serve as sites for thrombus formation or as initiation sites of calcification.

The fatigue test for the sample after immersion in a lipid solution was carried out in air. However, there is some debate as to whether drying cracks develop upon removal of the specimen from the lipid solution. To eliminate these effects, fatigue tests were carried out in a lipid solution. Figure 3.5 shows the variation of E' for the PCL(2000)EDA with time during the fatigue process. The sample for fatigue testing was immersed in a lipid solution for 30 and 96 days. The E' of PCL(2000)EDA in the lipid solution is lower than that in air. This is attributed to the plasticization effect of lipids or water. The fatigue lifetime of SPUU decreased with an increase in lipid solution immersion time. This is a similar trend to that observed in air. These results may indicate that absorption of lipids under cyclic straining did not induce the reduction in fatigue strength. Lipids which absorbed and diffused into hard-segment domains during the long-term exposure to the lipid solution were the cause of the reduced fatigue strength.

### Influence of Hydrolytic Enzymes on Fatigue Strength of SPUU

Enzymes are able to catalyze the degradation of synthetic polymers. Cell-polymer interactions may lead to cellular activation and enhanced enzyme exocytosis by the inflammatory cells [12]. Thus, estimation of the fatigue strength of polymers after exposure to a hydrolytic enzyme solution is important from the viewpoint of medical applications.

To characterize the state of degradation, the weight change of the specimen after exposure to an enzyme solution was investigated. The weight change for SPUUs was measured after exposure to a pepsin solution for 14 days. The weight decrease of PEG(1000)Y was higher than other SPUUs. Since PEG is hydrophilic and the absorbed water content of

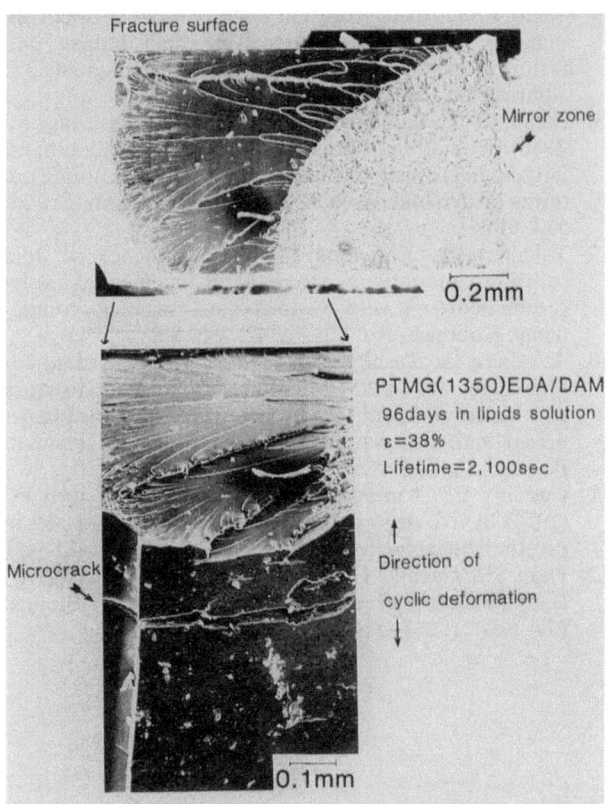

**Fig. 3.4.** Scanning electron micrograph for the fatigue fracture surface of PTMG (1350) EDA/DAM after exposure to a lipid solution for 96 days. The fatigue test was carried out under the conditions of the imposed strain amplitude of 38% and an ambient temperature of 295K

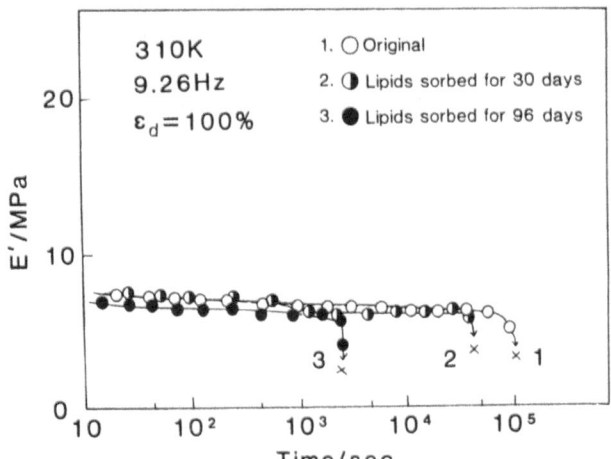

**Fig. 3.5.** Variation of E′ with time during the fatigue process for PCL (2000) EDA in a lipid solution at 310K. Fatigue test was carried out after immersion under the condition of the imposed strain amplitude of ca.100%

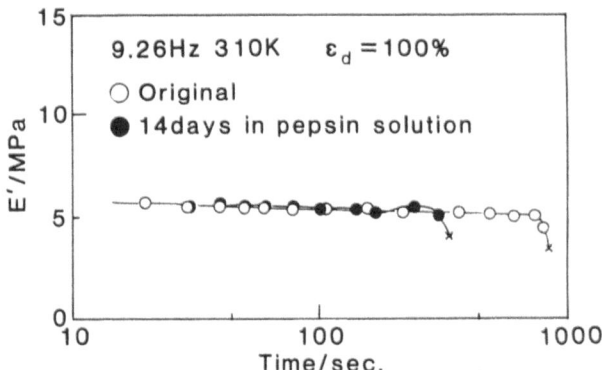

**Fig. 3.6.** Variation of E′ with time during the fatigue process for PEG (1000) TriMDA after immersing in a pepsin solution (pH = 2.0) for 14 days. The fatigue test was carried out under the conditions of the imposed strain amplitude of ca.100% and the ambient temperature of 310K

PEG(1000)Y is greatest among the SPUUs, pepsin can easily penetrate into the water-swollen PEG-(1000)Y. Measurement of the solution viscocity of the sample after exposure to the enzyme solution revealed that the molecular weight of the specimen decreased after interaction with the enzyme.

Figure 3.6 shows the variation of E′ with time during the fatigue process for PEG(1000)TriMDA before and after immersion in a pepsin solution for 14 days. The fatigue lifetime for PEG(1000)TriMDA decreased after immersion in the pepsin solution, but that for PEG(1000)EDA did not. This is attributed to the difference in the microphase separated state. Since the fraction of partial phase mixing between the hard and soft segments in PEG(1000)TriMDA is greater than that in PEG(1000)EDA, PEG(1000)-TriMDA was easily hydrolyzed by pepsin compared with PEG(1000)EDA. Since the SPUUs composed of hydrophobic soft segments do not swell in water, the hydrolytic enzyme cannot attack the urethane or urea group in such SPUUs. Thus, SPUUs with hydrophobic soft segments did not show any degradation by pepsin.

## Conclusion

The amount of lipid sorption by an SPUU depended on the aggregation strength of the hard segment. The relations between fatigue strength under various pseudobiological environments and the aggregation state of SPUUs were investigated. The SPUU with ordered hard segments did not show any degradation due to lipid sorption. The hydrolytic resistance of SPUUs with hydrophobic polyether soft segments is better than those with hydrophilic soft segments. An SPUU with sufficient fatigue strength in a biological environment can be prepared from hydrophobic soft segments and ordered hard segments.

## References

1. Reid JS, Rosenberg G, Pierce W (1985) Transmission of water through a biocompatible polyurethane: Application to circulatory assist device. J Biomed Mater Res 19: 1181–1202
2. Martz H, Beaudoin G, Paytner D, King M, Marceau D, Guidoin R (1987) Physicochemical characterization of a hydrophobic microporous polyurethane vascular graft. J Biomed Mater Res 21: 399–412
3. Lyman DJ, Seare Jr. WJ Albo Jr. D, Bergman S, Lamb C, Metcalf LC, Richards K (1977) Polyurethane elastomers in surgery. Int J Polym Mat 5: 211–229
4. Zartnack F, Dunkel W, Affeld K, Bucherl ES (1978) Fatigue problems in artificial blood pumps. Trans Am Soc Art Intern Organs 24: 600–605
5. Coleman DL, Lim D, Kesseler T, Andrade JD (1981) Calcification of nontextured implantable blood pumps. Trans Am Soc Art Intern Organs 27: 97–104
6. Lelah MD, Lambrecht LK, Young BR, Cooper SL (1983) Physicochemical characterization and in vivo blood tolerability of cast and extruded Biomer. J Biomed Mat Res 17: 1–22
7. Takahara A, Tashita J, Kajiyama T, Takayanagi M (1985) Effect of aggregation state of hard segment in segmented poly(urethaneureas) on their fatigue behavior after interaction with blood components. J Biomed Mat Res 19: 13–34
8. Takahara A, Yamada K, Kajiyama T, Takayanagi M (1980) Evaluation of fatigue lifetime and elucidation of fatigue mechanism in plasticized poly(vinyl choride) in terms of dynamic viscoelasticity. J Appl Polym Sci 25: 597–614
9. Takahara A, Kajiyama T (1985) Influence of lipid sorption on fatigue strength of segmented poly(urethaneureas) with various hard segment components. Kobunshi Ronbunshu 42: 793–801
10. Takahara A, Tashita J, Kajiyama T, Takayanagi M, Macknight WJ (1985) Microphase separated structure and blood compatibility of segmented poly(urethaneureas) with different diamines in the hard segment. Polymer 26: 978–986
11. Cuddihy EF, Moacanin J, Roschke EJ, Harrison FC (1976) In vivo degradation of silicone rubber poppets in prosthetic heart valves. J Biomed Mat Res 10: 471–481
12. Phau SK, Castillo E, Anderson JM, Hiltner A (1987) Biodegradation of a polyurethane in vitro. J Biomed Mat Res 21: 231–246

# Discussion

*Cooper* (University of Wisconsin): The degradation of segmented polyurethaneureas with a polyethyleneglycol soft segment in a biological environment may caused by two factors, such as oxidation by peroxides and hydrolysis by hydrolytic enzymes. Which factor caused degradation in this case?

*Takahara* (Kyushu University): We observed the degradation of segmented poly urethaneureas with polyethyleneglycol under the action of hydrolytic enzymes. Possible degradation caused by oxidation was not confirmed by the characterization method we used.

# 4. In vitro and ex vivo studies of the antithrombogenicity of polyether-segmented nylon 610 of crystalline-amorphous microstructure

Nobuhiko Yui, Kazunori Kataoka, and Yasuhisa Sakurai[1]

**Summary.** The interaction of platelets with polypropylene oxide-segmented nylon 610 surfaces was investigated by two distinct approaches. First, an in vitro simulation test of thrombosis on copolymer surfaces was performed by continuous flow of recalcified platelet-rich plasma through polymer columns to clarify the relation between platelet activation and thrombosis on these surfaces. Second, an ex vivo test of the polymers was carried out using an arteriovenous shunt in rabbits to estimate the number and adhesiveness of circulating platelets in a living body with an implanted shunt. The results obtained suggest that a copolymer surface with a microstructure composed of crystalline and amorphous phases minimizes the activation of adsorbed platelets, resulting in excellent thromboresistance.

**Key words:** Antithrombogenicity—Polyether-segmented nylon 610—Crystalline-amorphous microstructure—Platelet activation

The exposure of blood to artificial surfaces results in platelet interactions, which trigger the sequence of steps resulting in thrombosis [1]. Therefore, in making artificial organs and surgical prosthetic devices with high performance, it is indispensable to design material surfaces which minimize adverse platelet interactions [2].

We have carried out systematic studies on the antithrombogenicity of various polycondensation polymers in terms of estimating platelet adhesion on their surfaces [3–8]. Throughout these studies, we found that the platelet adhesion on polypropylene oxide (PPO)-segmented polyamides with various polyamide segments was closely related to their microstructure, which was composed of crystalline and amorphous phases. Platelet adhesion was minimized at the surfaces of the copolymers with a long period of 12–13 nm and a crystallite thickness of 6.0–6.5 nm [6–8]. This result suggested that the balance of crystalline and amorphous phase distribution was an important factor in eliminating platelt adhesion and activation on these surfaces. Moreover, we employed

X-ray photoelectron spectroscopy to investigate the surface chemical composition of a series of PPO-segmented nylon 610 copolymers and showed that the surface which minimized platelet adhesion had the same chemical composition as the interior of the copolymer [9]. This result supported our belief concerning the importance of having a surface microstructure composed of crystalline and amorphous phases to eliminate platelet adhesion and activation. In previous papers, we evaluated the in vivo antithrombogenicity of PPO-segmented nylon 610 copolymers and suggested that their crystalline-amorphous microstructure was responsible for the excellent antithrombogenic character [10, 11].

This paper deals with the interaction of platelets with PPO-segmented nylon 610 copolymer surfaces. Two distinct approaches were used—an in vitro test of surface thrombosis and an ex vivo arteriovenous shunt test in the rabbit.

## Materials and methods

In the in vitro simulation test, nylon 610 and two kinds of PPO-segmented nylon 610 with a different PPO content were used. The structural formula of the copolymer is as follows:

$$\left[ O(\underset{\underset{CH_3}{|}}{CH}CH_2O)_l C[\underset{\underset{O}{\parallel}}{N}(CH_2)_6 \underset{\underset{H}{|}}{N}C(CH_2)_8 \underset{\underset{O}{\parallel}}{C}]_m \right]_n $$

:PPO-segmented nylon 610

The synthesis and characterization of the copolymers have been previously reported [4, 9], and the structural parameters of nylon 610 and the copolymers used in this study are summarized in Table 4.1. These copolymers are designated by a three-sequence code, such as 61P3-25, where "61" refers to nylon 610, "P3" to PPO with a molecular weight of 3000, and "25" to the weight percentage of PPO in the copolymer. The copolymer which minimized platelet adhesion in the previous test using fresh canine blood was 61P3-25, which has a long period of approximately 12 nm, and a crystallite thickness of 6.5 nm [5–8]. In that test, the

[1]Institute of Biomedical Engineering, Tokyo Women's Medical College, 8-1 Kawada-cho, Shinjuku-ku, Tokyo, 162 Japan

**Table 4.1.** Structural parameters of PPO-segmented nylon 610

| Code | PPO content[a] (wt.-%) | Degree of crystallinity[b] of nylon 610 region | Long period[c] (nm) | Crystallite thickness[d] (nm) |
|------|------------------------|------------------------------------------------|---------------------|-------------------------------|
| Nylon 610 | 0 | 0.67 | 9.9 | 6.3 |
| 61P3-25 | 25 | 0.67 | 11.6 | 6.5 |
| 61P3-47 | 47 | 0.75 | 14.6 | 7.1 |

[a] PPO content was determined by elemental analysis.
[b] Degree of crystallinity of nylon 610 region was estimated by density method.
[c] Long period was measured from small-angle X-ray scattering.
[d] Crystallite thickness was measured from wide-angle X-ray diffraction.

amount of adhering platelets on the polymer surfaces increased in the following order—61P3-25, 61P3-47, nylon 610.

The in vitro simulation test of thrombosis on polymer surfaces was carried out using a modified microsphere column method previously reported in detail [10]. The procedure is summarized only briefly here. Platelet-rich plasma (PRP; platelet concentration ca. $2-3 \times 10^8$ cells/cm³) was prepared from the citrated blood of male Japanese white rabbits. $CaCl_2$ aqueous solution (2 weight percent) was added to the PRP so that the concentration of $Ca^{2+}$ in the PRP was 5.5 mmol/l. The recalcified PRP was continuously added to a polyvinyl chloride column (3 mm inner diameter and 10 cm long) packed with 1 g of polymer-precoated glass beads (48–60 mesh) until the column was occluded by thrombosis or all of the PRP in the syringe was consumed. The flow rate of PRP was maintained at 0.2 cm³/min with the use of an infusion pump (Precidol, model 5003). The thrombosis time of each polymer column was defined as the time when the platelet count in the column effluent became zero and was determined as the intercept of the effluent curve of platelets on the time axis. The simulation test using recalcified PRP with sodium azide was also examined by adjusting the concentration of sodium azide in the PRP to 20 mmol/l.

For the ex vivo test, tubing of commercial segmented polyether polyurethane (SPU), made from polytetramethylene oxide, 4,4'-diphenylmethane diisocyanate, and 1,4-butanediol, 1.4 mm inner diameter and 20 cm long, was coated on its internal and partially on its external surface with the PPO-segmented nylon 610(61P3-25) or poly-(2-hydroxyethyl methacrylate) (PHEMA). The details of polymer coating on the tubing were reported previously [10]. Three kinds of tubing, 61P3-25, PHEMA, and non-coated SPU, were implanted in a male Japanese white rabbit by forming an arteriovenous (AV) shunt, i.e., surgically connecting the carotid artery to the jugular vein via the tubing. During the AV shunt

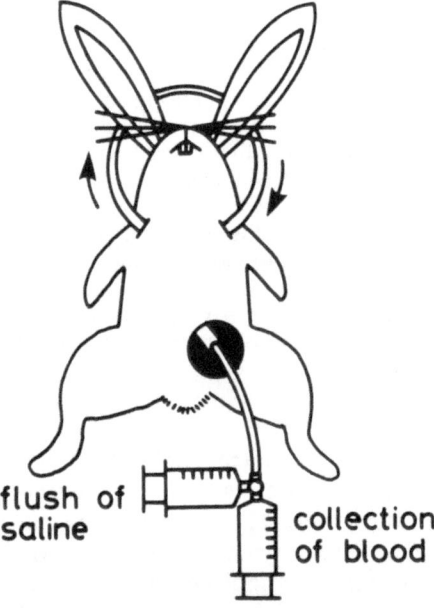

**Fig. 4.1.** Procedure for ex vivo arteriovenous shunt test in a rabbit

experiment, a small volume of fresh blood at prescribed times was collected through a polyvinyl chloride catheter cannulating the femoral artery. The blood sample was used to estimate changes in the number and adhesiveness of the circulating platelets with tubing-implant time. The adhesiveness of platelets was determined by passing the blood through a column packed with polystyrene-precoated glass beads. The procedure of the ex vivo AV shunt in a rabbit is illustrated in Fig. 4.1.

## Results and discussion

First, we performed the in vitro thrombosis test on the copolymer surfaces using recalcified PRP. It should be noted that the sequential steps for thombosis, includ-

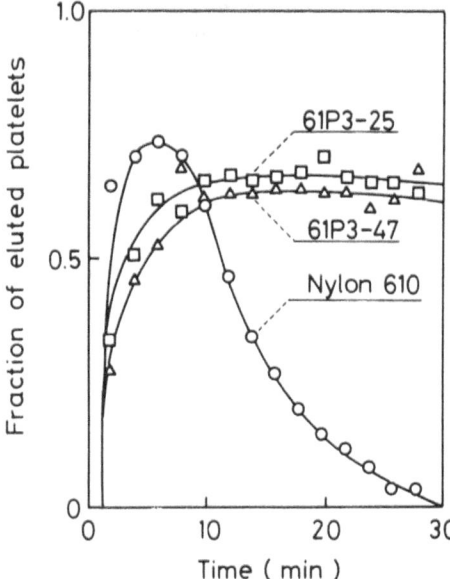

**Fig. 4.2.** Representative curves of platelet elution from polymer columns. Initial concentration of platelets—$3.22 \times 10^8$ cells/cm³

**Table 4.2.** Results of the in vitro simulation test of thrombosis on PPO-segmented nylon 610 surfaces

| Code | Thrombosis time (min) | | | | |
|---|---|---|---|---|---|
| | 0–10 | 11–20 | 21–30 | 31–40 | 41– |
| Nylon 610 | 2 | 0 | 2 | 4 | 0 |
| 61P3-25 | 0 | 0 | 0 | 3 | 5 |
| 61P3-47 | 1 | 1 | 2 | 1 | 3 |

Initial concentration of platelets in PRP: $(3.17 \pm 0.20) \times 10^8$ cells/cm³

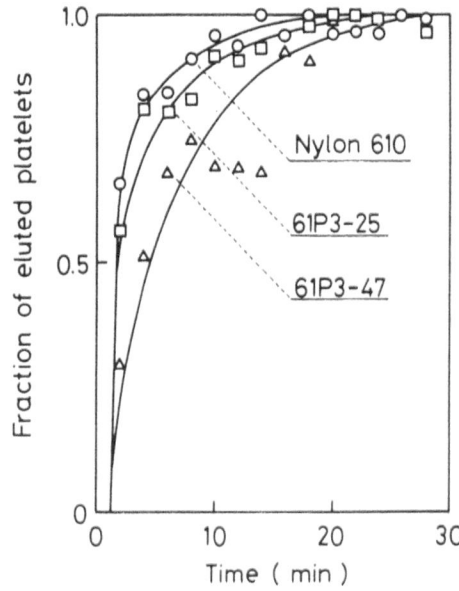

**Fig. 4.3.** Representative curves of platelet elution from polymer columns using PRP with sodium azide. Initial concentration of platelets—$2.00 \times 10^8$ cells/cm³

ing platelet activation and aggregation as well as the cascade of coagulation factors, occurs in the presence of calcium ions. Figure 4.2 shows representative curves of platelet elution from the polymer columns. Here, the platelets in the column effluent were counted as a measure of thrombosis in the column. The nylon 610 column showed a rapid decrease in platelet elution in the first 10 min and was occluded within 30 min due to thrombosis. In contrast, the 61P3-25 and -47 columns showed almost constant platelet elution over 30 min. This figure indicates that adsorbed platelets on these copolymer surfaces were not so activated to accelerate thrombosis as those on the nylon 610 surface. Table 4.2 summarizes the results of these in vitro simulation tests for each polymer column. In Table 4.2, the thrombosis time divided into 10-min intervals was obtained from eight separate experiments. As shown in this table, 61P3-25 had the longest thrombosis time of all the polymers evaluated and exhibited an average thrombosis time of over 40 min. In previous platelet adhesion tests using canine fresh blood, platelet adhesion was minimized in those copolymers containing a particular crystalline-amorphous microstructure. This microstructure corresponds to the 61P3-25 copolymer. The results obtained previously were considered to include the whole interaction of blood with the material surface, including both the initial adsorption of platelets and the subsequent platelet activation process. Thus, the results in Table 4.2 are consistent with those obtained in the canine platelet adhesion test.

To clarify the role of platelets in thrombosis, we added sodium azide to the recalcified PRP in the in vitro column experiment. Sodium azide is known to be an inhibitor of the energy metabolism of platelets. Upon adding sodium azide to the PRP, neither depression of platelet elution nor thrombosis was observed (Fig. 4.3). This result indicates that platelets undergo a sequence of activation processes due to changes in their energy metabolism, resulting in thrombosis. Therefore, enlongation of the thrombosis time in the 61P3-25 column presented in Table 4.2 is considered to be due to suppression of the activation process of adsorbed platelets rather than merely reducing the physicochemical adsorption of platelets on the surface.

We next examined the ex vivo antithrombogenicity of several polymers using the AV shunt test in order

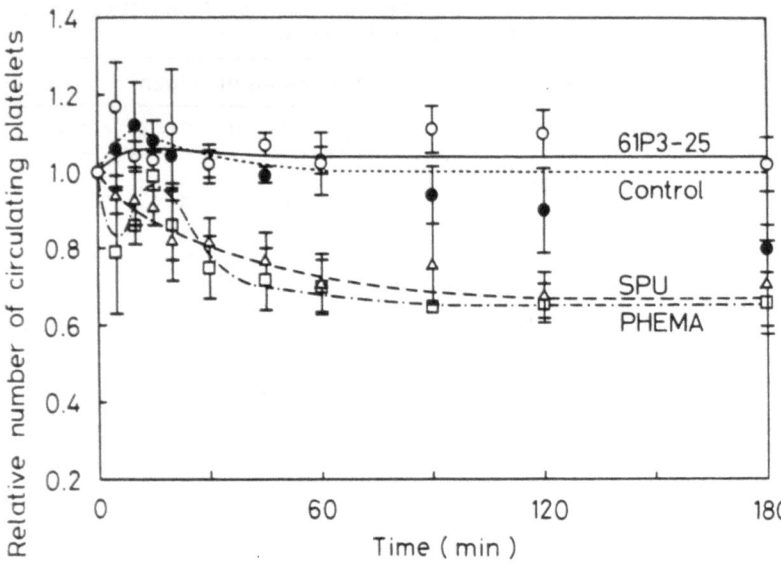

**Fig. 4.4.** Change in the relative number of circulating platelets with shunt-implant time

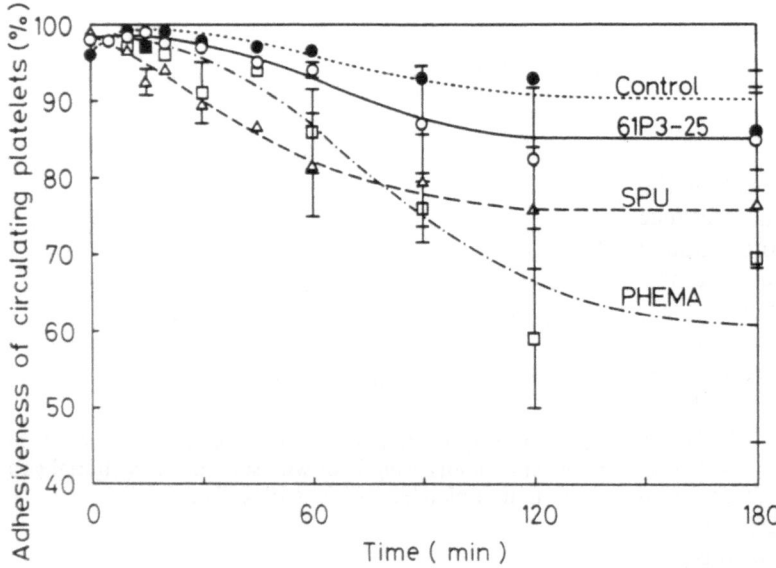

**Fig. 4.5.** Change in the adhesiveness of circulating platelets with shunt-implant time

to confirm the above hypothesis. The changes in the relative number and adhesiveness of circulating platelets with tubing implant time are shown in Figs. 4.4 and 4.5, respectively. Here, the adhesiveness of the circulating platelets was estimated as one of the platelet functions in vivo. PHEMA and noncoated SPU tubings showed a relatively great decrease in both the relative number and adhesiveness of the circulating platelets compared with the control. The control involved cannulation of the rabbit femoral artery with the PVC catheter. These results indicate depression of the function and number of platelets through their contact with or deposition on these polymer surfaces. On the other hand, the relative number and adhesiveness of circulating platelets for 61P3-25 were almost the same as in the control. These results strongly support the suggestion that the 61P3-25 surface minimizes the activation of adsorbed platelets.

In conclusion, the results of the in vitro and ex vivo studies suggest that copolymer surfaces with a certain microstructure composed of crystalline and amorphous phases exhibit excellent antithrombogenicity because of their ability to eliminate the activation of adsorbed platelets on the surface. Therefore, control of surface microstructures composed of crystalline and amorphous phases is a promising concept for the molecular design of antithrombogenic materials.

**Acknowledgments.** The authors are grateful to Profs. N. Ogata and K. Sanui, Sophia University, for their cooperation in the research presented in this paper. Thanks are also due to Mr. A. Takahashi, Mr. Y. Kashiwagi, Mr. F. Endo, Terumo Co., and Mr. T. Aoki, Sophia University, for their help in part of these experiments. This research was financially supported by the Japan Research Promotion Society for Cardiovascular Diseases.

# References

1. Anderson JM, K-Marchant K (1985) Platelet interaction with biomaterials and artificial devices. CRC Crit Rev Biocompat 1: 111–204
2. Yui N, Kataoka K, Sakurai Y (1986) Microdomain-structured polymers as antithrombogenic materials. In: Akutsu T, Koyanagi H, Pennington DG, Poirier VL, Takatani S, Kataoka K (eds) Artificial heart 1. Springer, Tokyo, pp 23–30
3. Yui N, Takahashi Y, Sanui K, Ogata N, Kataoka K, Okano T, Sakurai Y (1981) Effect of crystallinity of polymeric materials on antithrombogenicity. Jpn J Art Org 10: 1070–1073
4. Yui N, Tanaka J, Sanui K, Ogata N (1984) Polyether-segmented polyamides as a new designed antithrombogenic material: Microstructure of poly(propylene oxide)-segmented nylon 610. Makromol Chem 185: 2259–2267
5. Yui N, Tanaka J, Sanui K, Ogata N, Kataoka K, Okano T, Sakurai Y (1984) Characterization of the microstructure of poly(propylene oxide)-segmented polyamide and its suppression of platelet adhesion. Polym J 16: 119–128
6. Yui N, Oomiyama T, Sanui K, Ogata N, Kataoka K, Okano T, Sakurai Y (1984) Polyether-segmented polyamide as a new antithrombogenic material: Relationship between platelet adhesion and microstructure of poly(propylene oxide)-segmented aliphatic polyamides. Makromol Chem 5: 805–809
7. Yui N, Sanui K, Ogata N, Kataoka K, Okano T, Sakurai Y (1986) Effect of microstructure of poly(propylene oxide)-segmented polyamides on platelet adhesion. J Biomed Mat Res 20: 929–943
8. Yui N, Kataoka K, Okano T, Sakurai Y, Sanui K, Ogata N (1986) Microstructure of polyether-segmented polyamides and its role in antithrombogenicity. In: Christel P, Meunier A, Lee AJC (eds) Biological and biomechanical performance of biomaterials. Advances in Biomaterials 6. Elsevier, Amsterdam, pp 309–314
9. Yui N, Kataoka K, Sakurai Y, Sanui K, Ogata N, Takahara A, Kajiyama T (1986) ESCA study of new antithrombogenic materials: Surface chemical composition of poly(propylene oxide)-segmented nylon 610. Makromol Chem 187: 943–953
10. Yui N, Kataoka K, Sakurai Y, Aoki T, Sanui K, Ogata N (1988) In vitro and in vivo studies on antithrombogenicity of poly(propylene oxide)-segmented nylon 610 in relation to its crystalline-amorphous microstructure. Biomaterials 9: 225–229
11. Aoki T, Ogata N, Yui N, Kataoka K, Sakurai Y (1987) Antithrombogenicity of segmented nylon 610 with crystalline-amorphous microstructure. Jpn J Art Org 16: 1395–1398

# Discussion

*Cooper* (University of Wisconsin): What are the physical properties of the semicrystalline amorphous block polymers compared with the urethanes? Can they be use in the same applications by simple substitution?

*Yui* (Tokyo Women's Medical College): We have examined the physical properties, such as viscoelasticity and stress-strain measurements and found that these segmented polyamides are superior to the polyurethanes in terms of strength and modulus; they have a modulus of the order of $10^9$ to $10^{10}$ dynes/cm$^2$ at room temperature. Another advantage with this polymer is that it can be processed by injection molding. Segmented polyurethane ureas have relatively good thromboresistance but have the disadvantage that they must be processed from solution.

*Cooper:* I have studied the physical property correlations of the polyether-polyester copolymers, which in the USA are called Hytrel. They have a semicrystalline hard segment of poly(tetramethylene teraphthalate) The main difference between these materials and urethanes is a higher hysteresis in stress cycling. Thus, I think that in the area of fatigue, the semicrystalline segmented polymers may have many characteristics which are different to those of polyurethanes. More testing is necessary to clarify this situation.

# 5. Design and synthesis of blood-compatible polyurethane derivatives

Yoshihiro Ito, Takashi Kashiwagi, Shu Qin Liu, Lin Shu Liu, Yasuhiro Kawamura, Yuichiro Iguchi, and Yukio Imanishi[1]

**Summary.** Polyurethanes carrying fluoroalkyl, sulfonic acid, carboxylic acid substituents, or quaternary ammonium groups, or which have poly(ethylene glycol) or poly-dimethylsiloxane graft chains, or which are ionically or covalently heparinized, have been synthesized. The water contact angle of these polyurethane derivatives ranged from 0° to 110°.

Heparinized polyurethanes were highly blood compatible. The other polyurethane derivatives were more blood compatible than usual polyetherurethaneureas. It was concluded that hydrophilization and hydrophobilization of the surface are effective for improving the blood compatibility of polyurethanes, which are relatively blood compatible because of their characterisitic surface structure.

**Key words:** Blood compatibility—Polyurethane—Heparin —Wettability

Polyurethanes are the most useful materials for medical devices because of their excellent mechanical properties and relatively high blood compatibility [1]. But the blood compatibility is not high enough for clinical use as small-diameter vascular prostheses.

There are three possible ways to improve the blood compatibility of polyurethanes. The first is chemical modification, the second is combination with biological anticoagulants, and the third is endothelialization.

For the first approach, we designed and synthesized polyurethane derivatives with different wettabilities. For the second approach, heparinized polyurethanes were synthesized by appropriate methods. Interactions of these polyurethane derivatives with blood components, such as platelets or blood coagulation factors, were investigated.

## Materials and methods

### Polymer syntheses

#### Conventional polyurethane
The polyurethane is made of polytetramethylene glycol (PTMG, molecular weight 2020), 4,4'-diphenylmethane diisocyanate (MDI), and 1,2-diaminopropane (PDA)—1:2:1.

### Polyurethanes containing fluoroalkyl substituents
Figure 5.1 shows the method for synthesizing poly-urethanes containing fluoroalkyl groups in the hard (PEUU-FH) or soft segments (PEUU-FS) [2–4]. In the former, PTMG and MDI were reacted to yield a prepolymer. F-528, which is a dihydroxyl compound containing a fluoroalkyl substituent, was then added to extend the prepolymer to a high molecular weight polyurethane. The content of fluorine ranges from 7.0 to 24.0 wt%.

In the case of PEUU-FS, polyether [P (FAPO)], which is a copolymer of fluoroalkyl epoxide (FAPO) and propylene oxide, as shown in Fig. 5.2, was reacted with MDI and PDA to yield polyure-thaneurea.

### Polyurethanes containing polydimethylsiloxane as side chains
Partially epoxidized polybutadiene (molecular weight 3020, HO-PEBD-OH), which contains hydroxyl groups at both ends of the chain, MDI, and diethylene glycol (DEG) were reacted to yield a polyurethane containing epoxide groups in the soft segments [5]. The epoxide groups were converted to hydoxyl groups by reaction with an alcohol. At this stage, the poly-urethane was cast into a film. Hydroxyl groups on the surface of the film were reacted with excess MDI and then with polydimethylsiloxane (molecular weight 7000) containing a primary amine group at one end of the chain to yield a polyurethane containing poly-dimethylsiloxane side chains (Fig. 5.3).

### Polyurethanes containing NHSO$_3$H and COOH substituents
Polybutadiene (molecular weight 3070), which contains hydroxyl groups at both ends of the chain, was reacted with MDI to yield a urethane prepolymer [6]. PDA was added to extend the prepolymer. The un-saturated polyurethane was reacted with chlorosul-fonyl isocyanate and hydrolyzed to yield polyurethane carrying NHSO$_3$H and COOH groups, as shown in Fig. 5.4.

[1] Department of Polymer Chemistry, Kyoto University, Yoshida Honmachi, Sakyo-ku, Kyoto, 606 Japan

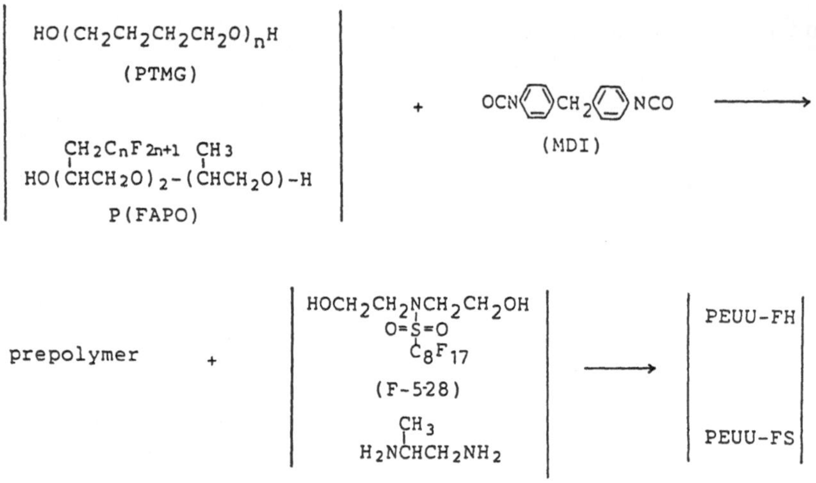

HO(CH$_2$CH$_2$CH$_2$CH$_2$O)$_n$H

(PTMG)

$$\begin{array}{c} CH_2C_nF_{2n+1} \quad CH_3 \\ HO(CHCH_2O)_2-(CHCH_2O)-H \end{array}$$

P(FAPO)

$+$ OCN⟨ ⟩CH$_2$⟨ ⟩NCO $\longrightarrow$

(MDI)

**Fig. 5.1.** Synthetic method of polyurethanes containing fluoroalkyl groups in hard or soft segments

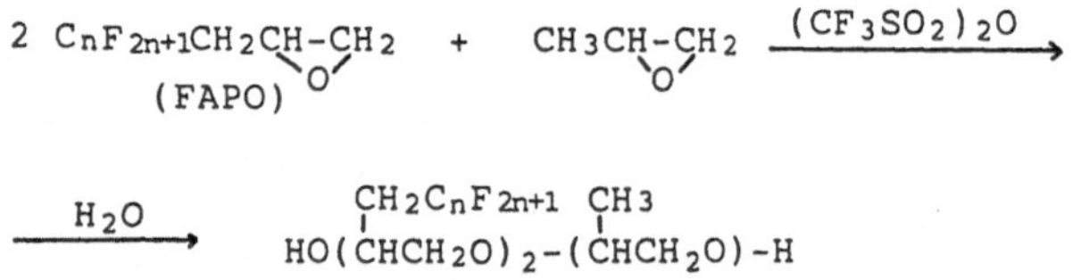

prepolymer $+$

$$\begin{array}{c} HOCH_2CH_2NCH_2CH_2OH \\ O=S=O \\ C_8F_{17} \end{array}$$

(F-528)

$$\begin{array}{c} CH_3 \\ H_2NCHCH_2NH_2 \end{array}$$

$\longrightarrow$

PEUU-FH

PEUU-FS

$$2\ C_nF_{2n+1}CH_2CH-CH_2 \ + \ CH_3CH-CH_2 \xrightarrow{(CF_3SO_2)_2O}$$

(FAPO)  O                    O

**Fig. 5.2.** Synthetic route of P (FAPO)

$$\xrightarrow{H_2O} \begin{array}{c} CH_2C_nF_{2n+1} \quad CH_3 \\ HO(CHCH_2O)_2-(CHCH_2O)-H \end{array}$$

| n | composition of FAPO (%) |
|---|---|
| 4 | 2 ± 1 |
| 6 | 52 ± 4 |
| 8 | 30 ± 4 |
| 10 | 10 ± 2 |
| 12 | 3 ± 1 |
| 14 | 1 ± 0.5 |

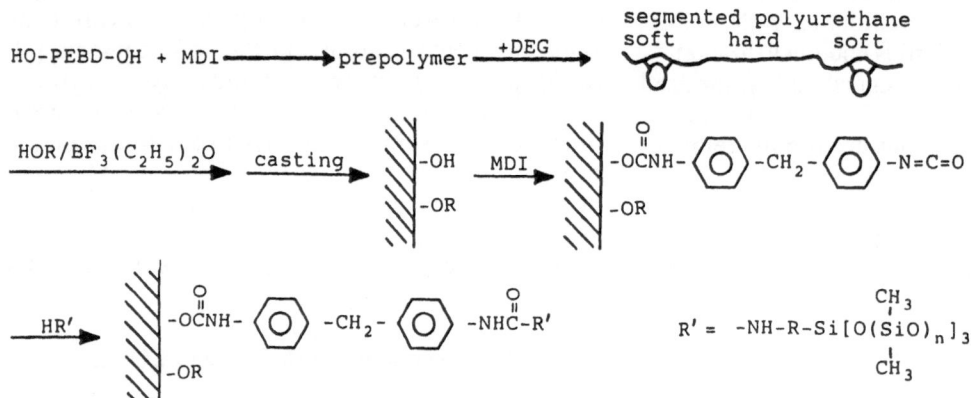

HO-PEBD-OH + MDI $\longrightarrow$ prepolymer $\xrightarrow{+DEG}$ segmented polyurethane

$\xrightarrow{HOR/BF_3(C_2H_5)_2O}$ casting $\longrightarrow$ [-OH / -OR] $\xrightarrow{MDI}$ [-OCNH-⟨ ⟩-CH$_2$-⟨ ⟩-N=C=O / -OR]

$\xrightarrow{HR'}$ [-OCNH-⟨ ⟩-CH$_2$-⟨ ⟩-NHC-R' / -OR]

$$R' = -NH-R-Si[O(SiO)_n]_3 \quad \begin{array}{c} CH_3 \\ | \\ | \\ CH_3 \end{array}$$

**Fig. 5.3.** Synthetic method for polyurethanes containing polydimethyl siloxane as side chains

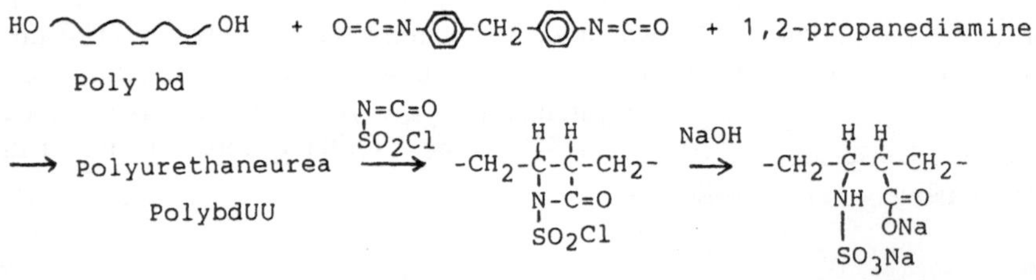

HO ∿∿∿ OH $+$ O=C=N-⟨ ⟩-CH$_2$-⟨ ⟩-N=C=O $+$ 1,2-propanediamine

Poly bd

$\longrightarrow$ Polyurethaneurea $\xrightarrow[SO_2Cl]{N=C=O}$ -CH$_2$-C-C-CH$_2$- $\xrightarrow{NaOH}$ -CH$_2$-C-C-CH$_2$-

PolybdUU

**Fig. 5.4.** Synthetic method for polyurethanes containing NHSO$_3$H and COOH substituents

**Fig. 5.5.** Synthetic method for polyurethanes containing SO$_3$H or COOH

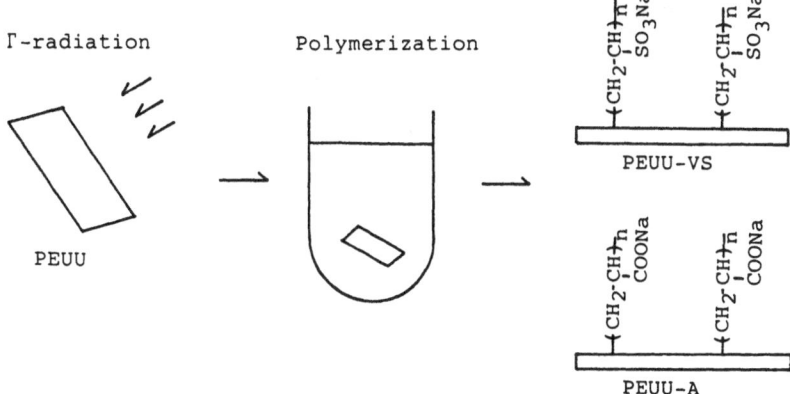

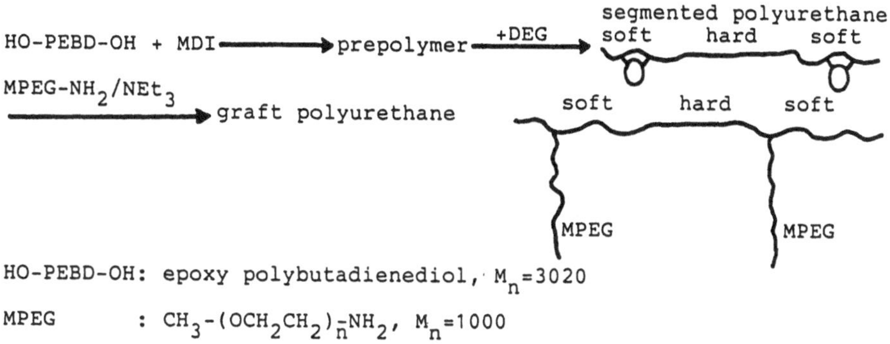

**Fig. 5.6.** Synthetic method for polyurethanes containing polyethylene glycol as side chains

HO-PEBD-OH + MDI ⟶ prepolymer $\xrightarrow{+DEG}$ segmented polyurethane

MPEG-NH$_2$/NEt$_3$ ⟶ graft polyurethane

HO-PEBD-OH: epoxy polybutadienediol, $M_n$=3020

MPEG    : CH$_3$-(OCH$_2$CH$_2$)$_{\overline{n}}$NH$_2$, $M_n$=1000

## Polyurethane containing SO$_3$H or COOH substituents

The conventional polyurethane was preirradiated by [60]Co gamma rays, and then vinyl sulfonate or acrylate was grafted on the surface, as shown in Fig. 5.5 [7].

## Polyurethanes containing polyethylene glycol as side chains

Partially epoxidized polybutadiene (molecular weight 3070), which possesses hydroxyl groups at both ends of the chain, MDI, and diethyleneglycol were reacted to yield a polyurethane containing epoxide groups in the soft segments [8]. the epoxide groups of the polyurethane were reacted with polyethyleneglycol (molecular weight 1000), containing a primary amine group at one end of the chain, in the presence of triethylamine as a catalyst to yield the polyurethane shown in Fig. 5.6. The content of polyethyleneglycol is 66.5 wt%.

## Polyurethanes containing quaternary ammonium groups in the main chain or side chains

Polymers of this type are represented by Q-PAEUU in Fig. 5.7 [9]. A polyether bearing a tertiary amine group in the main chain or side chains was synthesized. Mixtures of the amine-containing polyether and PTMG in various molar ratios were reacted with MDI to yield prepolymers. The chain extension with PDA yielded polyetherurethaneurea containing tertiary amine groups in the main chain or side chains. The content of tertiary amine group is 4.04 wt%. The amine groups were quaternized by alkyl halides to yield Q-PAEUU.

## Heparinized polyurethanes

The Q-PAEUU was ionically heparinized by immersion in a solution of 1 wt% sodium heparinate, as shown in Fig. 5.7 [9–11].

Polyurethanes carrying carboxylic acid ester groups were synthesized by the reaction of PTMG, MDI, and L-Lys-OMe, as shown at the top of Fig. 5.8. The surface of the polyurethane film was hydrolyzed and neutralized with citric acid. A polyurethane film on which carboxylic acid groups were introduced was synthesized, as shown at the bottom of Fig. 5.8. Heparin was coupled to the carboxylic acid groups of the polymer using 1-ethyl-3-(3-dimethylaminopropyl) carbodiimide, which is a water-soluble carbodiimide (WSC). The amount of immobilized heparin is 24.5 $\mu$g/cm$^2$.

Figure 5.9 shows the insertion methods of heparinizing polyurethanes with different kinds of spacer groups such as 1,6-diaminohexane, 1,12-diaminododecane, polyallylamine (molecular weight 10 000, 60 000) or caproic acid. Heparin was connected to the polyurethane through the free amine or carboxyl groups of the spacer arm.

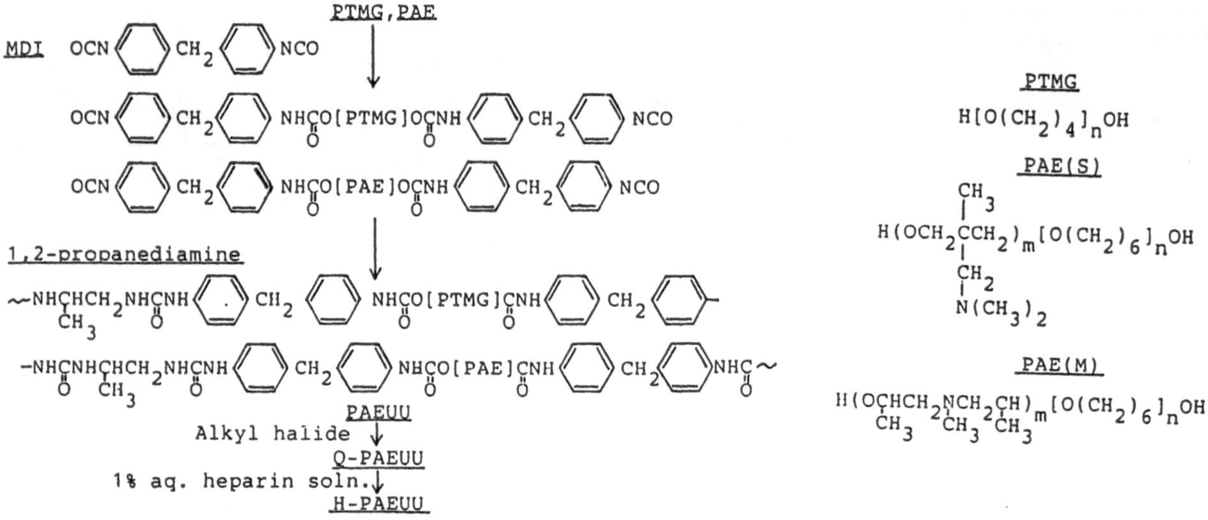

**Fig. 5.7.** Synthetic method for polyurethanes containing quaternary ammonium groups in main chain or side chains and ionically heparinized polyurethanes

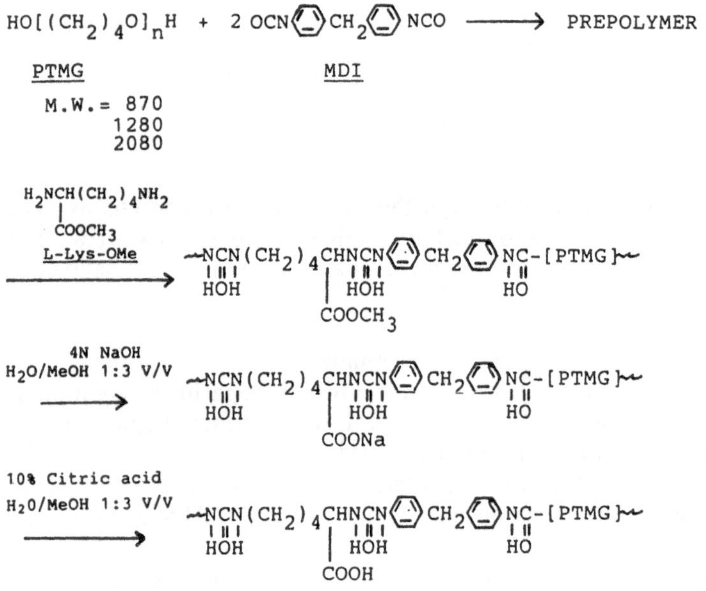

**Fig. 5.8.** Synthetic method for covalently heparinized polyurethanes

## Wettability of polymers

Wettability was evaluated by water contact angle. The water contact angle was measured by putting a sessile droplet of distilled water on the surface of the polymer film in contact with the air [10].

## In vitro blood clotting test

Canine blood was placed on the sample and aqueous $CaCl_2$ was added [9]. After 15-min contact incubation at 37°C, the thrombus that formed on the sample was weighed. The amount of thrombus that formed on the glass was taken as the standard.

## Platelet adhesion

Platelet-rich plasma (PRP) was prepared from canine blood and platelets were labeled with $Na_2$ $^{51}CrO_4$ and $^3H$-serotonin [12]. $^{51}Cr$ was found in the plasma membrane and cytoplasm of the platelet, and $^3H$-serotonin in the amino-storage granule. Labeled PRP was placed on a polymer film for 10 min at 37°C. The radioactivity of adherent platelets was counted. From the $^{51}Cr$ radioactivity, the number of adhering platelets was determined. From the $^3H$ radioactivity, the amount of released serotonin from adhering platelets was determined.

**Fig. 5.9.** Synthetic method for heparinized polyurethanes with intervening different spacer groups

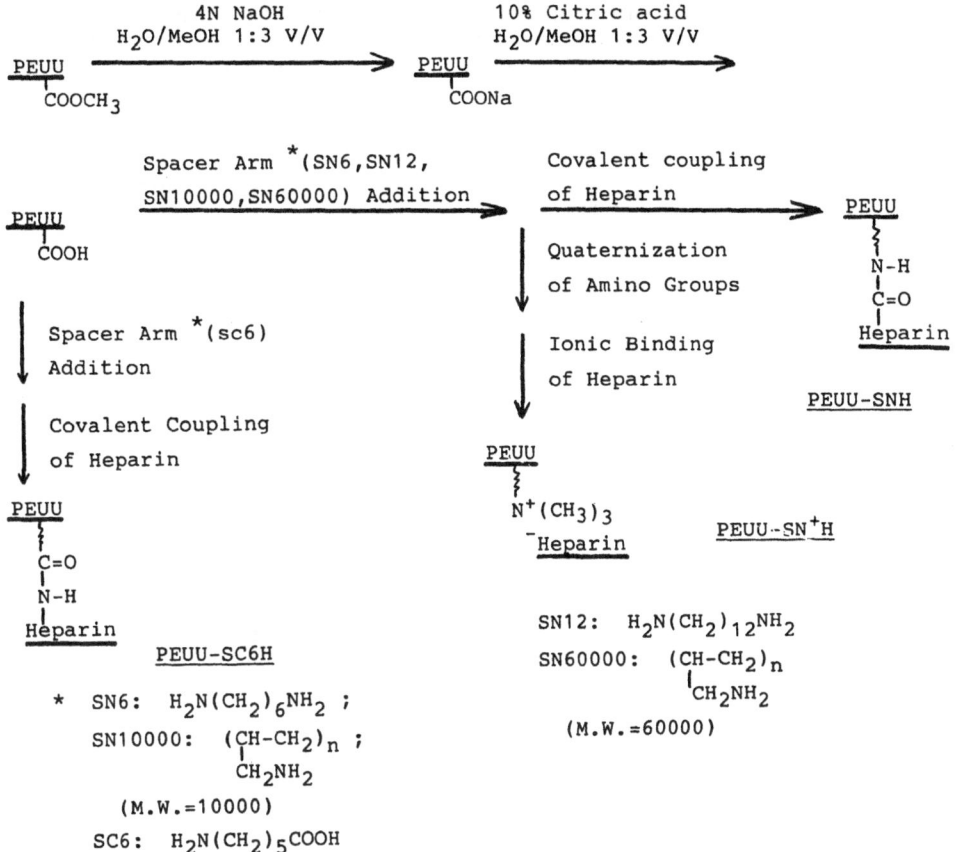

## Activated partial thromboplastin time, recalcification time, and thrombin time

**Activated partial thromboplastin time (APTT).** Platelet-poor plasma (PPP) and an aqueous solution of rabbit-brain phospholipid were mixed in a polymer-coated test tube and incubated for 5 min at 37°C [6, 7]. Then aqueous $CaCl_2$ solution was added. The time required for fibrin formation (APTT) was determined.

**Recalcification time (RCT).** The same procedure as above was used in the absence of rabbit brain phospholipid [8]. The time required for the formation of a fibrin network was determined.

**Thrombin time (TT).** The same procedure as used for the APTT experiment was carried out except that thrombin was added instead of $CaCl_2$ and phospholipid [10]. In this case, a coagulation time was measured.

## In vivo test

Sutures of the polyurethanes were spun by a wet spinning method and implanted into canine veins. The left and right jugular veins and the femoral veins were ex-

posed and a 19-gauge needle was inserted into the vein. The implant material was introduced through the needle into the lumen of the vessel. After the needle was withdrawn, the suture was ligated to the vessel. After 3 months, the suture was taken out and observed by scanning electron microscopy (SEM).

## Results and discussion

Table 5.1 shows the polyurethane derivatives synthesized in this investigation in decreasing order of water contact angles. The results of the evaluation of the materials antithromobogenic character are also shown.

The water contact angle of the polyurethanes containing 7 wt% fluorine content (PEUU-FH) was $106° \pm 2°$. The contact angle did not increase very much, even thought the content of fluoroalkyl groups in the polyurethane increased. This indicates that most of the fluoroalkyl groups tend to be exposed to the surface of the polymer at a low overall content. The fluoroalkyl groups suppressed the biological interaction of the polyurthane surface with blood components, resulting in a relatively high blood compatibility.

**Table 5.1.** Wettability and in vitro antithrombogenicity of synthesized polyurethane derivatives

| Substituents in Polymer | Water contact angle (°) | Thrombus formed (%) | Platelet adhesion | | APTT, RCT, or TT (s) |
|---|---|---|---|---|---|
| | | | Adhesion ($10^3$ $\mu m^2$) | Serotonin release (%) | |
| Fluoroalkyl (PEUU-FH) | 106–109 ± 2 | 55–60 | 10 ± 1 | 15 ± 7 | — |
| Polydimethylsiloxane | 98 ± 3 | 65–70 | 10 ± 2 | — | 145 ± 5[a] |
| —(conventional) | 68 ± 5 | 83–95 | 20 ± 2 | 30 ± 4 | 124 ± 2 |
| $NHSO_3H$ and COOH | — | 50–80 | 15 ± 2 | — | 194 ± 5 |
| SO$_3$H | 58 ± 3 | 60–70 | 17 ± 2 | — | 181 ± 4 |
| COOH | 50 ± 3 | 65–75 | 13 ± 2 | — | 147 ± 4 |
| N$^+$ (CH$_3$)$_3$ | — | 47–93 | 16 ± 2 | 25 ± 2 | — |
| Ionically heparinized | — | 0 | 4 ± 2 | 15 ± 4 | — |
| Covalently heparinized | 20 ± 3 | 0 | 15 ± 2 | 20 ± 2 | >200[b] |
| Polyethylene glycol | 0 | 53 | 9 ± 1 | — | 182 ± 5[a] |
| (glass | 0 | 100 | 30 ± 2 | — | 90 ± 5>) |

*APTT* activated partial thromboplastin time, *RCT* recalcification time, *TT* thrombin time
[a]RCT
[b]TT

In the case of the polydimethylsiloxane-grafted polyurethane, the contact angle was 98° ± 3°, which is very similar to the value of silicone rubber. The antithrombogenicity is intermediate between those of the fluoroalkylated polyurethanes and conventional polyurethanes.

The wettability of all polyurethanes having ionic groups was high. The difference in contact angles between polyvinyl sulfonate-grafted and polyacrylate-grafted polymers can be ascribed to different amounts of grafting. Interactions of the ionic polyurethanes with blood depended on the kind and the concentration of ionic groups. Interactions of cationic groups of the polymer, such as quaternary ammonium groups, with anionically charged biocomponents were so strong that the higher the surface concentration of cationic groups, the lower the antithrombogenicity of the material. On the other hand, anionic groups suppressed the biological interaction of the polymer with blood. The polyurethane containing $NHSO_3H$ or $SO_3H$ groups prolonged the thrombin time. This experimental result is interesting, because similar functional groups are found in heparin.

Heparinization decreased the water contact angle and strongly enhanced the antithrombogenicity of the polyurethanes. It has been reported that heparin deactivates thrombin by complexing with antithrombin III. The prolongation of the thrombin time of the covalently heparinized polyurethane suggests that the immobilized heparin can deactivate thrombin. Moreover, ionically heparinized polyurethane suppressed the platelet adhesion and activation of adhered platelets. Heparinized polyurethanes with intervening spacer arms also exhibit antithrombogenicity in spite of the relatively small amount of immobilized heparin. The introduction of a spacer enabled heparin to be released slowly.

The polyurethane having polyoxyethylene side chains was the most wettable among those investigated. The water contact angle of the swollen material was almost zero, but the swelling prohibited a precise determination of the value. This finding suggests exposure of polyoxyethylene chains on the surface. This material was the most blood compatible except for the heparinized polyurethanes.

From the above results, it is concluded that the heparinized polyurethanes possess the highest in vitro blood compatibility. These polymers were tested for in vivo biocompatibility. Figure 5.10 shows SEM images of the sutures implanted in a canine vein for 90 days. The surface of the ionically heparinized polyurethane suture is very clear without any attachment of a thrombus. On the other hand, on the covalently heparinized polyurethane suture, the growth of endothelial cells was observed. As described before, ionically bound heparin suppressed the adhesion of platelets, but covalently bound heparin was less effective in suppressing platelet adhesion. It is suggested that a moderate stimulation of adhered platelets by bound heparin leads to the secretion of platelet-derived growth factor (PDGF) from its alpha granules, resulting in the growth of endothelial cells. In any event, the heparinized polyurethanes are highly blood compatible both in vitro and in vivo.

The antithrombogenicity/wettability relation of the present polyurethanes is summarized in Fig. 5.11. Short-term blood compatibility can be obtained by heparinization. Approaches to long-term blood compatibility remain a subject for future research.

**Acknowledgments.** This research was supported by the Ministry of Education, Science, and Culture and the Japan Society for the Promotion of Science for Japanese Scientists.

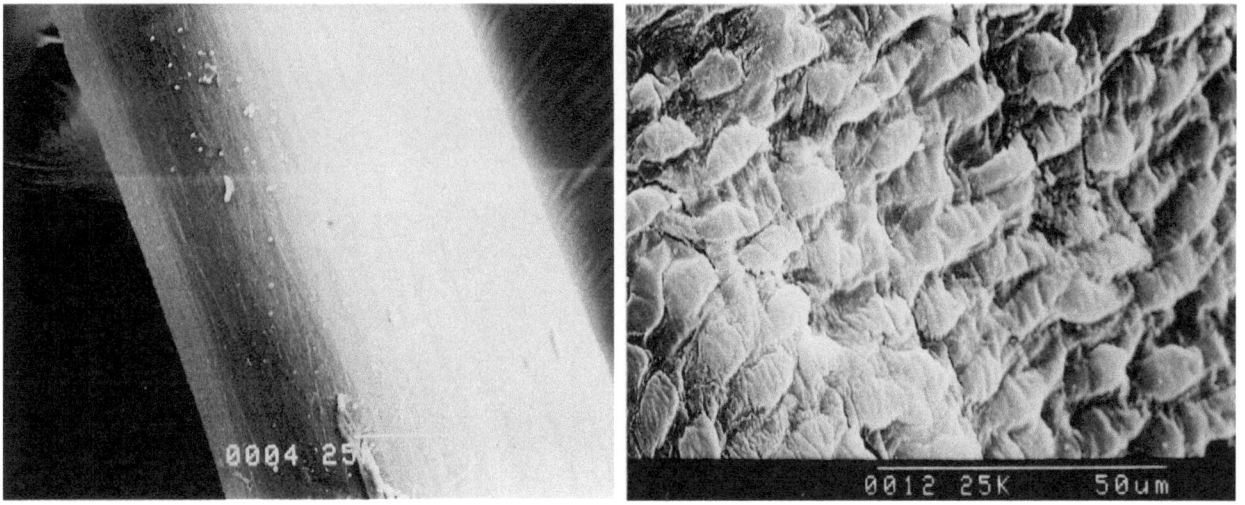

**Fig. 5.10a, b.** Scanning electron micrographs of **a** ionically or **b** covalently heparinized polyurethanes after 90 days' implantation

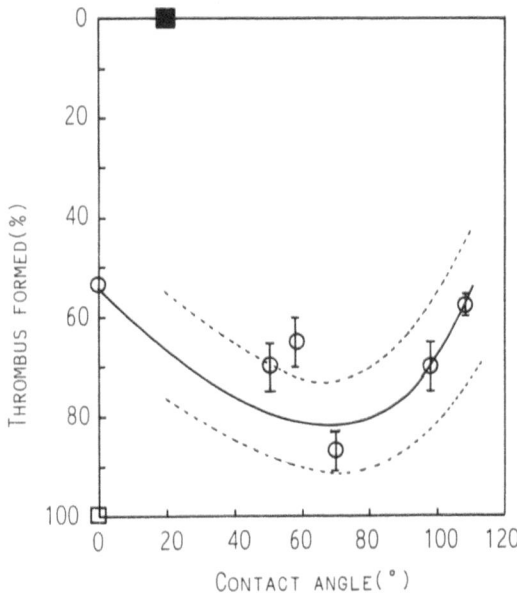

**Fig. 5.11.** Relation between the water contact angle and thrombus formation on the polyurethane derivatives synthesized in this investigation. ■ heparinized polyurethanes, ○ nonheparinized polyurethanes, □ glass

# References

1. Lehal MD, Cooper SL (1986) Polyurethanes in medicine. CRC, Boca Raton
2. Kashiwagi T, Ito Y, Kang IK, Sisido M, Imanishi Y (1985) Synthesis of fluorinated polyurethane and its evaluation as antithrombogenic material. Polym Prepr Jpn 34: 582 (in Japanese)
3. Kashiwagi T, Ito Y, Sisido M, Imanishi Y (1987) Synthesis of fluorinated polyurethane and its evaluation as antithrombogenic material. Polym Prepr Jpn 36: 818 (in Japanese)
4. Kawamura Y, Ito Y, Sisido M, Imanishi Y (1986) Synthesis of polyetherurethaneurea bearing long fluoroalkyl chains in the soft segments, its oxygen permeability and antithrombogenicity. Kobe Polym Symp 32: 61 (in Japanese)
5. Liu SQ, Ito Y, Sisido M, Imanishi Y (1987) Synthesis and biocompatibility of segmented polyurethane having PDMS side chains grafted on the surface. Polym Prepr Jpn 36: 819 (in Japanese)
6. Iguchi Y, Ito Y, Sisido M, Imanishi Y (1986) Synthesis of heparinoid polyurethane and its interaction with blood components. JSB Prepr 8: 30 (in Japanese)
7. Iguchi Y, Ito Y, Sisido M, Imanishi Y (1987) Synthesis and interaction with blood components of heparinoid polyurethane. Polym Prepr Jpn 36: 822 (in Japanese)
8. Liu SQ, Ito Y, Sisido M, Imanishi Y (1986) Synthesis and biocompatibility of segmented polyurethane with poly(ethylene glycol) side chains. Polym Prepr Jpn 35: 534 (in Japanese)
9. Ito Y, Sisido M, Imanishi Y (1986) Synthesis and antithrombogenicity of polyetherurethaneurea containing quaternary ammonium groups in the side chains and of the polymer/heparin complex. J Biomed Mater Res 20: 1017–1033
10. Ito Y, Sisido M, Imanishi Y (1986) Synthesis, antithrombogenicity, and interactions with plasma proteins of anionic polyurethanes and heparin-bound polyurethanes. J Biomed Mater Res 20: 1157–1178
11. Liu LS, Ito Y, Sisido M, Imanishi Y (1986) Study on the antithrombogenicity of covalently or ionically heparinized polyetherurethaneurea with spacer arms. Polym Prepr Jpn 35: 536 (in Japanese)
12. Mori A, Ito Y, Sisido M, Imanishi Y (1986) Interaction of polystyrene/poly (γ-benzyl L-glutamate) and poly(methyl methacrylate)/poly(γ-benzyl L-glutamate) block copolymers with plasma proteins and platelets. Biomaterials 7: 386–392

# Discussion

*Kim* (University of Utah): One of the methods you use to attach heparin to the surface is ionic bonding. How does the ionic exchange then operate?

*Ito* (Kyoto University): Sodium heparinate was used. With ionically heparinized polyurethane, heparin is released. But in the initial stages of contact between polyurethane and blood, if the initial antithrombogenic surface is completed it is not necessary to release heparin.

*Miyama* (Technological University of Nagaoka): In the case of ionically bound heparin, the release rate of heparin is very critical in preventing thrombus formation: If it is too fast or too slow, the heparinized system is ineffective. What is the release rate of heparin in your case?

*Ito:* We have not measured this under flow conditions.

# 6. Improved blood compatibility of heparin immobilization and PEO-PDMS-heparin triblock copolymer coating on surfaces of segmented polyurethaneurea

Teruo Okano[1], David Grainger[1], Ki Dong Park[1], Chisato Nojiri[1], Jan Feijen[2], and Sung Wan Kim[1]

**Summary.** New heparin-immobilized polyurethaneurea surfaces utilizing hydrophilic spacer systems have been developed for in situ surface modification. Surface modification both by hydrophilic grafting of polyethylene oxide (PEO) and PEO-heparin as well as by heparinized amphiphilic block copolymer coatings significantly improves the nonthrombogenicity of the polyurethaneurea surface without changing the bulk mechanical properties. Heparin immobilization by grafting and coating provides levels of bioactivity that are successful in suppressing contact activation of the intrinsic cascade as well as inhibiting platelet adhesion in vitro. Ex vivo evaluation of these systems in whole blood shunts under conditions of low flow rate and low shear show an impressive ability of immobilized heparin to prolong shunt patency over control materials.

Key words: Surface modification—Immobilized heparin—PEO grafted surface—Blood-compatible polyurethaneurea—Heparin triblock copolymer

Polymeric materials have contributed significantly to the development and improvement of devices and systems in artificial organs. Segmented polyurethaneureas have been used in many prosthetic applications, specifically in vascular grafts and the artificial heart, owing to their inherent nonthrombogenic and suitable mechanical properties. However, the blood compatibility of these segmented polyurethaneureas is not acceptable for the further development of ideal artificial organs in contact with blood. This paper includes new methods for the improvement of the blood compatibility of polyurethaneureas by in situ surface modifications without changing the bulk properties of the existing segmented polyurethaneurea substrate. Ebert and Kim have previously reported that heparin-immobilized surfaces with alkyl spacers prevented fibrin net formation by means of heparin's bioactive catalytic effect in inactivating thrombin [1]. These surfaces, however, activated platelets because of the hydrophobicity of the alkyl spacers [2] and, perhaps, heparin itself [3], resulting in platelet aggregation. Thus, while the system produced the desired nonthrombogenic effects, involving suppression of the intrinsic cascade activation, the spacer system together with heparin also induced undesirable platelet activation, resulting in thrombosis. To improve nonthrombogenicity of the heparinized surfaces, therefore, it is necessary to establish a method not only of maintaining the bioactivity of immobilized heparin but also of preventing heparin-induced platelet activation and aggregation.

This paper describes the development of heparin-immobilized segmented polyurethaneurea surfaces using hydrophilic, long polyethylene oxide (PEO) chains as spacers. Previously described highly dynamic motions of PEO spacers at blood-material interfaces [4, 5] are expected to contribute to an increase in heparin bioactivity and a reduction in platelet adhesion. Spacer length effects for heparin-immobilized segmented polyurethaneurea surfaces are discussed in relation to this strategy.

Okano and colleagues have previously proposed that hydrophilic/hydrophobic microdomain surfaces maintain a unique interaction with blood components [6, 7]. Platelet adhesion and activation on microdomain surfaces were significantly suppressed in both in vitro and ex vivo experiments, mediated by the existence of an organized protein layer [8]. Covalent addition of bioactive heparin microdomains to the hydrophilic/hydrophobic block copolymer microdomains is intended by synthesis of heparin-PEO-polydimethylsiloxane (PDMS) triblock copolymers. From this perspective, heparin bioactivity and platelet adhesion and activation were studied and discussed.

[1] Center for Controlled Chemical Delivery and Department of Pharmaceutics, University of Utah, Salt Lake City, UT 84112, USA
[2] Biomaterials Section, Dept. of Chemical Technology, Twente University of Technology, Enschede, The Netherlands

## Materials and methods

### Heparin immobilization on segmented polyurethane surfaces

Heparin has been immobilized onto the surface of Biomer (commercial segmented polyetherurethane-urea, Ethicon Co. Sommerville, NJ, USA) using hydrophilic spacer groups, specifically polyethlene oxides (PEO) with molecular weights of 200, 1000, and 4000. The reaction process is shown in Fig. 6.1 [9]. The synthetic scheme involves the coupling of a telechelic diisocyanate-derivatized PEO to Biomer through an allophanate/biuret reaction. The free isocyanate remaining on the spacer group is then coupled through a condensation reaction to functional groups (-OH, -NH$_2$) on heparin.

The first step in the procedure is to derivatize the PEO polymers with isocyanate functional groups. This is accomplished by reacting toluene 2 4-diisocyanate (TDI) and PEO in a 2:1 molar ratio. TDI is first dissolved in benzene and PEO slowly added dropwise. This is done to assure a continual excess of TDI and to prevent inter- or intramolecular oligomerization between PEO polymer units. The reaction proceeds under N$_2$ gas for 2–3 days at 60°C. The TDI-PEO-TDI molecule is then purified through repeated precipitation in diethylether.

The TDI-PEO-TDI spacer groups are grafted onto the Biomer surface through an allophanate/biuret reaction between the urethaneurea-nitrogen proton and the isocyanate-derivatized PEO, as shown in Fig. 6.2a. Glass beads (200 $\mu$m diameter), used as a model substrate, are first acid-cleaned and dried and then coated with Biomer (0.5% DMAC). The Biomer-coated beads are then thoroughly washed and dried (60°C under vacuum). Telechelic isocyanated-PEO spacers are coupled to the surface of the Biomer beads in the presence of a catalyst—0.1 v/v % dibuty-ltindilaurate (DBTDL)—in benzene at 60°C. The reaction is carried out over different times to vary the amount of PEO surface grafting. The PEO-grafted beads are then thoroughly washed with benzene to remove unreacted, unbound PEO.

A portion of the isocyanate PEO-grafted surfaces have been immersed in methanol to block the isocyanate groups remaining on the free ends of the PEO grafts. These PEO-Biomer surfaces are used as controls in in vitro surface experiments. The amount of PEO grafted on the surface, as measured by acid-base back titration of the free isocyanate groups, has been measured to be between $0.4 \times 10^{-8}$ to $2.5 \times 10^{-8}$ moles NCO/cm$^2$ bead surface and is dependent on the reaction time.

Heparin is covalently bound to the isocyanate-PEO-Biomer surfaces through a coupling reaction be-

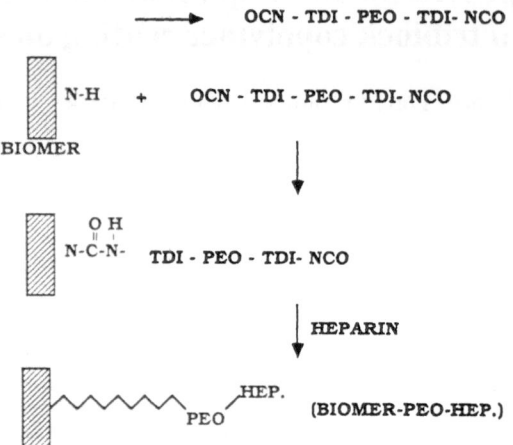

**Fig. 6.1.** Heparin immobilization onto Biomer surfaces

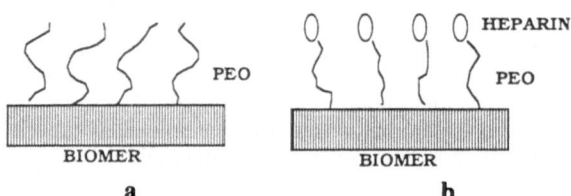

**Fig. 6.2a, b.** Heparin immobilized surfaces of Biomer

tween the free hydroxyl or amine groups on heparin and the free isocyanate group on the PEO spacer, as shown in Fig. 2b. Heparin is first dissolved in formamide, followed by the addition of DBTDL (0.05 v/v %) and the isocyanate-PEO-Biomer beads. The bead solution is gently stirred at room temperature for 3 days. The heparin-PEO-Biomer beads are thoroughly washed with acetone and water to remove unreacted materials and solvents.

The surface concentration of immobilized heparin is determined by the toluidine blue chromogenic method of Smith and co-workers [10] and has been determined to be $0.31 - 0.7$ $\mu$g/cm$^2$ bead surface.

This method of surface modification has also been successful in the coating of films, tubes (shunts), and other polyurethane devices.

### Heparin-PEO hydrophobic chain triblock copolymer coating

Heparin-PEO-PDMS triblock copolymers have been synthesized by the procedure shown in Fig. 6.3 [11]. Semitelechelic amino-PDMS (Petrarch Systems, Bristol, PA, USA) is first coupled to amino telechelic PEO in toluene under nitrogen at room temperature via two different diisocyanate coupling agents—TDI and methylene diphenyl diisocyanate (MDI)—

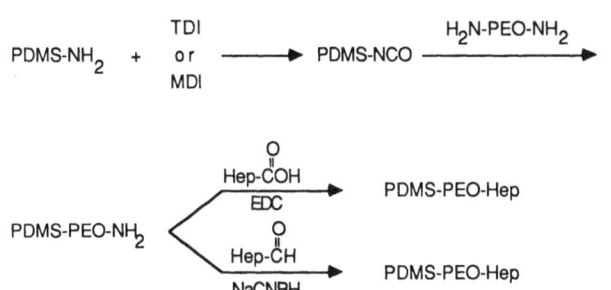

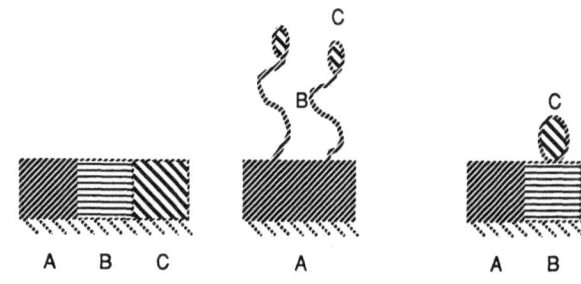

**Fig. 6.3.** Synthetic scheme for triblock copolymers of heparin-PEO-PDMS

**Fig. 6.4.** Coating morphologies for heparin-PEO-PDMS block copolymers. **A** hydrophobic domain (PDMS), **B** hydrophilic domain (PEO) **C** heparin domain

creating a diblock copolymer having one free amino group at the PEO chain terminus. This amino group is functionally used in two different coupling procedures to covalently link heparin to the diblock copolymer in solution coupling reactions. The well-known carbodiimide method (EDC), using heparin's carboxylic groups, and the selective reduction amination procedure, using sodium cyanoborohydride to reduce a Schiffs base between heparin and the diblock copolymer, both yield bioactive triblock copolymers (heparin-PEO-PDMS).

To make heparin soluble in THF: water solution with PDMS-PEO-NH$_2$ for coupling, heparin is first cation-exchanged with trimethyl ammonium bromide in water to form a heparin salt with enhanced organic solubility (Triton B heparin). For EDC-activated coupling, this modified Triton B salt is dissolved in water and THF is slowly added with stirring until a 1:4 water: THF mixture is formed. PDMS-PEO-NH$_2$ is dissolved in a similar mixture and the two solutions are mixed and the pH brought to 5.0. EDC in THF:water is added in eight portions at 30-min intervals and the reaction is maintained by stirring at room temperature for 12 h. The reaction is then kept at pH 7.5 for 24 h and finally terminated by removing the solvents by evaporation, lyophilization, and thorough rinsing of the resulting solid with water to yield the triblock copolymer.

Derivatized heparin is prepared by nitrous acid hydrolysis followed by Triton-B treatment to provide an organically soluble, bioactive heparin containing one aldehyde group per molecule. This heparin derivative is coupled to PDMS-PEO-NH$_2$ by reductive amination. The fresh copolymer is dissolved in THF:water with sonication and heparin is similarly dissolved in separate THF:water mixtures. The two solutions are mixed and the pH adjusted to 6.5. Sodium cyanoborohydride (dissolved in THF:water) is added and the entire solution is stirred at room temperature for 7 days at pH 6.5. The reaction products are recovered by removing THF by evaporation, lyophilization, and subsequent thorough rinsing

of the white solid with water to remove unreacted heparin and reducing agent.

The heparin-PEO-PDMS triblock copolymers form stable, thin layers by coating over hydrophobic substrates, such as silastic rubber, polystyrene, polyvinylchloride, and polyurethane. For in vitro assessments, the triblock copolymer was coated over cleaned glass beads (230 $\mu$m diameter). Schematic structures of these triblock copolymer coatings are shown in Fig. 6.4.

## In vitro evaluations

### Plasma preparation

Fresh platelet-rich (PRP) and platelet-poor plasma (PPP) was prepared by collecting blood from male rabbits (New Zealand White, 2.5 kg) via catheterized femoral artery exsanguination into plastic syringes containing 3.8% sodium citrate solution (final dilution 1:9). Blood was carefully transferred to Falcon tubes, centrifuged at 200 × g for 10 min at 4°C and the PRP supernatant collected. The pellets were further centrifuged at 1500 × g for 20 min at 4°C, and PPP supernatant was mixed with the PRP to give a PRP with a final platelet concentration of 3 × 10$^5$/ml. After mixing, platelets were equilibrated at room temperature for 60 min and used within 4 h.

### In vitro assay components

Antithrombin III (ATIII), S-2222, and factor Xa (KabiVitrum, Molandal, Sweden) were reconstituted from lyophilized vials with sterile water according to supplier's instructions (Helena Labs, Beaumont, TX, USA) and stored frozen. Thrombin (Thrombinair, Armour Pharmaceutical Comp., Kanakakee, IL, USA; 1000 units/vial) was diluted with sterile water to 10 units/ml and stored frozen.

### Factor Xa assay

Surface-immobilized heparin was analyzed for Factor Xa bioactivity by a chromogenic assay (Kabi Vitrum). A heparin standard curve was made using solution heparin concentrations of between 0.1 and 0.7 units/ml.

Heparin standards (0.1 ml) were diluted with 0.1 ml AT III and 0.8 ml buffer. Aliquots of this solution (0.2 ml) were incubated at 37°C for 3 min and factor Xa (0.1 ml, Kabi Vitrum, room temperature) was added and incubated for an additional 30 S. S-2222 (Kabi Vitrum, 37°C) was then added and incubated at 37°C for 3 min. The reaction was terminated by adding 0.3 ml 50% acetic acid and mixing. Samples were monitored spectrophotometrically at 405 nm using a Perkin-Elmer Lambda-Vis 7 spectrophotometer against water blanks.

To evaluate immobilized-heparin surfaces, heparin-immobilized beads (0.06 g) were incubated with 0.2 ml solution (AT III: buffer = 1:9 v/v) for 3 min at 37°C. Factor Xa, S-2222, and acetic acid were then added over the same time-course and in identical quantities as for the heparin standards. Aliquots were monitored for absorbance at 405 nm and compared with the heparin standard curve. The systems were also assayed for nonspecific adsorption of FXa using PEO-grafted Biomer surfaces.

### Activated partial thromboplastin time

Activated partial thromboplastin time (APTT) was determined using a Fibrosystem fibrometer with the following procedure. Heparinized PPP (0.1 to 0.5 units/ml, 0.1 ml) was incubated with 0.1 ml Activated Thrombofax Reagent (Sigma) for 2 min, after which 0.1 ml 0.02 $M$ CaCl$_2$ was added and the time for a fibrin clot to form (mechanical end point) was recorded.

This procedure established a heparin standard curve to evaluate heparin-immobilized surfaces. Coated beads (0.02 g) were used to evaluate heparin-immobilized surfaces in place of heparinized PPP. The subsequent steps are the same as previously described for the heparin standards and the bioactivity of immobilized heparin was obtained by comparison of end points with the heparin standard curve.

### Thrombin times

Inhibition of thrombin generation by heparinized surfaces was compared with heparin standards by the procedure of Sirridge and Shannon [12] modified to monitor coated beads. Beads coated with cross-linked PDMS, PDMS-PEO, and heparin-PEO-PDMS block copolymers (20–50 mg) were weighed into Fibrosystem Fibrocups and incubated for 10 min at 37°C with PPP (0.1 ml). Thrombin (0.1 ml, 10 units/ml) was added and clotting times measured on a Fibrosystem Fibrometer. These results were compared with results from heparinized plasma standards (0.05–0.25 units/ml).

### Platelet adhesion to polymer surfaces

Quantities of coated beads (140 mg) were carefully weighed into plastic disposable 3-ml syringes and equilibrated with 2 ml PBS buffer (pH = 7.40) overnight prior to adhesion studies. Buffer was squeezed out and 0.5 ml PRP introduced via another syringe and the syringes then tapped to remove air bubbles. The syringes were sealed with Parafilm and rotated through a water bath at 37°C so that the beads were constantly exposed to PRP. Sets of syringes were arranged for adhesion time intervals of 15, 30, 45, and 60 min of PRP incubation. At each time point, the syringes were quickly removed from the rotating bath, emptied into Falcon tubes, and counted immediately with the Coulter Counter. A control sample of PRP incubated without beads was used as a reference for each time point. The adhered platelet number was expressed as a percentage of control PRP at each time point. Figure 6.5 shows a schematic illustration of the in vitro beads experiment.

### Ex vivo A-A shunt model

Commercialized polyester-polyurethane tubing (1.5 mm outer diameter × 1.5 inner diameter, 30 cm length, Miki Sangyo Co. Ltd., Tokyo, Japan) was coated on its luminal surface with 1% w/v solution of

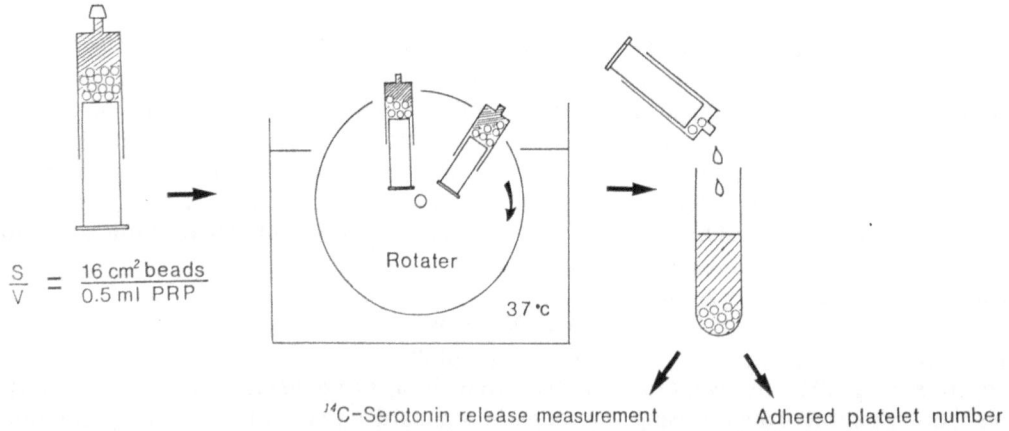

$$\frac{S}{V} = \frac{16\ cm^2\ beads}{0.5\ ml\ PRP}$$

Rotater

37°C

$^{14}$C–Serotonin release measurement          Adhered platelet number

**Fig. 6.5.** In vitro platelet adhesion experiment

various polymeric test materials. Tubing was coated by pumping polymer solutions through the tubing with a peristaltic pump for 30 s followed by 2-h drying under peristaltically pumped air and 24-h vacuum-drying at 40°C. This procedure was usually repeated to ensure uniform coating. After drying, the coated tubes were then equilibrated overnight with phosphate-buffered saline (PBS; pH = 7.4, 0.15 mol/l). Male rabbits (New Zealand white, 2–3 kg) were anesthetized with ketamine/promethazine and the right femoral and right carotid arteries were carefully exposed surgically. A catheter (5 F, Desert Medical) was inserted into the femoral artery to monitor systemic blood samples for platelet count and ADP-induced platelet aggregation and hematocrit. The coated tubing was rinsed and carefully inserted into the clamped ligated carotid artery of the rabbit. At time $t = 0$, the clamp was removed and shunt flow was started. An ultrasonic flow meter (Transonic Systems, model T201, Ithaca, NY, USA) was placed distal to the A-A shunt around the carotid artery and the flow rate was controlled to 2.5 ml/min (shear rate = 126 $s^{-1}$) using a suture tourniquet. Flow rate within the shunt was monitored continuously and the occlusion time was defined as the time for flow to decrease to zero.

### Systemic blood monitoring

Periodically, throughout the course of the shunt experiments, 2 ml blood was removed via the femoral catheter using a double-syringe technique and identical volumes replaced with buffer. Hematocrit was plotted as a funtion of shunt implant time. Mixed 9:1 with citrate, PRP and PPP were made by conventional centrifugation methods. Platelet counts were monitored using a Coulter Counter (Model ZBI) and platelet aggregability was monitored by ADP-induced aggregation.

## Results and discussion

### Surface bioactivity of immobilized heparin

Table 6.1 summarizes total amounts of immobilized heparin on the Biomer surfaces, as measured by the toluidine blue method and resulting calculated heparin bioactivities determined by $Fix_a$ assay and thrombin time measurement. Heparin catalytically potentiates the action of ATIII to inactivate thrombin, a critical process in suppressing the intrinsic blood coagulation cascade. Heparin contains specific binding sites for ATIII and thrombin, among other coagulation factors. Therefore, the orientation and exposure of heparin binding sites significantly affects the bioactivity of immobilized heparin. Generally, the bioactivity

of heparin decreases after immobilization onto all surfaces studied, possibly because of chemical modifications or physical inaccessibility of heparin's binding sites for coagulation factors. However, ex vivo results demonstrate that even such a small fraction of bioactive immobilized heparin can have a significant effect on improving implanted shunt performance. By using a hexamethylene ($C_6$) spacer between the substrate and the bound heparin, immobilized heparin maintained $0.81 \pm 0.06 \times 10^{-2}$ international units/cm$^2$ bioactivity, which translates to 5.3% of free heparin, as determined by ATIII complexation. The use of hydrophilic PEO spacers demonstrates that the bioactivity of immobilized heparin is consistently higher than that of the $C_6$ alkyl spacer system. In addition, heparin bioactivity increases with increasing PEO spacer length. The heparin-immobilized surface using PEO 4000 maintained the highest bioactivity at approximately $1.06 \pm 0.02 \times 10^{-2}$ international units/cm$^2$ C19%, even though it possessed the least amount of heparin on the surface as detected by toluidine blue. These results suggest that the increasingly mobile nature of longer spacer chains permits a more bulklike environment for heparin binding and influences the observed bioactivity of immobilized heparin.

### In vitro results for heparin-PEO-PDMS

The bioactivity of coated films of heparin-PEO-PDMS triblock copolymers assessed by toluidine blue, thrombin times, and factor Xa assays are summarized in Table 6.2. A reliably linear relation ($r^2 = 0.960$) exists between the amounts of heparinized block copolymer-coated beads in the toluidine blue determinations and resulting absorbance at 631 nm. Blanks containing beads compared well with blanks containing only 0.2% NaCl, demonstrating that nonspecific dye-binding was minimal. Calculation of coated bead dye-binding correlated with the heparin standard curve indicated a surface-immobilized heparin content of $41.5 \pm 14.8$ $\mu$g heparin/g of beads or, assuming a bead diameter of 230 $\mu$m and a reported glass bead density of 2.5 g/cm$^3$, 0.55 $\mu$g/cm$^2$ surface concentration.

In thrombin time measurements, 50 mg unheparinized PDMS and PDMS-PEO coated beads showed no prolongation of clotting times ($13 \pm 1.1$ s) while 50 mg heparinized copolymer beads prolonged clotting in the Fibrocup in excess of 200 s. Smaller quantities of heparinized beads (20 mg) averaged clotting times of $46.73 \pm 7.3$ s. This bioactivity corresponded to a heparin concentration of 0.33 units/ml if compared with the heparin standard curve. If compared with the actual amounts of heparin within each standard (by recalculating the standard curve in terms of amounts of heparin instead of concentrations), then 20 mg

**Table 6.1.** Nonthrombogenic activity of heparin immobilized surfaces

| Spacers | Heparin amount[a] ($\mu$g/cm$^2$) | Bioactivity ($\times 10^{-2}$; int. units/cm$^2$) | Fix assay (%) | Bioactivity ($\times 10^{-2}$; int. units/cm$^2$) | Thrombin time[b] (%) | Occlusion time[c] (min) |
|---|---|---|---|---|---|---|
| C$_6$ | $0.85 \pm 0.12$ | 0.81 ($\pm 0.06$) | 5.32 | 0.75 ($\pm 0.02$) | 4.93 | 80 ($\pm 3$) |
| PEO 200 | $0.65 \pm 0.04$ | 0.86 ($\pm 0.03$) | 7.38 | 0.81 ($\pm 0.03$) | 6.96 | 90 ($\pm 10$) |
| PEO 1000 | $0.50 \pm 0.04$ | 1.03 ($\pm 0.02$) | 11.50 | 0.95 ($\pm 0.02$) | 10.60 | 130 |
| PEO 4000 | $0.31 \pm 0.05$ | 1.06 ($\pm 0.02$) | 19.09 | 0.97 ($\pm 0.02$) | 17.47 | 185 ($\pm 25$) |

Values are means + SEM ($n = 3$–5)
[a] Toluidine blue method after washing thoroughly with PBS
[b] Bioactivity ratio of immobilized heparin to the total amount bound
[c] Arterio-arterial rabbit shunt test

heparinized copolymer-coated beads represents 0.04 units of heparin or, assuming a total 20-mg surface area of 1.51 cm$^2$, a heparin surface concentration of $2.65 \times 10^{-2}$ units/cm$^2$.

Factor Xa results correlate well with thrombin time data. The method involves analyzing heparin as a bioactive complex of heparin and ATIII and its ability to bind and neutralize a known amount of factor Xa. Unbound, excess factor Xa then catalyzes the release of a chromogenic molecule, p-nitroanaline (pNA) from a substrate (Bz-Ile-Glu-Gly-Arg-pNA) and the amount of pNa detected photometrically is inversely proportional to the amount of bioactive heparin present. Unlike the toluidine blue assay, which detects all heparin able to bind the dye, the factor Xa assay detects only the heparin on the surface which is bioactive, forming complexes with both ATIII and factor Xa.

In the factor Xa analysis, the heparin standard curve for the chromogenic assay demonstrated reliable linearity ($r^2 = 0.970$); sample absorbances of less than 0.120 $A$ were assumed to deviate from this linearity and were discarded. For this reason, amounts of heparin-PEO-PDMS copolymer-coated beads in excess of 5 mg exhibited heparin bioactivities giving absorbances in this range and could not be included in the assay. However, control beads coated with cross-linked PDMS and PDMS-PEO were assayed in amounts up to 20 mg. PDMS beads showed absorbance corresponding to baseline levels of blank standards for all quantities of beads. PDMS-PEO copolymer beads (20 mg) demonstrated absorbances corresponding to 0.004 units of heparin ($2.65 \times 10^{-3}$ units/cm$^2$), indicating some nonspecific absorption of factor Xa to this coating. Smaller amounts of these beads, however, gave absorbances equivalent to the blanks. Heparinized block copolymer-coated beads (5 mg) resulted in absorbances which when correlated to the standard curve corresponded to 0.010 units of heparin or $2.66 \times 10^{-2}$ units/cm$^2$, nearly an order of magnitude greater than its unheparinized analogue.

**Table 6.2.** In vitro quantitation of surface-immobilized heparin on coated beads

| Substrate | Heparin surface concentration[a] | | |
|---|---|---|---|
| | Tol. blue ($\mu$g/cm$^2$) | Thrombin (units/cm$^2$) | Factor Xa (units/cm$^2$) |
| PDMS | 0 | 0 | 0 |
| PDMS-PEO | 0 | 0 | $2.65 \times 10^{-3}$ |
| PDMS-PEO-Heparin | 0.55 | $2.65 \times 10^{-2}$ | $2.66 \times 10^{-2}$ |

[a] Average of six samples, assuming bead diameter of 230 $\mu$m and bead density of 2.5 g/cm$^3$

Given the experimentally determined activity of the heparinized copolymer surface ($2.66 \times 10^{-2}$ units/cm$^2$) and the original activity of the immobilized heparin sodium salt (165.4 units/mg) [11], the calculated amount of bioactive immobilized heparin is 0.16 $\mu$g/cm$^2$. The toluidine blue assay, which measures heparin whether bioactive or not, indicates nearly 3.5 times this amount on the surface, implying that only one in three or four surface-immobilized heparin molecules is bioactive.

**Platelet adhesion to heparinized surfaces**

Figure 6.6 demonstrates the relation between platelet adhesion and PEO spacer length for PEO-grafted Biomer surface and heparin-immobilized PEO-Biomer surfaces. In the case of PEO-grafted surfaces, platelet adhesion was decreased compared with Biomer controls. Alkyl (C$_6$)-grafted surfaces were shown to increase platelet adhesion. Platelet adhesion exhibits a minimum at a PEO molecular weight of 1000. Mori and Nagaoka [4] reported a decrease in platelet adhesion with increasing PEO chain length up to a PEO molecular weight of 2500, where adhesion leveled off to a constant value. The different conditions between those experiments and ones described here are that our PEO grafts had different terminating end groups and our platelet experiments utilized longer incubation times with platelets. Platelet adhesion in our experiments may include two phases of platelet response, namely platelet attachment (passive adhesion) and platelet shape change and activation (active adhesion).

After immobilization of heparin, platelet adhesion is still decreased compared with Biomer surfaces. Platelet adhesion is nearly the same for different PEO spacer systems and, thus, a specific spacer length effect is not observed. These results suggest that the main interactions between platelets and heparin-immobilized surfaces are caused by heparin itself, which may cover the surface and mask other surface characters. However, compared with the alkyl spacer system, PEO spacer systems did show consistently lower platelet adhesion, suggesting that the PEO spacers, in general, pacified platelet adhesion in contrast to the alkyl spacer system.

Platelet adhesion to heparin-PEO-PDMS monitored by depletion of platelets from PRP at 37°C is shown in Fig. 6.7 for various time intervals. Although previously published data for platelet adhesion and blood clottability on PDMS are inconsistent [13–16], cross-linked PEO, PDMS, and heparin-PEO-PDMS all show very low platelet adhesion compared with Biomer control surfaces. In addition, although no quantitative analysis was obtained, platelet aggregates in the bulk fluid phase were qualitatively noted from Coulter Counter distributions to increase over time for the PEO and Biomer systems and remain surprisingly low in both PDMS and heparin-PEO-PDMS systems.

## Ex vivo evaluation by a new A-A shunt model

Nonthrombogenicity of modified polymer surfaces in whole blood was evaluated ex vivo by our newly developed low-flow-rate A-A shunt method [17]. The procedure involves connecting coated or control tubing (1.5 mm inner diameter × 30 cm length) as a shunt in the carotid arteries of male rabbits. The experiment measures the time needed for the formation of a stable, nonembolized thrombus large enough to occlude the blood flow in the tube and is referred to as the occlusion time. After shunt implantation, other hematological parameters are simultaneously monitored, including platelet number, platelet activation and aggregation, and APTT. These results show that none of the systemic hematological parameters are affected by shunt implant and infer that heparin is covalently attached to the surface and not released in detectable quantities in the blood. Figure 6.8 shows the occlusion time for Biomer and heparin-immobilized Biomer surfaces using different mole-

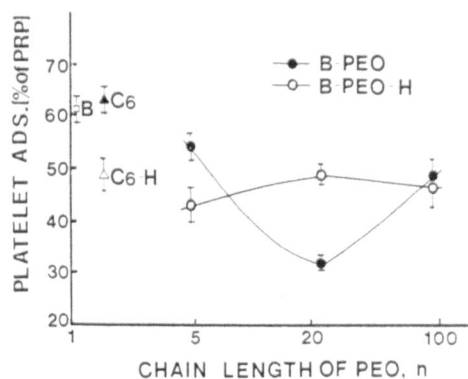

**Fig. 6.6.** Effect of chain length of PEO on platelet adhesion. Amount of PEO on PEO grafted surfaces is 12 $\mu$g/cm$^2$ for all systems. Amount of heparin is 0.31, 0.50, and 0.6 $\mu$g/cm$^2$ for 4000, 1000, and 200 PEO grafted Biomer surfaces, respectively

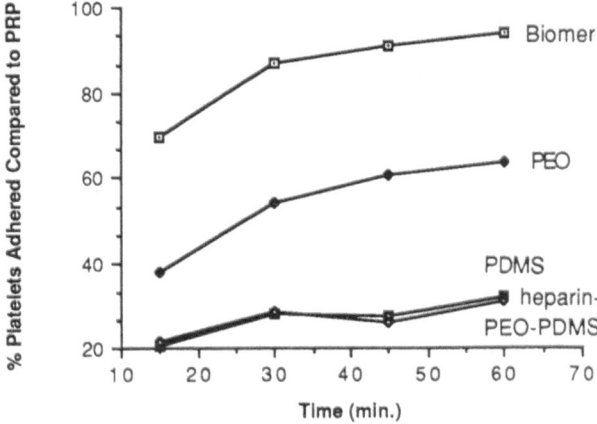

**Fig. 6.7.** Platelet adhesion in vitro to heparin-PEO-PDMS block copolymers

cular weights of PEO. Heparinized surfaces demonstrate significant prolongation of occlusion times while PEO-grafted surfaces without heparin did not prolong occlusion time significantly, even if these surfaces reduce platelet adhesion in vitro (Fig. 6.6). These results suggest that surface-induced coagulation in whole blood under conditions of low flow rate and low shear forms stable thrombus masses on the surface as a result of a synergistic or cooperative, complementary actions of fibrin net formation together with platelet aggregation. Without platelet deposition, the thrombus mass would amount to very little—hardly enough to occlude the shunt. Also, without contact activation and fibrin net stabilization of the thrombus mass, embolization would result in no occlusion at all. Therefore, some critical, stable thrombus mass, composed of a platelet plug reinforced with insoluble fibrin, must from in every shunt to cause complete and irreversible occlusion. Heparinized surfaces appear to be effective in suppressing both of these responses (fibrin and platelet deposition) to remain potent longer while PEO grafts do not suppress at least one of these responses in ex vivo conditions. Mori and Nagaoka [4] and Merrill and Salzman [5] have proposed that PEO-grafted surfaces are less thrombogenic due to decreased protein adsorption and platelet adhesion as a result of high dynamic motion of PEO chains. However, even if thrombus is not observed on their PEO-grafted surfaces, there is the possibility of generating microemboli detached from the surface of prevailing, low-cohesive forces between the forming thrombus and the PEO surface. By contrast, similar PEO-grafted surfaces generated extensive blood coagulation under the low-flow conditions of our A-A shunt experiments, where embolization is unlikely, demonstrating that more complex or significant thrombogenic events are occurring at the interface to promote thrombosis beyond simple surface PEO mobility. These effects include contact activation, fibrin formation, platelet adhesion, and stable thrombus formation. More detailed metabolic effects (active adhesion) of blood proteins and cells ex vivo or in vivo should be important in discussing real-time nonthrombogenic properties of PEO-grafted surfaces in whole blood.

Biomer-PEO surfaces immobilized with heparin show longer occlusion times than Biomer, as shown in Fig. 6.8. A significant generalized hydrophilic spacer effect is observed, that is, PEO spacers prolong patency. In addition, hydrophilic PEO spacers prolong occlusion times over hydrophobic alkyl spacers. Also, the occlusion time is increased with increased PEO spacer length, indicating specific spacer length effects. Although platelet adhesion in vitro does not appear to be influenced by PEO spacer length in heparin-immobilized systems, the nonthrombogenic activities

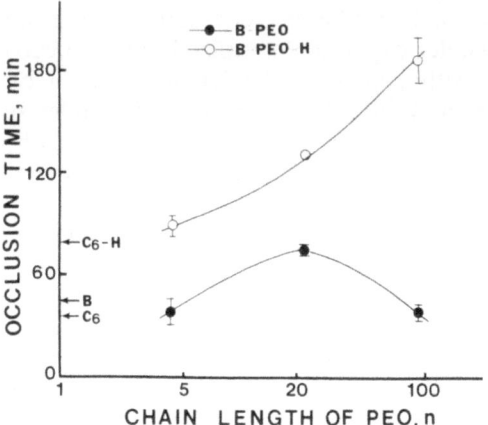

**Fig. 6.8.** A-A shunt occlusion times for immobilized Biomer surfaces

witnessed ex vivo for different spacer length systems are attributed primarily to differing effects of spacer lengths on the whole blood bioactivity of heparin. The efficacy of hydrophilically immobilized heparin is demonstrated despite decreases in apparent bioactivities upon surface immobilization.

Occlusion times for the heparin-PEO-PDMS system and controls are shown in Fig. 6.9. Control surfaces (Biomer, PDMS, PEO) perform poorly in the shunt, all demonstrating occlusion times of less than 50 min. Heparin-PEO-PDMS remains patent, even under these extreme flow conditions, for over 200 min. These results suggest that heparin may suppress fibrin net formation, thereby either suppressing thrombus formation or allowing platelet thrombus embolization, with subsequent prolongation of occlusion time. Based on low levels of platelet adhesion detected in vitro, however, it is likely that patency is a function of low platelet adhesivity and heparin bioactivity.

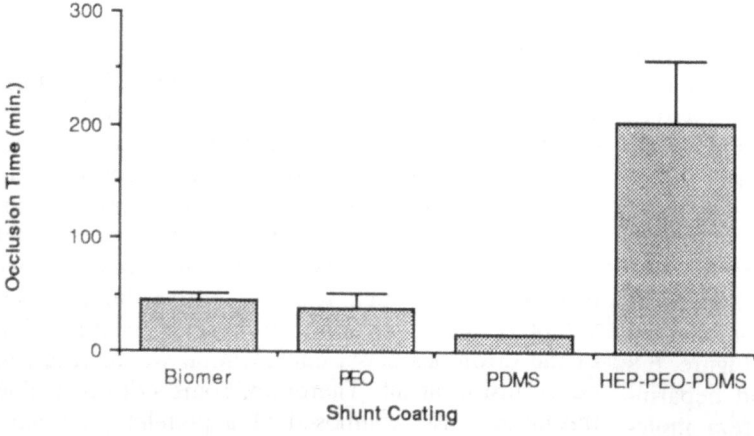

**Fig. 6.9.** A-A shunt occlusion times for heparin-PEO-PDMS copolymer system

## Conclusions

In summary, heparinized surfaces—both those immobilized in bulk and those immobilized in situ at the surface of polyurethaneureas—demonstrate advantages as coatings over current, popular blood-contacting materials. Immobilized bioactivity of heparin is shown to be a function of PEO spacer length, yet immobilized heparin demonstrates no chain-length effect on platelet adhesion. PEO grafts on Biomer surfaces show minimal platelet adhesion at a molecular weight of 1000. Phase-separated triblock copolymers of heparin-PEO-PDMS show low levels of platelet adhesion compared with Biomer and homopolymer controls. Heparin's bioactivity in this system demonstrates prolongation of thrombin times and a significant ability to bind factor Xa.

In ex vivo shunt experiments under low flow, low shear conditions, all heparinized surfaces exhibit prolonged occlusion times compared with controls, indicating the ability of immobilized heparin to inhibit thrombosis in whole blood.

**Acknowledgment.** This work was supported by NIH grants HL20251-10 and HL17623-13.

## References

1. Ebert CD, Kim SW (1982) Immobilized heparin: spacer arm effects on biological interactions. Thromb Res 26: 43–57
2. Heyman PW, Cho CS, McRea JC, Olsen DB, Kim SW (1985) Heparinized polyurethanes: *in vitro* and *in vivo* studies. J Biomed Mat Res 19: 419–436
3. Brace LD, Fareed J (1985) An objective assessment of the interactions of heparin and its fractions on human platelets. Sem Thromb Haemostas 11: 190–198
4. Mori Y, Nagaoka S (1982) A new antithrombogenic material with long polyethylene oxide chains. Trans Am Soc Art Int Org 28: 459–463
5. Merrill EW, Salzman EW (1983) Polyethylene oxide as a biomaterial. ASAIO J 6: 80–84
6. Okano T, Nishiyama S, Shinohara I, Akaike T, Sakurai Y, Kataoka K, Tsuruta T (1981) Effect of hydrophilic and hydrophobic microdomains on mode of interaction between block polymer and blood platelets. J Biomed Mat Res 15: 383–402
7. Okano T, Shimada M, Aoyagi T, Shinohara I, Kataoka K, Abe K, Sakurai Y (1986) The hydrophilic-hydrophobic microdomain surface having the ability to suppress platelet aggregation and their *in vitro* antithrombogenicity. J Biomed Mat Res 20: 919–927
8. Okano T, Kataoka K, Abe K, Sakurai Y, Shimada M, Shinohara I (1983) *In vivo* evaluation of antithrombogenicity of block copolymers with hydrophilic and hydrophobic microdomains by arteriovenous shunts. Prog Org 2: 863–866
9. Park KD, Okano T, Nojiri C, Kim SW, Heparin immobilization on polyurethane surfaces-effect of hydrophilic spacers. J Biomed Mat Res (in press)
10. Smith PK, Mallia AK, Harmanson GT (1980) Colormetric method for the assay of heparin content in immobilized heparin preparations. Anal Biochem 109: 466–473
11. Grainger D, Kim SW, Feijen J (1988) Poly(dimethylsiloxane)-poly(ethylene oxide)-heparin block copolymers: I. Synthesis and characterization. J Biomed Mat Res 22: 231
12. Sirridge MS, Shannon R (1983) Evaluation of thrombin formation. Laboratory evaluation of hemostasis and thrombosis, 3rd edn. Lea and Febiger, p 161
13. Weathersby PK, Kolobow T, Stool E (1975) Relative thrombogenicity of polydimethylsiloxane and silicone rubber constituents. J Biomed Mat Res 9: 561–568
14. Zapol WM, Bloom S, Carvalho A, Wonders T, Skoskiewicz M, Schneider R, Snider M (1975) Improved platelet economy using filler-free silicone rubber in long-term membrane lung perfusion. Trans ASAIO 21: 587–591
15. Yates WG, Schaap RN, Baumann GC (1978) Effects of filler-free silicone rubber on platelets during bovine extracorporeal membrane oxygenation. Trans Am Art Int Org 24: 644–648
16. Nyilas E, Kupski EL (1970) Surface microstructural factors and blood compatibility of silicone rubber. J Biomed Mat Res 4: 369–432
17. Nojiri C, Okano T, Grainger D, Park KD, Nakahama S, Suzuki K, Kim SW (1987) Evaluation of nonthrombogenic polymers in a new rabbit A-A shunt model. Trans Am Soc Artif Int Org 33: 602

# Discussion

*Kataoka* (Tokyo Women's Medical College): I see from your slide that there is an optimum molecular weight of PEO and that an molecular weight of 1000 is better than 3000.

*Kim* (University of Utah): That is based on the thrombin activity test; the result does depend to a certain extent on the test employed.

*Kataoka:* How about with in vivo and ex vivo tests? Is there an optimum molecular weight?

*Kim:* Yes. We are carrying out these tests at present.

# 7. Blood compatibility of polyacrylonitrile containing ethyleneoxide and dimethylamino side chains

Hajime Miyama[1], Kazuhito Ikegami[1], Yoshio Nosaka[1], Kazunori Kataoka[2], Nobuhiko Yui[2], and Yasuhisa Sakurai[2]

**Summary.** Polyacrylonitrile copolymer containing ethyleneoxide (EO) and dimethylamino (DA) side chains was synthesized. For the copolymer, the relation between adhesion of platelets on the copolymer surface and the DA content of the copolymer was examined by a "column method," whereby a platelet suspension was passed through a column of glass beads precoated with the copolymer.

Retention of platelets was 100% irrespective of DA content for the copolymer having almost the same water content. However, when rat serum albumin (RSA) or rat $\gamma$-globulin (R$\gamma$G) was added to the platelet suspension, the retention of platelets significantly decreased and was reduced to 0% when the DA content was low. A similar result was observed when the copolymer surface was previously coated with RSA or R$\gamma$G, instead of adding RSA or R$\gamma$G to the platelet suspension.

The adsorption of RSA or R$\gamma$G to the copolymer surface was examined in a batch system. Adsorption increased remarkably with a decrease in the DA content. It is concluded that the increase in the DA content decreases the adsorption of RSA and R$\gamma$G on the copolymer surface, resulting in an increase in the adhesion of platelets on the copolymer surface.

**Key words:** Nonthrombogenic polyacrylonitrile—Ethyleneoxide side chain—Dimethylamino side chain—Adsorption of serum albumin—Adsorption of serum globulin

Previously, it was reported that polyvinylchloride [1] or polyacrylonitrile [2] containing ethylene oxide (EO) side chains showed excellent nonthrombogenicity. Recently, we synthesized a polyacrylonitrile copolymer containing EO and dimethylamino (DA) side chains [3]. We found from an in vivo test that the copolymer shows excellent nonthrombogenicity at a low DA content and that the nonthrombogenicity decreases with an increase in DA content. To clarify the mechanism of the phenomenon, the relation between adhesion of platelets on the copolymer surface and DA content of the copolymer was examined by a "column method," which was developed by Kataoka et al. [4].

[1] Department of Chemistry, Technological University of Nagaoka, Kamitomioka, Nagaoka, 940-21 Japan
[2] Institute of Medical Engineering, Tokyo Women's Medical College, 8-1 Kawada-cho, Shinjuku-ku, Tokyo, 162 Japan

## Materials and methods

### Synthesis of copolymer

Since the synthesis of the copolymer was described in detail previously [2, 3], the method will be described briefly. The trunk polymer was synthesized by the photopolymerization of acrylonitrile with carbontetrabromide as an initiator in dimethylsulfoxide (DMSO). The obtained polymer was photosensitive and contained bromine atoms and will be abbreviated as "PANBr." At various feed ratios, PANBr, methoxypolyethyleneglycol methacrylate (M23G; prepared by Shin-Nakamura Chemical Co., Ltd.),

$$CH_2 = \underset{\underset{O = C \ (\ OCH_2CH_2 \ )_{23} OCH_3}{|}}{C} - CH_3$$

and dimethylaminoethyl methacrylate (DAEM),

$$CH_2 = \underset{\underset{O = C - OCH_2CH_2 - N(CH_3)_2}{|}}{C} - CH_3$$

were dissolved into DMSO. DAEM and other reagents were of reagent grade. The mixture was photoirradiated from the outside of the vessel at 25°C for 6 h in nitrogen flow with a 100-W high-pressure mercury lamp. The reacted solution was concentrated at reduced pressure and poured into a large quantity of aqueous methyl alcohol. The precipitated polymer was thoroughly washed with distilled water and methyl alcohol at 50°C and dried at 40°C. the copolymer was purified twice by reprecipitation.

### Evaluation of polymer properties

The molecular weight of PANBr was measured by gel permeation chromatography (Waters, GPC-224) using an $N,N$-dimethylformamide (DMF) solution, with calibration using polystryrene standards. The composition of the copolymer was determined by [1]H-NMR spectroscopy (JEOL, JNM-GX270), where spectra were measured by using 10 mg of each polymer dissolved into 0.5 ml DMSO-$d_6$ in an NMR tube (outer diameter 5 mm). The water content of the copolymer was determined from the difference between the weight of the copolymer film soaked in distilled water for more than 48 h and that dried in a vacuum at 60°C for 10 h, expressed by the ratio (%) of the water content to the weight of the wet film. Interfacial free energy $\gamma_{sw}$ between the graft-copolymer film and water was calculated according to the equation of Andrade et al. [5] from the contact angle between an air bubble and the film and that between an octane bubble and the film. Values of the contact angles were obtained in water kept at 25°C using a contact angle goniometer of CA-A type of Kyowa Kagaku Co., Ltd.

### Measurement of platelet adhesion

Details of the method were reported previously [4]. The polymer was coated on glass beads (48–60 mesh, Toshiba Ballotini Co.). Then, 1 g of precoated beads was closely packed in a poly vinyl chloride tube (10 cm length and 3 mm internal diameter).

Blood was withdrawn by cardiopuncture from a Wistar male rat into 0.25% sodium citrate aqueous solution. Platelet-rich plasma (PRP) was separated by centrifugal operation for 20 min at 900 rpm. From the PRP, platelets were precipitated by centrifugal operation for 15 min at 2000 rpm. The platelets were suspended in Hanks' balanced salt solution (HBSS), to which N-2-hydroxyl-N'-2-sulfoethylpiperazine (HEPES) was added to keep the pH at 7.3. The platelet concentration in the solution was ca. $1 \times 10^7$ cells/ml. When RSA or RγG was added to the solution, a 0.1% solution of each in HBSS was added keeping the same cell count and pH (7.3). Here, RSA (Sigma, Fraction V) and RγG (Sigma, Fraction II, III) were used.

The platelet suspension from a disposable syringe was passed through the column with the use of a Precidol Model 5003 infusion pump for 3.5 min at a flow rate of 0.4 ml/min. The column had been primed with HBSS to exclude a liquid-air interface. The number of platelets in the solution before and after the elution was determined by a Coulter counter (Coulter Electronics Inc.). Retention (percentage) of the platelets was calculated according to the following equation:

$$(1 - [P]/[P]_0) \times 100$$

where $[P]_0$ and $[P]$ were concentrations of the platelets before and after the elution. The retention value was an average of four runs. Morphology of the platelets adhered on polymer surface was observed by scanning electron microscopy (JEOL, JXA-733) on the glass beads after the elution, where the platelets were fixed by immersing into a saline solution of glutaraldehyde.

**Table 7.1.** Composition and water content of graft-copolymers

| Sample no. | Composition (wt%) | | | Water content (wt%) |
|---|---|---|---|---|
| | Trunk polymer | M23G | DAEM | |
| 1 | 70.6 | 29.4 | 0.0 | 32 |
| 2 | 61.9 | 36.7 | 1.4 | 34 |
| 3 | 64.0 | 29.8 | 6.3 | 29 |
| 4 | 62.4 | 30.0 | 7.6 | 31 |
| 5 | 66.3 | 25.2 | 8.5 | 29 |
| 6 | 66.4 | 21.8 | 11.9 | 24 |
| 7 | 56.3 | 24.1 | 19.6 | 33 |

### Measurement of adsorbed proteins

About 2 g of glass beads (150–250 mesh) precoated with the polymer were immersed into 10 ml HBSS-HEPES, containing 0.2 mg RSA or RγG and incubated at pH 7.3 for 6 h at 30°C. Concentration of the proteins were measured before and after the incubation by adding Coomassie Brilliant Blue G-250 to the solution and measuring absorption at 595 nm. The amount of the proteins adsorbed was calculated from the difference in the protein concentrations before and after the incubation.

### Results

Composition and water content of the graft copolymers are shown in Table 7.1, where the average molecular weight of the PANBr used for the photography was in the range of $7.3 \times 10^5 - 8.1 \times 10^5$.

Figure 7.1 shows the relation between the platelet retention and the DAEM content of the polymer at pH 7.3. When RSA was absent both in the platelet suspension and on the coated polymer, the retention was almost 100% irrespective of the DAEM content. When RSA was present on the polymer surface or both in the solution and on the polymer surface, the retention was almost zero for the polymers with a low DAEM content and increased with an increase in DAEM content for polymers with a DAEM content higher than 1.4 wt%. Here, RSA was precoated by immersing the glass beads in the 0.1% protein solution and rinsing with buffer solution. When RγG was present, a similar tendency was observed, as shown in Fig. 7.2.

The scanning electron-microscopic (SEM) picture in Fig. 7.3 shows that the platelets were appreciably adhered and deformed even for polymers with a zero

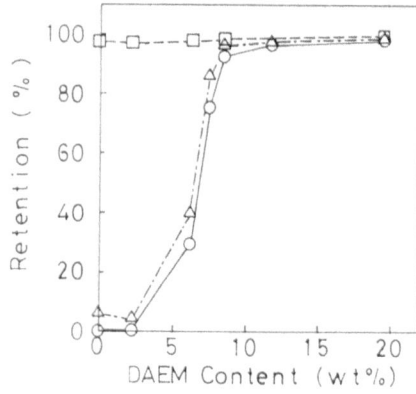 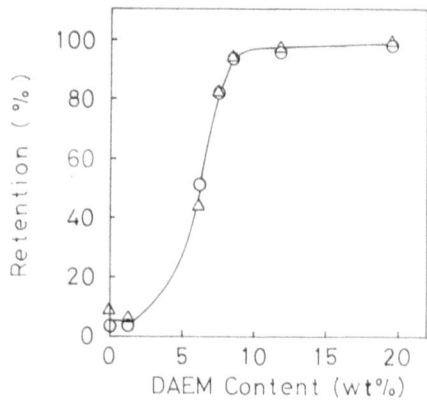

**Fig. 7.1.** Effect of RSA on the relation between platelet retention and DAEM content. *Squares* no RSA is present either in solution or on polymer surface; *triangles* no RSA is present in solution but is present on surface; *circles* RSA is present both in solution and on surface

**Fig. 7.2.** Effect of RγG on the relation between platelet retention and DAEM content. *Triangles* no RγG is present in solution but is present on polymer surface, *circles* RγG is present both in solution and on polymer surface

a, b 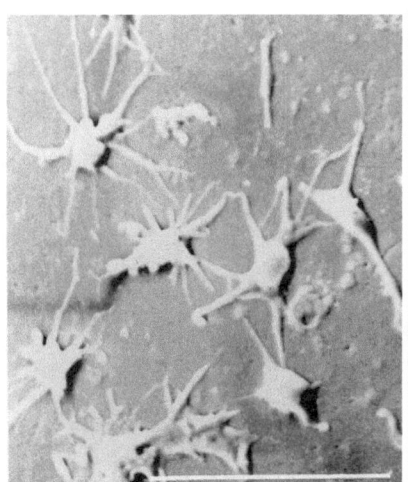 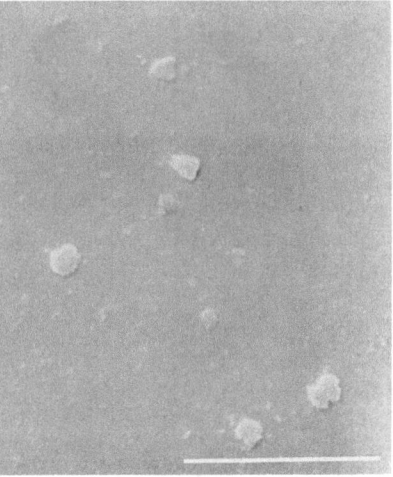 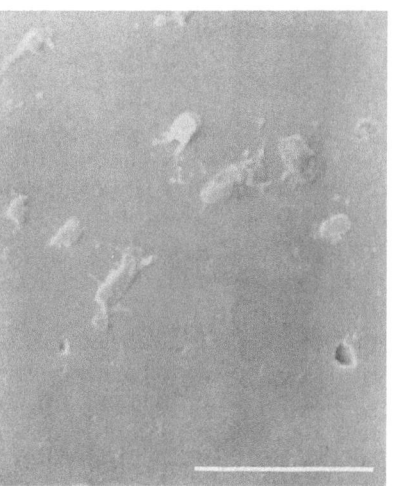 c

**Fig. 7.3a–c.** SEM pictures of platelet adsorbed on the polymer surface. **a** No RSA is present in solution and DAEM content of polymer is 0%; **b** RSA is present in solution and DAEM content is 0%; **c** RSA is present in solution and DAEM content is 19.6%. *Bar* indicates 10 μm

DAEM content when RSA was absent. However, when RSA was present, there was little adherence and deformation for polymers with a low DAEM content and appreciable adherence and deformation for polymers with a high DAEM content.

As shown in Fig. 7.4, the interfacial free energy between the polymer and water increased with an increase in DAEM content.

As shown in Figs. 7.5 and 7.6, the adsorption of proteins on the polymer surface reached a maximum when the DAEM content was 1.4% and decreased gradually thereafter. However, the decrease became steep above a content of 8% DAEM.

## Discussion

As shown in Figs. 1 and 2, the retention of platelets is 100% for polymers of any DAEM content without protein treatment, but it is almost zero for the polymer with a DAEM content of less than 1.4% when RSA or RγG is present in the solution or on the polymer surface. Figure 7.3 shows that the presence of the protein markedly affects the adhesion and deformation of the platelets. These results indicate that the presence of RSA or RγG is necessary to prevent platelet adhesion. Figures 7.5 and 7.6 show that the adsorption of both RSA and RγG on the

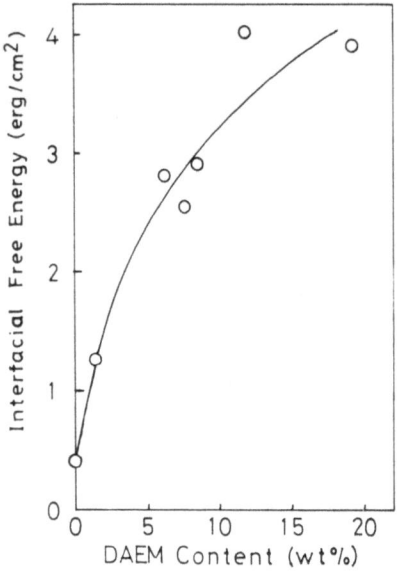

**Fig. 7.4.** Relation between interfacial free energy and DAEM content of polymer

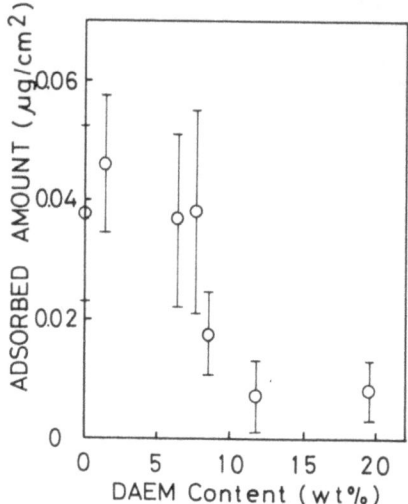

**Fig. 7.5.** Relation between amount of RSA adsorbed on unit area of polymer surface and DAEM content of polymer

polymer surface is high when the DAEM content is low, and vice versa. The adsorption also shows a maximum when the DAEM content is 1.4%, which coincides with the start of the increase in platelet retention seen in Figs. 7.1 and 7.2.

From these results, the following important conclusions are obtained: (a) The presence of plasma proteins is required to prevent platelet adhesion on the surface of polymers having polyethyleneoxide (PEO) chains; (b) the proteins adsorbed on the polymer surface are responsible for the prevention of the platelet adhesion. To explain the minimal platelet adhesion on PEO-derivatized surfaces, Mori et al. [1] proposed that the motion of the PEO side chains with water molecules bound to the PEO units causes microscopic water flow, which prevents the local stagnation of blood components and the adhesion of platelets. Later, Miyama et al. [2] proposed from the evaluation of a graft copolymer having PEO and DAEM side chains that the DAEM parts of the graft polymer are localized on the polymer surface, which leads to an increase in $\gamma_{sw}$ (Fig. 7.4). This may prevent the motion of the PEO chains and the microscopic water flow on the surface and accelerate the stagnation of the blood components. However, scarce attention has been given to the role of the adsorbed protein in PEO-derivatized surface. It has been believed that protein adsorption is negligible on PEO-derivatized surfaces because of high dynamic motion of PEO chains and that high dynamic motion of the PEO chains is itself responsible for repulsing platelets from the surface. However, our present results are inconsistent with

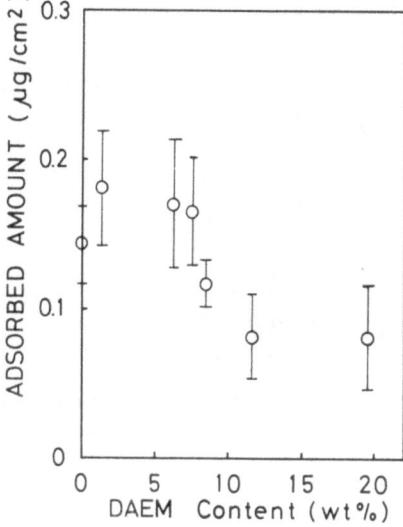

**Fig. 7.6.** Relation between amount of RγG adsorbed on unit area of polymer surface and DAEM content of polymer

this mechanism and indicate the crucial role of adsorbed proteins in decreased platelet adhesion on PEO-derivatized surfaces. As a result of the extended conformation of hydrated PEO chains, PEO-derivatized surfaces seem to have a diffused interface with water. Thus, it is likely that the adsorbed proteins penetrate into the PEO layer to form a micro-heterogeneous PEO/protein layer. These penetrating proteins may retain their native conformation in consequence of the weak interaction with the PEO chain. This consideration of the formation of the penetrating protein layer is consistent with the previous finding of Mori et al. [1] that two layers mixed with PEO side chains were formed on the PEO-derivatized surface implanted in canine veins. This proteinaceous layer plays a part in the prevention of the adhesion of the platelets probably owing to the decrease in interfacial free energy and/or to the mobility of the PEO side chains.

The increase in platelet adhesion with an increase in DAEM content seems to be due to the decrease in protein adsorption at a high DAEM content, which leads to the direct interaction between PEO side chains and the platelets themselves. Considering the amphiphilic nature of PEO, there is a possibility that PEO chains may penetrate into the hydrophobic moieties of platelet membrane. The reason for the increase in DAEM content reducing the protein adsorption may be related to the surrounding ionic strength.

Since the $pK_a$ of the DAEM side chain of the present polymer is 7.1, about 40% of the DAEM is protonated under the present experimental conditions (pH 7.3). Because of the high ionic strength ($\mu = 0.15$) in the experiment, the DAEM attracts small inorganic anions in solution, which may prevent the adsorption of proteins. The effect of ionic strength as well as the effect of counter ion species on the adsorption of proteins on the polymer surface is now being examined to support this hypothesis.

## References

1. Mori Y, Nagaoka S, Takeuchi H, Kikuchi T, Noguchi N, Tanzawa H, Noishiki Y (1982) A new antithrombogenic material with long polyethylene side chains. Trans Am Soc Art Org 28: 459–463
2. Miyama H, Kuwano A, Fujii N, Nagaoka S, Mori Y, Noishiki Y (1985) Synthesis, physical properties and blood compatibility of polyacrylonitrile copolymer containing polyethylene oxide side chains. Kobunshi Ronbunshu 42: 623–528
3. Miyama H, Fujii N, Hokari N, Toi H, Nagaoka S, Mori Y, Noishiki Y (1988) Nonthrombogenicity of polyacrylonitrile graftcopolymer containing polyethyleneoxide and dimethylamine side chains. J Bioact Compat Polym 2: 222–231
4. Kataoka K, Maeda M, Nishimura T, Nitadori Y, Tsuruta T (1980) Estimation of cell adhesion on polymer surfaces with the use of "column-method". J Biomed Mat Res 14: 817–823
5. Andrade JD, King RN, Gregonis DE, Coleman DL (1982) Surface characterization of poly(hydroxethyl methacrylate) and related polymers: I. Contact angle method in water. J Polym Sci Polym Symp 66: 313–336

## Discussion

*Kim* (University of Utah): Without protein you showed a lot of platelet adhesion and release on the surface. What were the experimental conditions? Did you suspend the platelets in buffer solution without proteins?

*Miyama* (Technological University of Nagaoka): Yes.

*Kim:* So I suppose that with a change in the environment the cells could lyse or swell in the absence of protein. This perhaps causes a very large amount of cell deposition on the surface due to the changes in the nature of the cells. Did you carefully check the cell morpholoy?

*Miyama:* No we did not because it is very difficult to do this with suspended platelets.

*Kim:* Again, if you suspend the platelets in buffer without any proteins I would expect the bound glycoproteins to be released quickly since the platelet cell surface consists of bound glycoprotein, so if there is protein in the plasma it is well equilibrated. After glycoprotein is removed from the surface of the cell, it is expected that the dense granules inside the platelets will be easily released. This may cause spreading of adhered platelets on the surface. That is just my speculation.

*Kataoka* (Tokyo Women's Medical College): Prof. Miyama shows that even in the platelet suspension if we coat the protein on the polymer surface there is a drastic reduction in platelet adhesion down to almost 0%. Namely, protein addition in the buffer is not always necessary to decrease platelet retention. So, a change in the platelet property, if any, due to the absence of proteins in the medium seems to have no serious effect on the experimental results.

*Cooper* (University of Wisconsin): Do you mean that this is right for all proteins?

*Miyama:* No. Just albumin and gammaglobulin.

# 8. A reconstituted vessel's wall model on microporous substrates as a small-caliber artificial graft

Takehisa Matsuda, Setsuo Takaichi, T. Kitamura, Hiroo Iwata, Hisateru Takano, and Tetsuzo Akutsu[1]

**Summary.** This paper deals with the development of a biological model which mimics the intima and media of the natural vessel wall. the essential feature of the vessel organ reconstruction system designed and developed here is a multiphasic heterocellular structure with a high degree of hierarchy. The structuring components are a polymer matrix, a collagen gel layer, a smooth muscle cell (SMC) multilayer, an artificial basement membrane, and an endothelial cell (EC) living. In vitro step-by-step architecture resulted in the development of a viable vessel wall model in terms of structural hierarchy, morphology, and metabolic function. It is hoped that this prototype will serve as a hybrid-type small-caliber artificial graft as well as a physiological and pharmacological research tool.

**Key words:** Endothelial cell—Smooth muscle cell—Hybrid artificial graft—Artificial basement membrane

There is a continued need for a small internal diameter artificial vascular graft for diseased peripheral and coronary arteries. In this application, thrombosis persists as a major early complication. A very promising approach is a hybrid artificial graft lined with endothelial cells. Extensive studies based on an endothelial cell lining approach have been conducted mainly in the USA for the past several years [1–5]. These studies are based on the fact the nonthrombogenicity of natural vessels is imparted by biochemical functions of endothelial cells present at the inner layer of the vessels. Endothelial cells (ECs) synthesize and secrete a variety of biologically active substances, such as prostacyclins, heparan sulfate, antithrombin III, and tissue plasminogen activator. These serve as potent antiplatelet agents, coagulation inhibitors, and fibrinolysis activators.

In this paper, we report preliminary results on a type of organ vessel wall reconstruction technology and the development of a biological model which resembles the natural blood vessel intima and media in terms of structure, morphology, and function. The essential feature of the system, as schematically shown in Fig. 8.1, is a multiphasic cellular assembly with a hierarchical structure. The graft consists of a polymer matrix, a collagen gel layer, a smooth muscle cell (SMC) multilayer/extracellular matrix layer, an artificial basement membrane, and an endothelial cell monolayer lining.

## Methods and materials

### Harvesting, culturing, and seeding

ECs were harvested from the bovine thoracic aorta by either mechanical scraping or by using the enzyme collagenase. SMCs were harvested from bovine and Wister rat thoracic aortas either by using the enzymes collagenase and elastase or by using an explant outgrowth method. The culture of the primary and several passages was carried out in Dulbecco's modified Eagle's medium (DEM) supplemented with 15% fetal calf serum (FCS). The heat-inactivated FCS was used for culturing SMC. The number of adhered cells was quantitatively determined by using a Coulter-Counter (Model ZB) after trypsinization.

### Artificial basement membrane

Various types of bovine collagen (types I, II, III, and IV) purchased from Nitta Gelatin (Osaka) were screened for use of the artificial basement membrane. Bovine type I collagen, which was supplied in a Dulbecco's modified Eagle's medium solution and could easily form a gel upon incubation at 37°C, was kindly donated from Japan Biomaterials Research Institute (T. Miyata, Tokyo). This type I collagen complexed with mucopolysaccharides and was used for the artificial basement membranes. Mucopolysaccharides, including heparin, heparan sulfate, dermatan sulfate, chondroitin sulfate, and hyaluronic acid, were purchased from Seikagaku Kogyou (Osaka).

[1]Department of Artificial Organs, National Cardiovascular Center Research Institute, 5-7-1 Fujishiro-dai, Suita, Osaka, 565 Japan

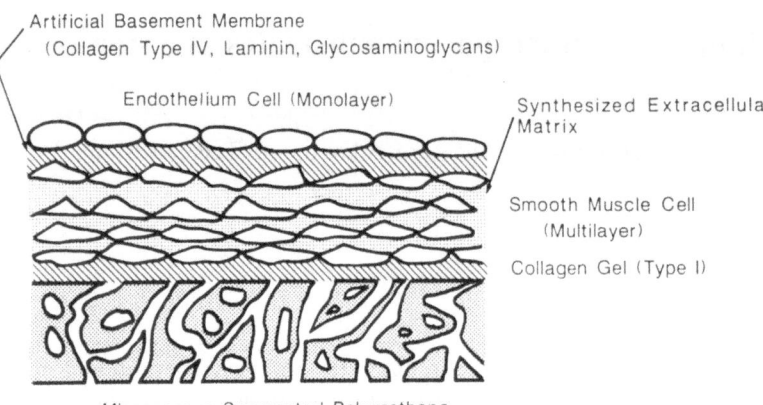

## Matrix polymer

The matrix polymers used were Dacron graft (knitted Cooley double velour, 24 mm in diameter; Meadox Medical. Inc., USA) and microporous segmented polyurethane graft (siliconized segmented polyurethane, developmental product; Kanegafuchi Chemicals, Japan). This elastomeric vascular graft was developed by K. Kira (Kanegafuchi, Japan) and H. Matsumoto (Saitama Medical College, Japan).

## Morphology

Scanning electron microscopy (SEM), transmission electron microscopy (TEM), and phase-contrast microscopy were used to analyze the surface and cross-sectional cellur morphology of cultured cells and the cellular assembly.

## Results

### Adhesion and growth characteristics of ECs

ECs, which were derived from the bovine thoracic aorta either by enzymatic treatment or mechanically scraping methods, adhered well on both collagen and fibronectin-coated dishes. Upon seeding, ECs adhered to the surfaces within a few hours and grew to form a confluent monolayer after culturing for several days. The "cobblestone" morphology characteristic of confluent ECs was observed under a phase-contrast microscope (Fig. 8.2). The identification of ECs was determined by fluorescence staining of the EC low-density lipoprotein (LDL) receptor using a fluorescence-labeled LDL antibody. On the other hand, little fluorescence staining was observed for SMCs. The cell population at the confluent state was found to be around $2 \times 10^5$ cells/cm$^2$. Although no overgrowth in terms of cell population was noticed

upon culturing beyond the confluent monolayer state, a morphological change was observed. The SEM image indicates that at the near confluent state, a cell-to-cell gap was still observed (Fig. 8.3c, d), but further culturing resulted in the formation of a tight junction between adjacent cells (Fig. 8.3a, b), resulting in a morphology resembling that of a natural vessel's endothelium. The adhesion and growth characteristics of ECs on various types of collagen were as follows: Types I and IV were the most adhesive collagens, followed by type III. The least adhesive protein was collagen type II. The very high adhesion found for type IV collagen was in good agreement with the fact that the basement membrane of natural vessels contains mostly type IV collagen. Although some difference in adhesion characteristics between the types of collagen was observed, little significant difference was observed for the growth characteristics (doubling time, $18.0 \pm 1.2$ h), irrespective of the collagen type.

### Adhesion and growth characteristics of SMCs

The identification of SMCs derived from the thoracic aorta was determined by the fluorescene staining of cells using a myosin antibody. Smooth muscle cells adhered well from primary culture and grew on the collagen and fibronectin-coated dishes. The SMCs in the confluent state showed the "hills and valleys" morphology clearly under phase-contrast microscopy (Fig. 8.4). The addition of a vasocontraction hormone, angiotensin II, on primary cultured cells induced a morphological change from a flattened to a contracted round shape, indicating that the contraction function, which is one of the major functions of SMC, was present at least in primary culture. Further culturing resulted in overgrowth of SMCs with a build-up of multilayered SMCs (Fig. 8.4d). This was directly observed by cross-sectional observations using TEM, as shown in Fig. 8.5. The TEM image in Fig. 8.5a shows that around 14 layers built up in this

**Fig. 8.2a–d.** Endothelial cell growth and confluent monolayer formation. Cobblestone morphology is seen in **d**

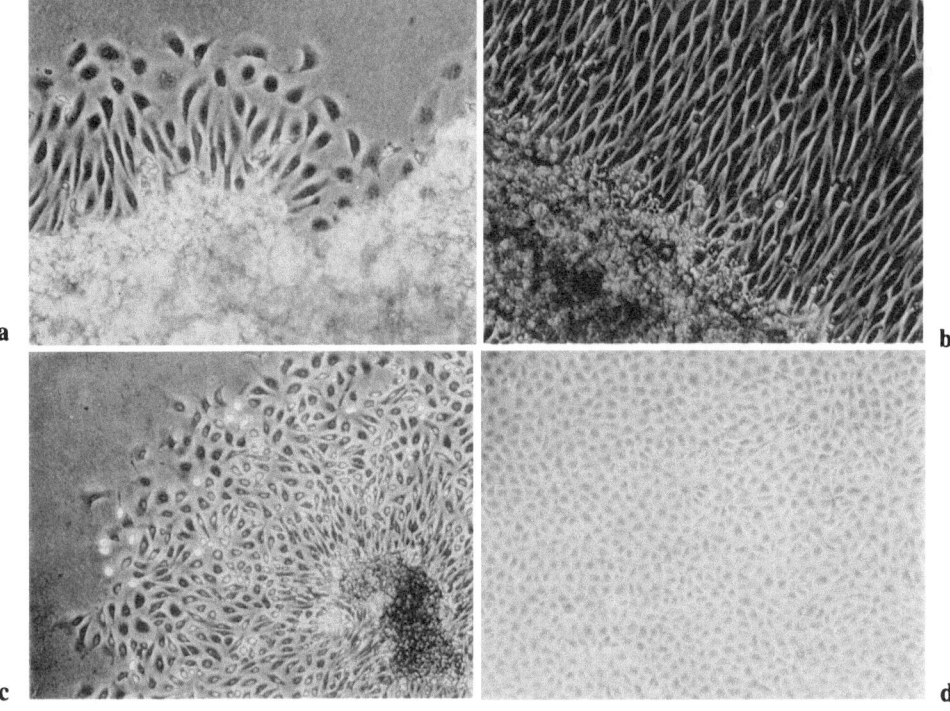

**Fig. 8.3a, b.** Scanning electron micrographs of endothelial cell monolayer at **a** the near confluent and **b** maturer confluent states

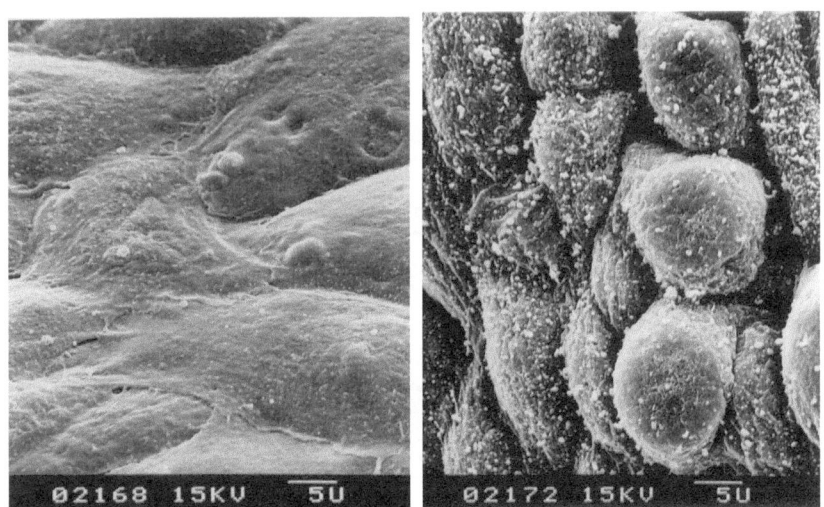

particular case, which was continuously cultured for almost 1 month. The morphological structure of the SMC is very clear (Fig. 8.5b). The layer-to-layer space between two adjacent layers was around 0.5–1 μm and seemed to be filled with an extracellular matrix probably synthesized and secreted from the SMCs. It is speculated that the formation of the self-organized multilayering arrays is due to the inherent nature of the growth characteristics of SMCs. This is in marked contrast to the growth characteristics of endothelial cells, which exhibit contact inhibition at the con-fluence of the monolayers. The growth curve of vascular cells plotted against the incubation period clearly differentiates the growth patterns between these vascular cells; there was no overgrowth after the confluent monolayering for ECs, whereas SMCs became multilayered (Fig. 8.6). Upon longer culturing of SMCs, necrosis observed by TEM occurred in the deeper layers. This was probably due to an insufficient supply of nutrients and oxygen, suggesting that in selecting a substrate for an artificial graft a porous substrate is required to supply these nutrients to the

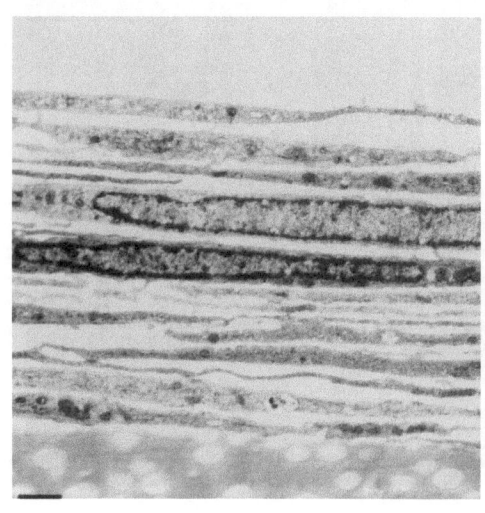

Fig. 8.4a–d. Smooth muscle cell growth. "Hills and valley" morphology at the confluent state is seen in **b**

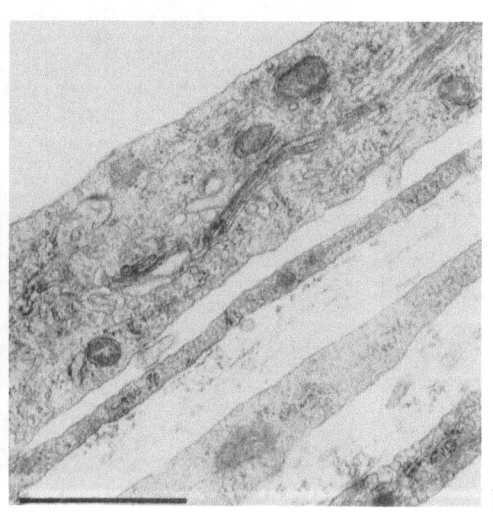

Fig. 8.5a, b. Cross-sectional view of SMC multilayers under transmission electron micrography

deeper layers through the surrounding tissues.

The adhesive protein dependency of SMCs on adhesion and growth characteristics was a follows: The adhesion rate was highest for collagen types I and II, followed by type III; the least adhesion was found for type IV. This is reasonable since the major type of collagen found in the extracellular matrix present at the media is type I collagen. However, the growth rate as measured by the doubling time was almost same, irrespective of the type of collagen (19.2 ± 0.8 h).

## Hierarchical structure of cellular assembly

The ECs were seeded onto the multilayered SMCs, which were cultured for 48 days, but no apparent adhesion and subsequent growth was observed even after coculturing for several days. The seeded ECs remained round and no pseudopod formation was observed. When a collagen type I gel was overlayered on multilayered SMCs, it dramatically enhanced the EC adhesion and growth. An SEM image shows the formation of the confluent monolayered ECs, which were overgrown on the SMC multilayer (Fig. 8.7). The morphology showed tight junctions and resembled the lumen surface of a natural graft. The preliminary coculturing study of the cellular assembly showed that the overlayered ECs seem to regulate overgrowth of SMCs, probably as a result of intercellular communication between SMCs and ECs. The cross-sectional view of the step-by-step cocultured system under TEM showed a hierarchical structure composed of the EC monolayer lining, basement membrane, the SMC multilayer with extracellular matrix, and collagen substrate layer. Based on the organ reconstruction technology developed here, this prototype vessel wall model mimics the intima and media of a natural vessel wall. It is hoped that this construction will serve as a small-caliber artificial graft as well as a pharmacological and physiological research tool for studying the transport and physiological functions of blood vessel walls.

### Verification of non-thrombogenicity of EC lining

To verify the nonthrombogenicity of the cultured ECs, platelet adhesion and aggregation behavior were studied by incubation of bovine platelet-rich plasma (PRP) on the cell-lined or collagen-lined dishes. The collagen type I substrate served as a control and exhibited massive platelet aggregates with an extensive pseudopod formation and flattening, indicating that collagen is a very potent thrombogenic surface, as expected. It is well known that collagen plays a vital role in primary hemostasis when a vessel wall is injured in vivo. On the other hand, the SMC-lined surface showed much reduced platelet adhesion; the flattened SMCs did not induce adhesion or aggregation of platelets, whereas newly divided SMCs, which had

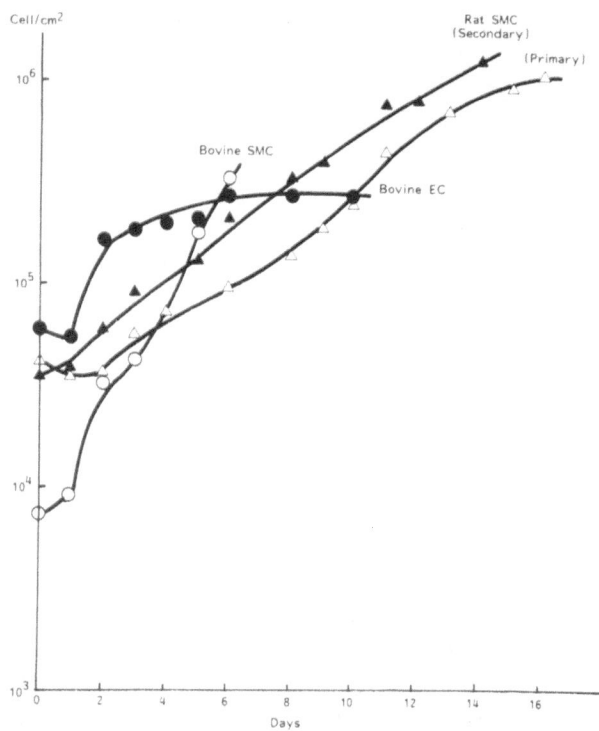

**Fig. 8.6.** Growth patterns of vascular cells. *EC* endothelial cell monolayer, *SMC* smooth muscle cell multilayer

microvilli on their cell membrane, trapped platelets within microvilli but did not induce aggregation or a change in shape. The least thrombogenic surface was the EC-lined surface. Little adhesion was observed except that a single platelet occasionally adhered to the EC monolayer (Fig. 8.8). Further study of the effect of coagulation, platelet and white blood cell systems in relation to pharmacologically active substances, such as prostacyclin, antithrombin III, and

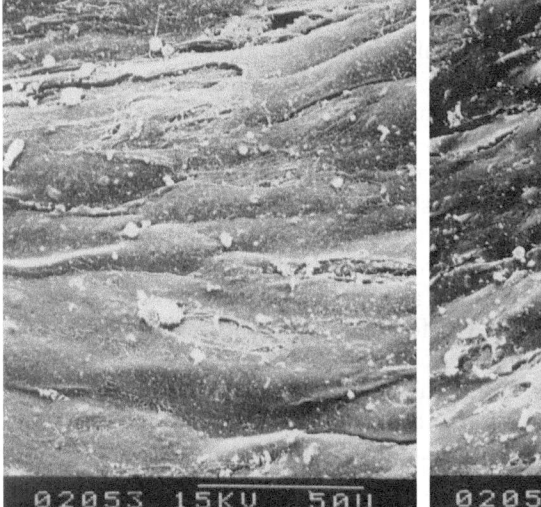
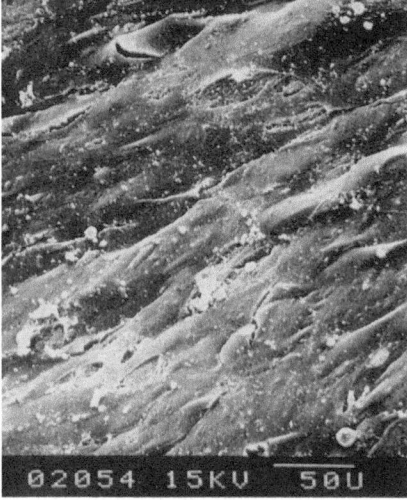

**Fig. 8.7a, b.** Endothelial monolayer formation on collagen type I gel overlayered on smooth muscle cell multilayer

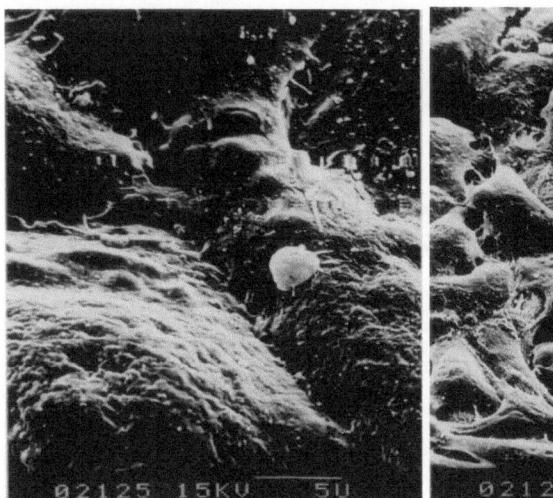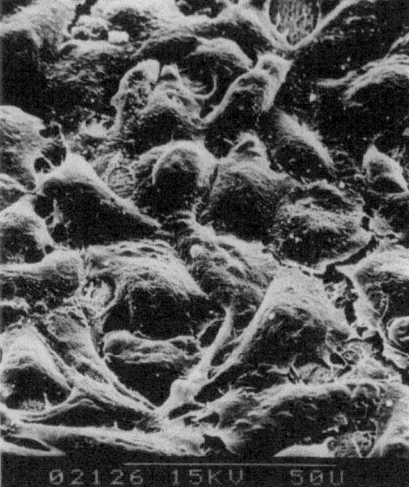

a                                                                                                      b

**Fig. 8.8a, b.** Platelet adhesion on endothelial cell monolayer. A single platelet occasionally adheres to the endothelial cell monolayer

tissue plasminogen activator, which it is believed are secreted from ECs, should be carried out. This will allow better understanding of the detailed function of ECs in antithrombogenicity. It is hoped that this approach toward creating a viable endothelial cell lining as a lumen surface of small-caliber grafts will be clinically useful.

## Design of artificial basement membrane

The basement membrane (BC) has at least three functions in vivo. First, the BC serve to anchor and adhere ECs. Second, it serves as a barrier separating the intima from the media, where SMCs dominate. If SMCs migrate into the intima, atherosis might be induced. Third, the BC plays a role in hemostasis. This is especially important in vessel wall injury. In the EC/SMC assembled vessel wall model, the first two functions are definitely required. However, in terms of the third function, the total reverse is demanded of the artificial basement membrane, because extremely high antithrombogenicity is necessary once the basement membrane is directly exposed to blood owing to the shear-induced delamination of ECs. Therefore, the essential requirements of an artificial basement membrane are: (a) very good adhesion and growth characteristics for ECs; (b) high adhesion strength to provide resistance to the blood shear stresses; (c) extremely high antithrombogenicity; and (d) control of SMC growth in the EC/SMC conjugated cellular assembly system [6]. The design of artificial basement membranes incorporating these four requirements is essential to the development of a hybrid artificial graft. The major components of the basement membrane of natural graft walls are collagen, laminin, and mucopolysaccharides. Collagen is suitable as a basement matrix from the point of view of its gelling capability as well as its adhesivity, but it is not suitable

**Table 8.1.** Cellular adhesion to artificial basement membrane

| Artificial basement membrane[a] | Platelet adhesion[c] (% control) | Endothelial cell adhesion (% control) |
|---|---|---|
| Control[b] | 100 | 100 |
| Chondroitin | 95 | 93 |
| Chondroitin-6-sulfate | 65 | 70 |
| Dermatan sulfate | 75 | 299 |
| Hyaluronic acid | 9 | 103 |
| Heparan sulfate | — | 235 |

[a] Complex of collagen type I and mucopolysaccharide (1:1 by weight)
[b] Collagen type I as control
[c] After Kasai and Akaike [7]

in terms of antithrombogenicity. Indeed, collagen triggers the activation of both platelets and the coagulation system. However, some mucopolysaccharides present in the vascular wall are potent anticoagulants; these include heparan sulfate and dermatan sulfate. The combination of collagen and mucopolysaccharide may be a promising composite material for an artificial basement membrane. Kasai and Akaike previously reported the platelet adhesion characteristics of collagen/mucopolysaccharide complexes [7]. The combination with hyaluronic acid gave the least platelet adhesive surface in their limited experiments. Our preliminary study [8] aiming at an optimal design of the artificial basement membrane showed that the combination of collagen type I with dermatan sulfate or heparan sulfate and/or hyaluronic acid both enhances cell adhesion and antithrombogenicity (Table 8.1). A more detailed study is now underway.

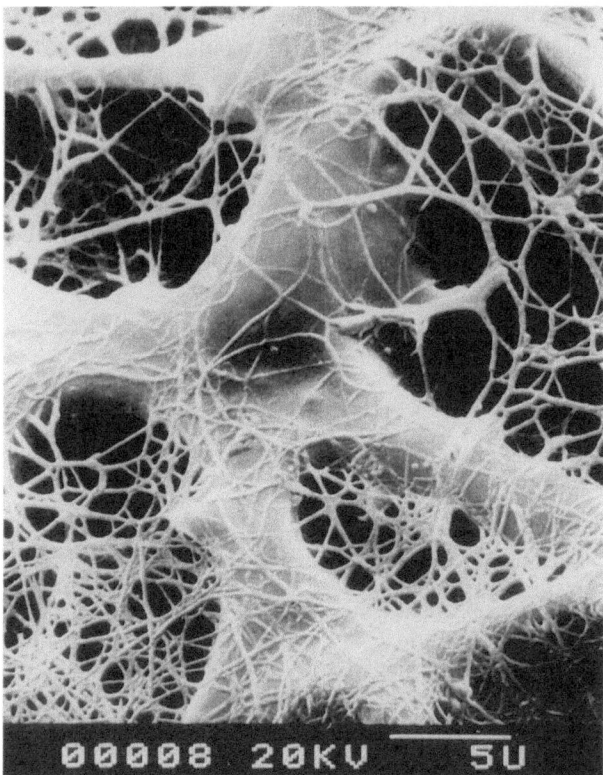

**Fig. 8.9.** Formation of artificial basement membrane on microporous artificial vascular graft with open-cell structure

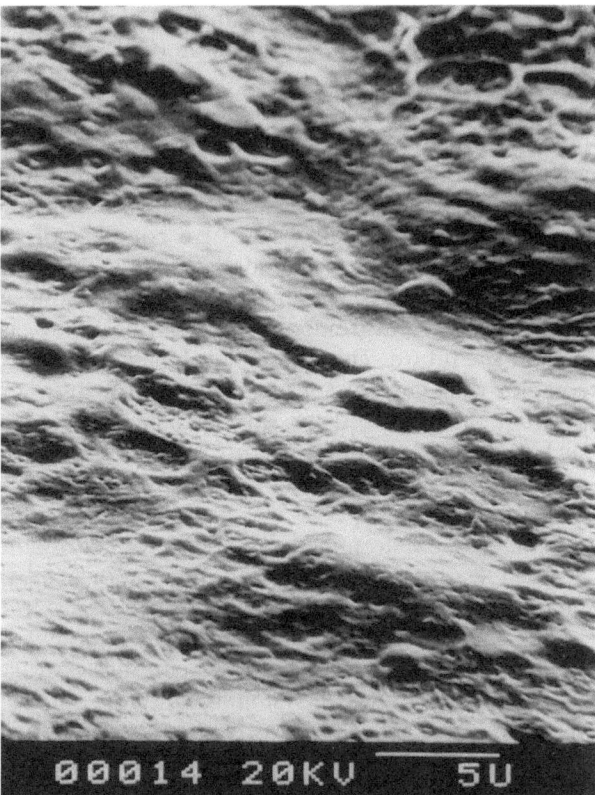

**Fig. 8.10.** "Cobblestone" morphology of endothelial cell monolayer formed on artificial graft overlayered with artificial basement membrane

## Endothelial cell seeding on artificial vascular graft

The requirements of a matrix polymer suitable for small-caliber artificial grafts are flexibility and an open-cell microporous structure (unpublished data). The former is especially important to small-caliber artificial grafts, because a large compliance mismatch with the host graft reduces patency rates. Therefore, elastomeric properties close to those of the vascular wall are required. The open-cell microporous structure facilitates the supply of nutrients and oxygen from the surrounding tissues to the adhered cell layers as well as provides a mean for suturing at the host/graft junction. In these experiments, a Dacron-knitted double-velour graft of 24 mm internal diameter and a microporous segmented polyurethane graft with an internal diameter of 3 mm were used as matrix polymers. The polyurethane was silicon containing and had a microporous open cell structure. Figure 8.9 is an SEM image of the artificial basement membrane-coated microporous elastomeric graft, showing the fibrous collagen/heparan sulfate complex entrapped on the microporous surface. Upon EC seeding on the gelled layer of these grafts and culturing, the morphology resembles the lumen sur-

face of natural vessels (Fig. 10). The cellular assembly technology developed here was also successfully applied to the porous polyurethane. Thus, reconstruction technology based on an endothelial cell monolayer lining, a smooth muscle cell multilayer, and an artificial basement membrane has been successfully accomplished.

## Discussion

Endothelial cell seeding techniques have been extensively studied by Herring et al. [1, 2]. This technology was further advanced by rotational seeding techniques [5] for monolayer culturing on the lumen surface of artificial vascular grafts. Recently, Weinberg and Bell reported in their short paper that a blood vessel model constructed from cultured vascular cells was successfully developed [4]. This preliminary report on a hybrid artificial graft includes several important aspects of cell incorporation. First, organ reconstruction technology of a vessel wall and a prototype that mimics the intima and media of the vessel wall was developed. Although it is still in an early stage, the prototype model is a viable, compliant, morphologically and metabolically reconstructed hybrid vascular graft. The model developed here should impart nonthrombogenicity as found in the vessel wall. The design criteria for an artificial basement membrane were defined. These are particularly important for developing a hybrid artificial graft, irrespective of the EC monolayer lining or the EC/SMC conjugated cellular assembly. The optimal design of a complex of collagen and mucopolysaccharide maximally satisfying such requirements as adhesion, growth, adhesive strength, and antithrombogenicity will be a key subject for the future. The system developed here is more complex than current approaches using EC linings on polymer matrices with or without adhesive proteins such as collagen and fibronectin. Whether the cellular assembly technique forming the hierarchical structure described here is superior to conventional EC linings remains to be determined. The conventional method is much less time- and labor-consuming; however, the method presented here is much closer to the natural vessel wall in terms of structure, morphology, and function. Future comparisons between these two systems will indicate which system is superior. Although the developed model is mostly composed of bovine vascular cells and collagen, it is expected that a human cell-based system could also be achieved with atherocollagen which has the least angiogenicity. The biodegradation of an artificial basement membrane could occur upon long-term implantation. However, it is expected that a basement membrane forming in situ owing to synthesis and secretion from ECs could serve as a real basement membrane.

Another facet of the system developed here is that the cellular assembly system can potentially serve as a pharmacological, physiological, and cell biological research tool. In vitro studies of drug-induced vasoconstriction/dilation, vascular permeability, intercellular interaction, and vascular diseases such as atherosclerosis and thrombosis are feasible. A cell using double-chambered filter wells in which the cellular assembly is formed on microporous filters is currently being used for these purposes.

## References

1. Herring M, Gardner A, Glover J (1978) A single-staged technique for seeding vascular grafts with autogenous endothelium. Surgery 84: 498
2. Herring MB, Dilley R, Gardner AL, Glover J (1982) Seeding of mechanically derived endothelium on arterial prostheses. In: Stanley JC (ed) Biologic and synthetic vascular prostheses. Grune and Stratton, New York, p 62
3. Dilley RS, Herring MB (1984) Endothelial seeding of vascular prostheses. In: Jaffe EA (ed) Biology of endothelial cells. Martinus Nijhoff, Boston
4. Weinberg CB, Bell E (1986) A blood vessel model constructed from collagen and cultured vascular cells. Science 231: 397
5. Takagi A, Tada Y, Idezuki Y (1986) Jpn J Art Org 15: 1795
6. Matsuda T, Takaichi S, Iwata H, Kitamura T, Takano H, Akutsu T, Art Org 87
7. Kasai S, Akaike T (1983) Jpn J Art Org 12: 327
8. Matsuda T, Kitamura T, Iwata H, Takaichi S, Takano H, Akutsu T, Jpn J Art Org

# Discussion

*Takahara* (Kyushu University): How does the size of the pore of the polyurethane affect the layer structures?

*Matsuda* (National Cardiovascular Center): It depends on the fabrication technique. The pore size of the samples I use is about 5–10 $\mu$m. The pore is not homogeneous isn size but ranges from 2–15 $\mu$m.

*Takahara:* What kind of change occurs with a small pore diameter with regard to the interface?

*Matsuda:* I think that the size of the pore is important for anchoring the gel layer, the so-called adhesion basement membrane. I believe that the smaller the pore, the better the adhesion or anchoring achieved.

*Hayashi* (Hokkaido University): What is the role of the smooth muscle in the system? Is it different from that in the natural artery?

*Matsuda:* That is an interesting question. Researchers in the USA use only endothelial cell lining; they do not use smooth muscle cells. I think that cell to cell interactions may be very important for the metabolic function of the hybrid types; endothelial cells secrete some kind of biologically active substance to control the smooth muscle cells. Another aspect of this study is that this technology can also be used in pharmacological, physiological, and cell-biological research, for example, vascular permeability and the effects of vasoconstriction, vasodilation, and drugs.

*Hayashi:* In the natural artery, there is a very thick elastic lamina between the endothelial cell and the media. Therefore, it could be that there is no interaction between endothelial cells and smooth muscle cells.

*Matsuda:* There are many problems involved here that need to be answered in the future.

# 9. A small-caliber vascular graft for aortocoronary artery graft with temporarily artificial and permanently natural antithrombogenicity and natural vessel compliance

Yasuharu Noishiki[1], Teruo Miyata[2], Chisato Nojiri[3], and Hitoshi Koyanagi[3]

**Summary.** A small-caliber vascular graft was developed and evaluated as a carotid artery replacement and aortocoronary artery graft in animal experiments. Canine carotid arteries were obtained, soaked in distilled water, and then sonicated bring about cell destruction. In this way, a natural tissue tube composed of collagen and elastic laminae was obtained. The tube with a protamine sulfate solution inside was cross-linked with polyepoxy compounds, which made the graft white, hydrophilic, soft, and pliable. The graft was dipped into a heparin solution, which allowed heparin to bind ionically. Eighty grafts (3 mm inner diameter, 6 cm in length) were implanted in the carotid arteries of 40 dogs and resected 1–389 days after implantation. Three grafts were occluded by graft infection and 77 were patent (96% patency). Sixteen control grafts, in which the tissue tube was cross-linked with glutaraldehyde but was not heparinized, were implanted in eight dogs. All of them were occluded within 1 week. Aortocoronary bypass grafting was also performed using the heparinized graft in eight dogs for periods up to 4 months. All the grafts were confirmed to be patent by autopsy or graft angiography. Measurement of the heparin content revealed that about 90% of it was released within 1 month. After the release of heparin, the surface of the graft was completely covered with endothelial cells. The graft wall kept its soft and pliable properties even after the long-term implantation. These results indicate that the antithrombogenicity produced by the combination of the slow release of heparin and endothelialization, together with the natural vessel compliance in the graft, were the major reasons for its success as a small-caliber graft.

**Key words:** Small-caliber vascular graft—Polyepoxy compounds — Heparinization — Endothelialization — Aortocoronary bypass grafting

Recently, large-caliber vascular grafts have shown satisfactory clinical results. However, middle-sized grafts have some problems and no satisfactory small grafts for long-term use have as yet been developed. For small-caliber vascular grafts less than 5 mm, both the antithrombogenic and compliant properties are essential to the long-term patency. Numerous pilot studies have been performed, but in only a few grafts made of either synthetic polymers, such as segmented polyurethane, or biological materials has some improvement been seen. It is, however, very difficult to give permanent antithrombogenic and compliant properties to graft materials. For example, prosthetic surfaces, which seem to have excellent antithrombogenicity in an artificial heart application, become covered with biological substances such as plasma proteins when used as vascular substitutes. Because of this response, good initial results in vascular grafts are often short-lived. To solve this problem, we developed a new heparinized vascular graft made of a hydrophilic polyurethane [1] and discussed its advantages and disadvantages. Our current interests have been focused on a graft made of biological material. In general, biological materials have an affinity to the host tissue. To adapt the biological materials for medical use, one needs to perform some modification, except when the tissues are used autologously. Until now, only glutaraldehyde (GA) has been used for this purpose, but GA treatment completely changes the native properties of the material. A heparinized canine carotid artery graft [2] was treated with GA, yet showed excellent antithrombogenicity. Despite this, we were dissatisfied with the graft because of its poor compliance. Because of this, a new cross-linking method for biological materials was developed, and the previously reported carotid artery graft was made soft and pliable by the use of polyepoxy compounds. Consequently, the graft had both antithrombogenicity from slow heparin release and natural vessel compliance. The graft was evaluated as a carotid artery replacement and a coronary bypass graft in experimental animals.

[1]Division of Surgery, Department of Rehabilitation Medicine, Medical School, Okayama University, Misasa, Tottori, 682-02 Japan
[2]Japan Biomedical Material Research Center, 11-21 Nakane 2-chome, Meguro-ku, Tokyo, 152 Japan
[3]Tokyo Women's Medical College, 10 Kawada-cho, Shinjuku-ku, Tokyo, 162 Japan

## Materials and methods

### Cross-linking reagent used

The cross-linking reagents used were polyepoxy compounds (PC), such as polyethylene glycol diglycidyl ether, glycerol polyglycidyl ether, polyglycerol polyglycidyl ether, and sorbitol polyglycidyl ether (Nagase Chemical, Ltd., Osaka, Japan). In this study, polyglycerol polyglycidyl either (PGPGE) was used. Its molecular structure and cross-linking reaction with collagen molecules are illustrated in Fig. 9.1. The cross-linking reaction can be performed at room temperature, and the specimens cross-linked with PCs become hydrophilic.

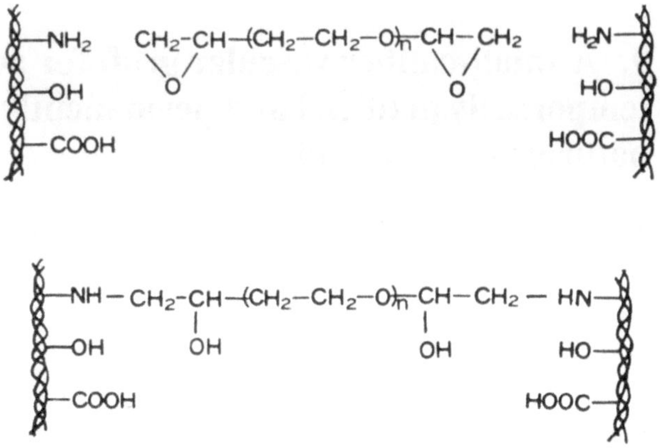

### Basic material of graft

A fresh carotid artery with an inner diameter of 2.5–3.0 mm was obtained from dogs. The artery was soaked in distilled water for 1 h and sonicated at 28 kilocycles for 20 s to produce cell destruction. Cell debris was then removed by washing with distilled water. In this way, a natural tissue tube composed of collagen and elastic laminae was obtained.

### Heparinization method

A 2% protamine sulfate solution at pH 5.9 was poured into the natural tissue tube graft lumen, and the graft was inflated with air at a pressure of 80–100 mmHg for 30 min to force the protamine into the graft wall.

The graft inflated with air pressure was treated with a 5% PC solution in 50% ethanol and 0.1 $M$ $Na_2CO_3$ at pH 10.0 for 5 h to cross-link the tissue and covalently immobilize protamine impregnated into the wall. The graft was then washed with distilled water.

The graft was soaked in a 1% heparin solution at pH 7.0 for 5 h at 45°C and repeatedly washed with distilled water.

The graft was then preserved and sterilized in a 70% ethanol solution (Fig. 9.2a).

### Control graft

For the control experiment, nonheparinized grafts treated with either GA or PC were prepared. Carotid arteries obtained from dogs were cross-linked with 1% GA solution, inflated at 80–100 mmHg air pressure for 5 h after sonication to remove the cell components and used for mechanical property measurements and animal studies. The PC-treated control was prepared by the method described in the preceding section without using protamine or heparin. This control was used for mechanical property measurements.

**Fig. 9.1.** Molecular structure of polyethyleneglycol diglycidyl ether (PC) and cross-linking reaction of PC with $\varepsilon$-NH2 groups of collagen molecules

The number of $\varepsilon$-NH$_2$ groups of the collagen molecules in each graft which had reacted with the reagent was analyzed using the trinitro-benzene sulfonic acid (TNBS) methd [3].

### Mechanical properties

#### Strength
Fresh canine GA cross-linked, PC cross-linked, PC cross-linked, and heparinized carotid arteries were used. Cylindrical specimens were fixed longitudinally and tensile strength measurements were performed. The elongation and tensile strength were measured on each specimen.

#### Stiffness and elastic behavior
Each cylindrically shaped specimen was placed in an evaluation system developed by Hayashi et al. [4]. The relation between the intraluminal pressure and external radius of each specimen was plotted as the logarithm of pressure ratio versus distension ratio.

### In vivo experiments

Two kinds of in vivo experiments were peformed using the prepared graft.

#### Carotid artery replacement
Fifty-six mongrel dogs weighing 8–12 kg were used for the experiment. About 6 cm of both carotid arteries was harvested and a 6-cm long by 2.5- to 3.0-mm internal diameter segment of heparinized graft was implanted end to end. Penicillin (500 mg) was given, but no anticoagulants were used at any time. Eighty heparinized grafts were implanted, as well as 16 GA-treated control grafts. The experimental animals had

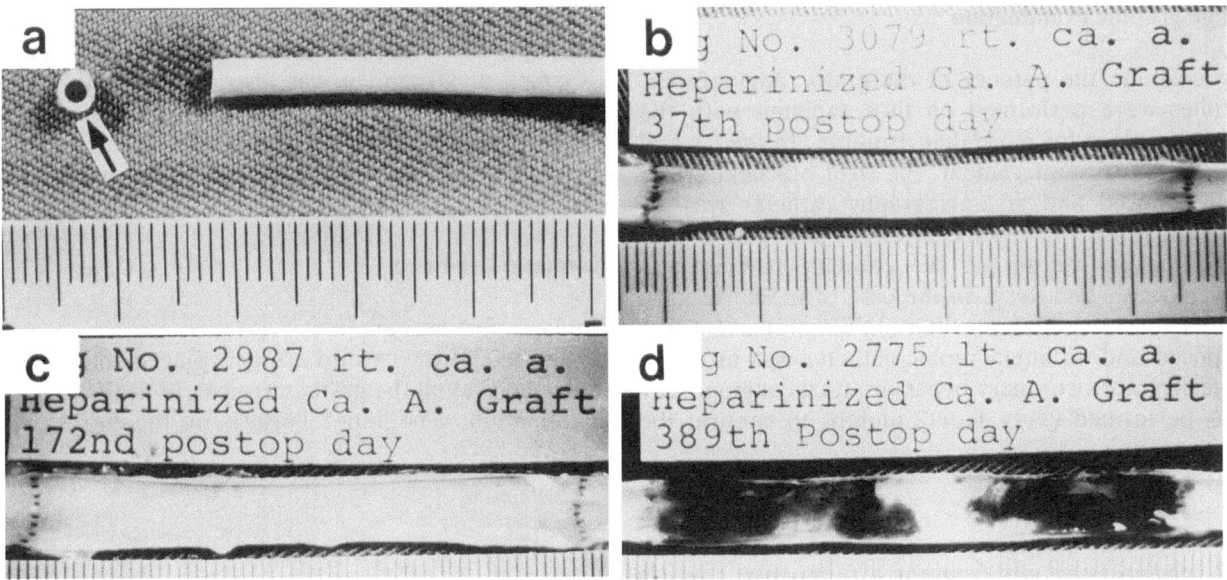

**Fig. 9.2a.** Before implantation. The *arrow* indicates a cross-sectional view of the graft. **b–d** The luminal surface of the grafts removed at 37, 172, and 389 days after implantation

free access to standard dog food and water. The animals were killed electively at appropriate time intervals. The implantation periods ranged from 1 h to 389 days.

## Aortocoronary bypass grafting

Eight mongrel dogs weighing 16.5–21 kg were anesthetized with intravenous sodium pentobarbital and mechanically ventilated with a Bird MK8 respirator. Aortocoronary bypass grafting with a 3-mm internal diameter graft was performed through a right or left lateral thoracotomy according to the following procedures, without cardiopulmonary bypass (Fig. 9.3). The proximal side-to-end anastomosis to the ascending aorta was performed with interrupted 6-0 polypropylene sutures with the aorta partially clamped. After a coronary artery was exposed, it was ligated just below its origin. A temporary shunt from an internal mammary artery to the coronary artery was instituted with a 23-gauge polyethylene tube to prevent myocardial ischemia during distal anastomosis while the heart was beating. Then, the distal end of the graft was anastomosed to a longitudinal coronary arteriotomy by interrupted 7-0 polypropylene sutures and the temporary shunt tube was removed. Before proximal anastomosis, heparin at 1 mg/kg was given intravenously. The wound was then irrigated with saline solution and closed with 4-0 silk sutures. Prophylactic antibiotics were given intravenously during the operation and continued subcutaneously for 7 postoperative days. Anticoagulants were not given postoperatively. The dogs were allowed to survive for long-term evaluation.

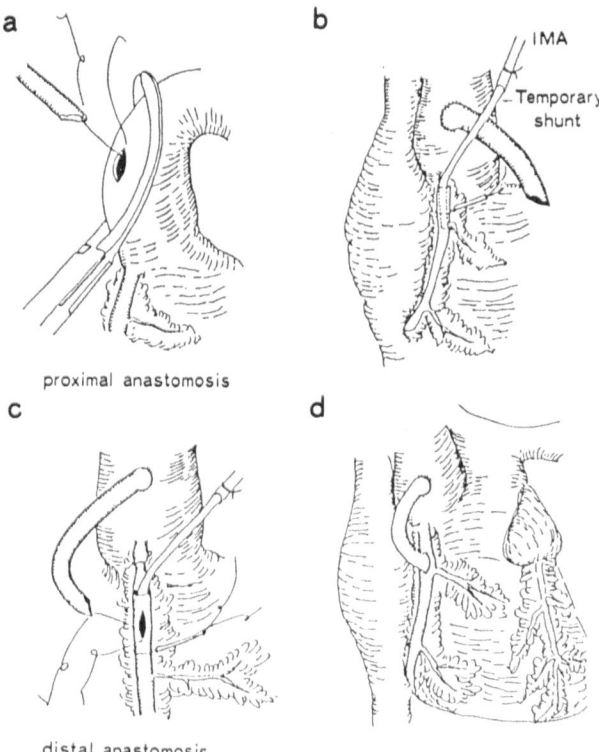

**Fig. 9.3a–d.** Surgical procedure of aorta-right coronary artery bypass grafting without cardiopulmonary bypass. *IMA* internal mammary artery

## Angiographic examination

To examine the patency of the grafts, angiographic studies were performed on those animals with the grafts in place for more than 1 month. In the case of carotid artery replacement, the right bracheal artery was exposed and an angiography catheter was inserted, contrast media was injected, and X-rays were taken when the tip of the catheter reached the brachiocephalic artery. In the case of the aortocoronary bypass experiment, the right femoral artery was exposed and an angiographic catheter was inserted. Selective aortocoronary bypass graft cineangiography was performed every 1 or 2 months to confirm the graft patency.

## Observations

All specimens excised from the experimental animals were subjected to macroscopic, microscopic, and scanning electron-microscopic observations after routine handling [2].

### Determination of heparin concentration in graft

Heparin concentration in the whole graft wall was measured using the method of Lagnoff and Warren [5].

### Measurement of blood flow

Blood flow within each graft was measured before wound closure in the aortocoronary bypass grafting experiment with an electric flowmeter, 2-mm transducer (Nihon-Koden Co. Ltd.).

## Results

### Mechanical properties of graft

Using the method of Hayashi et al., the stiffness parameter "$\beta$" (quantitative comprehensive wall

stiffness) of each specimen was calculated [4]. From these results, the vascular compliance of each specimen at 90 mmHg was also calculated [6]. The strength and elongation of each specimen was measured. These results are shown in Table 9.1. The reaction rate of the $\varepsilon$-NH2 groups of each specimen is also shown.

## Animal experiment

### Angiographic examination

In the case of the carotid artery replacement, X-rays indicated that all the grafts were patent at the time of examination. The inner surface of the grafts was

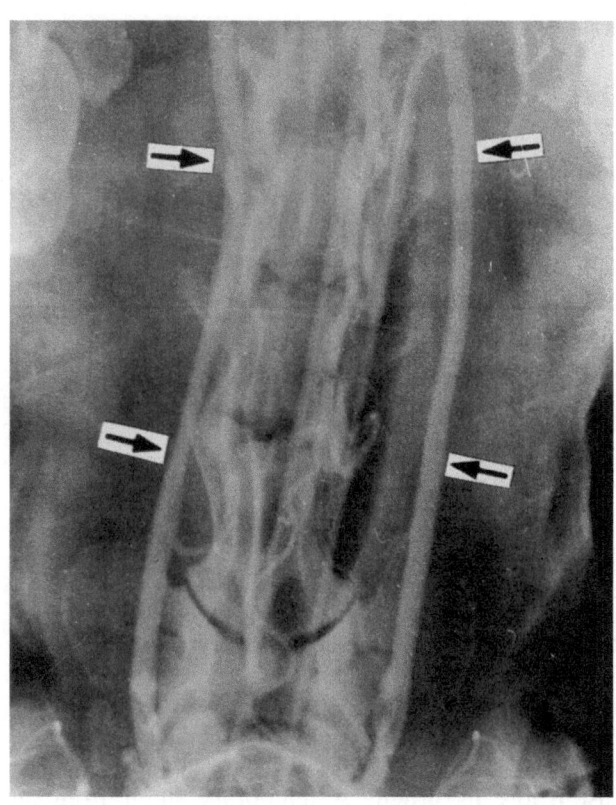

**Fig. 9.4.** Angiography of carotid artery grafts implanted for 144 days. The grafts are located between the *arrows*

**Table 9.1.** Mechanical properties of dog carotid arteries

| Treated arteries | Tensile strength (g/mm²) | Elongation rate (%) | Stiffness parameter "$\beta$" | Compliance at 90 mmHg ($\times 10^{-3}$ mmHg$^{-1}$) | Reaction rate of $\varepsilon$-NH$_2$ (%) |
|---|---|---|---|---|---|
| Native artery | $207 \pm 27$ | $116 \pm 15$ | 16.8 | 2.33 | 0 |
| GA crosslinked artery | $175 \pm 39$ | $57 \pm 12$ | 38.1 | 0.80 | $41 \pm 6$ |
| PC crosslinked artery | $199 \pm 97$ | $127 \pm 11$ | 21.1 | 1.70 | $53 \pm 7$ |
| PC, protamine crosslinked artery heparinized | $215 \pm 82$ | $84 \pm 37$ | 25.4 | 1.40 | $45 \pm 8$ |

*GA* glutaraldehyde, *PC* polyepoxy compounds

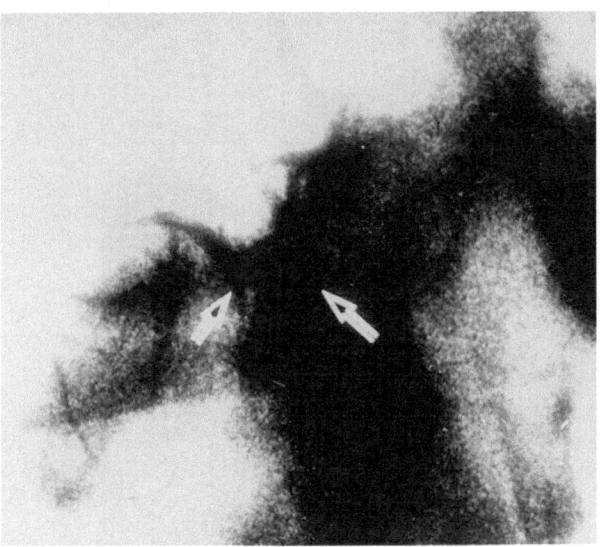 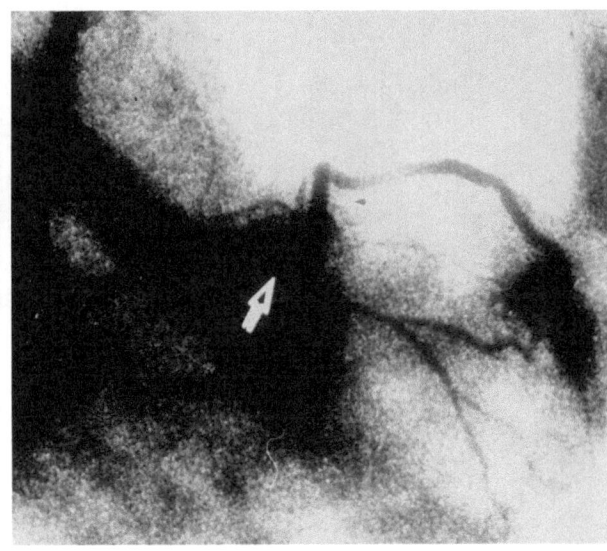

a                                                                                                                                b

**Fig. 9.5a, b.** Cineangiograms of the graft from the aorta to the right coronary artery 113 days after implantation, showing the patent graft (between *arrows*). **a** Left anterior oblique projection; **b** right anterior oblique projection

smooth throughout its length, and no stenosis or aneurysmal dilatation was observed in any of the grafts (Fig. 9.4). In the case of the aortocoronary bypass grafting experiment, cineangiography was performed. Figure 9.5 shows the cineangiogram at 113 days after aortocoronary artery bypass grafting. Figure 9.6 shows the graft to the circumflex artery at 21 days. The graft was patent and showed a smooth luminal contour.

### Implantation of grafts

Heparinized grafts were white, pliable, and more elastic than the yellowish controls. The inner surface of both grafts was shiny and smooth, but the heparinized grafts were easier to suture and match to the host arterial wall. There was no blood leakage through the grafts wall on implantation, and no kinking occurred even when the graft was bent.

### Blood flow measurement

In the aortocoronary bypass grafting experiment, blood flow within the graft was measured. The flow ranged from 25 to 35 ml/min within the grafts to the right coronary artery and 75 to 100 ml/min within those to the left anterior descending artery or circumflex artery. These flows were equivalent to those of normal coronary arteries.

### Removal of grafts

At necropsy, the dogs were anesthetized with intravenous sodium pentobarbital, and heparin 2 mg/kg was given intravenously to prevent clot formation. After exposure of the graft, patency was evaluated by palpation. The graft was perfused with normal saline

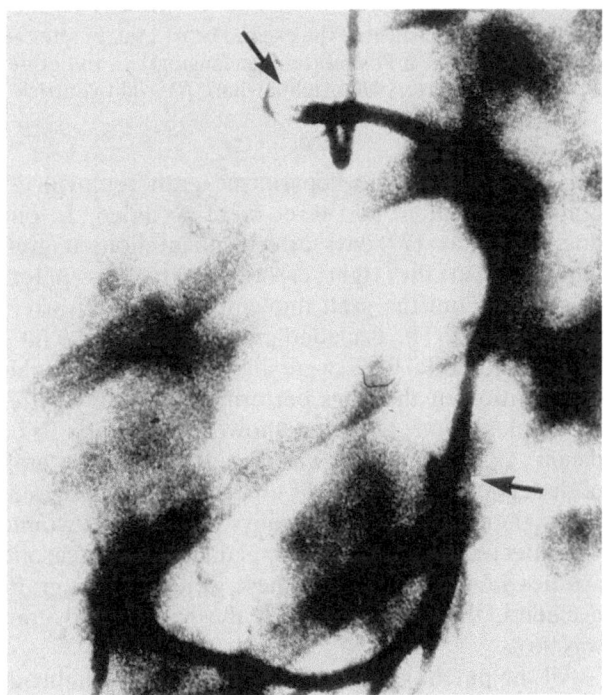

**Fig. 9.6.** Cineangiogram of the graft from the aorta to the left circumflex artery 21 days after implantation. The graft was patent and showed a luminal contour including anastomotic sites (between *arrows*)

via a cannula inserted into the proximal natural vessel. Further perfusion in situ with 1% buffered glutaraldehyde solution was used to preserve the original anastomotic area and to fix any biological debris on the luminal surface.

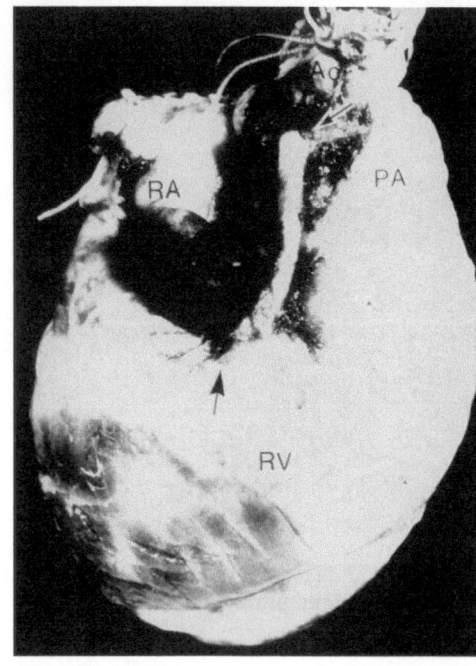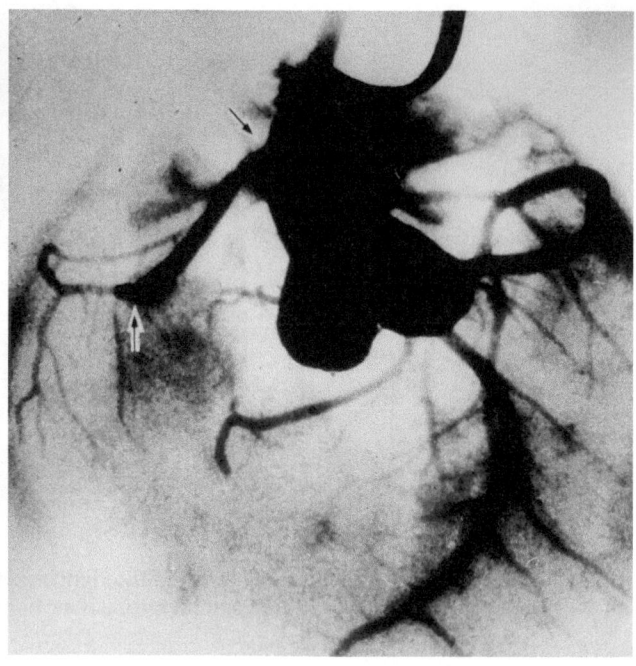

a                                                                                                      b

**Fig. 9.7a.** Gross aspect of the excised heart 14 days after aortocoronary bypass grafting to the right coronary artery (graft is between *arrows*). **b** Postmortem cineangiogram, the graft (between *arrows*) was found to be patent. *Ao* ascending aorta, *PA* pulmonary artery, *RA* right atrium, *RV* right ventricle

At the time of the heparinized graft removal, 77 grafts were patent and three were occulded. In one dog, killed at 172 days after implantation, a graft implanted in the right carotid artery was patent (Fig. 9.2c), but the graft implanted in the left artery was occluded. The occluded graft was soft and white, but anastomotic lines were hard. An angiographic examination of the dogs performed at 40 days after the implantation, however, showed both grafts to be patent. Consequently, it was considered that the graft occluded a certain period of time after the angiogram. In another dog, killed at 11 days, the cervical wound was infected and the grafts implanted in both carotid arteries were occluded. As these were the only grafts occluded, the patency rate of the heparinized graft was 96%.

All the patent grafts were still as soft and pliable as the native artery. Within 100 days after implantation, the inner surfaces were completely free from thrombus deposition (Fig. 9.2b). The surfaces were as shiny, white, smooth, and glistening as those of the host arterial intima (Fig. 9.2c). In the case of those grafts that remained in place for more than 100 days, slightly yellowish or whitish and semitransparent small spots were sporadically observed on the surface.

One dog, killed at 389 days after a fight with another dog, had a bite wound in the neck. The removed grafts showed severe bleeding inside the graft walls, and the inner surfaces were red, but there was no thrombus deposition on the graft surfaces, and the

grafts walls were soft and pliable (Fig. 9.2d).

The control grafts were occluded within 1 week after implantation, and they were very hard and dark down in color.

In the case of the aortocoronary bypass, at necropsy the heart was excised en bloc. The cannula for the buffered GA solution perfusion was placed in the ascending aorta via one of the neck vessels, and the aorta was ligated distally. Then the graft was harvested with the host vessels and postfixed with 1% GA solution for 24 h. Within an eight-dog aortocoronary experimental series, three dogs died of viral infection, 3, 5, and 14 days after the procedure. At necropsy, all dogs had patent grafts. One was killed because of an misdiagnosis of graft occlusion, but postmotern cineangiograms revealed that the graft was patent. Figure 9.7 shows the excised heart and the cineangiogram of the graft 14 days after the implantation. The graft was clean without thrombi. Four dogs were allowed to survive for long-term evaluation. All their grafts showed 100% patency when examined cineangiographically at time intervals of 21–113 days.

**Scanning electron-microscopic observations**

Scanning electron microscopy (SEM) revealed the inner surface of the heparinized grafts before implantation not to be smooth, but to have a naked elastic lamina with many holes and wrinkles on the surface.

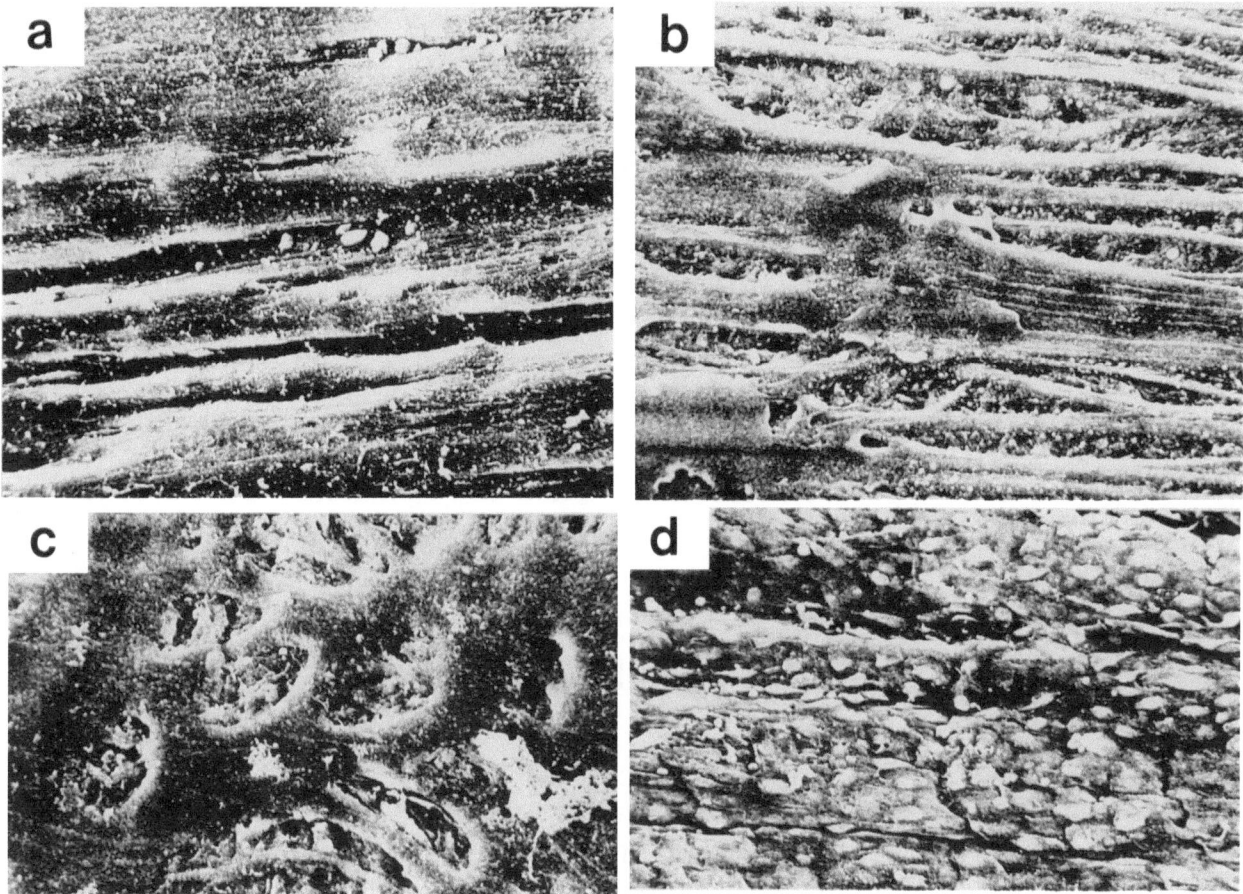

**Fig. 9.8a–d.** Scanning electron micrographs of the luminal surfaces of the grafts. **a** Before implantation, × 1000; **b** 23rd postoperative day, × 300; **c** 172nd postoperative day, fibrin deposition was noticed, × 300; **d** 389th postoperative day, × 300

No endothelial cells were seen (Fig. 9.8a). After implantation, the surface was covered with a layer of protein that was so thin that the structure of the elastic lamina could be observed through it (Fig. 9.8b). On the surface of the grafts removed at less than 100 days, there was neither fibrin deposition nor platelet aggregates, and the surfaces were rough due to the wrinkles in the elastic lamina. At the anastomotic line, pannus was first observed at 37 days and was noticed at each anastomotic line in all the grafts left in place for more than 37 days. The size of the pannus was not longer than 1 mm beyond the anastomotic line. The pannus was completely covered with endothelial cells. After 106 days, there were small fibrin deposits on the graft surface at the lines formed by the elastic lamina (Fig. 9.8c). Endothelial cells were not observed on the inner surface of the center areas of any grafts after periods as long as 172 days (Fig. 9.8c). However, in the case of the graft which remained in situ for 389 days, the whole inner surface was covered with endothelial cells (Fig. 9.8d).

**Microscopic observations**

Microscopic observations confirmed that there was neither thrombus nor fibrin deposition on any graft before 81 days. The luminal surface was composed of the internal elastic membrane, with no endothelial cells on the surface. At the early stage, there was no foreign body reaction giant cell infiltration on the outer surface of the graft (Fig. 9.9a). A small number of plasma cells were observed a short period of time after implantation. At the anastomotic lines of grafts implanted for more than 37 days, there were small panni covered with endothelial cells seen by SEM to be adherent to the graft surface. A representative pannus is shown in Fig. 9b. At more than 30 days, some macrophages were noticed in the interelastic luminal spaces near the luminal surface (Fig. 9.9a). Before implantation, these spaces were occupied by disrupted smooth muscle cells, collagen, and elastic fibrils. After implantation, macrophages gradually phagocytized the sonicated smooth muscle cells. After more than 2 months, spaces containing only collagen

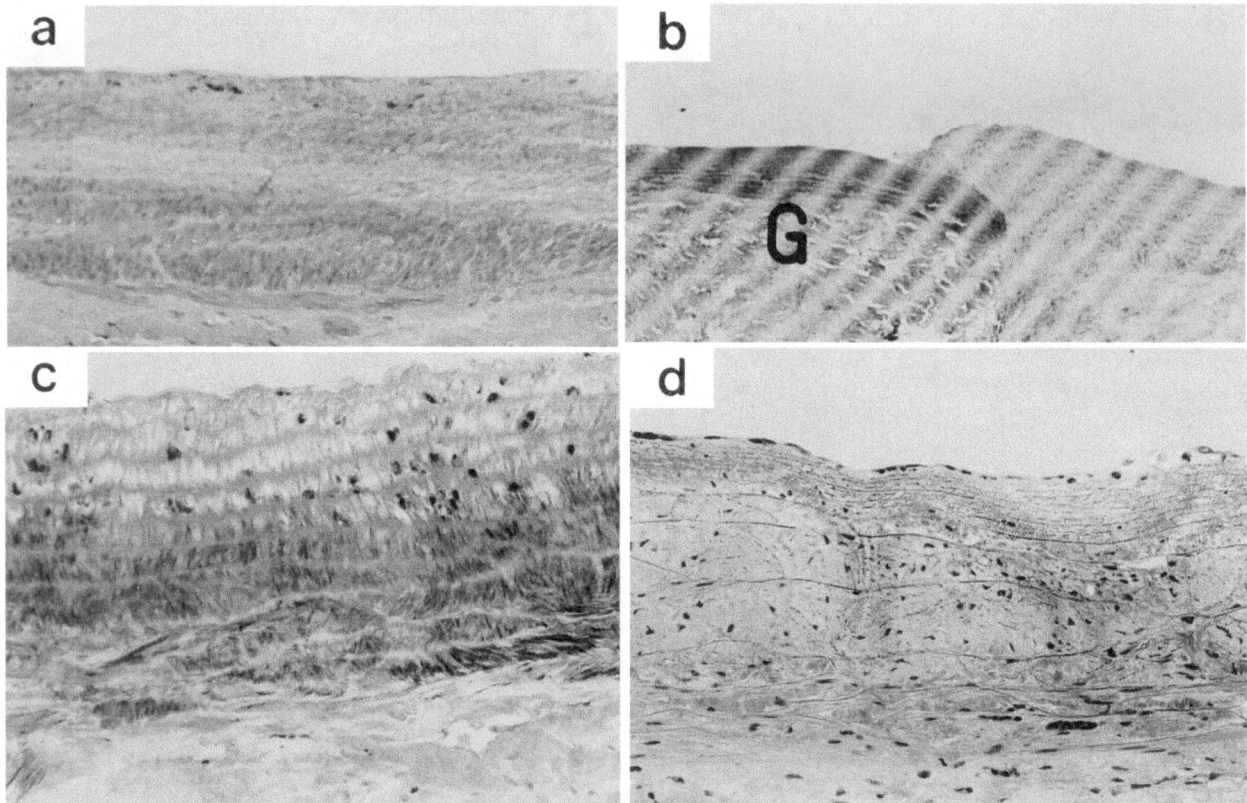

**Fig. 9.9a–d.** Photomicrographs of cross sections of the grafts removed. Hematoxylin-eosin. **a** 45th postoperative day, macrophages are seen near the luminal surface, × 80; **b** 172nd postoperative day, **c** 172nd postoperative day, × 300; **d** 389th postoperative day, × 200; *G* grafts

and elastic fibrils were observed (Fig. 9.9c). After more than 6 months, smooth muscle-like cells infiltrated these spaces from the adventitia side. In the walls of long-term grafts, cells filled the spaces completely. In 75% of the spaces near the luminal surface, these elongated cells were arranged circumferentially. The rest were oriented longitudinally. After 389 days, the central part of the inner surface was covered with endothelial cells, which impinged directly on the surface of the elastic lamina (Fig. 9.9d). The structure of the graft following long-term implantation closely resembled that of the native arterial wall, and near the anastomotic line at 389 days a think layer of pannus with an endothelial cell lining covered the surface. The thickness of the pannus was about 30 μm. There was no foreign body reaction in the long-term specimens and no degenerative changes such as hyalinization, calcification, or arteriosclerosis.

### Concentration of heparin in graft

Before and after the implantation, the total amount of heparin in the graft was measured. The results indicated that the amount before implantation was about 7.0 units/cm², but in specimens in place for more than

80 days, there was no heparin in the graft wall. This was confirmed for grafts in place for 106, 153, 172, and 389 days. The rate of release of the heparin from the graft wall is shown in Fig. 9.10.

### Discussion

Antithrombogenicity and compliance are both important factors in small-caliber vascular grafts. We previously developed a method that would afford antithrombogenic properties to collagenous biomaterials, such as vascular grafts made from carotid arteries [2] and ureters [7]. This method was very effective in preventing thrombus formation for both small caliber arteries and large vein vascular grafts. The mechanism is as follows. Heparin is bound ionically to protamine that has been previously covalently linked to the materials, so that the heparin is slowly released following implantation. This slow release of heparin can prevent fibrin formation on the graft surface. As the heparin is gradually desorbed, the graft becomes naturally antithrombogenic because endothelial cells begin to cover the graft surface. Consequently, the graft can remain permanently antithrombogenic by

**Fig. 9.10.** Amount of heparin remaining in the grafts as a function of implantation time

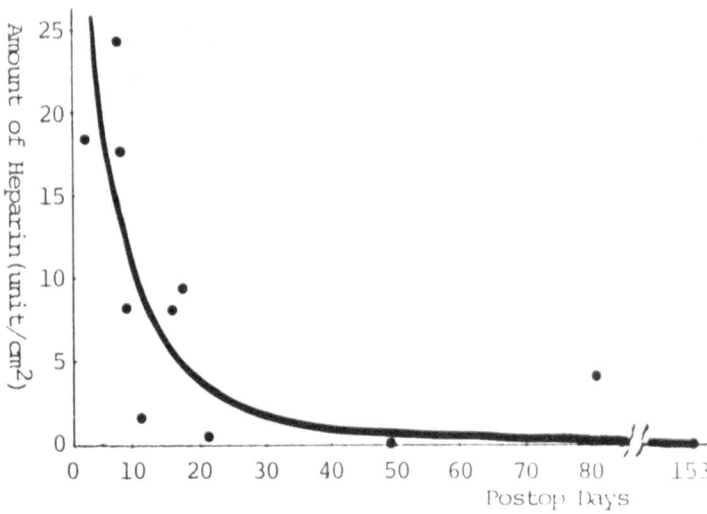

endothelialization. Animal experiments reveal that this method produces stable antithrombogenicity in small-caliber arterial grafts. In previous preparations of this heparinized graft, the protamine impregnated into the graft wall was cross-linked with GA under conditions of graft inflation, and although the graft showed no thrombus formation on its surface following implantation, the graft became less pliable and yellow with time. These changes occurred because when the graft was treated with GA to cross-link the protamine to its wall, it also cross-linked the protamine to the collagen molecules inside the graft wall. While GA cross-linking makes the materials less biodegradable, insoluble, and less antigenic, it makes the materials less flexible. Recently, other adverse effects of GA treatment have been reported.

To overcome these difficulties, a new cross-linking method was introduced. A remarkable difference in appearance between materials treated with GA and PC is their color: GA treatment makes the materials yellow, but PC makes them white. There are also remarkable differences in their softness and elasticity. In long-term animal experiments, the grafts treated with PC maintained their elasticity. This natural compliance during implantation seems to be very important in obtaining permanent patency of small-caliber vascular grafts. Another characteristic of the PC treatment is the hydrophilic property imparted to the material, which is important for its affinity with the host tissue and makes the graft more nonthrombogenic.

The strength of the graft treated with PC is also noteworthy because despite its softness it has sufficient strength to withstand mechanical stresses associated with vascular graft applications. The absence of aneurysmal dilatation in any graft following long-term implantation indicates the stability of the graft in vivo. The finding of no foreign body reaction

around the graft wall also indicates that this cross-linking method is quite safe for implant applications.

Reconstruction of an arterial wall with the graft was most successful with smooth muscle-like cells infiltrating the graft wall. We observed the healing process of the implanted vascular graft and noted that the smooth muscle cells infiltrated the neointima of the graft and were arranged parallel to the direction of the tensile stress placed upon the graft wall [8]. If the tensile stress is not present, smooth muscle cells seldom appear. The appearance of such cells in the graft treated with PC suggested that there is enough compliance of the graft to induce the migration of these cells. In the case of GA-treated grafts, the environmental condition in the graft wall is considered to be insufficient for the infiltration of the smooth muscle-like cells. The grafts cross-linked with GA become yellowish and lose their elastic characteristics. By contrast, PC cross-linked grafts maintain their natural vessel compliance and are stronger than the original vessels, thus providing excellent suturability and compliance match. Futhermore, the PC cross-linked grafts are hydrophilic because of hydroxyls in the molecular structure (Fig. 1), while the GA cross-linked grafts are hydrophobic. In this respect, the PC cross-linked graft has superior antithrombogenic characteristics because the high hydrophilicity may give the material antithrombogenicity [9]. Mori et al. [9] clarified that materials which were given hyperhydrophilic properties with polyethylene glycol became antithrombogenic. Our graft cross-linked with PC, which contains polyethyleneglycol in its molecular structure, has high hydrophilic properties. It has another merit with regard to antithrombogenicity in that it became weakly negatively charged after the cross-linking. This was because $\varepsilon$-$NH_2$ groups in the collagen molecules were used for the cross-linking, and these increased the carboxy groups relatively. The weak charge in negativity contributes to the antithrombogenicity of the materials because of the prevention of platelet aggregation on the negatively charged surface. A basic study we made on a graft cross-linked with PC without heparinization showed antithrombogenicity on the surface. This experiment will be reported in the near future. Therefore, in terms of antithrombogenicity, as well as compliance match, PC cross-linked grafts are superior to GA cross-linked grafts when applied as small-caliber vascular substitutes.

Aortocoronary bypass grafting with this graft resulted in 100% patency, although the graft was handicapped with a low-flow rate and flow turbulence induced by the side-to-end anastomosis. By comparison, in carotid replacements, the flow rate was higher and the anastomosis was end-to-end.

It has been reported that the patency rate of human aortocoronary saphenous vein bypass grafts dropped dramatically during the 1st year. In 30% of cases, occlusion occurred within the 1st month because of mural thrombosis overlying areas without an endothelial cell lining, which were damaged by intraoperative manipulation and distension pressures above 100 mmHg [10, 11]. Furthermore, late graft failure related to progressive intimal hyperplasia of the vein wall may be due to the organization of early intimal thrombi after the initial endothelial damage [12]. Therefore, the anticoagulant or antiplatelet therapy is usually instituted after aortocoronary bypass grafting [13]. However, bleeding complications are not rare and sometimes they are fatal. The present graft has the advantage that no anticoagulation or antiplatelet therapy is necessary after the operation. From the results of aortocoronary bypass grafting to the right coronary artery, in which flow within the graft was very low because of the hypoplastic right coronary artery of dogs, it appears that the graft can be applied to a coronary artery having poor run-off.

Endothelialization was delayed because heparin inhibits cell adhesion and fibrin deposition on the luminal surface. However, in these preliminary animal experiments, the PC cross-linked heparinized grafts showed excellent patency, suggesting that the graft will be a potentially promising graft applicable to aortocoronary bypass or vascular surgery below the knee.

Infection was the most likely cause of graft occlusion in this study because only one graft became occluded in the absence of infection. In this case, the anastomotic area had a scar around the graft, suggesting the presence of microinflammation around the anastomotic line. Therefore, if infection can be eliminated, the graft patency rate should be very high.

From these results, we can conclude that the combination of short-term antithrombogenicity of slowly released heparin followed by the more permanent antithrombogenicity of endothelialization, together with the natural tissue compliance of these grafts, were the major reasons for their success as small-caliber vascular grafts.

**Acknowledgments.** The authors would like to express their grateful thanks to Dr. Hayashi, National Cardiovascular Center, Japan, for his valuable suggestions and assistance in examining the graft compliance. The authors also would like to thank M. Morishima and K. Tanaka for their technical assistance with animal experiments, and K. Abe for his electron-microscopic examination.

# References

1. Noishiki Y, Nagaoka S, Kikuchi T, Mori Y (1981) Application of porous heparinized polymer to vascular graft. Trans Am Soc Art Int Org 27: 213–218
2. Noishiki Y, Miyata T (1985) Successful animal study of small caliber heparin-protamine-collagen vascular grafts. Trans Am Soc Art Int Org 31: 102–106
3. Wang CL, Miyata T, Weksler B, Rubin AL, Stenzel KH (1987) Collagen-induced platelet aggregation and release: I. Effects of side-chain modifications and role of arginyl residues. Biochim Biophis Acta 544: 555–567
4. Hayashi K, Handa H, Nagasawa S, Okumura A, Moritake K (1980) Stiffness and elastic behavior of human intracranial and extracranial; arteries. J Biomechanics 13: 175–184
5. Lagnoff D, Warren G (1962) Determination of 2-deoxy-2-sulfoaminmohexose content of mucopolysaccharides. Arch Biochem Biophys 99: 396–400
6. Baird RN, Kidson LG, L'Italien GJ, Abbott WM (1977) Dynamic compliance of arterial grafts. Am J Physiol 233: 568–572
7. Miyata T, Noishiki Y, Matsumae M, Yamane Y (1983) A new method to give an antithrombogenicity to biological materials and its successful application to vascular grafts. Trans Am Soc Art Int Org 29: 363–368
8. Noishiki Y (1978) Pattern of arrangement of smooth muscle cells in neointima of synthetic vascular prostheses. J Thorac Cardiovasc Surg 75: 894–901
9. Mori Y, Nagaoka S, Takiuchi H, Kikuchi N, Tanzawa H, Noishiki Y (1982) A new antithrombogenic material with long polyethyleneoxide chains. Trans Am Soc Art Int Org 28: 459–463
10. Fuchs JCA, Mitchener JS, Hagen PO (1978) Postoperative changes in autogenous vein grafts. Ann Surg 188: 1–15
11. Noishiki Y, Yamane Y (1977) On the expanding procedure of autogenous vein graft. J Jpn Coll Angiol 17: 145–148
12. Gundry SR, Jones M, Ishihara T, Ferrans VJ (1980) Intraoperative trauma to human saphenous veins: Scanning electron microscopic comparison of preparation techniques. Ann Thorac Surg 30: 40–47
13. Rajah SM, Salter MCP, Donaldosone OR, Rao RS, Boyde RM, Partridge JB, Watson DA (1985) Acetylsaline and dipyhridamole improve RM, Acetylsalicylic acid and dipyridamole improved the early patency of aorta-coronary grass bypass grafts. A double blind, placebo-controlled, randomized trial. J Thorac Cardiovasc Surg 90: 373–377

## Discussion

*Imamura* (Tokyo Women's Medical College): Is it correct that only epoxy compounds can allow the linkage of protamine to the arterial wall?

*Noishiki* (Okayama University): It is possible to use any kind of cross-linking reagent. At first we used glutaraldehyde for the impregnation of the protamine and its cross-linking. Heparin can ionically bind protamine sulfate. But in this case, the graft becomes very rigid and there is 90% loss in arterial compliance, so we decided to use a hydrophilic reagent.

*Imamura:* Epoxy compounds are antithrombogenic; heparin and protamine interaction is likewise antithrombogenic. Which is more effective in preventing thrombus formation?

*Noishiki:* I think that the hydrophilic nature is very important and the slow release of heparin is not effective for this purpose.

*Kim* (University of Utah): You have heparin released for up to 45 days and then the endothelial cells take over and the surface becomes antithrombogenic. Have you done any experiments without heparin with just the epoxy? What is the patency?

*Noishiki:* Yes we have carried out these tests and the results are almost the same. Without heparin the graft can be patent, but only if the diameter is greater than 3 mm. To achieve patency with a diameter of less than 3 mm, heparin must be used.

*Kim:* If heparin was not released from the surface but administered systemically every day, what results would you expect?

*Noishiki:* The amount of heparin released from the graft surface is very small. With systemic heparinization, only a very small amount of heparin reaches the graft surface. Thus, immobilization of heparin directly to the graft wall is more effective and lessens the side effects such as bleeding.

*Imamura:* There is a controversy concerning the methods for evaluating the patency rate in animals. Some authors believe that infection should be excluded from the patency rate, whereas others, like yourself, would include it. Could you comment on this?

*Noishiki:* I think that infection is the biggest problem with biological materials. I include everything.

*Imamura:* What about thrombus formation due to technical problems? The anastomosis is very narrow and turbulence can occur, leading to thrombogenesis.

*Noishiki:* Yes this is a major problem too. If there are technical difficulties, the area of the anastomosis is the first to be occluded. When problems do occur, the mid-part of the graft initially shows susceptibility to thrombus formation and becomes occluded.

*Cooper* (University of Wisconsin): Your treatment seems to be an advance over the glutaraldehyde treatment of natural materials, which is currently used in certain applications. This latter treatment seems to be prone to aneurysm development over a long period of time. Has your new treatment eliminated this as a serious problem or may it occur over longer periods of time? For example, have you done any physical property testing of the explanted arteries to see if the properties change with the implant time?

*Noishiki:* Unfortunately, today I cannot show the results of long-term experiments; I have just shown the results for 389 days, even though we have been carrying out experiments for more than $2\frac{1}{2}$ years. We have not observed any aneurysmal dilatation. The graft wall becomes more elastic and tougher with time because cells migrate into the graft wall and produce collagen and elastin. I include it, too.

**Part II**

**Ventricular Assist Device:
Research and Development**

# 10. The Novacor heart assist system: Development, testing and initial clinical evaluation

Peer M. Portner[1]

**Summary.** An electrically powered, implantable, permanent left ventricular assist system (LVAS) is at an advanced stage of development. A dual pusher-plate blood pump coupled to a spring-decoupled electromechanical drive is positioned preperitoneally in the left upper quadrant of the abdomen and connected to an intrathoracic volume compensator. A microprocessor-based electronic controller with rechargeable standby battery is implanted subcutaneously in the right subcostal region and provides power and extremely responsive control. Synchronous counterpulsation is achieved without physiological sensors. Primary power from an externally worn battery pack, data communication, and programming are accomplished by transmission across the intact skin, utilizing a belt skin transformer.

The LVAS has been well characterized in vitro and in vivo. Life testing of components, subsystems, and full systems over a period of many years has demonstrated excellent durability. Hemocompatability, minimal hemolysis, and high reliability have been demonstrated in vivo with no adverse physiological effects. Twenty pump/drive unit implants have exceeded 3 months, seven have exceeded 5 months, and the longest was nearly 8 months.

Clinical evaluation of a temporary configuration of the LVAS has been initiated for selected indications, including bridge to transplant. Total support of the systemic circulation for periods up to 90 days without embolic or other device-related complications has been achieved in 13 terminal patients. Six of these patients underwent transplantation and four are long-term survivors.

**Key words:** Permanent circulatory support—Left ventricular assist system—Dual pusher-plate blood pump—Solenoid energy converter—Transcutaneous power transmission—Bridge to transplant

## System design

The system configuration of the Novacor left ventricular assist system (LVAS) is illustrated, from an anatomical perspective, in Fig. 10.1. Implanted subsystems (Fig. 10.2) include the blood pump, energy converter, volume compensator, electronic control and power

(ECP) unit, and belt skin transformer (BST) secondary. The ECP contains a rechargeable battery, allowing a period of fully autonomous operation of the implanted system. Extracorporeal subsystems include the BST primary and external power source and status monitor (EPSM). A diagnostic and programming unit (DP), not shown in Fig. 10.1, facilitates periodic, more detailed, monitoring of system performance and reprogramming of operating parameters.

The blood pump and energy converter are physically integrated into the compact pump/drive unit and implanted preperitoneally in the left upper quadrant of the abdomen. The volume compensator is located in the left pleural space and coupled, through the diaphragm, to the pump/drive unit via a flexible tube. The pump inflow conduit traverses the diaphragm and cannulates the left ventricle at the LV apex. The outflow graft is directed to the thoracic or abdominal aorta.

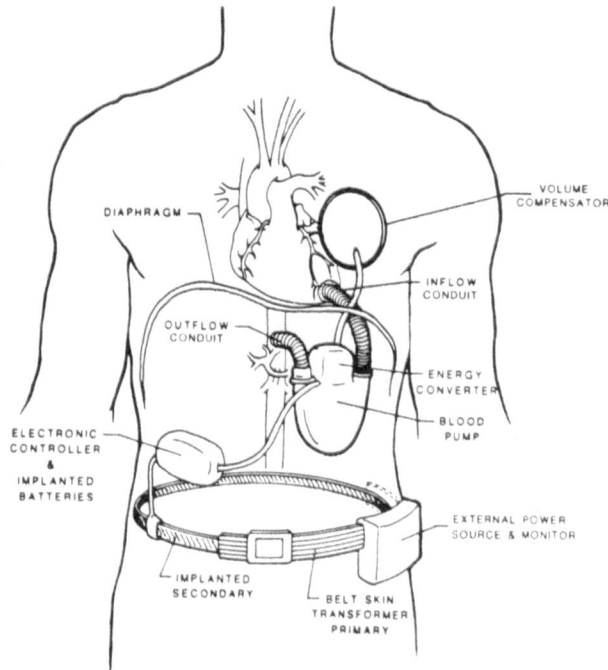

**Fig. 10.1.** Schematic representation of anatomical placement of the Novacor LVAS

[1]Novacor Medical Corporation and Stanford University Medical Center, 7799 Pardee Lane, Oakland, CA 94621, USA

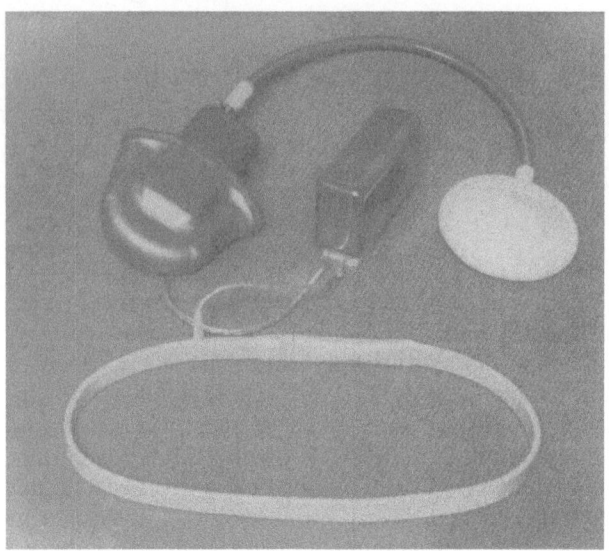

**Fig. 10.2.** Implantable components of the N120 permanent LVAS

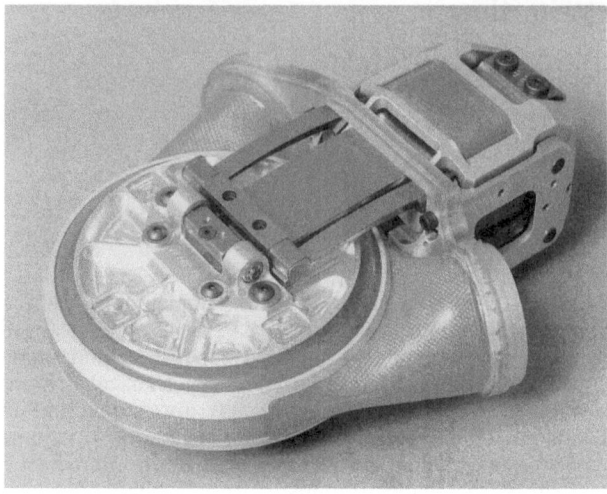

**Fig. 10.3.** N100 pump/drive unit, showing dual pusher-plate blood pump coupled to dual-armature solenoid energy converter

The ECP is implanted subcutaneously in the right subcostal region and is connected by flexible leads to the energy converter (in the pump/drive unit) and to the subcutaneous BST secondary. The BST transmits primary power, from the EPSM, across the intact skin to the implanted ECP. The BST also provides a bidirectional data link between the implanted and extracorporeal subsystems.

**Pump/drive unit**

Two sizes of the pump/drive unit are under development—the 70-ml N100 model and the 90-ml N120 model. The pump/drive unit (Fig. 10.3) is comprised of a dual pusher-plate sac-type blood pump closely coupled to a pulsed, dual-armature, solenoid energy converter.

The blood pump has a seamless polyurethane sac (Biomer™, Ethicon Inc.) that is epoxy-bonded between symmetric pusher plates [1]. Tangential inflow and outflow valve sections provide optimal flow characteristics and contain connectors for the pump conduits. The valves are clinical quality 25-mm porcine or 21-mm pericardial tissue valves (Edwards Laboratories, Baxter, Inc.) whose sewing ring is replaced by a silicone flange.

The seamless sac design eliminates flow discontinuities and regions of stasis or turbulence, substantially reducing thrombogenicity. The sac is solution-cast on a polished aluminum mandrel conformally coated with ultra-pure, silica-free, silicone, resulting in a microscopically smooth blood-contacting surface. In the N120 pump, fluid diffusion through the sac is minimized by a trilaminate design, consisting of a

butyl rubber layer sandwiched between Biomer layers.

Symmetric sac deformation maintains an optimal flow pattern throughout the pumping cycle. The increased pusher-plate area of the dual pusher-plate design results in improved pump-fill characteristics. The displacement of each pusher plate is half that of a single pusher-plate (or diaphragm) pump of equivalent dimension and stroke volume. This results in significantly reduced deformation and stress, substantially increasing sac flex life and minimizing the development of microscopic surface fissures that may potentiate calcification.

The solenoid energy converter has essentially only two moving parts [2]. These are identical armature assemblies that pivot symmetrically toward each other on miniature needle bearings. Each armature assembly consists of a laminated (Vanadium Permendur) C-core and a pair of copper coils epoxy-bonded into an aluminum armature carrier. Each armature carrier is integral with a matched, preloaded, titanium beam spring that actuates the blood pump through one of the pusher plates.

The function of the energy converter is illustrated in Fig. 10.4. The pump is shown initially (Fig. 10.4a) in end diastole with the solenoid gap open and the preloaded beam springs exerting no force on the pusher plates. The subsequent segment (Fig. 10.4b) shows the start of pump systole following solenoid energization, closure, and latch. Solenoid closure transfers energy to the main springs, which separate from the preload stops and exert a force on the pump pusher plates. The final segment (Fig. 10.4c) shows the end of pump systole; the main springs have expended their

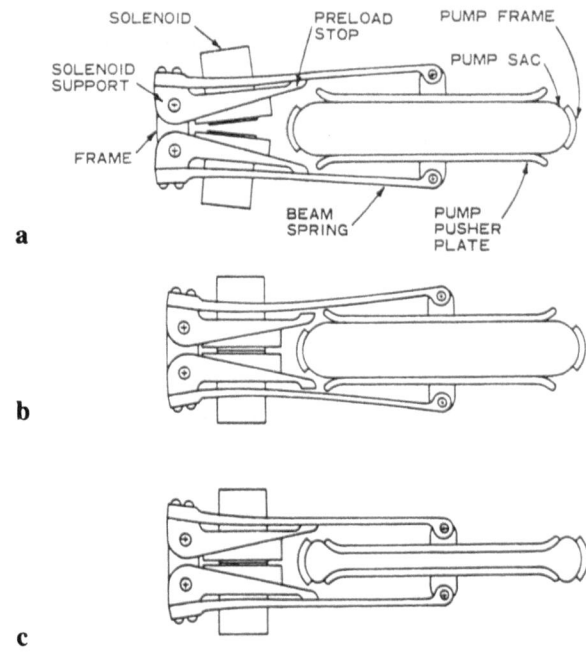

**Fig. 10.4a–c.** Energy converter operation. **a** Pump filled; **b** solenoid closed and magnetically latched—start of eject stroke; **c** end of eject stroke

energy in pump ejection and returned to the preload stops. The solenoid latching current is then terminated and the pump is ready to fill, passively, with the next ventricular systole.

All control information is derived from variable inductance displacement sensors within the pump/drive unit. The sensors monitor solenoid armature and main spring position, providing a continuous measure of solenoid gap and pump volume. This information allows the ECP to program solenoid energization and to control timing of the pump fill and eject cycles. LVAS operation, normally synchronous counterpulsation, is thereby accomplished without dependence on physiological transducers.

A unique feature of the Novacor pump/drive unit is its complete symmetry. The symmetric structure of the dual-armature solenoid energy converter results in balanced, reaction-free, operation. There is no transfer to adjacent tissues of reactive forces, torques, or gyroscopic effects.

## Volume compensator

The lenticular-shaped variable volume compensator is composed of a flexible diaphragm attached to a titanium housing, which communicates via a reinforced flexible tube with the enclosed space of the pump/drive unit. When implanted in the pleural space, diaphragm expansion against the lung accommodates

the cyclic volume displaced by the blood pump.

The compensator diaphragm and flexible tube utilize a trilaminate Biomer/butyl/Biomer construction for diffusion control. A magnesium chloride desiccant, encapsulated within a silicone rubber matrix, absorbs the reduced quantity of water diffusing into the enclosed space. The entire compensator is covered with Dacron velour to encourage tissue fixation.

## Electronic control and power

All LVAS control functions, including timing and energization of solenoid cycles, are resident in the microprocessor-based ECP subsystem. Power circuits develop solenoid closure and latching excitation from transcutaneous energy or from an internal, rechargeable, battery.

A simplified block diagram of the ECP (Fig. 10.5) illustrates the principal components. The power hybrid circuit mediates the flow of power from the BST and charges the internal secondary battery. The two energy hybrid circuits are responsible for solenoid excitation. One efficiently charges an energy-storage capacitor via the inverter transformer. The other controls energy transfer from the storage capacitor to the solenoid, using a bridge configuration of power MOSFET switches, which allows bidirectional energy flow and enables servo control of solenoid closure.

Real-time solenoid servo control facilitates smooth, impact-free, solenoid closure required for high reliability [3]. Measured or derived values of solenoid armature velocity and excitation current are utilized to modify solenoid closure. High-speed nonlinear processing is accomplished with a dedicated CMOS integrated circuit. The solenoid latching current is also programmed to decrease during pump systole as the latch force declines.

The control surface-mount circuit board performs a variety of control tasks. The circuit is designed around a 6303 microprocessor with associated CMOS memories and a 10-bit multiplexed ADC. It contains semicustom ICs for control interface and logic, transducer interface, and solenoid servo. The primary mode of LVAS operation, synchronous counterpulsation, utilizes a Frank-Starling control mechanism responsive to fill. Control algorithms are based on pump fill and eject rates. Asynchronous operation at an externally programmed rate is an alternate mode.

A console-based extracorporeal ECP with integral physiological and diagnostic monitoring has been used for most animal studies to date, and it is utilized in all temporary clinical applications. It is connected to the implanted pump/drive unit via percutaneous leads. Circuitry is contained in redundant plug-in modules, and dual uninterruptible power supplies protect against line failure and allow patient transport.

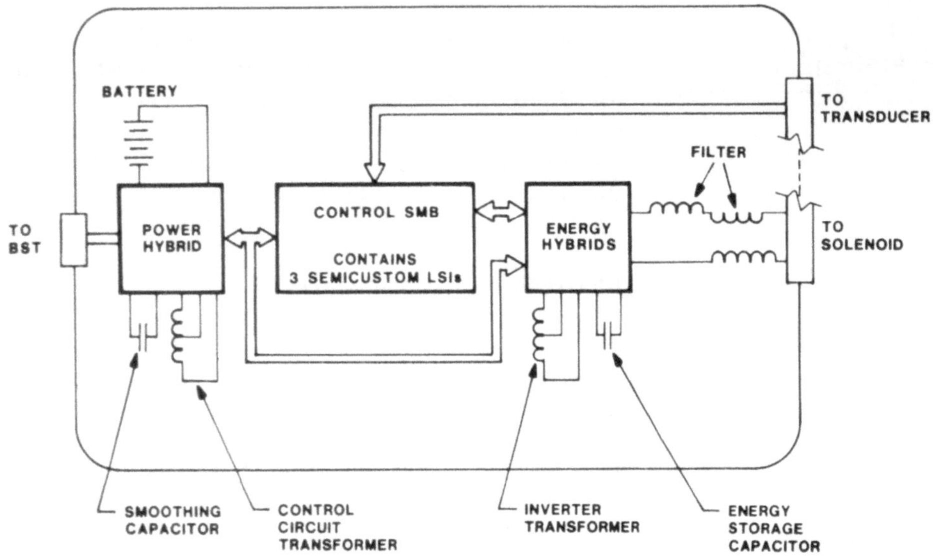

**Fig. 10.5.** Implantable ECP elements

## Belt skin transformer and external electronics

The BST provides a means for power transmission across the intact skin from the EPSM to the ECP [4]. It also provides a bidirectional communication link. The BST consists of a pair of flexible concentric coils positioned around the waist, the external primary overlying the subcutaneously implanted secondary. This geometry ensures stable coupling, insensitive to axial displacement, high efficiency and low field intensity.

The single-turn secondary coil consists of multiple, electrically parallel conductors with a flat helical shape encapsulated in a smooth silicone belt. The secondary connector is a tapered silver plug characterized by very low resistance. The five-turn continuous primary is connected to the EPSM.

The EPSM provides primary power to the BST and a limited set of status indicators. Its power converter drives the BST primary through a resonating capacitor. The phase-locked driver circuit utilizes pulse width modulation to control power output. Operating frequency adjusts around 80 kHz to compensate for changes in coupling. A rechargeable, 12-h, silver-zinc battery pack provides primary DC power for the EPSM.

## In vitro testing

In vitro testing encompasses characterization studies and endurance testing. Characterization studies are carried out on a standard instrumented NIH mock circulatory system modified by the addition of a motor-driven analog left ventricle. Loop parameters

**Table 10.1.** LVAS performance characteristics

|                                    | N100 |    | N120 |
|------------------------------------|------|----|------|
| Stroke volume (ml)                 | ≤ 70 |    | ≤ 90 |
| Pump rate (bpm)                    | > 200 |   | > 200 |
| Pump output (l/min)                | > 10 |   | > 12 |
| Energy converter efficiency[a]     | 49%  | to | 62%  |
| Blood pump efficiency[b]           | 84%  | to | 92%  |
| Pump/drive efficiency[c]           | 45%  | to | 52%  |

[a] Mechanical energy out to electrical energy in
[b] Hydrodynamic work out to mechanical work in
[c] Hydrodynamic work out to electrical energy in

can be changed to vary independently rate, preload, and afterload.

LVAS performance characteristics are summarized in Table 10.1. Synchronous counterpulsation with substantial ventricular unloading has been demonstrated over a wide range of hemodynamic variables. Because control is history-independent, the system is inherently highly responsive to extreme changes in rate, preload, and afterload.

Extensive endurance testing has been carried out at the component, subsystem, and system level to document durability and reliability. Blood pumps have been tested on multistation, cam-driven testers, accumulating more than 60 years. Four pumps continue on test after more than 5 years. No pumps of the current design have failed. Blood pumps and energy converters are simultaneously subjected to endurance testing in pump/drive unit or total system tests. Such subsystem tests have accumulated more than 20 years in vitro.

Formal, monitored, endurance testing for the N120 total system is currently underway as part of the NIH

Preclinical Device Readiness Testing program [5]. Nine of the planned twelve systems have been placed on test. Individual, instrumented mock circulatory loops (Fig. 10.6) are utilized for each system, under conditions designed to simulate in vivo environment. Pump flows are automatically cycled over a range of 6–9 l/min on a diurnal basis, and physiological pressures are maintained within prescribed limits. Continuous on-line data acquisition and processing is accomplished with a dedicated microcomputer-based monitoring system. Two systems have been on test longer than 9 months, and a total of more than 3 years of testing has been accumulated to date without failure.

Critical, highly stressed, components such as energy-converter springs and energy-storage capacitors have been tested at accelerated rates on special testers. Springs have accumulated an average of 59 equivalent years and capacitors an average of 15 years without failure.

## Animal testing

More than 150 animal experiments have been carried out since 1972 to evaluate the performance and physiological effect of the evolving LVAS (Table 10.2). Since 1979, these implants have utilized the Novacor dual pusher-plate pump. Sixty of these experiments, with durations extending to nearly 8 months, have been conducted with N100 and N120 pump/drive units. Additional experiments have been designed to evaluate separately the volume compensator and the BST.

Until 1983, the calf was used in all pump/drive implants and the dog was used in BST studies. Since 1984, all in vivo experiments have been carried out in the adult ovine, avoiding the problems of high growth rate, accelerated valve calcification, and pseudoneointimal proliferation encountered in the immature bovine [6].

The pump/drive unit is positioned in the ventrolateral abdominal wall inferior to the diaphragm. The

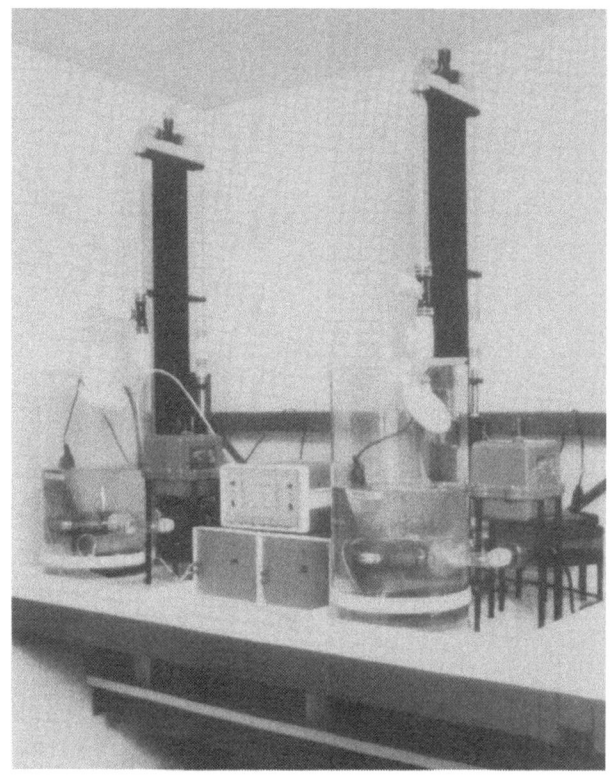

**Fig. 10.6.** Instrumented mock circulatory loop for Preclinical Device Readiness Testing program

outflow graft is anastomosed to the mid-descending thoracic aorta and the inflow conduit placed, via the apex, into the left ventricular chamber. Implantation is accomplished without cardiopulmonary bypass, utilizing inflow occlusion.

Experimental animals are instrumented for left and right ventricular and aortic pressures, as well as pulmonary artery flow and electrocardiogram. On-line data acquisition and reduction are performed by a dedicated microcomputer, providing real-time hemodynamic analysis. More than 40 hemodynamic and pump parameters are calculated, displayed, and stored for later processing [7].

**Table 10.2.** Summary of in vivo experiments: Pump/drive unit

| Period | Energy converter | Blood pump | Number of experiments | | | Longest duration (days) |
|---|---|---|---|---|---|---|
| | | | Model | Acute | Chronic | |
| 1972–79 | MK16, 19, 20 | NIH[a] | 9 | 35 | 25 | 129 |
| 1979–83 | MK20, 22 | II, III | 1 | 5 | 26 | 161 |
| 1982–present | N100 | N100 | 0 | 8 | 37 | 175 |
| 1983–present | N120 | N120 | 1 | 0 | 14 | 236 |

Data shown are through September 1987
[a] Blood pumps obtained through NIH from other investigators

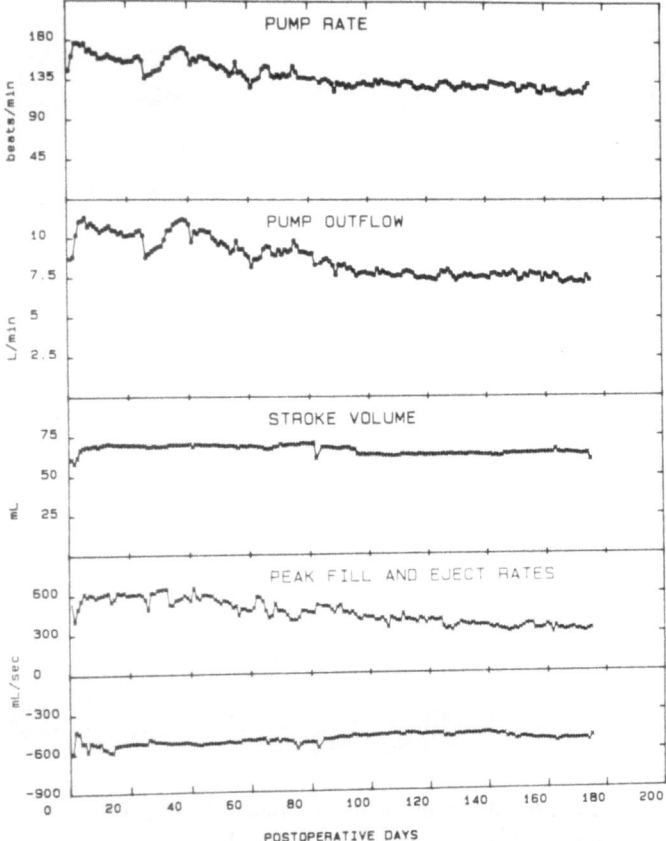

**Fig. 10.7.** Pump flow trends for ovine experiment

Acute studies have been utilized extensively to characterize performance of the pump/drive unit, to evaluate and optimize control algorithms of the ECP, and to document the physiological effect of LVAS operation. These studies have demonstrated that synchronous counterpulsation results in significantly superior support for the failing heart when compared with asynchronous operation [2]. Excellent responsiveness over a wide range of physiological variables, including severe arrhythmias, has been documented. Support of the entire systemic circulation has been documented during profound myocardial failure and even ventricular fibrillation.

Chronic LVAS studies have been utilized to investigate long-term physiological effects and to document in vivo durability and reliability. Implants of progressively longer duration have been achieved, with more than twenty exceeding 3 months and seven exceeding 5 months.

The duration of bovine studies was severely limited by pseudoneointimal (PNI) proliferation of the inflow conduit and accelerated valve calcification, resulting in progressive stenosis and rapidly declining flow. Inflow conduit stenosis has not been observed in the adult ovine and the incidence of valve calcification has been markedly reduced. Typical results of the

ovine experience are illustrated in the trend plots of Fig. 10.7, which show pump flow and fill and eject rates over the course of a 175-day experiment. The observed decline in pump flow and fill rate mirrors the decline in pump (cardiac) rate. There was no evidence of PNI or valvular stenosis at explant.

Anticoagulants and antiplatelet aggregating agents have not normally been utilized in chronic studies. Explanted blood pumps have, however, been free of thrombus and calcification. Except for transient changes in the early postoperative period, blood chemistry, hematology, electrolytes, and coagulation factors have remained in the normal range. Serum hemoglobin levels have consistently remained below 3 mg%, consistent with minimal hemolysis.

Chronic BST studies have been carried out in a series of more than sixty dogs and in three sheep. Six dogs and two sheep were followed for more than a year of continuous excitation, with the longest being $2\frac{1}{2}$ years (ongoing). In the absence of infection, the subcutaneous secondary belt was well tolerated for periods in excess of 2 years, without evidence of discomfort, inflammation, fibrous encapsulation, or belt degradation.

Chronic volume compensator studies have been conducted in four ovine experiments. In two, the

**Fig. 10.8.** N100 LVAS configuration for temporary clinical support. Console contains redundant ECPs and integrated physiology/LVAS monitor

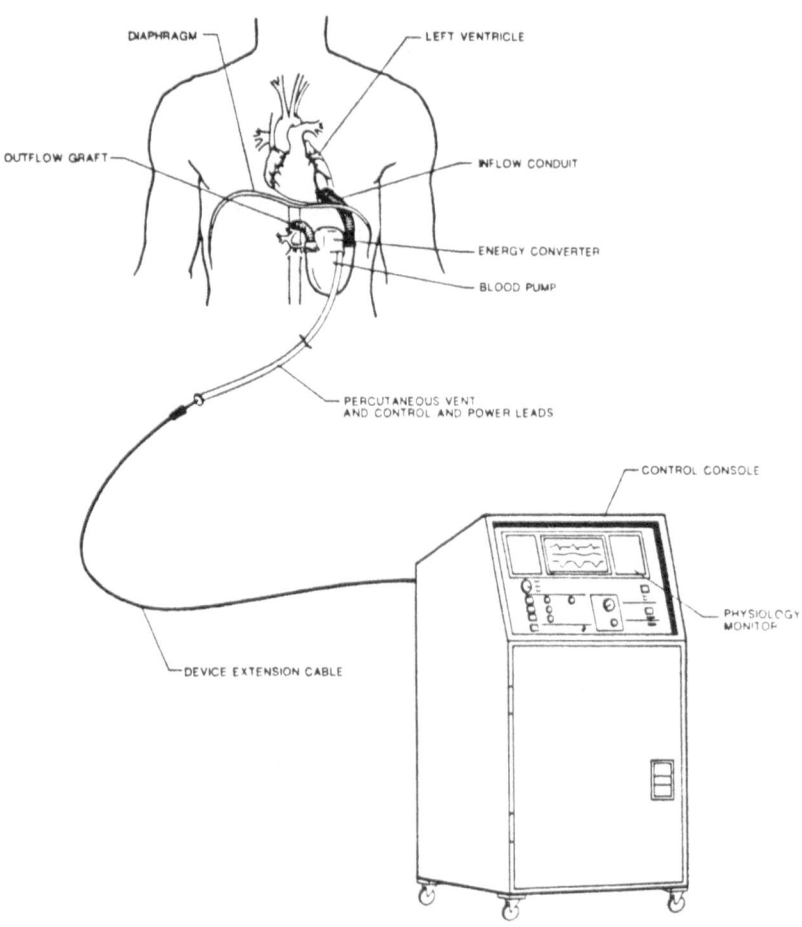

compensator was coupled to an operating N120 pump/drive system for periods longer than 200 days (202, 236). The other two were actuated by an external pneumatic driver (227, >550 days). The measured dynamic compliance (pressure excursion divided by stroke volume) remained essentially unchanged in the pump/drive system studies. The closed system remained sealed throughout the longer of these studies, and the measured humidity gradually increased to 50% over 8 months. Serial measurements of static compliance in the externally actuated compensators also remained unchanged for periods extending to $1\frac{1}{2}$ years (ongoing), suggesting minimal tissue ingrowth and encapsulation.

## Clinical experience

Following extensive preclinical evaluation, an investigational device exemption (IDE) was granted by the US Food and Drug Administration (FDA) for temporary implantation of the N100 system in patients with acute heart failure. The clinical trial was initiated at Stanford University Medical Center in September 1984 and was subsequently expanded to additional institutions in the USA and Europe. Eighteen implants have been carried out to date (through September 1987) in eight institutions—thirteen as bridge-to-transplant procedures and five for postcardiotomy failure. Six of these implants, all bridge to transplantation, were performed at Stanford. Overall, six bridge patients received an orthotopic cardiac transplant and four are long-term survivors.

The LVAS configuration in the current clinical study incorporates a console-based ECP connected to the implanted pump/drive unit via control and power leads contained in a percutaneous vent tube (Fig. 10.8). Implantation is carried out through a standard median sternotomy extended inferiorly to the umbilicus. Unlike the animal experiments, cardiopulmonary bypass is routinely utilized. A pocket for the pump/drive unit is fashioned, preperitoneally, within the abdominal wall or subcutaneously, depending on patient size and habitus. The percutaneous vent tube is tunneled subcutaneously, using a special trocar, from this pocket to the exit near the right anterior iliac crest.

Of the thirteen bridge patients, ten were male, three were femal, and ages ranged from 27 to 44 with a mean of 40.8 years. The preimplant etiology included ischemic end-stage heart disease (four patients), cardiomyopathy (four patients), postinfarction cardiogenic shock (three patients), acute viral myocarditis, and acute refractory rejection of a cardiac allograft. Typically, the patients were in cardiogenic shock with a cardiac index $<1.5$ l/min/m$^2$, unresponsive to maximal inotropic and IABP support.

The implant duration ranged from a few hours to 90 days with a mean of 20.2 days. The average duration for those transplanted was 24.0 days. Seven patients died prior to transplant. Causes of death included multiorgan failure, respiratory failure, acute rejection, peritoneal hemorrhage, and perioperative CVA (from a preexisting ventricular mural thrombus). Impaired renal function and hepatic congestion preimplantation were factors in several of these patients.

Total support of the systemic circulation, with substantial left ventricular unloading, was noted in all patients. Six patients were mobilized out of bed. One of these patients, a 47-year-old male at St. Louis University, was particularly notable. Donor procurement was complicated by a high preformed antibody level, requiring cross match and resulting in a 90-day implant. During this period, the patient was fully ambulatory, walking up to a mile each day, with assistance in moving the console. Completely incapacitated before receiving the Novacor LVAS, the patient (who was totally pump-dependent) was fully rehabilitated in the 1st month. Renal, hepatic, and pulmonary function were restored to normal, severe right heart failure was reversed, and muscle tone significantly improved. The patient's greatly improved condition at the time of transplant was reflected in a rapid recovery and hospital discharge after only 11 days.

There have been no thromboembolic or other device-related complications. All patients were partially anticoagulated, initially with low molecular weight dextran and, as chest drainage diminished, with low-dose heparin. At explant, the blood pump, valves, and conduits were free of thrombus and exhibited minimal fibrin deposition on the bioprosthetic valve struts.

Orthotopic cardiac transplantation was carried out in six patients. One of these patients died of presumed, but unconfirmed, septic shock a few days following transplantation. Another patient died of acute right heart allograft failure. Four patients are long-term survivors, 8 months to 3 years following transplantation.

## Discussion

Implantable, electrically powered, left ventricular assist systems are under development at several centers [8]. These permanent systems will provide extended, nontethered, circulatory support to patients with terminal heart failure. The Novacor LVAS was the first fully integrated system specifically designed for permanent application in humans [9, 10]. Components of this system have been under development since 1970 and animal experiments have been underway since 1972 [11].

The Novacor system is characterized by high efficiency and beat-to-beat responsiveness. Superior reliability and durability, documented both in vitro and in vivo, are a consequence of fundamentally sound design and meticulous quality control. Blood pumps have been tested in vitro for periods in excess of 5 years and pump/drive units for periods in excess of 3 years. Total system reliability testing under refereed test conditions is in progress with more than 3 years of accumulated experience without failure.

Implants in experimental animals of progressively longer duration have been achieved with pump/drive units. More than 20 have exceeded 3 months and the longest, nearly 8 months, utilized a closed system with a volume compensator. There has been no evidence, in these studies, of adverse physiological effect. Hemocompatibility and minimal hemolysis have been documented without routine use of anticoagulants or antiplatelet agents. A change in animal model from the immature bovine, used until 1983, to the adult ovine has eliminated many of the problems associated with these and other studies [6, 12]. Chronic BST studies have exceeded 1 year in six animals and 2 years in two, demonstrating tissue compatibility and minimal degradation of the implanted secondary. Volume compensator function has been evaluated in vivo for periods well in excess of 1 year without evidence of fibrous encapsulation or other functional compromise.

Initial clinical experience with an interim configuration of the Novacor LVAS, utilizing an external console, has further documented safety and efficacy of the system. Eighteen implants have been carried out, including 13 bridge-to-transplant procedures, for periods as long as 3 months. There have been no device-related complications and, in particular, no thromboembolic events. Total support of the systemic circulation was achieved in all cases with capture of the entire cardiac output and demonstrated pump dependence. Six of the bridge patients received orthotopic cardiac transplants and four are long-term survivors after implants ranging from 2 to 90 days. The first patient, alive and well 3 years after the procedure, was the first long-term survivor in the world of a bridge to transplant [13].

In addition to providing a life-saving therapeutic option for selected patients, the bridge-to-transplant experience provides a uniquely relevant opportunity to study LVAS performance and patient response. The bridge patient represents the ultimate candidate for a permanent LVAS. The early clinical results, particularly the demonstrated rehabilitation of patients to completely normal function and the absence of complications, offer a very encouraging view of the future for fully implantable permanent systems.

# References

1. Portner PM, Jassawalla JS, Chen H, Conley MG, Maeder PA, Oyer PE (1979) A new dual pusher-plate left heart assist blood pump. Proc 2nd Meeting Int Soc for Artif Organs. Art Org (Suppl) 3: 361–365
2. Portner PM, Oyer PE, Jassawalla JS, Chen H, Miller PJ, LaForge DH, Green GF, Shumway NE (1984) A totally implantable ventricular assist device for end-stage heart disease. In: Unger F (ed) Assisted circulation 2, pp 115–141
3. Brugler JS, LaForge DH, Lee J, Rising DL, Billich J, Miller PJ, Jassawalla JS, Portner PM (1985) Implanted control and power electronics for a left ventricular assist system. Proc Intersoc Energy Conv Eng Conf, pp 1613–1617, August 1985
4. Portner PM, LaForge DH, Pitzele S, Maeder PA, Lee J (1979) Trancutaneous energy for an implanted electrical circulatory support system using distributed inductive coupling. Proc Eur Soc Artif Organs, pp 109–112
5. Portner PM, Oyer PE, Jassawalla JS, Brugler JS, Ream AK, Miller PJ, Chen H, Daniel MA, LaForge DH, Lee J, Ramasamy N, Conley MG, Beering FK, Spahic B, Billingham ME (1986) Device readiness testing of the Novacor implantable permanent ventricular assist system. Proc Annu Contr Conf, Device and Technology Branch, NHLBI, p 33, December 1986
6. Ramasamy N, Miller PJ, Green GF, Oyer PE, Baldwin JC, Ream AK, Wyner J, Portner PM (1986) Long-term studies with an electromechanical ventricular assist system in the calf and sheep. In Nose Y, Kjellstrand C, Ivanovich P (eds) Progress in artificial organs 1985. ISAO Press, Cleveland, pp 456–463
7. Ream AK, Robinson DJ, Corbin SD, Griepp RB, Portner PM (1977) A minicomputer-based physiologic monitoring system. Proc San Diego Biomedical Symp, pp 225–232
8. Altieri FD (1983) Status of implantable energy systems to actuate and control ventricular assist devices. Art Org 7: 2–20
9. Portner PM, Oyer PE, Jassawalla JS, Miller PJ, Chen H, LaForge DH, Skytte KW (1978) An implantable permanent left ventricular assist system for man. Trans Am Soc Art Org 24: 98–102
10. Portner PM, Oyer PE, Jassawalla JS, Miller PJ, Chen H, LaForge DH, Green GF, Ream AK, Shumway NE (1983) An alternative in end-stage heart disease: long-term ventricular assist. Heart Transplant 3: 47–59
11. Portner PM, Dong E Jr., Jassawalla JS, LaForge DH (1973) Performance of an implantable controlled solenoid circulatory assist system. Trans Am Soc Art Int Org 19: 235–242
12. Portner PM, Green GF, Ramasamy N (1983) The blood interface at artificial surfaces within a left ventricular assist system. In: Surface phenomena in hemorheology: Their theoretical, experimental and clinical aspects. Ann NY Acad Sci, pp 471–503
13. Portner PM, Oyer PE, McGregor CG, Baldwin JC, Ream AK, Wyner J, Zusman DR, Shumway NE (1985) First human use of an electrically powered implantable ventricular assist system. 5th Congress of the Int Soc Artif Organs, October 1985

# Discussion

*Mitamura* (Hokkaido University): I am very much interested in the rechargeable nickel-cadmium battery. Could you explain this in further detail in terms of capacity and size? Did you encounter any problems with this battery such as leakage of liquid or gas?

*Portner* (Novacor Medical Corporation): I should first stress that we have not used that part of the system in the clinical studies that I reported. The rechargeable batteries represent a weak area of technology in these systems. We began using miniature batteries of the SAFT AF type and found that even the so-called high-reliability batteries were in fact very unreliable. So we changed at the last minute to a sub-C battery, which increased the size of the package significantly. We reduced the number of cells from ten to eight, but the battery was still of a fairly substantial size. We hope to be able to find a better battery before we take this system to the clinical stage. We are expending most of our efforts at present on investigating high-energy/density lithium batteries rather than nickel-cadmium. We are currently using Sanyo sub-C batteries, which have proven to be extremely reliable. In the long term, they are simply not small enough.

*Taenaka* (National Cardiovascular Center): Do you think it is advisable to insert a device intracorporeally instead of paracorporeally from the point of prevention of infection even for a short period of time such as 1–2 weeks? Did you experience any problems in compressing the abdominal organs during the assist?

*Portner:* I believe it is fundamentally true that an implanted device, particularly a passive, i.e., nonpulsating, percutaneous conduit has less likelihood of infection than a paracorporeal device, which either relies on a pulsating blood conduit or a pulsating air drive line. There are not enough data to establish this statistically as a fact. However, we know that all patients who have had a Jarvik implant for any extended period of time have become infected. We have not observed any evidence of infection in our patients, though this is a very limited series.

A more appropriate answer to your question may be that the primary purpose in carrying out these studies is not to provide a therapeutic tool but to allow the initial clinical evaluation of a permanent system which can be further developed. This system can be used to investigate the kind of problems you raised in your second question, which addresses the potential compromise of visceral organs by the intracorporeal placement of the device. To date, we have not seen any evidence of compromise. In our very first patient, there was a perforation of the bowel which occurred roughly 2 weeks after explant. At the time of exploration, it was the conclusion of the surgeon that the perforation was not directly related to the device implant. This of course cannot be ruled out except by further experience. That initial patient had had diverticular disease, which may have been a contributing factor. We have implanted the device in patients who were smaller than this patient using a preperitoneal location, which potentially involves the greatest compromise of internal organs and we have not seen subsequent problems. In some of the larger patients, e.g., two patients at Stanford who were almost 90 kg, we implanted the device in a subcutaneous position. So, we are still in somewhat of an exploratory period. A primary goal is to provide the initial clinical evaluation of the permanent system. I would not like to make any strong recommendations as to which systems should be used for the bridge to transplant. As I said earlier, I happen to believe that the bridge to transplant will be a transient phenomenon, which will largely disappear once a permanent system becomes available, because the donor situation is not going to improve and the only way to relieve this problem is to provide a mechanical alternative. At some point, there will be a need for those involved in the transplant field to try and group the patients into those who should receive mechanical devices and those who should receive transplants.

# 11. Electromechanically driven, computer-controlled implantable cardiac assist device

Takao Nakamura[1], Kozaburo Hayashi[1], and Junji Seki[2]

**Summary.** An electromechanically driven cardiac assist device has been developed for long-term implantation inside the body. The system is composed of a pusher plate-type blood pump and an actuator with a DC brushless motor and ball screw. For the reliability of the system, a minimal number of sensors are incorporated. Sixteen-bit and eight-bit microprocessors are used for the pump operation and motor speed control, respectively. The motor is driven by a width-modulated, pulsed signal of the sinusoidal voltage wave having variable voltage and fixed duty ratio. An open-loop control method has been developed and its performance was tested in vitro. Although the system fulfilled the design specifications, the efficiency was rather low due to the open-loop control. To overcome this problem, we decided to use the back electromotive force of the motor as a feedback signal. The hardware and software have been redesigned and are being tuned.

**Key words:** Back electromotive force—Cardiac assist device—Microprocessor—Motor—Pusher plate-type blood pump

Pneumatically driven total artificial hearts and left ventricular assist devices have been developed successfully to the stage of clinical application. The current pneumatic systems, however, are not suitable for long-term use due to the lack of portability of the drive unit, the risk of infection, and so on. Totally implantable systems are being developed to overcome these problems. The final goal is to implant permanently all the components inside the body, including the blood pump, actuator, energy converter, energy source, and electronics package.

We have been developing an electric motor-driven, totally implantable left ventricular assist system operated by two microprocessors. The width-modulated, pulsed signal of the sinusoidal voltage wave is used to drive the motor with a variable voltage and fixed duty ratio operation. In this paper, we describe the outline of the system and show the in vitro performance test

data. In addition to the basic system, we are developing a novel control algorithm using the back electromotive force (EMF) signal of the motor as a feedback signal, aiming to improve the system efficiency and controllability. This new method is also presented here.

## Pusher plate-type blood pump

A pusher plate-type blood pump was used for this system because it is easily actuated by mechanical methods. The pump has the capability of rational control for physiological requirements by monitoring the position of the pusher plate with attached sensors.

We designed a pusher plate-type left ventricular assist pump based on mechanical analyses for the long-term reliability [1]. Figure 11.1 shows a cross section of the pump coupled with the electric motor-driven actuator described below. The stroke and net stroke volume of the pump are 15 mm and 60 ml, respectively. The pump housing is now made of an epoxy resin because of the ease of fabrication. The diaphragm, inflow and outflow cannulae of the pump are made of segmented polyether polyurethanes, and the pump inner surface is covered with the same material [2]. In vitro and in vivo experiments showed good pump performance without failure in the diaphragm [1].

To detect the position of the pusher plate, a magnet and a Hall effect sensor were attached to the pusher plate and pump back plate, respectively. No additional sensors are needed for the basic control of the system.

## Motor-driven actuator

To drive the pusher plate-type pump, we have designed an implantable electric motor-driven actuator consisting of a brushless DC motor and a ball screw [3, 4]. Figure 11.1 shows the cross section of the actuator attached to the pump. The motor utilized is of a brushless, three-phase, delta-wound, 14-pole type, having a maximum input power of 101 W. Such

[1]Section of Biomedical Controls, Research Institute of Applied Electricity, Hokkaido University, Kita 12, Nishi 6, Kita-ku, Sapporo, 060 Japan
[2]Department of Biomedical Engineering, National Cardiovascular Center Research Institute, 5-7-1 Fujishiro-dai, Suita, Osaka, 565 Japan

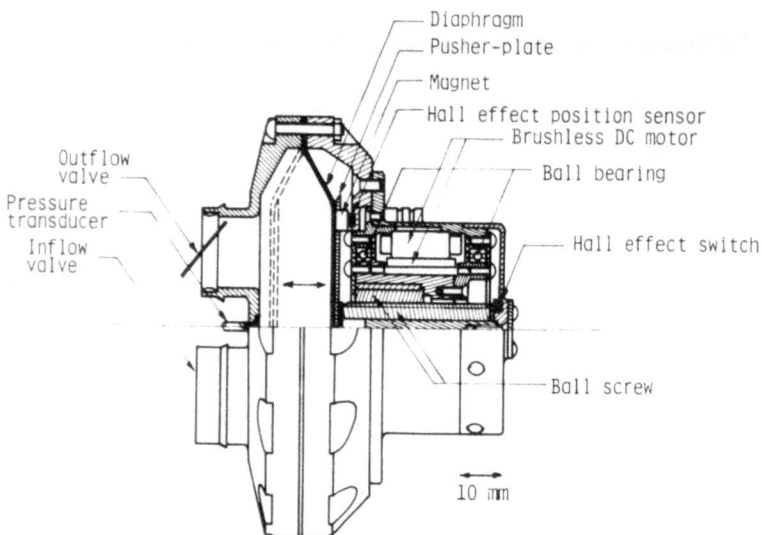

Diaphragm
Pusher-plate
Magnet
Hall effect position sensor
Brushless DC motor
Ball bearing

Outflow valve
Pressure transducer
Inflow valve

Hall effect switch

Ball screw

10 mm

**Fig. 11.1.** Cross section of the electric motor-driven, pusher-plate-type blood pump and actuator. After Hayashi et al. [1]

a high-power motor is used in present system in order to avoid excessive temperature elevation in the actuator. The motor is driven by width-modulated, pulsed signals of three sinusoidal waves with different phases. The ball screw used to transform the motor rotation into the axial linear motion consists of a screw shaft 12 mm in diameter, a threaded nut with a 4-mm lead, and small balls. Since the pusher plate is detached from the shaft end, the pusher plate moves together with the shaft in the pump systolic phase, and then the plate goes back by the pump preload during the diastolic phase. If one more pump is attached to the opposite end of the actuator, this device can be used as a total artificial heart.

The total weight of the actuator, mostly made of stainless steel, is around 480 g; it is about 50 mm in diameter and 30 mm in length. The weight of the pump and actuator assembly is around 620 g.

## Drive algorithm of motor

In the electromechanical systems developed by other groups [5, 6], the input voltage to the motor was controlled by changing the duty ratio of the width-modulated pulsed signal, with the voltage amplitude kept at a constant level. The pulse-width modulation (PWM) with the fixed voltage amplitude and variable duty ratio has a disadvantage in low-power operation: The signals with long intermittent periods between pulses cannot generate smooth motor torque. To avoid this drawback, we have proposed a new method: The input power to the motor is controlled by the PWM signal with fixed duty ratio and variable voltage amplitude [3, 4]. A digitally programmable switching regulator has been designed to change the voltage amplitude with high efficiency.

## Control-drive system

### Hardware

The block diagram of the control-drive system is shown in Fig. 11.2. This system is composed of three subsystems: pump controller, motor speed controller, and motor driver.

The 16-bit microprocessor (MC68000)-based, pump controller computes the speed and applied voltage to the motor from the stroke and other preset values, such as the end-diastolic and end-systolic positions of the pusher plate, and sends this information to the motor speed controller. The eight-bit microprocessor (Z80A)-based, motor speed controller receives this information and sends the rotational phase and voltage instructions to the motor driver. The phase is controlled by an interval timer with an interrupt operation. The motor driver generates PWM signals using a D-A converter and triangle-wave oscillator and switches the transistor-matrix circuit to apply the PWN voltage signals to the motor.

### Control algorithm

We have studied the performance of the actuator with a newly developed torque tester [7]. The maximum beat rate and pump afterload were assumed to be 120 bpm and 150 mmHg, respectively. Based on the experimental results and predetermined specifications, an open-loop control algorithm has been developed [8].

The relations between the motor condition (speed and voltage) and the pusher-plate position during pump systole, and between the motor condition and the elapsing time from the start of pump diastole were determined by preliminary experiments; they were

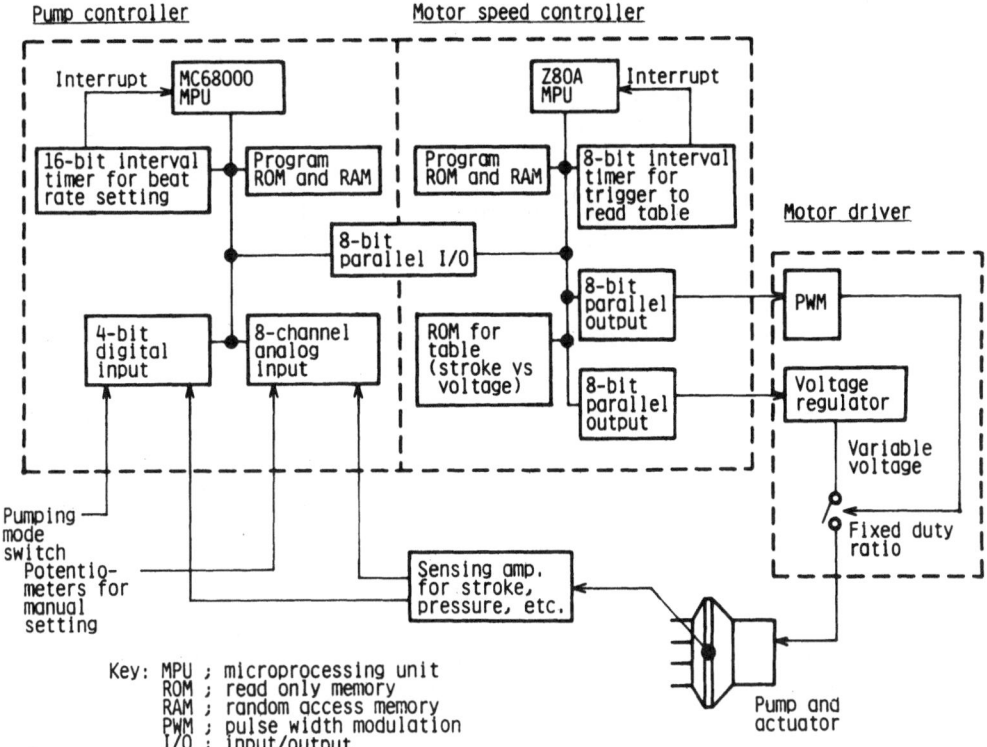

**Fig. 11.2.** Block diagram of the prototype control-drive system. After Hayashi et al. [1]

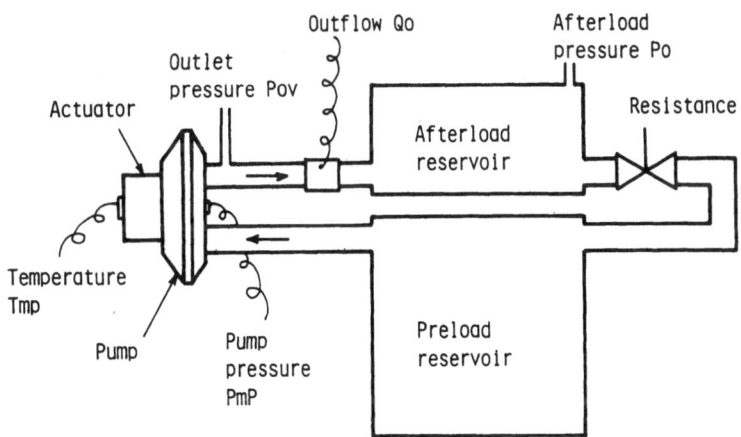

**Fig. 11.3.** Mock circulatory system used for in vitro performance test

stored in the read-only memory of the pump controller. In the pump systolic period, the speed and voltage of the motor are controlled in reference to these relations. In the pump diastole, the motor condition is changed every 2.5 ms because the load applied to the motor is constant as a result of the detachment of the pusher plate from the shaft of the ball screw.

The designed drive modes are: (a) electrocardiogram-synchronous mode; (b) constant rate mode; (c) constant stroke mode; and (d) manual (on-off) mode.

**In vitro performance**

The in vitro performance of the system was studied by a mock circulatory system, schematically shown in Fig. 11.3. The results are shown in Fig. 11.4. The pump-ventricular pressure was around 30 mmHg higher than the afterload pressure due to the pressure loss in the outflow valve (Bjork-Shiley, 21XAP). The pump output was around 6 l/min for the three-quarters full stroke. The decrease in the pump outflow with the increase in the preload may be attributable to the regurgitation through the inflow valve during the valve closure period in the early pump systole.

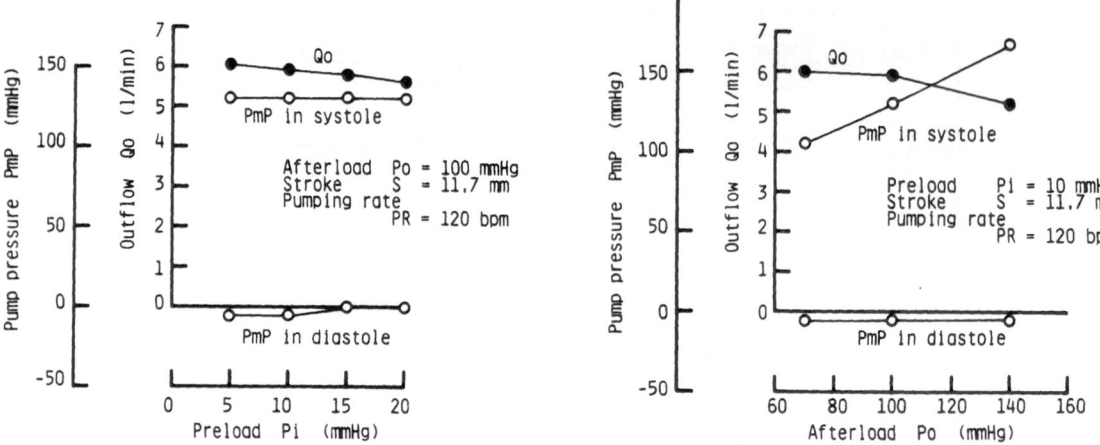

**Fig. 11.4.** In vitro performance of the electric motor-driven left ventricular assist device

Although the system showed the designed performance, the total system efficiency calculated between the motor input power to the fluid dynamic outflow work was fairly low (around 6%), indicating that the system could not be optimally operated by the open-loop control method. To improve the function of the system, a closed-loop control method has been newly developed, which is explained in the following section.

## Design of revised system

### Control method

To drive the motor in a more stable manner and to improve the efficiency and controllability of the system, the rotation of the motor or the load of the actuator has to be detected and utilized for the control. We are redesigning the prototype system mentioned above. In the new version, the input power to the motor is controlled with reference to the signal from the rotor position as a feedback. The rotor position is detected by the back EMF signal, which is generated by the rotor motion and produced in the motor windings. Although there are many methods to detect the rotor position, the back EMF signal is the most advantageous because no additional sensors are required for the operation. This method may be the most reliable.

The back EMF signal yields two types of information—the amplitude and the phase—given by the motor speed and rotor position, respectively. In our system, only the phase information is used to control the motor input power. The efficiency is highest when the rotational magnetic field on the motor windings is out of phase by 90° to that of the back EMF.

The control method with the back EMF signal has

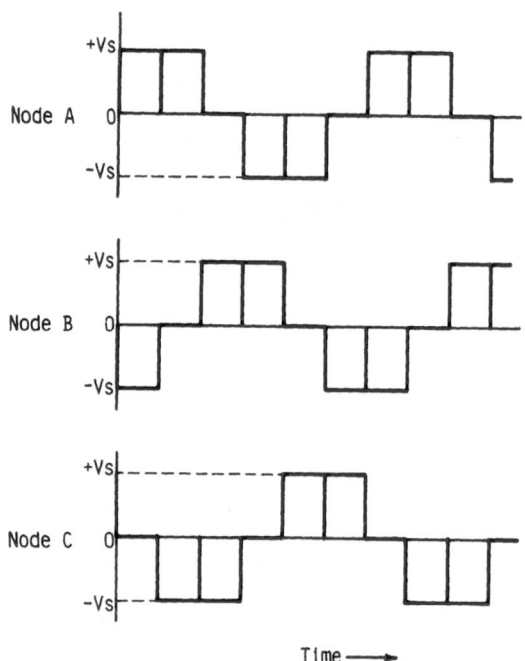

**Fig. 11.5** Waveforms applied to the nodes of the motor. *Vs* supply voltage

been reported by Chambers et al. [9] and Jarvik et al. [10]; they applied PWM to two-phase motors. Application of the back EMF signal to the three-phase, delta-wound motor does not seem to be possible because it is very difficult to combine three PWM signals which are out of phase 120° to each other. It does become possible, however, if we use the variable voltage-type PWM method developed in this study. Typical waveforms of the applied voltage to the three nodes of the motor are shown in Fig. 11.5. A combination of rectangular waveforms with a phasic duration of 60° is used for the current system.

**Fig. 11.6.** Block diagram of
eight-bit microprocessor-based
motor speed controller and motor
driver for the revised system

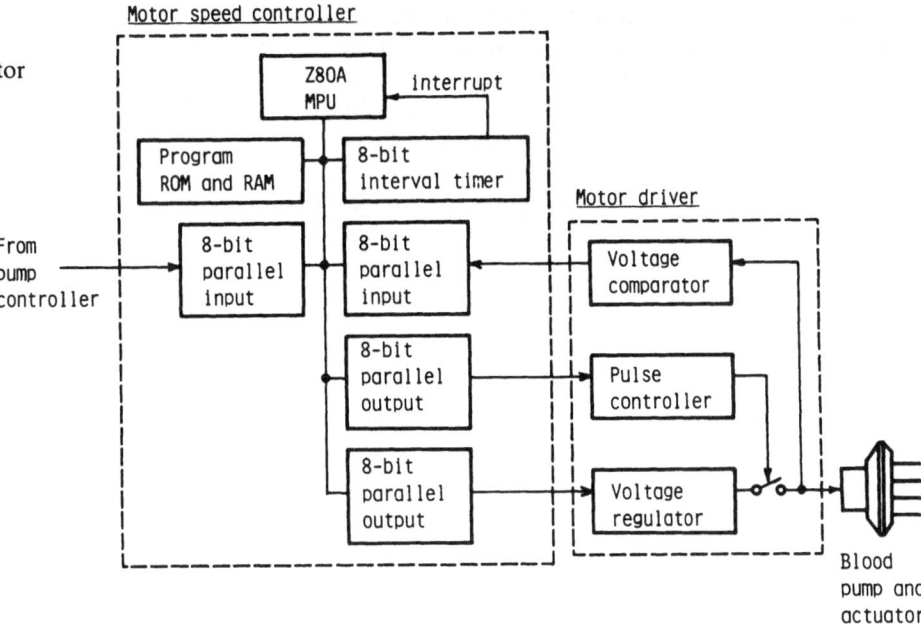

**Fig. 11.7a, b.** Flow chart of the
software for the motor speed controller in the revised system. **a**
Main and **b** interrupt routines.
*EMF* electromotive force

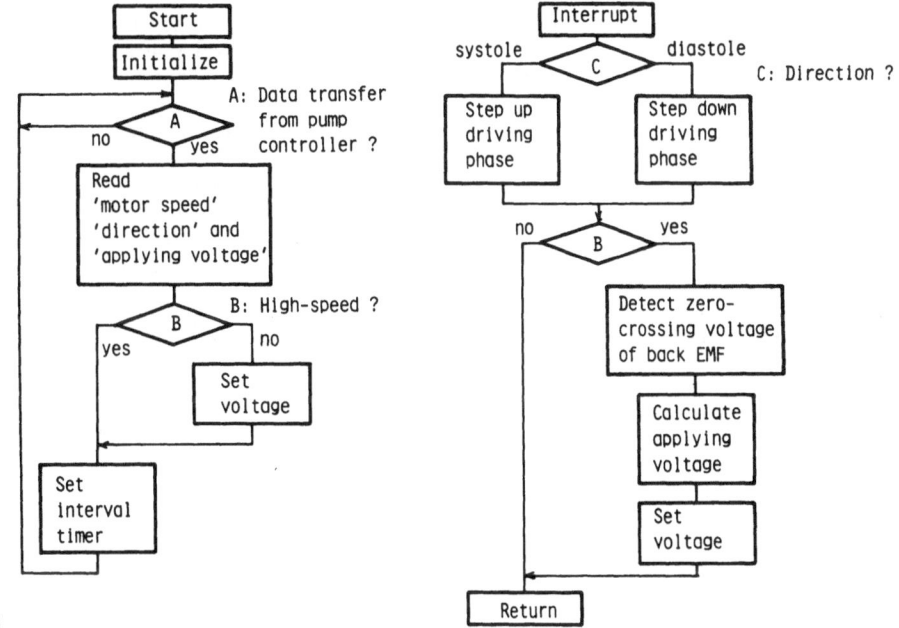

## Control drive system
## (hardware and control algorithm)

The control drive system developed previously [3, 4, 7] has been revised for the new algorithm. The motor speed controller and the motor driver have been changed (Fig. 11.6) to control the actuator according to the waveforms shown in Fig. 11.5. The phase of the back EMF is detected by a programmable digital timer and a newly incorporated voltage comparator. To monitor the phase, the timer in the motor speed controller is used. A parallel input port is added to the motor speed controller to obtain the phase informa-

tion of the back EMF signal acquired by the voltage comparator. Two parallel output ports are used to control the voltage amplitude and switch the power-transistor matrix.

The relations among supplied voltage, generated torque, and phase have been studied. The results show that they have excellent linearity, which means that the motor input power can be controlled linearly by the phase information. Based on these results, prototype software has been developed. The flowcharts of the motor speed controller are shown in Fig. 11.7.

The pump controller performs the same operations as in the previous system. The motor speed controller receives the information from the pump controller and decodes it to set the interval timer and control the voltage regulator. The timer interrupts the processor to change the rotational phase of the motor every 60° of the drive signal. Thus, the signal applied to the motor nodes is changed every 60° of the signal. Two of the three nodes are driven by the positive and negative voltages having the same amplitude, while the back EMF signal is detected from the remaining node.

Since the amplitude of the back EMF signal is small when the motor speed is low, the control method using the back EMF signal can be used when the motor speed is high. The open-loop control algorithm described previously is used to drive the motor when the speed is low.

The revised system is now being tested and tuned using the torque tester to improve the system stability and efficiency. After tuning the software, in vitro and in vivo tests will be carried out to study the system performance.

**Acknowledgments.** This work was supported financially in part by a Grant-in-Aid for Developmental Scientific Research from the Ministry of Education, Science and Culture, and by a Research Grant for Cardiovascular Disease (60-A) from the Minstry of Health and Welfare in Japan.

# References

1. Hayashi K, Nakamura T, Takano H, Umezu M, Taenaka Y, Matsuda T (1984) Design of pusher-plate-type left ventricular assist device based on mechanical analyses. Art Org 8: 204–214
2. Hayashi K, Matsuda T, Nakamura T, Umezu M, Takano H (1986) Mechanical and ESCA studies of segmented polyether polyurethanes with various molecular weights for blood pump application. In: Nose Y, Kjellstrand C, Invanovich P (eds) Progress in Artificial Organs—1985. ISAO Press, Cleveland, pp 989–993
3. Hayashi K, Seki J, Nakamura T, Fukumasu H (1986) Portable drive unit for artificial heart: Toward a totally implantable system. In: Akutsu T (ed) Artificial heart 1. Springer, Tokyo, pp 97–102
4. Nakamura T, Hayashi K, Seki J (1985) Computer-controlled, implantable cardiac assist device. Proceedings 38th Annual Conference on Engineering in Medicine and Biology, 30 Sept–2 Oct 1985, Chicago, p 319. Alliance for Engineering in Medicine and Biology, Washington DC
5. Rosenberg G, Snyder W, Weiss W, Landis DL, Geselowitz DB, Pierce WS (1982) A roller screw drive for implantable blood pumps. Trans Am Soc Art Int Org 28: 123–126
6. Mitamura Y, Okamoto E, Hirano A, Mikami T (1987) Development of motor driven assist pump systems. Proceedings 9th Annual Conference of IEEE Engineering in Medicine and Biology, 13–16 Nov 1987, Boston, pp 184–185. Institute of Electrical and Electronic Engineers, Piscataway
7. Nakamura T, Hayashi K, Seki J (1986) Microprocessor-controlled motor driven implantable cardiac assist device—Design of driving and control algorithm. Jpn J Art Org 15: 669–672 (in Japanese)
8. Nakamura T, Hayashi K, Seki J (1987) Motor-driven implantable cardiac assist device—Software development for drive and control. Jpn J Art Org 16: 175–178 (in Japanese)
9. Chambers JA, Davies LA, Mahler LM, Yen TT (1978) Development of an electrical energy converter for circulatory devices. NIH Contract/Grant Report NO1-HV-2906. National Technical Information Service, Springfield
10. Jarvik RK, Lioi AP, Isaacson MS, Orth J, Nielsen SD, Kessler TR, Olsen DB, Kolff WJ (1982) Development of reversing electro-hydraulic energy converter for left ventricular assist device. NIH Contract/Grant Report NO1-HN-72975. National Technical Information Service, Springfield

# 12. Development of nutating centrifugal blood pump

Teruaki Akamatsu, Tomohiro Shiroyama, and Hiroyuki Fukumasu[1]

**Summary.** Conventional centrifugal blood pumps have drawbacks: blood degeneration at hot spots in the bearing in closed magnetic coupling drive and infection and contamination through the shaft seal in direct motor drive. To overcome these problems, Baurmeister and Affeld proposed and developed a centrifugal pump with a nutating (non rotating) impeller, the so-called tea spoon pump. However, a great reduction in hydrolysis is necessary with this pump. Pump performance, therefore, had to be improved. This was done by the following: (a) annular flow passage surrounded with an inner guide wall and outer housing wall; (b) contoured inlet and outlet passage. These amendments serve to achieve rectified flow in the same manner as a piston (impeller) pushing blood in an endless cylinder (annular passage). Centrifugal force as a result of rotating blood flow sustains the pressure difference between the outlet and inlet.

Initially, we tried to make a simplified two-dimensional prototype and then proceeded with three-dimensional models. We experimentally examined the optimum size of the impeller and optimum contour of the housing. To adjust the pump characteristics according to flow rate, we also tried to adopt a flexible outlet diffuser with variable cross section. By means of hemolysis tests compared with results with the roller pump, pump performance is still undergoing improvement.

**Key words:** Centrifugal blood pump—Pump characteristics—Nutating motion—Fluid dynamic pump design

As centrifugal blood pumps are compact and easy to handle compared with pumps of a displacement type (air-driven diaphragm or sack-type artificial ventricle), various types of centrifugal pumps have been utilized as extracorporeal assist pumps. Conventional centrifugal blood pumps, the impeller shaft of which is directly connected to the motor shaft, has several drawbacks involving infection and contamination through the shaft seal. With the other type of blood pump, the impeller of which is magnetically coupled with the rotating shaft of the motor, the seal problem can be avoided, but there is the shortcoming of blood degeneration due to overheating and shear stress at the shaft bearing.

To overcome this problem, Baurmeister and Affeld proposed and developed a nutating centrifugal pump (tea spoon pump). Here, an axisymmetric impeller is set on the end of the nutating rod. The flexible membrane is attached to the rod at the nutation center, allowing the rod to nutate, not rotate, and separating the inside of the pump from the outside.

Though conventional centrifugal pumps have many impellers, this tea spoon pump, owing to its nutating motion, is unable to have more than one impeller with an axisymmetric shape; it is thus poor in pump pressure and efficiency. To improve the pump performance, the authors developed a nutating cetrifugal pump with a core portion.

The present paper deals with our recently developed nutating centrifugal pumps and the two-dimensional prototypes.

## Structures of nutating centrifugal pumps

The authors developed a structure with the core portion installed as shown in Fig. 12.1. This creates an annular passage, which has the same effect as the many impellers of the conventional pump. Inside the core, a streamlined inlet port is made. Across the annular passage, an outlet port and adjacent diffuser of well contour is set up. The impeller and annular passage resembles a set of piston cylinders without inlet and outlet valves. Centrifugal force due to fluid rotation supports the pressure difference between the outlet and inlet. A vent hole bored in the core portion serves to wash out the blood near the membrane.

Our recently developed pumps are shown in Fig. 12.2. Large roller bearings support a rotating disc, in which small roller bearings hold the nutating rod. The flexible membrane is attached to the rod at the center of nutating motion and its flexibility allows the rod to nutate without rotation. A motor shaft is set in a hole at the right end of the rotating disc.

The annular passage is 40 mm in outer diameter, and 20–27 mm in inner diameter according to the size

[1] Department of Mechanical Engineering, Kyoto University, Yoshida Honmachi, Sakyo-ku, Kyoto, 606 Japan

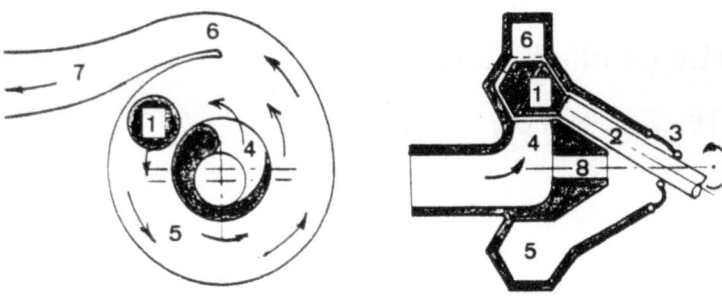

**Fig. 12.1.** Nutating centrifugal pump with core portion. *1* impeller, *2* nutating rod, *3* membrane, *4* inlet, *5* annular passage, *6* outlet, *7* diffuser, *8* vent hole

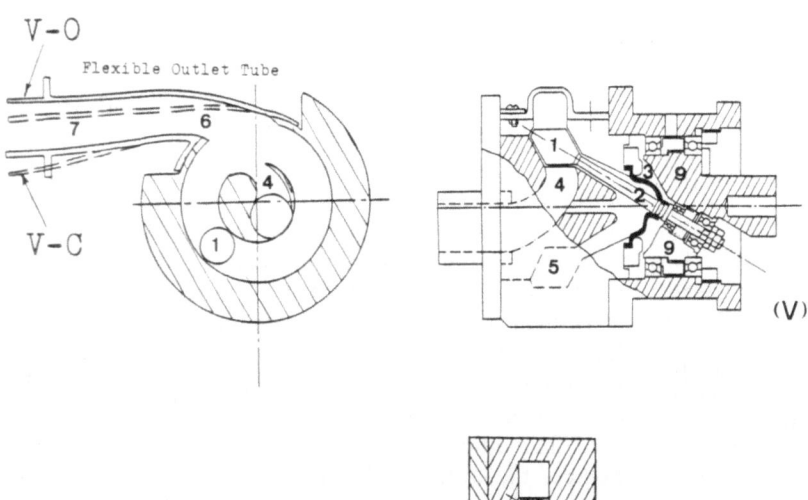

**Fig. 12.2.** Recently developed nutating centrifugal pumps models *II*, *IV*, *Vo* with flexible outlet tube, and *Vc* with the tube clamped. *Numbers* as in Fig. 1. *9* rotating disc

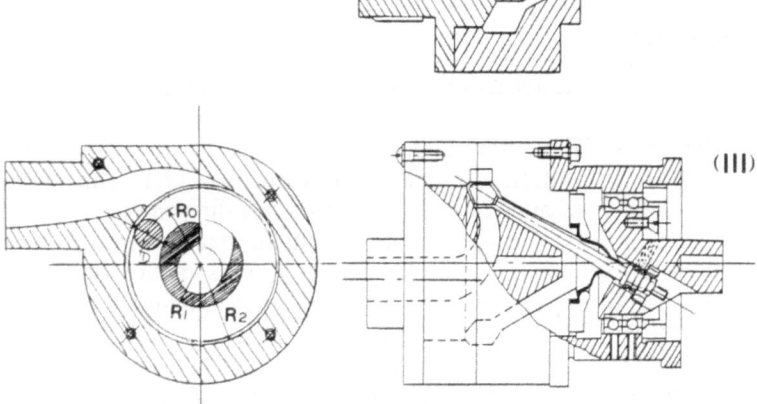

of the impeller. The rod, made of titanium, tilts 30° against the pump axis, and the impeller, made of plastic, is of a combined truncated-conical shape. Figure 12.2 presents three kinds of recently developed models—II, IV, and V—that differ in the shape and size of the impeller. The pump housings are made of acrylic resin or polycarbonate.

Generally, the profile of the outlet diffuser greatly affects the pump characteristics and the conversion efficiency of dynamic pressure to static pressure. To examine whether the pump characteristics alter with the flow rate by adjusting the profile of the outlet diffuser tube, we made the tube of flexible silicone rubber in model V. By clamping with contoured plates, the profile of the outlet tube was modified from the original shape shown by the solid lines in Fig. 12.2 (V) to that shown by the dotted lines.

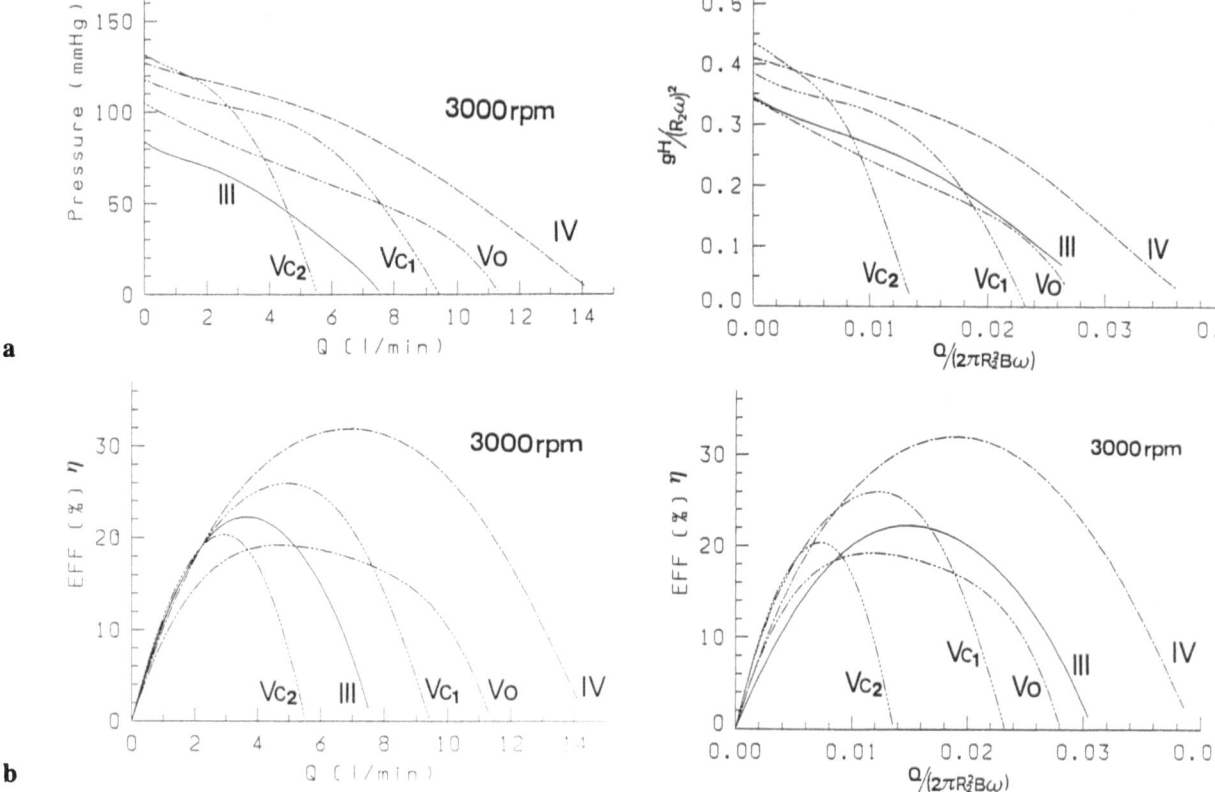

**Fig. 12.3a, b.** Relations of **a** pressure versus flow rate and **b** efficiency versus flow rate at 3000 rpm compared in models II, IV, and V

**Fig. 12.4a, b.** Nondimensional relations of **a** pressure versus flow rate and **b** efficiency versus flow rate

## Experiments and results

A torque meter was set between the pump and motor. The pressure and flow rate were measured at the inlet and outlet. The flow patterns in the outlet diffuser were occasionally visualized by a tracer method. The working fluid used was water except in the hemolysis test. The relations of pressure versus flow rate and pump efficiency versus flow rate at the impeller rotational speed of 3000 rpm are shown in Fig. 12.3 and compared in models II, IV, and Vo, with no clamp, and $Vc_1$ and $Vc_2$, with a slight and deep clamp (the flow passage in $Vc_2$ is narrower than that in $Vc_1$).

Model II has the lowest observed pressure and is rather low in pump efficiency. Model IV is the highest in both pressure and efficiency. In model V, with the flexible outlet tube, the pump characteristics show a sensitive shift according to modifications in the outlet tube profile, but the efficiency is not as high as expected in spite of the large impeller. (A half year later, this low efficiency was observed to have been caused mainly by the inadequate profile of the inlet port.) Better adjustment of the profile of the outlet tube is necessary.

Fig. 12.4 shows nondimensional expressions of the relations of pressure versus flow rate and efficiency versus flow rate. The abscissa is nondimensional flow rate, which is the average radial flow velocity $Q/2\pi R_2B$ divided by the peripheral velocity of the impeller $R_2\omega$ at the outlet radius $R_2$. The ordinate in Fig. 12.4 is nondimensional pressure, which is pressure head gH divided by the square of peripheral velocity $(R_2\omega)^2$. On the nondimensional graphs, each measured value for different rotational speeds of the impeller approximately coincides with a single curve: where H is pressure head, Q flow rate, $R_2$ outer radius of pump room, $R_0$ center radius of annular passage, A cross-sectional area of annular passage, B outlet port width, $\omega$ angular velocity, g gravity acceleration, and $\eta$ pump efficiency.

Figure 12.5 shows alternative expressions for the relations of pressure versus flow rate and efficiency versus flow rate. The abscissae are the nondimensional flow rate Q divided by the displacement stroke volume by impeller $AR_0\omega$. Their reciprocals indicate the number of rotations of fluid in the annular passage. The ordinates in Fig. 12.5 are the same as in Fig. 12.4. Models II, IV, and V pump the fluid at the highest efficiency after about three, four, and seven turns in the annular passage, respectively. A small number of turns is desirable to reduce the dwell time in high shear stress.

Preliminary hemolysis tests indicate that this centrifugal pump is twice higher than the roller pump. In any event, it is important to improve the pump in terms of efficiency and pressure. The higher the efficiency, the lower the required rotational speed of the impeller and the greater the reduction in hemolysis.

Of course, operation of the physiological pulsatile flow mode is possible by low inertia of the impeller and motor by controlling the rotational speed of the latter.

## Two dimensional prototype of centrifugal pump

Before we designed the present nutating centrifugal pumps, we tested two-dimensional models, as shown in Fig. 12.6, which simply simulated the rotational motion of the axisymmetric impeller. Cylindrical impellers were set on a rotating disc. In this case, the impeller did not nutate, but the flow outside the thin boundary layer on the disc and the impeller was similar to that induced by nutating motion. We initially chose two-dimensional structures because they are easy to make and modify.

Various kinds of pump casings (Fig. 12.7) were tested: circular type (C), spiral type (S), double spiral type (DS), endless simple piston-cylinder type (PC), and piston-cylinder with tangential outlet type (T-PC). The latter T-PC type is an improvement on the outlet profile of the PC-type, where flow separation was observed in the outlet. Cylindrical impellers of 15 and 22 mm in diameter and a tilting truncated-conical impeller (ST type in Fig. 12.7) were also tested.

The nondimensional relations of pressure versus flow rate and efficiency versus flow rate are shown in Fig. 12.8 for types S, C, PC, and T-PC. From experiments with the two-dimensional models, we judged the T-PC type to be the best. Peripheral positioning of the inlet port relative to the outlet port as in the T-PC type (Fig. 12.7) proved to have minimum fluctuations of inlet suction pressure and the highest desirable pressure head. We decided to develop this T-PC type as a nutating centrifugal pump and aimed to extend the pump operation region at the highest pressure.

## Discussion

Pressure in displacement-type artificial heart pumps (roller pump and air-driven ventricle type) is pro-

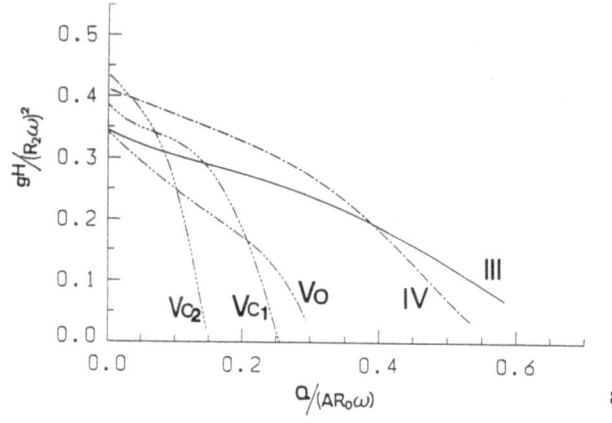

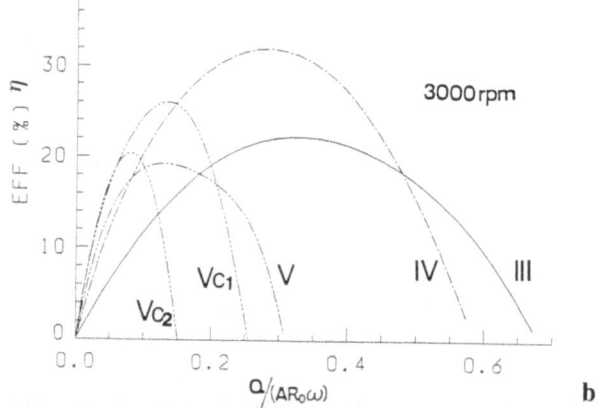

**Fig. 12.5a, b.** Alternative nondimensional relations of **a** pressure versus flow rate and **b** efficiency versus flow rate

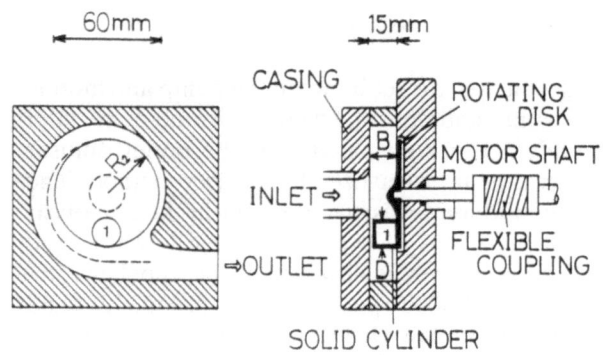

**Fig. 12.6.** Two-dimensional prototypes for nutating centrifugal pump. *1* impeller

duced by the simple displacement motion of the vessel wall, whereas pressure in centrifugal pumps is generated from kinetic energy of the rotating fluid. In our pump, after the fluid pushed by the impeller rotates several times in the annular passage, it flows away through the outlet diffuser. This is one of the main differences between this pump and conventional centrifugal pumps. The fluid dynamic design principle for the conventional centrifugal pump has been virtually

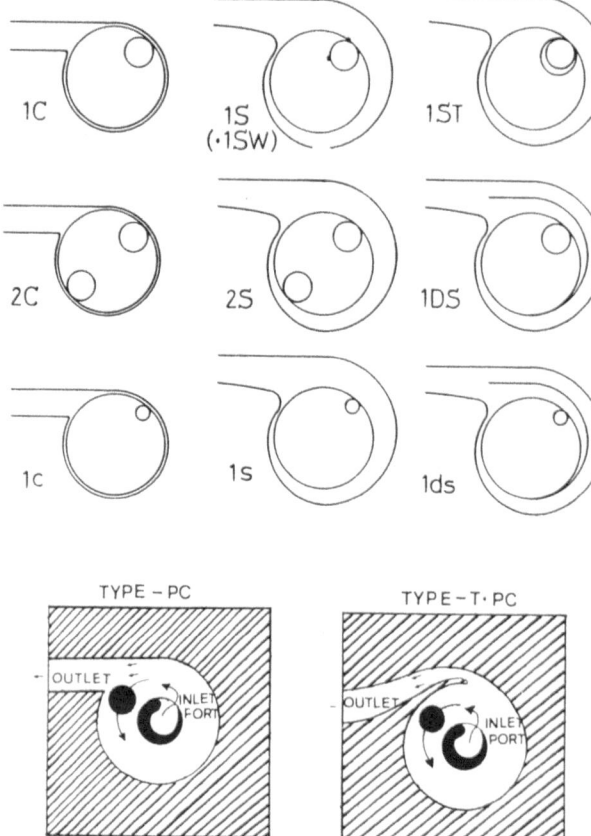

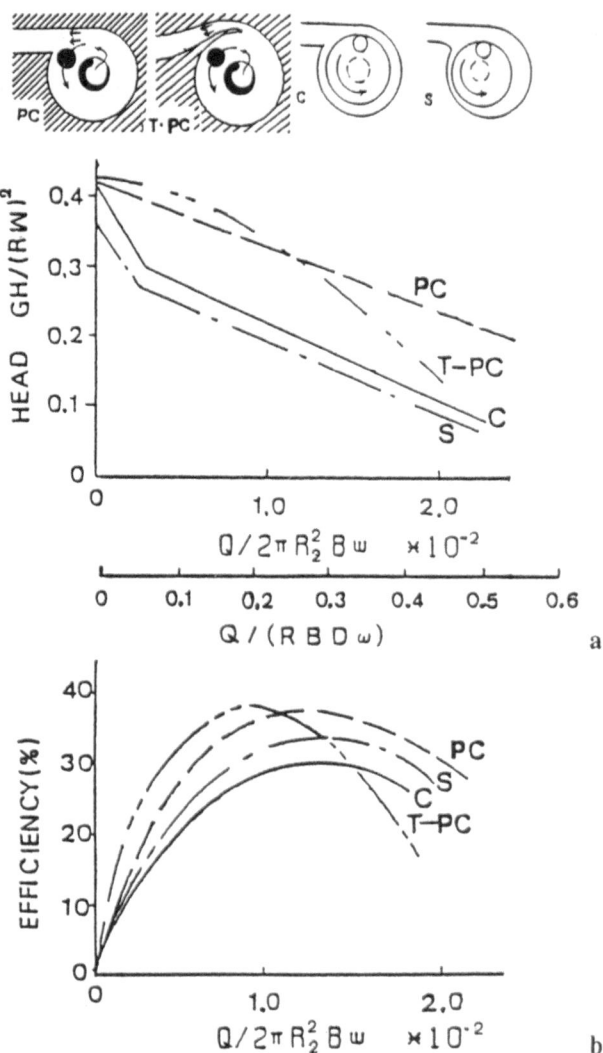

**Fig. 12.7.** Various kinds of pump casings of two-dimensional prototypes for nutating centrifugal pumps. *1* a single cylinder (one impeller), *2* double cylinders (two impellers), *T* truncated cone, *W* cylinder with trapping wires, *C* circular casing, *S* spiral casing, *DS, ds* double spiral, *PC* simple piston-cylinder type, *T-PC* piston cylinder type with tangential outlet

**Fig. 12.8a, b.** Nondimensional relations of **a** pressure versus flow rate and **b** efficiency versus flow rate compared in types T-PC, PC, C, and S

established, but with this nutating centrifugal pump there are new problems to be solved: fluid dynamic problems in the inlet, annular passage, outlet, and diffuser; the mixing process of fluids just entering the system with those already rotating; wall friction in the annular passage; shear stress in the narrow clearance between the impeller and annular wall (relevant to hemolysis); energy loss in the outlet and diffuser; and the effect of the vent hole on washing out the blood. Optimum size of the impeller and annular passage and optimum profile of the outlet tube will have to be determined in order to improve the pump performance. Moreover, there are other problems to be solved—fabrication and blood-compatible materials.

## Conclusion

Our experience in developing a nutating centrifugal pump has been described briefly from the two-dimensional prototype to the recently developed three-dimensional types. This pump was first investigated by Affeld's group at the Free University of Berlin, West Germany and by Wildevuur's group at the University of Groningen, Netherlands. The problem still remains of elucidating the flow inside the pump and improving the performance.

**Acknowledgments.** The authors wish to express their thanks to present and former students M. Matsushita, S. Murata, F. Beppu, N. Yamada, and A. Okabayashi for their assistance in these experiments over the past 5 years. The authors greatly acknowledge also the financial support of a Grant-in-Aid for Developmental Scientific Research of the Japanese Educational Ministry (62850034, 1987).

## References

1. Baurmeister U, Affeld K, Berger E (1982) The "tea spoon pump" a new centrifugal blood pump. ASAIO Abstracts vol 11-1
2. Affeld K, Baurmeister U, Berger E, Frank J (1981) Entwicklungsarbeiten und Blutkreise Pumpen. Freie Universität Berlin, Arbeits- und Ergebnisbericht, pp 17–57
3. Matsushita M, Akamatsu T, Murata S, Shiroyama T, (1983) Basic investigation of the flow in a nutating centrifugal blood pump. Preprints of the conference of Japanese Society of Mechanical Engineers 830–837, pp 37–39 (in Japanese)
4. Shiroyama T, Akamatsu T, Fukumasu H (1986) Improvement of tea spoon pump characteristics. Jpn J Art Org 15-2: 482–485 (in Japanese)
5. Akamatsu T, Shiroyama T, Matsushita M (1987) Studies on a nutating centrifugal blood pump, Jpn J Turbomachin 15-2, 73–78 (in Japanese)

# Discussion

*Portner* (Novacor Medical Corporation): Have you examined the flow in regions other than the impeller itself? Are you concerned about the possibility of stasis in the connecting rod area or is just the motion around enough to insure adequate washing in that region?

*Akamatsu* (Kyoto University): We are checking that at present. The plastic is transparent and by using fluids with the same refractive index we are able to examine the washing. We expect results soon on this.

*Portner:* I assume you have not done any animal experimentation yet.

*Akamatsu:* Not yet.

# 13. Technical considerations in the development of clinical systems for temporary and permanent cardiac support

David M. Lederman[1]

**Summary.** Fundamental distinctions exist between systems designed for temporary (<15 days) and long-term (>2 years) ventricular support. These are illustrated with a description of two ABIOMED systems: an extracorporeal system ("the BVS") designed for short-term in-hospital use and an implantable system ("the VAS") designed for long-term ambulatory use. In the last decade, temporary support to either or both ventricles has moved from the research laboratory to the clinical arena. During this same period, devices designed for permanent assist or total replacement have entered an intensive reliability testing phase with some limited clinical trials. Temporary systems are indicated for postcardiotomy ventricular dysfunction, post-MI cardiogenic shock, and as a bridge to cardiac transplantation. Indications for permanent support are essentially identical to those for cardiac transplantation, namely: end-stage cardiomyopathies of ischemic, viral, or unknown etiology. The BVS system, currently undergoing clinical trials, was developed for in-hospital temporary use following technical considerations designed to expand clinical applicability of cardiac support beyond research and teaching hospitals. The VAS system, currently undergoing reliability tests, was developed following technical criteria designed to minimize the risks of thromboembolism, infection, and other potential complications in permanently implanted ambulatory recipients.

**Key words:** Temporary ventricular support—Permanent ventricular support—BVS System 5000—ABIOMED VAS

During the past 5 years, clinical trials have been increasingly conducted with a variety of cardiac support systems [1–5]. Many of these devices were originally designed for long-term outpatient cardiac support but have been predominantly used, to date, for temporary inpatient support. These trials have included patients with postcardiotomy ventricular dysfunction, in postinfarction cardiogenic shock, and in patients for whom cardiac assist served as a bridge to transplantation either by intent or as a medical consequence.

Excluding the bridge-to-transplantation patients, results from clinical trials in the USA indicate that approximately half of the patients can be weaned from mechanical support and 60% of those are subsequently discharged from the hospital [6]. These are very positive results, especially since these devices have been generally used only after balloon counterpulsation and conventional medical measures have failed and where the prognosis, without mechanical assist, was death. The typical time on assist for these patients, whether weaned or not, has averaged $3\frac{1}{2}$ days, with the majority receiving cardiac support for less than 1 week [6]. These times are consistent with experimental data on myocardial cellular recovery from ischemia [1, 5, 7]. The results indicate that for certain patient categories, temporary cardiac support (typically less than 1 week) can be a life-saving modality.

A separate and small number of clinical trials have been conducted, since late 1982, using air-driven, tethered, artificial hearts implanted in patients with cardiomyopathies and for whom permanent mechanical circulatory support was the intent. These trials have highlighted the fact that design options are significantly more limited for permanent cardiac support systems than for those intended for short-term use. For example, in permanent systems, a considerable number of components, and perhaps the entire system, is implanted to reduce long-term infection risks. In contrast, devices intended for temporary support are ideally completely extracorporeal except for the cannulae. Technical considerations related to intracorporeal systems intended for lifetime support of the recipient include size, anatomical fit, power source and transmission, long-term reliability, and the risks of infection, thromboembolic phenomena and calcification.

Since the technical issues facing development of clinical cardiac support systems are so strongly dependent on the intended duration of assist, they are best illustrated by describing the key features and developmental status of two systems developed at ABIOMED, Inc.—one intended for temporary ventricular support (the "BVS") and one intended for permanent ventricular support (the "VAS").

[1]ABIOMED, Inc., 33 Cherry Hill Drive, Danvers, MA 01923, USA

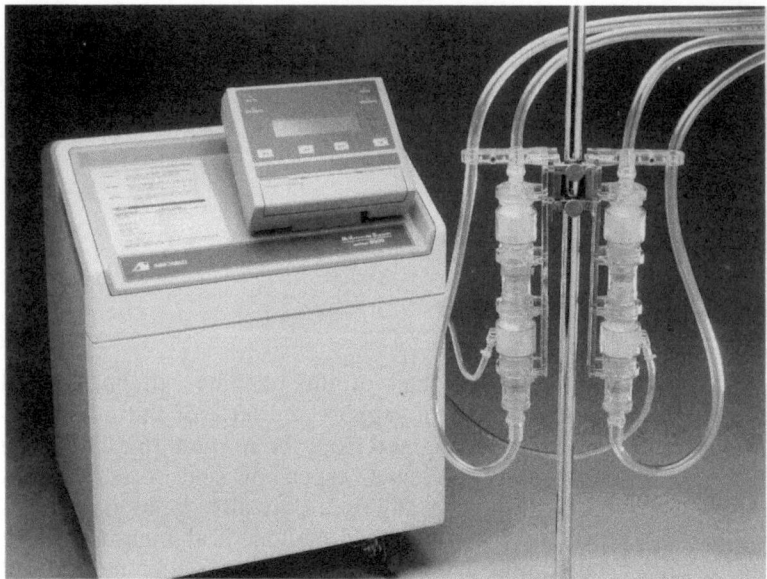

**Fig. 13.1.** BVS System 5000 console can operate two blood pumps for biventricular assist with minimal operator involvement (107 cm high, 91 kg weight)

## Temporary cardiac support—The BVS™

A new system, the BVS System 5000, has been recently introduced to clinical trials specifically for short-term use. The BVS has been under development and experimental evaluation for more than four years [8–10]. The focus was to develop a clinically oriented device as opposed to a research-oriented system. The main technical considerations were to develop an extracorporeal, pulsatile assist system that is atraumatic and safe, simple to use, and whose cost and complexity do not limit its clinical applicability to research and teaching hospitals.

### Materials

The BVS System 5000 consists of an automated electromechanical console that controls and provides pneumatic power to either one or two single-use disposable blood pumps (Fig. 13.1). The drive console is a microprocessor-controlled pneumatic drive system that operates one or two blood pumps. Beat rates and systolic/diastolic intervals are determined automatically by sensing gas flow to and from the blood pumps. The pumps are run in essentially a "fill-to-empty" mode. Beyond a common source of compressed air, the console drives and adjusts the left and right blood pumps completely independently of each other.

Normal use involves little operator involvement to reduce operator training and the chance of errors during assist. Once the pump is properly primed and connected, the console requires only that the console be turned on to provide maximum assist. Except for "on" and "off" buttons, the only other control is for

weaning and allows lowering the level of assist by dialing the desired pump flow. The system continuously displays pump beat rate and flow.

To maximize safety, the console provides several levels of redundancy. Batteries provide approximately 1 h of operation for emergency and patient transport conditions. Audible and visible alarms are automatically activated in the event of device malfunction or abnormal pressure or flow conditions. The microprocessor is backed by a hard-wired system that can automatically continue pumping at a fixed rate. Complete electrical or mechanical failure is backed by a foot-operated mechanical pump that allows continued support.

The disposable blood pump (Fig. 13.2) is a pneumatically driven device designed to support either side of the heart. It is placed externally to the patient with blood inflow to the pump from the left or right atrium and return flow to the aorta or pulmonary artery, respectively. Like the natural heart, the blood pump consists of two chambers. An inflow chamber (artificial atrium) acts as a compliant reservoir and empties into a pumping chamber (artificial ventricle), which is situated between two ABIOMED-developed trileaflet valves, whose cost is a very small fraction of that of current clinical prosthetic valves. Each of the two chambers consists of an elastomeric bladder which, like the valves, are entirely made from smooth-surfaced Angioflex polyurethane. This configuration effectively isolates the natural atrium from the pumping chamber.

To avoid atrial collapse, or suction of air, the inflow chamber fills continuously from the natural atrium by gravity alone. No vacuum can be generated by the console so that negative pressures can never be exerted on the blood pump. The pumping chamber is collapsed by a pulse of positive pressure from the console ejecting whatever comes into it and effectively acting as a bypass to the natural ventricle. The air line is the only connection between the drive console and the blood circuit. All necessary information to run and control the device is obtained through the air line [10].

The disposable blood pump is mounted on an I.V. pole and is connected to the heart via medical-grade tubing connected to inflow and outflow cannulae by means of blood-handling connectors designed specifically for the BVS. These connectors are critical safety components of the blood pump circuit and were designed to minimize risks at junctions between soft tubing and cannulae, which are sites where thromboembolic complications tend to occur.

The inflow and outflow cannulae are made from wire-reinforced medical-grade PVC and the exterior surfaces incorporate a dacron velour sleeve at the skin interface. The atrial cannula incorporates a lighthouse tip. The return cannula consists of a low-porosity graft for end-to-side anastomosis to either the aorta or pulmonary artery.

## Methods

In vitro characterization studies were conducted using a mock loop. This mock loop allowed independent variation of arterial and venous compliances and impedances. Reliability tests were conducted using 0.9% NaCl solutions at an average temperature of 37°C. Seven consoles and 14 blood pumps were put on test with each console running a pair, one blood pump operated under simulated left ventricular conditions (12 mmHg filling pressure, 97 mmHg outflow pressure) and one under simulated right ventricular conditions (12 mmHg filling, 35 mmHg outflow pressure). Systems were run for approximately 50% of the time under the normal operating mode and under the weaning mode (flow reduced to 65%–70% of normal) for the remainder of the test duration. In addition, a battery test of 30-min duration was performed twice a week.

Following 21 developmental animal experiments, a series of eight consecutive 28-day-duration calf experiments were conducted to evaluate system efficacy and safety prior to clinical application. The animals were initially anticoagulated with heparin IV to maintain activated clotting times (ACT) at approximately twice the normal level. The chronic anticoagulation regimen was started on the 1st operative day with weaning from heparin after 3–4 days and subsequent anticoagulation with coumadin, persantine, and aspirin to maintain prothrombin times at approximately twice normal.

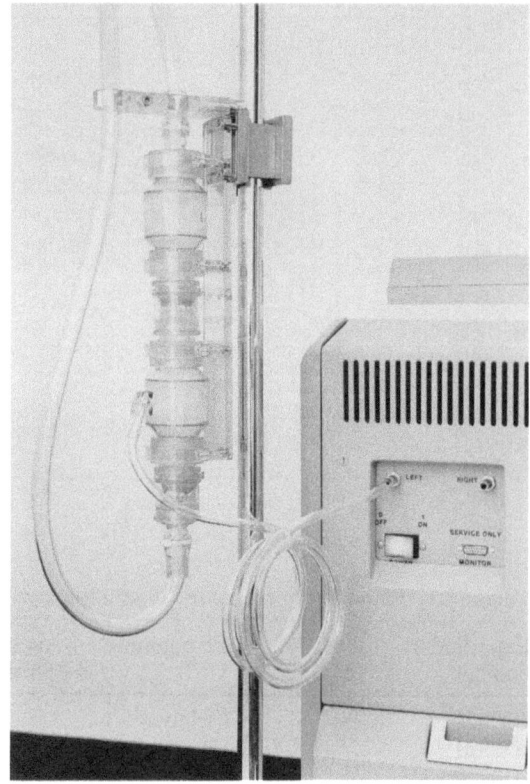

**Fig. 13.2.** Disposable blood pump incorporates an artificial atrium and can be mounted on an IV pole. Inflow from the heart is at the top, and blood return tubing is at the bottom. Connection to the console is by a single pneumatic tube

Serial measurements involved pump flow, hematology, coagulation, biochemistry, and chemistry. Explants were performed under sterile conditions with complete autopsies. Explanted blood pumps and cannulae were carefully rinsed, photographed, and samples subjected to scanning electron-microscope (SEM) examination.

## Results

The pump response to filling pressure, at different systemic pressures, is shown in Fig 13.3. Up to approximately 15 mmHg filling pressure, the system flow is linearly proportional to this pressure and independent of the systemic pressure. Flows of 4.5–5.0 l/min can be obtained for mean arterial pressures of 90 mmHg and filling pressures of less than 15 mmHg. The pump alone can maintain flows in excess of 6 l/min. The pump dp/dt ranged from 1000 to 1200 mmHg/s and the control was stable to transient increases and decreases of filling and outflow pressures. Responses to filling pressure changes were virtually instantaneous because of the ability of the pump inflow compliance chamber to smooth transients.

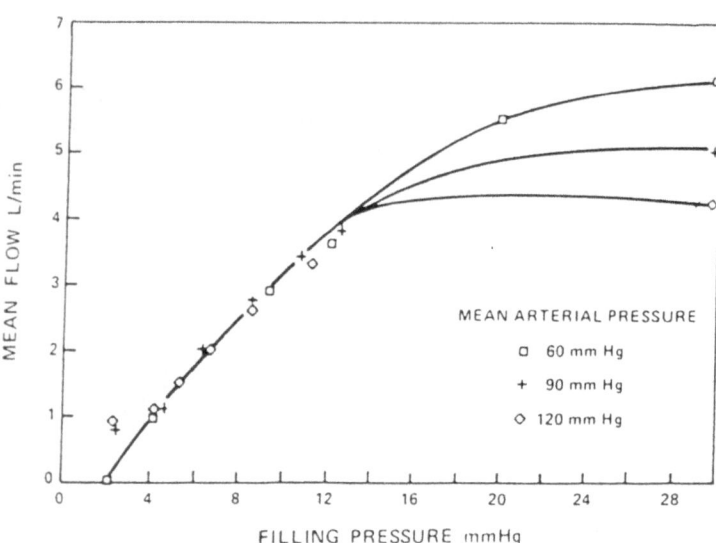

**Fig. 13.3.** Mean flows as a function of filling pressure at mean arterial pressures of 60, 90, and 120 mmHg. There is no vacuum used and pump inflow valve is at the same level as the tip of the atrial cannula

**Table 13.1.** Summary of six consecutive calf experiments

| Experiment number | Duration (days) | Termination | Average flow (l/min) | Platelet count ($10^3/\mu l$) | Urea nitrogen (mg/dl) | Plasma hemoglobin (mg/dl) |
|---|---|---|---|---|---|---|
| BVS-20 | 28 | Elective | 3.7 ± .2 | 680 ± 260 | 6.0 ± 1.5 | 1.1 ± 1.2 |
| BVS-21 | 28 | Elective | 3.7 ± .3 | 990 ± 530 | 5.5 ± 2.6 | 1.1 ± 1.2 |
| BVS-22 | 28 | Elective | 3.7 ± .2 | 774 ± 230 | 10.8 ± 3.7 | 3.7 ± 1.9 |
| BVS-23 | 28 | Elective | 3.7 ± .2 | 465 ± 100 | 8.4 ± 2.4 | 1.1 ± 0.9 |
| BVS-24 | 28 | Elective | 3.7 ± .3 | 580 ± 210 | 5.8 ± 2.2 | 1.0 ± 0.8 |
| BVS-25 | 28 | Elective | 3.7 ± .2 | 705 ± 320 | 11.0 ± 6.7 | 1.4 ± 1.2 |
| Abiomed controls | — | — | — | 651 ± 129 | 10.0 ± 3.0 | 2.0 ± 1.4 |

There were no blood pump failures of any kind in the reliability tests. Ten pumps were stopped after 28 days of continuous pumping. The remaining four pumps were left on test and have exceeded 8 months of failure-free operation. Characterization of the ten pumps showed no change or impairment of pump performance. The accumulated run time of approximately 24 000 h without failure projects a high level of reliability for the typical clinical application of less than 2 weeks (336 h).

All six animal experiments ran for exactly 28 days with no early terminations for any cause. The blood pumps performed uneventfully with no mechanical damage or malfunctions. Chronic anticoagulation maintained ACT between 1.5 and 2.0 times the normal level.

Selected data are summarized in Table 13.1. Control values were obtained from 21 preimplant animals. No significant changes in the average number of platelets, urea nitrogen, and plasma hemoglobin level were observed. No animal received a blood transfusion. Platelet counts (Fig. 13.4) showed no evidence of consumption. Urea nitrogen (Fig. 13.5) and plasma hemoglobin levels (Fig. 13.6) were unchanged from control values during the entire implant duration. Fibrinogen levels (Fig. 13.7) were elevated during the 1st postoperative week and gradually returned toward baseline values. Levels of albumin, creatinine, total bilirubin, lactate dehydrogenase (LDH), serum glutamic-oxaloacetic transaminase (SGOT), and white cell counts were unchanged from control.

Pump flows remained remarkably constant and were maintained by the system without the need of any operator involvement. The condition of the animals was unremarkable with no clinical evidence of cerebral or renal emboli. In one of the six experiments, the cannula connector restraints were physically dislodged by the animal and resulted in localized thrombotic deposits within the pump, but there was no clinical evidence of any organ dysfunction. The remaining five pumps underwent uneventful experimental procedures and were generally clean (Figs. 13.8–10). All cannula lumina were patent and free of thrombus. Connectors between the tubing and the

**Fig. 13.4.** Serial measurements of platelet counts for the six experiments

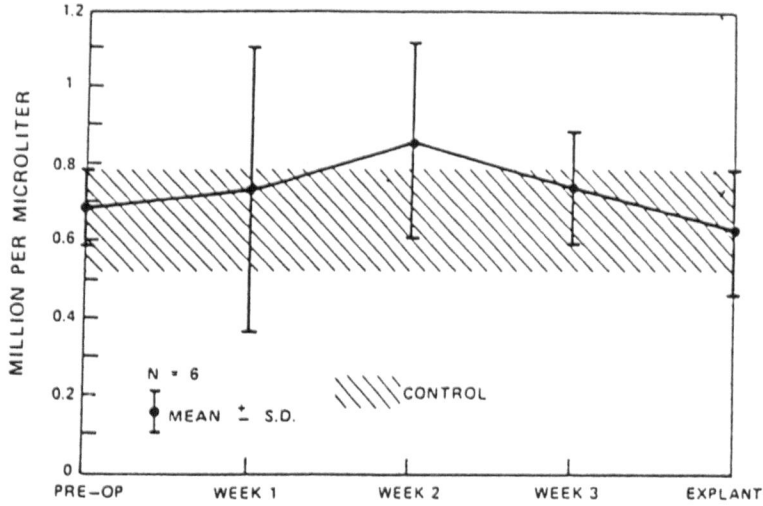

**Fig. 13.5.** Serial measurements of urea nitrogen for the six experiments

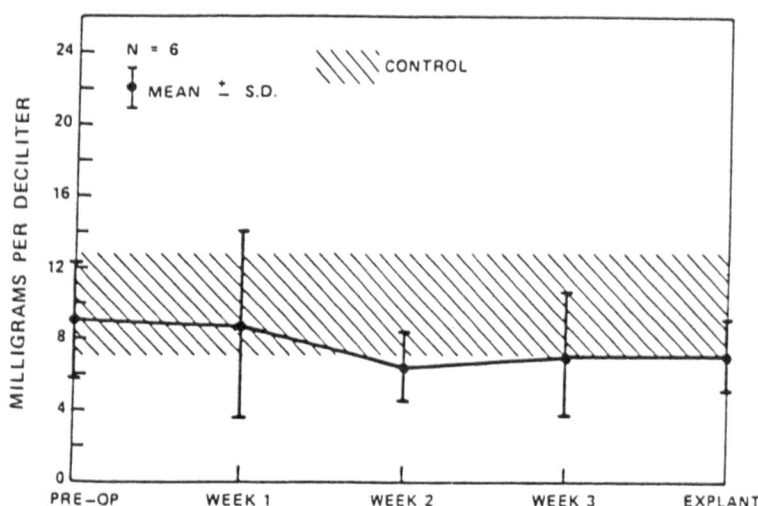

**Fig. 13.6.** Plasma hemoglobin measurements show no hemolysis

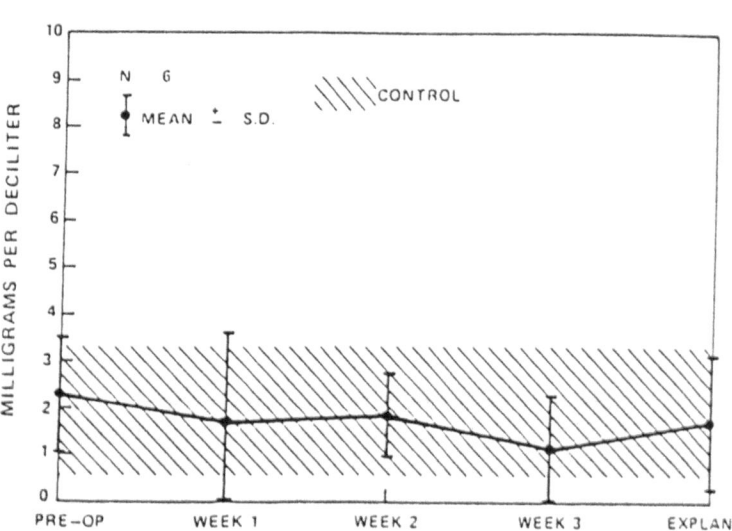

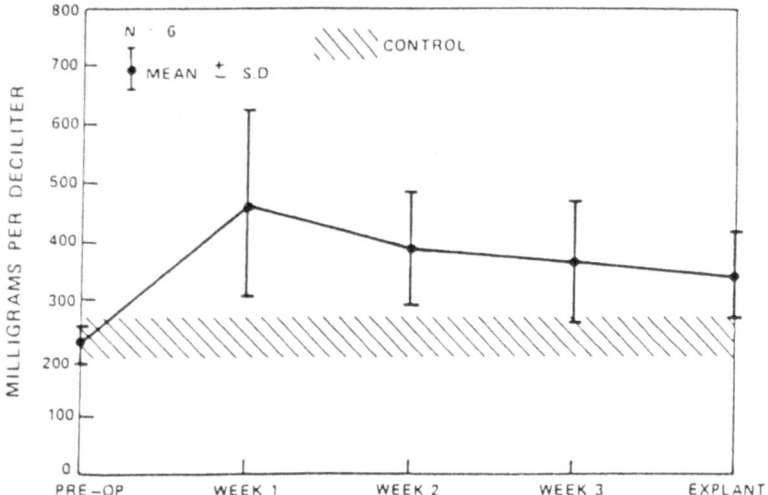

**Fig. 13.7.** Serial measurements of fibrinogen for the six experiments

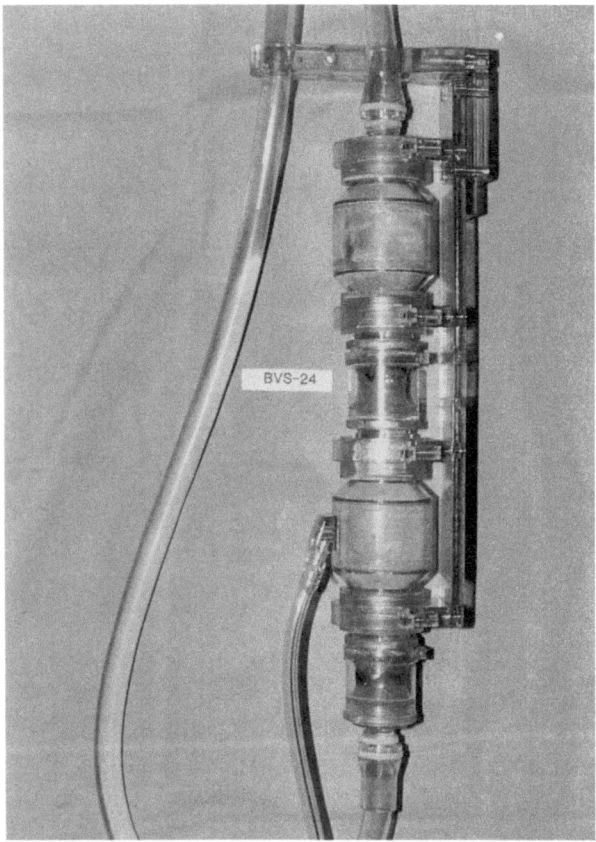

**Fig. 13.8.** Pump immediately after the experiment was completed and the pump had been gently rinsed with saline

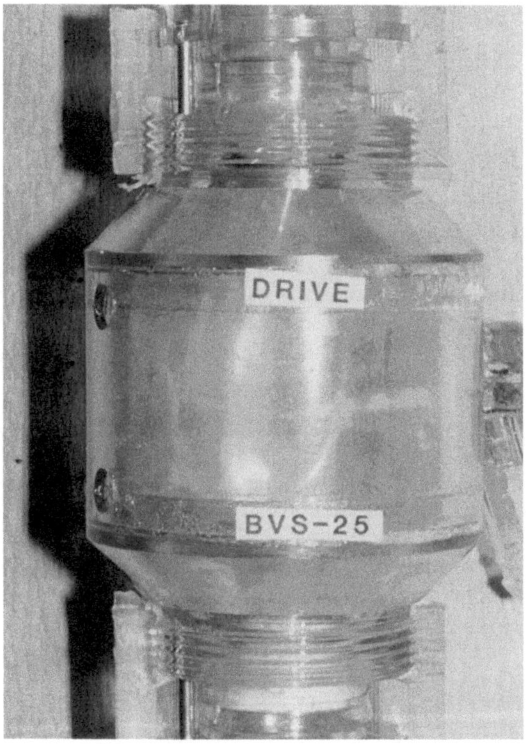

**Fig. 13.9.** Close-up of the Angioflex pumping bladder after 28 days of pumping

cannulae were remarkably free of junctional thrombi (Fig. 13.11). This is in contrast to the results obtained with conventional connectors, which show junctional thrombi after only a few hours of blood flow.

SEM images of all blood-contacting surfaces showed consistently minimal and sparsely populated areas of adherent platelets and leukocytes typical of smooth-surfaced inert materials.

Clinical trials have recently commenced and three patients have received BVS support through the mid-

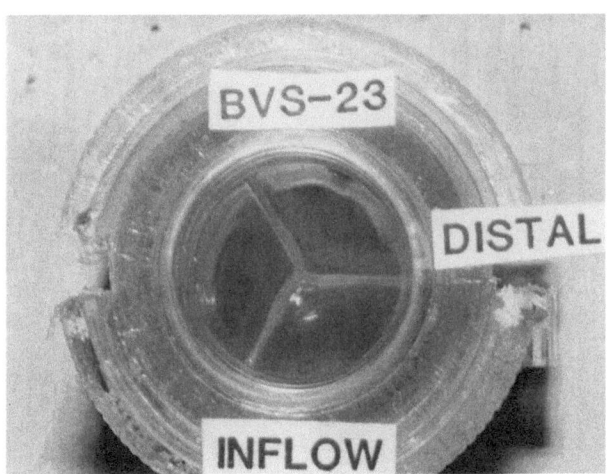

**Fig. 13.10.** A pump inflow Angioflex trileaflet valve after experiment completion and disassembly pump components

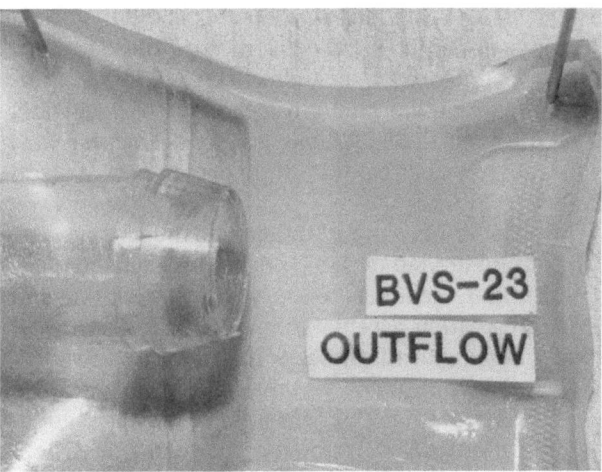

**Fig. 13.11.** A BVS connector after 28 days of in vivo operation. The connector-tube junction is free of deposits. Flow was from right to left

dle of 1987. Two patients in cardiogenic shock unresponsive to conventional therapies received biventricular support with the BVS and underwent heart transplants after 8.5 and 6.5 days of assist, during which their condition improved steadily to qualify them for transplantation. A third patient received biventricular support for 4 h after a failed transplantation but died due to bleeding complications unrelated to the BVS assist period. In all cases, the BVS provided adequate circulatory support with minimal operator involvement.

## Permanent cardiac support—The VAS

During the last decade, intensive research and development efforts in the USA have brought a number of permanent support and replacement systems to the reliability demonstration phase. The indications for permanent support are essentially identical to those for cardiac transplantation: end-stage cardiomyopathies of ischemic, viral, or unknown etiology. The excellent results obtained with heart transplants in recent years have set a standard that mechanical devices must attain before they become clinically acceptable. Systems intended for lifetime support must demonstrate acceptable reliability and an untethered lifestyle reasonably free of complications for the recipient.

It is estimated that for each donor heart that becomes available in the USA, there are approximately 20 recipients that require permanent cardiac assist. To address this need and with support from the National Institutes of Health, ABIOMED has been developing over the past 10 years a system designed for long-term

(>2 years) circulatory support. The primary impetus in the design of the ABIOMED VAS was to develop a totally implanted system which required no external venting and had no displacement volume problem [11–14]. A system that requires external venting cannot be considered totally implantable and subverts one of the key requirements in the development of totally implantable systems—the elimination of infection problems associated with percutaneous connections.

## Materials

The ABIOMED VAS (Fig. 13.12) is configured for abdominal implantation. As a left ventricular assist system, blood access is from the ventricular apex with ejection to the abdominal aorta proximally to the iliac bifurcation. It is designed to provide pulsatile flow without external venting or the use of a separate compliance chamber.

A block diagram of the system is shown in Fig. 13.13. It is designed to provide pulsatile flow without external venting or the use of a separate compliance chamber. The key components of the system are: (a) two free-diaphragm blood pumping chambers with one integrated trileaflet valve between the two chambers and one at the inlet to the pump; (2) an electrohydraulic energy converter consisting of a unidirectional axial flow pump and brushless DC motor, which drives a silicone hydraulic fluid shuttled between the two blood pump chambers by a two-position sliding sleeve valve; and (c) hybrid miniaturized electronics with a CMOS microprocessor-based controller, which synchronizes the system to the natural ventricle by sensing the ECG R-wave and controls the level of assist by sensing pressures in the hydraulic chambers and adjusting the DC motor drive.

The system components are integrated into a compact unit, which has contoured external surfaces and no sharp corners. The specific gravity of the system is approximately 1.1 so that it approximates neutral buoyancy.

The blood pumps are of the flexing membrane type with a strain limited design. Inflow into each chamber is tangential, leading to a swirling motion and shear rates within acceptable limits for prevention of blood trauma and thrombus formation [15] ($10 \text{ s}^-$ to $2\,000 \text{ s}^{-1}$). The pump is fabricated with a single polyurethane (Angioflex elastomer) as the blood-contacting surface with no steps or seams anywhere from the apical inflow to the aortic outflow. The pumps incorporate sinus-contoured trileaflet valves [16] as integral components. Thus, the entire blood circuit is made from the same material and without any seams or junctions anywhere along the flow path.

The axial flow pump consists of a submerged titanium axial pump-rotor combination that is driven by a 12-V brushless DC motor, whose back electromotive force zero crossings are sensed and used to provide motor commutation. Radial stability of the pump is provided by nonslotted cylindrical hydrodynamic bearings, and thrust loads are taken by ball bearings.

Hydraulic flow is switched by a two-position four-way sleeve valve, which wraps around the axial flow pump and is actuated by miniature solenoids. Electric to hydraulic power conversion involves basically two mechanical moving parts—the axial pump-rotor and the sliding sleeve. The hydraulic fluid (silicone oil) is the lubricant for the moving parts.

Control and power electronics involve hybrid miniaturization and utilize CMOS technology to minimize power losses. The implantable electronics include an R-wave detector and signal conditioning for pressure transducers and temperature sensors.

The primary power source is an external 20 AH silver-zinc rechargeable pack contoured either as a belt pack or a shoulder bag. Internal batteries use NiCd 0.8 AH cells, which are charged directly by an external charging circuit and provide support for approximately 30 min. A chip regulator supplies 5 V logic power. The power conditioning circuits incorporate monitoring and alarms for battery status and excessive power drainage and are components of the external power packs. Normal system operation is at low voltages (12 V nominal) and physiological hydraulic pressures.

The principle of operation is illustrated in Fig. 13.14. The preferred mode of operation is synchronous copulsation. The term "copulsation" refers to the fact that the natural and assist system arterial pressure pulses have no phase lag. During ventricular

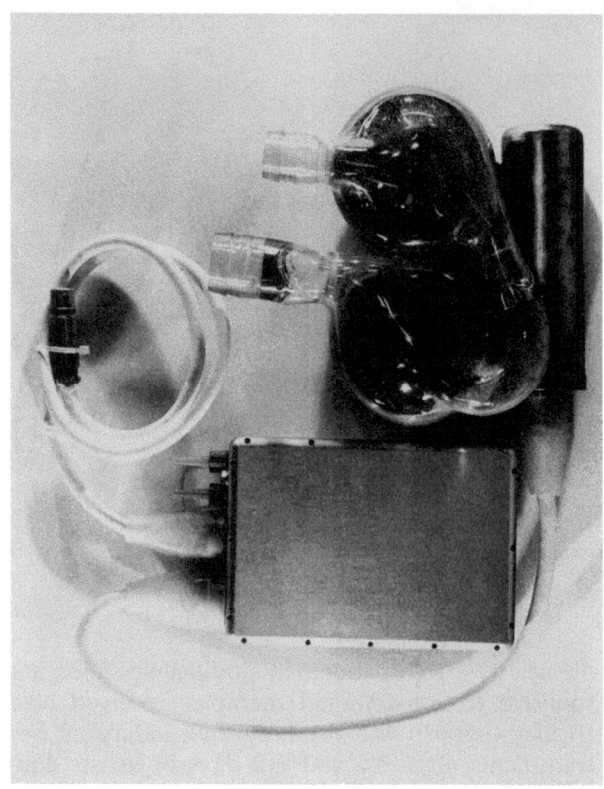

**Fig. 13.12.** ABIOMED VAS system showing the integrated blood pump, energy converter and implantable electronics

systole, fluid is withdrawn from the proximal blood chamber, A, and pumped into the distal chamber, B, thus lowering left ventricular outflow impedance and increasing aortic pressure. Hydraulic flow is reversed during ventricular diastole, returning the assist system to its initial state. Synchronization is achieved by R-wave detection and optimal assist is determined using simple control algorithms and sensing hydraulic pressure gradients. The system requires no external venting and has no displacement volume problem. Since pump filling is active, the ventricular and diastolic pressure can be preset to any desired level and ease of filling is essentially not an issue for this system. Hydraulic actuation dampens pressure transients in the blood system; maximum rates of pressure rise and fall are 1 000–1 200 mmHg/s.

In contrast to pusher-plate systems, this direct hydraulic drive approach lends itself readily to different configurations with no fundamental hardware changes. It leads naturally to a biventricular assist system (BVAS) or a total artificial heart (TAH) by decoupling and rearranging the two blood chambers with no change in the energy converter drive concept. The VAS, BVAS, and TAH configurations are shown in Fig. 13.15.

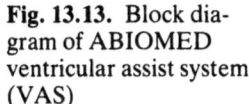

**Fig. 13.13.** Block diagram of ABIOMED ventricular assist system (VAS)

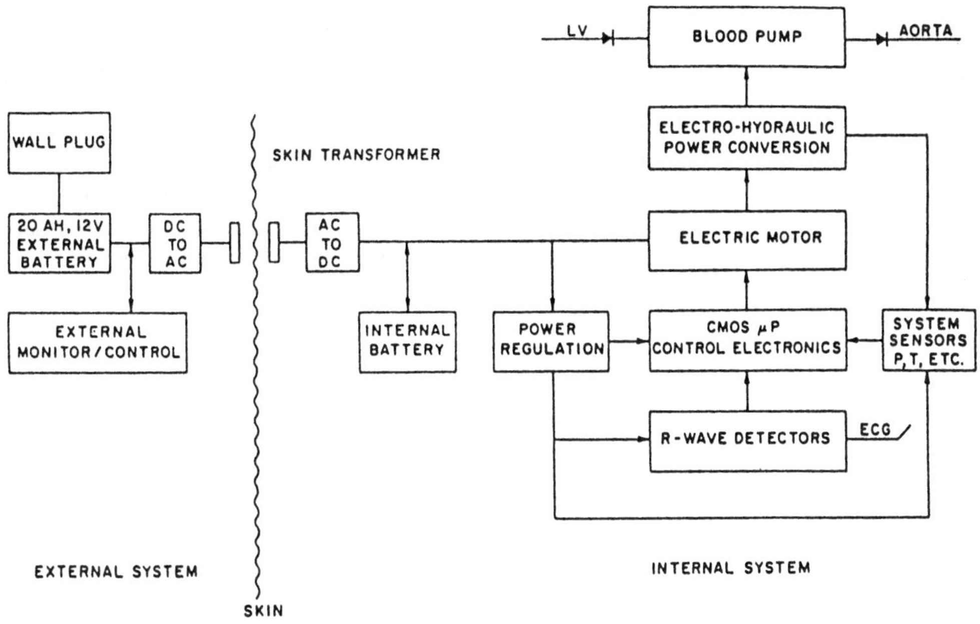

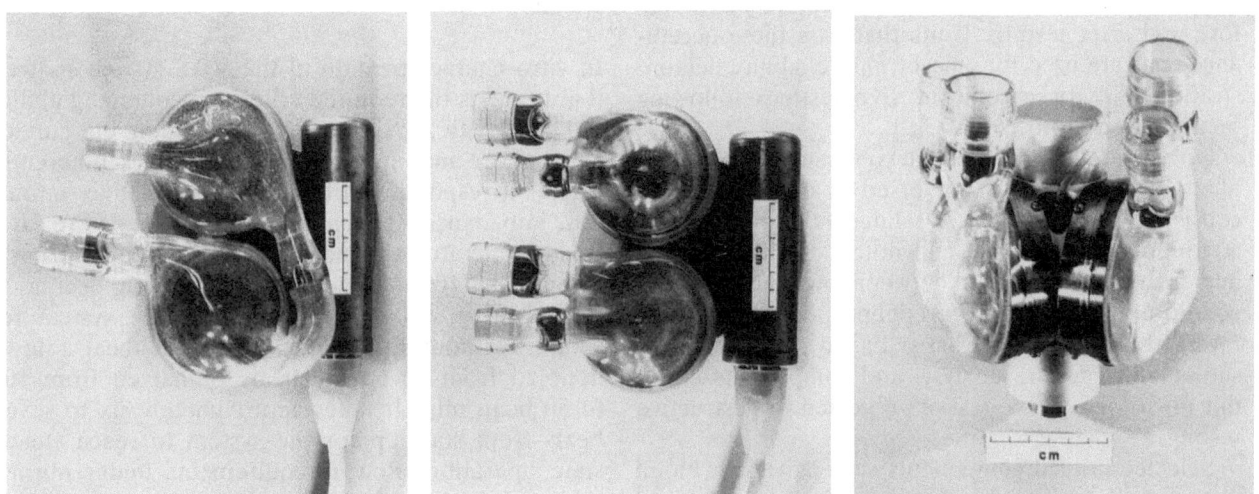

**Fig. 13.14a, b.** VAS principle of operation. With the 1:1 volumetric correspondence between blood and hydraulic fluid, a valve at the VAS outflow is not required or needed. **a** Left ventricular systole; **b** left ventricular diastole

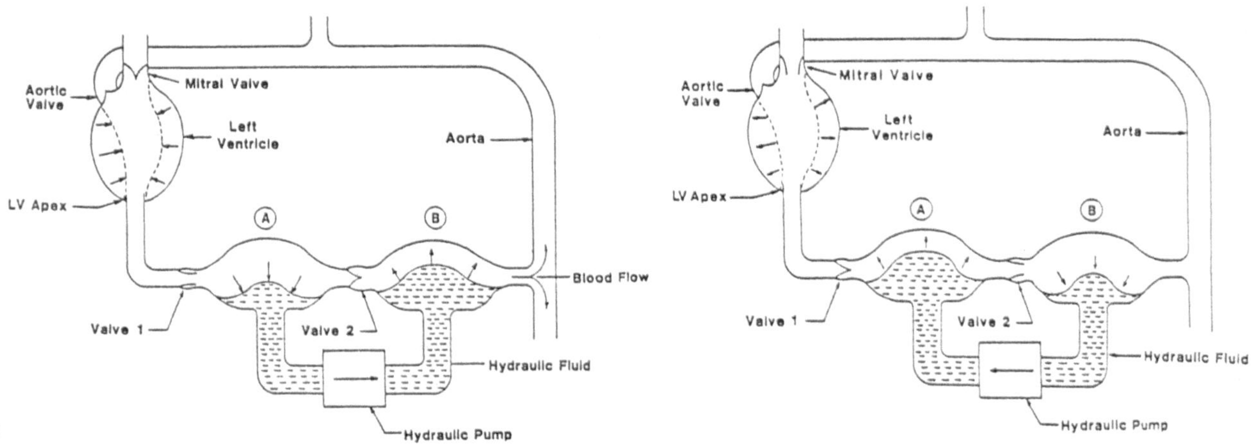

**Fig. 13.15. a** Ventricular assist device, **b** biventricular assist device, **c** total artificial heart. VAS, BVAS, and TAH. The three assist devices are identical in internal components but different in external configuration

## Methods

The primary task in the evaluation of a system intended for lifetime operation is to demonstrate long-term efficacy and reliability. The ABIOMED VAS has undergone extensive in vitro characterization studies under stimulated conditions in a standard mock loop. Data obtained include system output (flow, pressure) and input (power) as a function of filling pressure, aortic pressure, and beat rate. The time rate of change of pressure in the blood analog circuit and circulation patterns in the blood pumps are also documented. System response to transient changes in mock loop parameters assess the stability of control algorithms. Limited destructive testing serves to characterize system operation under some partial failure modes (incompetent valve, pin hole in diaphragm, loss of microprocessor control algorithm, high leakage path in sleeve valve assembly, steady loss of hydraulic fluid, etc.) with the objective of developing recognition criteria for these failures and defining optimal operation modes under these conditions.

Ongoing system reliability for 2-year operation will be determined by rigorous in vitro testing [17]. Chronic animal tests will qualify the system for clinical trials.

Upon fabrication, electromechanical components of each system are tested under conditions of higher electrical (increased temperature) and mechanical (increased loading) stresses to weed out early failures. Systems are put on mock loops for 168 h and a mean aortic to filling pressure difference of 130 mmHg. The filling pressure is kept sufficiently high so that the control algorithm forces the motor to run at its highest design speed. Failure is defined by changes in system output (loss or degradation of pumping) and by differences in operational characteristics (power input, temperature rise, etc.) at fixed operating points before and after testing. Units that pass these acceptance tests are used for efficacy and reliability demonstration and for chronic in vivo testings following preapproved protocols [17–19].

Ongoing reliability tests are conducted with the implantable components immersed in a blood analog consisting of physiological saline at 37°C. Data are continuously monitored and automatically recorded and each system is cycled between low- and high-flow conditions. Failures are predefined on a functional rather than operational basis. Failed systems will be subjected to failure analysis and components either put on continued life test or subjected to destructive testing.

Selected critical components such as valves, blood pumps, and sleeve valves have undergone accelerated or normal rate reliability testing to demonstrate that "wear out" is well beyond the 2-year operational life of the system. However, accelerated tests cannot simulate normal rate loads and their applicability is restricted to those aspects where the stress loading is higher than that obtained under normal conditions.

In vivo testing is the final step before clinical trials. Its principal objectives are to demonstrate system efficacy (i.e., capability to assume the ventricular workload in as normal a manner as possible without causing any additional physiological damage) and to qualify the system by showing that in vivo operation for many months does not have any adverse effect on system operation or components.

The animal model is the calf and detailed protocols define procedures and tests for determining the status of the device and of the animal model. Device pumping rate, pumping rate, flow, and power consumption are monitored under both synchronous and asynchronous operation. The battery operation and changing schedule simulates the expected conditions likely to be encountered during clinical trials. Animal monitoring includes ECG, heart rate, temperature, and hematology (coagulation times, cell counts, electrolytes, and plasma hemoglobin). The physiological condition of the animal ranges from rest to exercise (treadmill).

At explant, the blood-contacting surfaces are examined (naked eye, light microscope, SEM, and EDAX) for evidence of thrombus and calcification. The mechanical properties of pump diaphragms are assessed. Postmortem examinations include gross pathology of implanted sites, the heart, and aortic anastomosis and microscopic examination of the heart, lungs, liver, spleen, and kidneys. Other implanted and nonimplanted components of the system are examined for wear.

## Results

In vitro characterization of the VAS system showed that it meets the required criteria for pumping ability (10 l/min with AOP of 120 mm and filling pressure of 15 mmHg) and the control algorithm is inherently stable. It responds smoothly to rapid changes in outflow impedance, taking approximately 8 s to reach a steady state after the mean aortic pressure is abruptly raised from 100 to 200 mmHg or abruptly decreased from 200 to 100 mmHg. Similarly, the system responds without instabilities when the beat rate is doubled from 50 to 110 beats or halved from 100 to 50 beats/min. It takes approximately six to seven beats from start up for the system to reach steady state operation. Power requirements under normal loads (about 74 min, 100 mmHg pressure gradients) are 10–12 W.

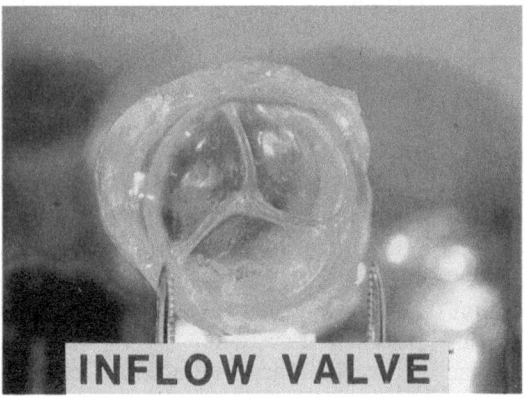 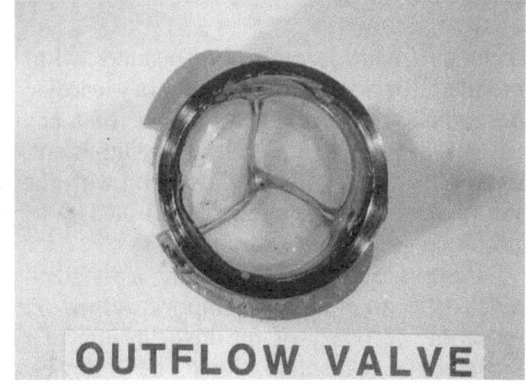

**Fig. 13.16.** Valves retrieved from a 3-month VAS implant. The leaflet and commissures were free of gross deposits

In vitro characterization experiments have demonstrated that the totally implanted dual-chambered VAS system operates with no external venting [12] or the need of volume compensation. Those studies defined the operational domain and control parameters and showed that high pump flows are maintained even at minimal assist levels [12]. These are important features, since continuously high flow through the blood pumps reduces the risk of thrombus formation.

The most extensive VAS component durability testing to date has been performed on the Angioflex polyurethane trileaflet valves. They have a demonstrated lifetime in excess of 420 million cycles under accelerated conditions and have been tested to 130 million cycles in real time. Blood pumps have been tested in real time for over 100 million cycles. The internal batteries have undergone about 200 charge/discharge cycles at the appropriate rates. Complete systems have accumulated in excess of 10 million cycles under in vitro reliability testing.

More than 30 valve implants in apicoaortic conduit configurations have been conducted in calves without the use of anticoagulant or antiplatelet therapy. The longest implant was 399 days and terminated electively due to excessive animal growth (360 kg). Calcification phenomena have been observed predominantly in leaflet regions of high mechanical strain, typically after 4–5 months of implantation. The potential and extent of calcification appear to correlate with circulating levels of calcium, phosphorus, and the calcium-binding protein osteocalcin [20]. Our measurements show that osteocalcin levels in growing calves are more than ten times higher than adult human values. Thus, while the potential for calcification of flexing blood-contact surfaces exists for recipients of permanent systems, it is difficult to assess its severity from animal data.

In vivo evaluation of the seamless blood pump components have involved approximately 65 experiments, including pumps driven pneumatically and hydraulically. These experiments have been conducted with and without anticoagulation and antiplatelet therapy. Prothrombin times were maintained at 1.5 times baseline level with Coumadin in those experiments in which therapy was used. The results of a 3-month, dual-chambered implant exemplify the long-term performance of the VAS blood pump. Throughout the experiment, the free hemoglobin level was less than 3 mg%, indicating no device-induced hemolysis. The flexing membranes and the stationary surfaces were found free of adherent thrombi. The valves and the inflow and outflow conduits were free of deposits (Fig. 13.6). No inflow pannus has been observed in any of the long-term implants. The outflow Dacron graft showed typically a stabilized pseudointima. Pathological and histological examinations were uneventful.

Vibration and noise characteristics of the VAS system have been measured. Noise at the skin level from an implanted VAS is less than 50 dB and arises entirely from the energy converter since the polyurethane blood pumps and valves are completely silent

Two-thirds of the waste heat generated by the drive electronics and by the energy converter is dissipated through the hydraulic fluid to the blood across the pumping chambers, and the remaining third through the system housing to the surrounding tissues. Adequate thermal dissipation of up to 30 W was demonstrated in long-term in vivo experiments. No signs of thermally induced thrombosis on blood-facing surfaces or necrosis on tissue-facing surfaces were observed. These results indicate that no thermal management problems exist.

## Discussion

Technical considerations associated with systems intended for long-term ambulatory cardiac support are radically different from those that characterize systems developed for temporary inpatient support. Some of these have been illustrated with the description of systems developed at ABIOMED for each of these two general categories.

Different types of ventricular assist devices have been used to support temporarily the circulation and allow recovery of the myocardium at risk or as a bridge to transplantation. These devices can be divided into two general groups: continuous flow devices adapted for extended (days) cardiac support, like roller and centrifugal pumps, and pulsatile systems some of which were developed for long-term support and adapted for temporary use. The continuous flow devices provide pulseless flow, have a lower disposable component cost, but require frequent replacement and continuous operator involvement. Pulsatile flow pumps are costly due to the requirement of two prosthetic valves per pump. Moreover, their drive mechanisms tend to be complex and operation typically requires well-trained personnel dedicated to the patient. The BVS System 5 000 was designed to combine the advantages of the two groups.

The design features incorporated in the ABIOMED VAS system exemplify one approach in dealing with the constraints that exist in the development of totally implantable systems intended for untethered ambulatory support. These are very much in contrast to the significantly broader design options that were available in the development of the BVS.

While some of the problems associated with cardiac assist, like the risks of thromboembolism and stroke, are generic to both temporary and permanent devices, the solutions are nevertheless different depending upon the intended duration of support. There are two options that can be combined for addressing these potential risks: pharmacological manipulation of the coagulation system and elimination of sites where thrombogenesis and embolization tend to occur. It is highly unlikely that any device can be implanted with no anticoagulation. However, the requirement to maintain an aggressive anticoagulation regimen on a carefully monitored patient receiving cardiac support in a hospital environment for a short period of time poses substantially lower risks than those associated with a strongly anticoagulated patient who is ambulatory and implanted with a permanent support system.

In the inpatient situation, the BVS represents a solution which incorporates the use of safe, single-use, disposable components designed to minimize the risks at common sites of thrombus formation like in-termaterial junctions. These disposable components were developed for use in combination with moderate levels of anticoagulation. For ambulatory permanent cardiac assist, the ABIOMED VAS eliminates all junctions, discontinuities, and regions of low flow which constitute potential sites for thrombus generation. This approach permits assist with minimal anticoagulation. The trade-off is obviously cost, since manufacturing totally seamless valved blood pumps is substantially higher and proportionate to the more demanding safety and durability requirements of a permanent system.

In summary, temporary cardiac support is increasingly becoming a life-saving clinical modality. No technical impediments remain. Permanent systems have advanced to the reliability demonstration phase with realistic goals defined in preparation for clinical trials. Two-year trouble-free operation is an achievable objective. For an electromechanical system, it represents the cycling equivalent of an automobile engine operating continuously for approximately 2 months. The primary technical issues that remain to be validated relate to long-term physiological effects on system integrity.

## References

1. Attar S (ed) (1985) New developments in cardiac assist devices. Praeger, New York
2. Under F (ed) (1984) Assisted circulation II. Springer, New York
3. Pae WE (1987) Temporary ventricular support, current indications and results. Trans Am Soc Art Int Org 33: 4–7
4. Park SB, Liebler GA, Burkholder JA, Maher TD, Benckart DH, Magovern GA Jr, Christlieb IY, Kao RL, Magovern GJ (1986) Mechanical support of the failing heart. Ann Thorac Surg 42: 627–631
5. Schoen FJ, Palmer DC, Berhard WF, Pennington DG, Handenschild CC, Ratliff NB, Berger RL, Golding LR, Watson JT (1986). Clinical temporary ventricular assist. J Thorac Cardiovasc Surg 92: 1071–1081
6. Conference on heart assist devices and heart replacement. Division of Thoracic and Cardiovascular Surgeons University of Maryland School of Medicine
7. Braunwald E, Kloner RA (1982) The stunned myocardium—Prolonged post-ischemic ventricular dysfunction. Circulation 66: 1146–1149
8. Singh, PI (1986) Technical considerations for clinical systems, presented at the University of Maryland Conference on Heart Assist Devices and Heart Replacement, Sept. 14–16
9. Singh PI, Bolt WJ, Cumming RD, Adams B, Snow J, Barak J (1987) Preclinical evaluation of a pulsatile ventricular assist device for short term support. International meeting on heart transplantation, total artificial heart and assist devices. Brussels, March 23–25
10. Bolt WJ, Singh PI, Cumming RD (1987) Closed loop control of a new pulsatile biventricular support system.

CECEC meeting. Paris, June 27

11. Singh PI, Adams BB, deSieyes DC, Cumming RD, Lederman DM (1982) Copulsation left ventricular blood pump. Trans Am Soc Art Int Org 28: 117–121

12. Kung RTV, Singh PI, deSieyes DC, Cumming RD, Adams BB Leicher FG, Magrassi P, Buckley MJ, Austen WG, Lederman DM (1983) Physiological characteristics of an electrohydraulic ventricular assist system. Proceedings Xth, European Society for Artificial Organs

13. Kung RTV, Singh PI, deSieyes DC, Adams BB, Cumming RD, Butler RG, Sevier FE, Buckley MJ, Boinia G, Bolt WJ, Gardner RA, Isaacson MS, Lederman DM (1985) Development of an electrohydraulic left heart assist system, final report. Contract No. NIH-NO1-HV-02913, Report No. NIH-NO1-HV-02913-10 (Available from the National Technical Information Service)

14. Kung RTV (1986) Electrohydraulic left heart assist system. NHLBI, devices and technology branch contractors meeting. US Government Printing Office

15. Lederman DM, Singh PI, Russell FB, Morgan RA, Cumming RD, Levine FH, Austen WG, Buckley MJ (1979) Discontinuity-free integrally valved left heart blood pump. Proc Eur Soc Art Org VI: 74–78

16. Russell FB, Lederman DM, Singh PI, Morgan RA, Levine FH, Austen WG, Buckley MJ (1980) Development of seamless trileaflet valves. Trans Am Soc Art Int Org 26: 66–70

17. Kung RTV (1985) Device readiness testing of an electrohydraulic VAS. NHLBI, devices and technology branch contractors meeting, p 82. US Government Printing Office

18. Request for proposal from the National Heart, Lung, and Blood Institute 84-1 (1984) Device readiness testing of implantable ventricular assist system. Bethesda

19. Altieri FD, Watson JT (1987) Implantable ventricular assist systems. Art Org 11: 237–246

20. Cumming RD, Snow JL, Singh PI, Romero LH, Harpster NK, Lian JB (1985) Mechanical etiology of calcification. NHLBI, devices and technology branch contractors meeting, p 104. US Government Printing Office

# Discussion

*Umezu* (National Cardiovascular Center): Could you tell us something about the fabrication of your polyurethane valves? In your long-term durability tests, what was the failure rate of the valves after 400 million cycles and what is the weakest point in the valves?

*Lederman* (ABIOMED): In answer to your first question, we manufacture our valves by solution-casting methods using our Angioflex polyurethane. Our valves are the result of over 10 years' experience. We have now reached the point where we can make valves with 90% acceptance by solution-casting techniques. The valve manufacturing could eventually be done automatically as was done with the intra-aortic balloon pump. We now plan to develop machines that can make the valves without manual involvement.

Among the important characteristics of our valves, I would emphasize the strain-limited design. Our data indicate that if the strain is limited to 8% during maximum flexure, gross calcification is not observed. In my opinion, the problem of calcification on synthetic materials can be overcome as long as it is a surface phenomenon. In our experience, this has always been the case; we have not seen biochemical degradation of the polyurethane. I should add that the animal model is very important. We have used calves and sheep in our valve studies. These studies have shown that sometimes the time before grossly calcified regions are observed is longer in sheep than in calves, but we have seen the same phenomenon in both animal models. We do not yet know how this relates to humans.

With regard to your second question, we have never experienced material failure in our trileaflet valves either in vitro or in animal experiments. There were some failures in the early part of our permanent VAS development program which were attributed to problems with hermetic seals and wire fractures. In general, early failures were found in mechanical rather than electrical components. In our system, the blood pump is the most reliable component; it also has the longest history. The energy converter is half as old in terms of our development history. I would say that with our VAS system, the most critical component is the electromechanical energy converter.

*Adachi* (Saitama Medical School): I completely agree with you that it is very important to deal with permanent use and temporary use separately. For the clinician, a simple, reliable, cheap device is needed. It is sometimes necessary to use a device for longer than we originally intended, especially in bridge transplantation, where we may have to wait a couple of months. Could we have your comments on this?

*Lederman:* In the USA, our temporary system is qualified to be used for 2 weeks. The FDA requirements are such that a system must be demonstrated to have performed reliably in preclinical trials for twice that length of time, i.e., 4 weeks, before approval for human trials is obtained. However, we have also carried out many experiments to qualify the system for longer term durations, such as may be expected in bridge to transplantation. At present, we have systems that have been running for over 8 months with no problems. The system could possibly operate for years, though it was designed to be used for 2 weeks or less. This is the case for the clinical trials to be carried out in the USA. As I have shown you, one of the systems was already used in a patient for 20 days outside the USA. I have no reservations about the reliability of this system.

*Adachi:* Do you think it may become necessary to replace the device?

*Lederman:* If the patient becomes pump-dependent, there are two options; heart transplantation or implantation of a permanent system. If the indications for initial use of the device are for temporary support and the patient is believed to have a chance of recovery, I think that the extracorporeal temporary system should be used. It is very simple and does not require more than 5 min of training to learn how to operate it. It is much easier to do cardiac support than it is to put a patient on the heart-lung machine, which is done very commonly. If the indications for patient selection have been well defined, any cardiac surgeon should be able to insert a temporary system without specialized training. Thus, the patient can be supported temporarily or if he becomes pump-dependent, one of the two permanent options can be considered.

# 14. Experimental and clinical evaluation of a sack-type ventricular assist device and drive system

Shin-ichi Nitta, Y. Katahira, T. Yambe, M. Tanaka, Y. Kagawa, T. Hongo, N. Sato, and M. Miura[1]

**Summary.** A newly designed ventricular assist device and driving system, including an automatic control system, is presented. The blood-contacting surfaces of the blood pump are coated with either Cardiothane or Cardiomat. The system was tested in experiments on goats, whereby only one of fifteen animals showed sudden thrombus formation after 34 pumping days. The system was also applied in three clinical cases for durations of 18 h, 2 days, and 5 days. In two of the cases, weaning could not be performed because of continued bleeding, and the other patient is still alive. No gross findings of thrombus formation were observed in any of the cases, except for a thin circular thrombus at the junction of the connectors and the sack of the blood pump.

**Key words:** Left ventricular assist—Antithrombogenicity—Driving system—Pump design

Following developments in the design, material, and performance of the ventricular assist device (VAD), the number of clinical applications has been increasing rapidly. Up to the end of November 1986, the total number of clinical applications in Japan was 51 cases [1], including our eight cases [2]. The incidence of cases weaned from VAD and long-term survivors were 61% and 22%, respectively. Though the development of VADs in engineering is remarkable, there still remain some problems in terms of the clinical aspects. Of these problems, nonthrombogenicity of the blood pump, especially at low flow rates, and easy operability of the driving system are important. To solve these problems, we have been engaged in the development and evaluation of the blood pump and driver system [3–6].

The purpose of this paper is to present our improved and developed blood pump and the driving system along with evaluation in the mock circulation, in animals, and in clinical cases.

## Pump design improvement using flow visualization and its quantitative analysis

The flow behavior within our several types of VAD were analyzed with a numerical method based on the quantitative flow visualization technique to obtain a thromboresistant VAD, which was evaluated in the adult-type mock circulatory loop [7, 8]. The length and location of aqueous soda polyachrylate pathlines on the flow visualization pictures were digitized with a tablet and input into a computer system. The Raynold number and the frequency parameter were 1415 and 19.54, respectively, in the test conditions [9].

As shown in Fig. 14.1 and Table 14.1, four types of our VADs were analyzed in this series. Types TH-1 and TH-2 were previously designed and developed as polyurethane transparent VAD [3]. Types TH-7A and TH-7B were recently designed and used in animal experiments and clinical cases. The basic difference in design between the earlier and current types is the distance between the inflow and outflow cannulae, as shown in Fig. 14.1. A newly developed connector with an artificial heart valve built in between the sac of the VAD and inflow and outflow cannulae, as shown in Fig. 14.2, was used in the mock loop and animal experiments. This valve built-in connector was used to evaluate different types of VAD, changing only the sac without changing the entire VAD, including the artificial heart valve in animal experiments. These separated inflow and outflow cannulae, valve built-in connector, and sac of VAD also enabled us to exchange only the failed part in the event of thrombosis or fracture.

Flow visualization images in early diastole using the solid tracer method in types TH-2 and TH-7B are shown in Fig. 14.3. In type TH-2 (Fig. 3a), the inflow stream causes minor and major vortices in early diastole. Separation ("S" in Fig. 14.3) and reattachment points ("R" in Fig. 14.3), as seen in the inflow side, are thought to be a possible cause of thrombus formation in the VAD.

However, there are no separation and reattachment points in the inflow area and there is only a large

[1]Research Institute of Chest Disease and Cancer and Department of Medical Engineering & Cardiology, Tohoku University, 2-1 Seiryo-cho, Sendai, 980 Japan

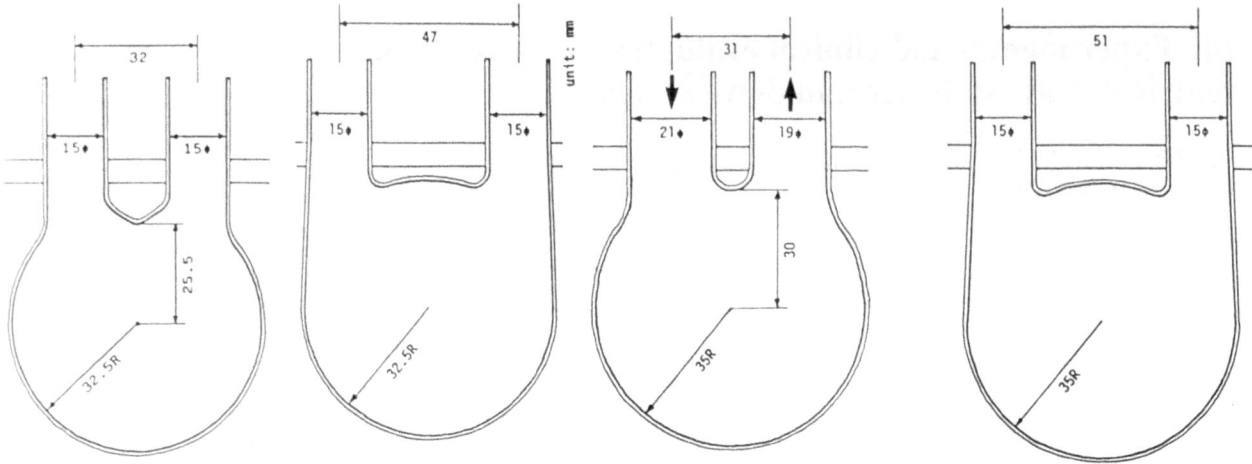

**Fig. 14.1.** Our four types of VAD

vortex in the center of type TH-7B (Fig. 14.3b) in the same drive conditions as TH-2.

### Improved blood pump and Cannulae

Experience with models TH-7A and TH-7B, both in vitro and in vivo, provided a firm basis for further development of these models. Figure 14.4 shows our pneumatically driven model TH-7B blood pump and connectors. The blood-contacting surfaces of the blood pump are coated with either Cardiothane or Cardiomat to obtain high antithrombogenicity. Both the inflow and outflow valves are fixed in a built-in fashion within the polycarbonate-made connector placed in between the blood pump and cannula.

Following our animal and clinical experience, the different types of inflow and outflow cannulae were developed as shown in Fig 14.5. These cannulae are also coated with either Cardiothane or Cardiomat on the side walls of the lumen. Four types of inflow cannulae, as depicted in Fig. 14.5, are used for direct insertion into the left atrium (LA) or right atrium (RA). Another cannula also shown in Fig. 14.5 was specially designed for transatrioseptal cannulation via the RA to the LA cavity to prevent air sucking around the insertion.

**Table 14.1.**

| Type of VAD | Sack volume | Stroke volume | Remarks |
|---|---|---|---|
| A (TH-1) | 88 | 65 | Previously designed type |
| B (TH-2) | 54 | 40 | 85% scale down of A |
| C (TH-7A) | 67 | 53 | Current type |
| D (TH-7B) | 54 | 40 | Current type |

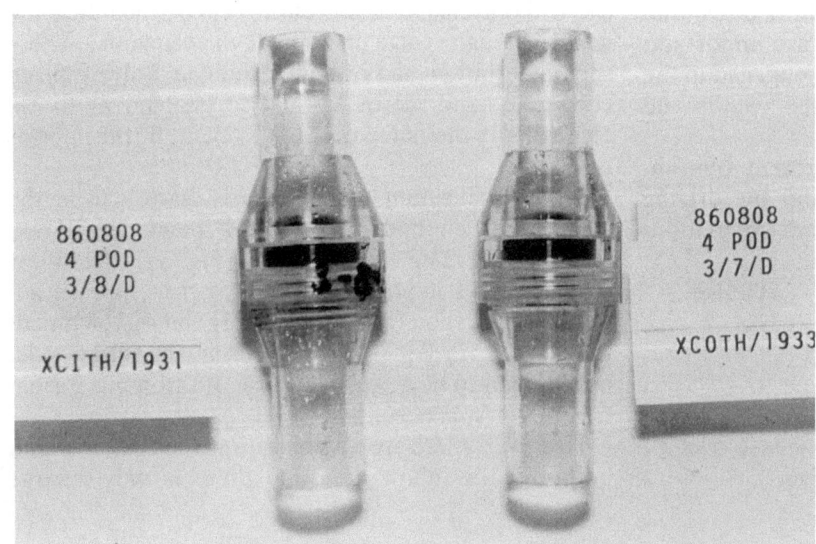

**Fig. 14.2.** Connectors with artificial valves built in between the cannulae and sac 4 days after use in chronic animal experiments

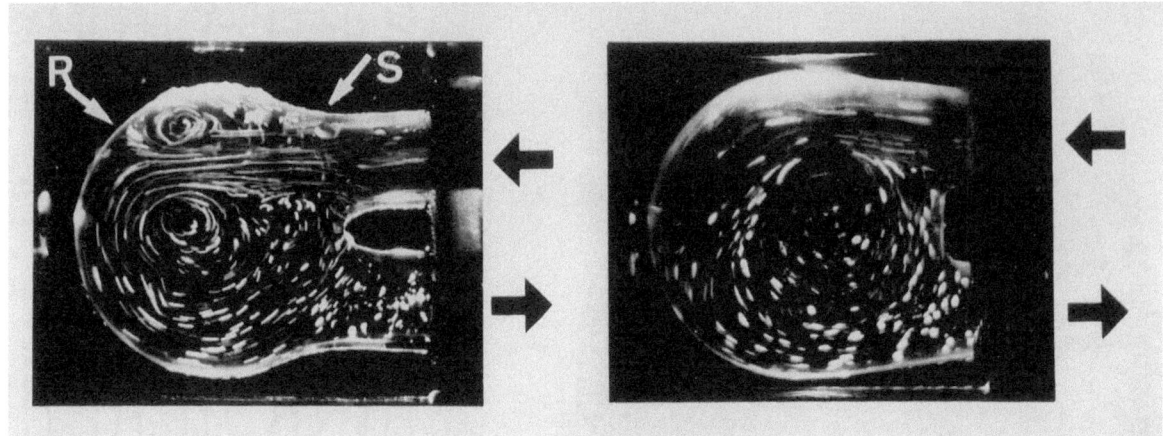

**Fig. 14.3a, b.** Flow visualization in **a** TH-2 and **b** Th-7B in early diastole. Exposure time, 1/60 s. Arrows show flow direction in VAD

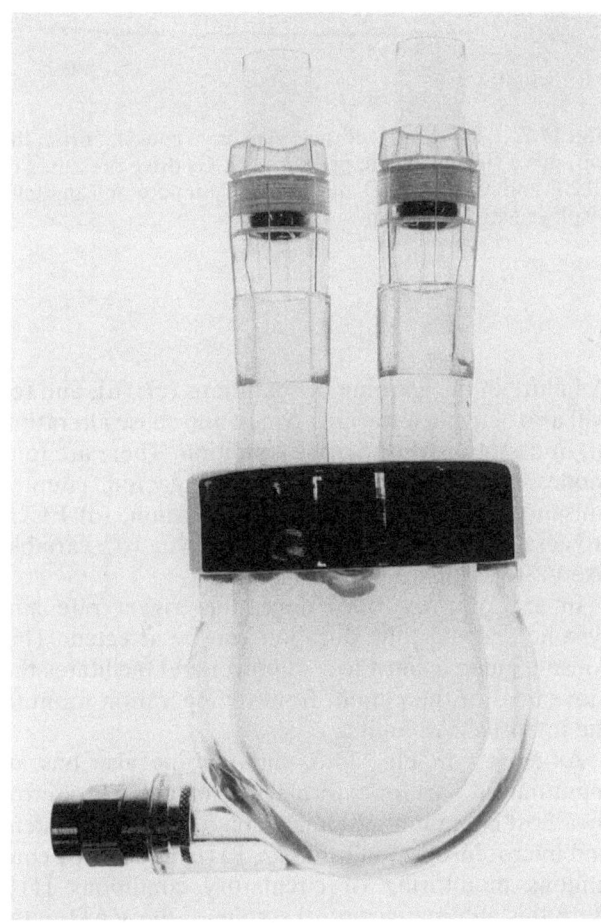

**Fig. 14.4.** Model TH-7B blood pump and connectors with Björk-Shirey valves

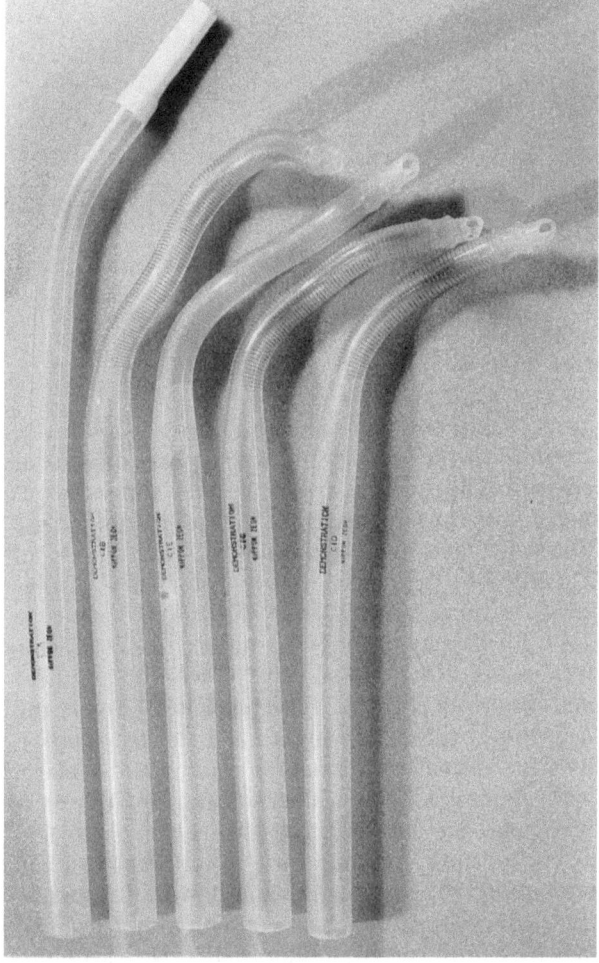

**Fig. 14.5.** Different types of four inflow cannulae (*extreme right to second from left*) and one outflow cannula (*extreme left*). The fourth inflow cannula was designed for transatrioseptal cannulation via the right atrium to the left atrial cavity under ECC support

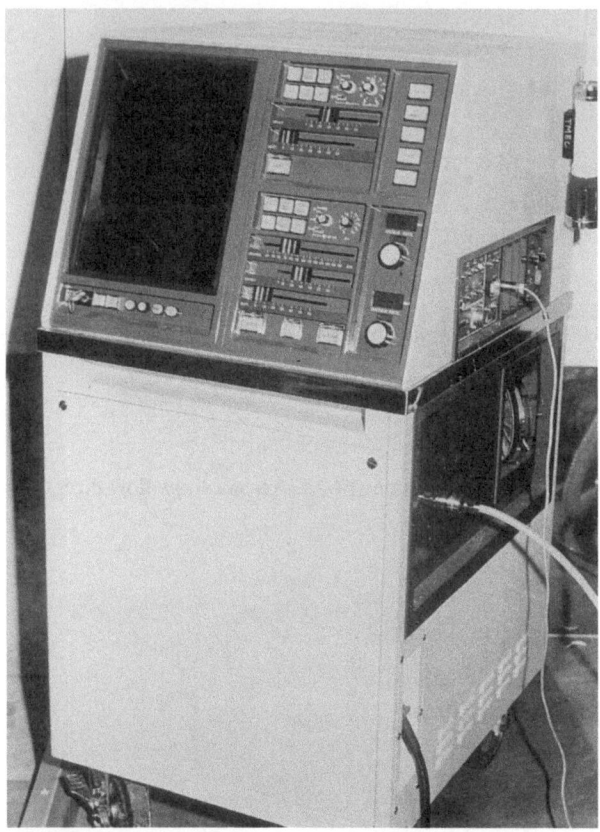

Fig. 14.6. Pneumatic drive console for clinical use

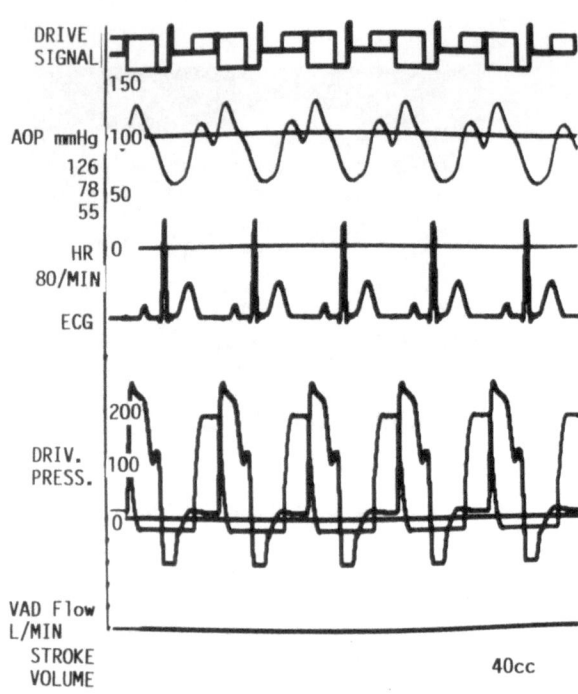

**Fig. 14.7.** CRT display of the VAD drive console. From the *top*, drive signals, aortic pressure, ECG, drive pressures of IABP and VAD, VAD output (liters/minute and digitally displayed stroke volume)

## Drive console

Figure 14.6 shows the pneumatic drive console for clinical use, which consists of two separate drivers, as seen in the upper right panel, so that simultaneous drive of both the left and right VADs or combined use of the IABP and VAD is possible [10]. On the upper left portion of the console, a big color CRT display and all warning lights appear. Figure 14.7 shows a color CRT display of the VAD drive console, tracing drive signals, aortic pressure, ECG with phasic drive signals in the colors of the two channels of driver, and VAD output (liters per minute and stroke volume). This CRT display also employs various audio alarm signals. Figure 14.8 is a block diagram of the electronic controller and monitor system, which provides fail-safe function for clinical use as follows: (a) ECG interruption; (b) loss of AC line power; (c) loss or excess external pneumatic power with either positive or negative pressure; (d) mechanical or electric failure of a subsystem; (e) reduced stroke volume from VAD.

When the ECG signal is interrupted, as in (a) or (b), the drive mode reverts to a fixed rate mode with a preset systolic appropriate warning light activated on the panel and a warning message appears on the CRT.

A failure in the warning of conditions (c), (d), and (e) will also activate a warning circuit and cause alteration in, or cessation of, the drive condition. There are four modes of operation: (a) ECG-triggered counter pulsation; (b) ECG-triggered copulsation; (c) ECG-triggered variable delayed time drive; (d) variable fixed-rate asynchronous pumping.

In any of these operations, the trigger rate and systolic and diastolic duration can be selected. This console guide against loss of power and facilitates the movement of the patient from the operation room to the intensive care unit.

As shown in Fig. 14.8, this console also has an input/output port for external automatic VAD control by a host computer system. A microcomputer system and microsensors (PO2, PCO2, PH) are used for continuous monitoring of circulatory conditions [11]. With this automatic control system of the VAD, integrated digital values of hemodynamic parameters can be obtained every systolic and diastolic period after recognition of the ECG, as shown in Fig. 14.9. These values can be used as a control for the following stroke according to the program of the VAD automatic control system by changing both the positive and negative pressure and systolic duration.

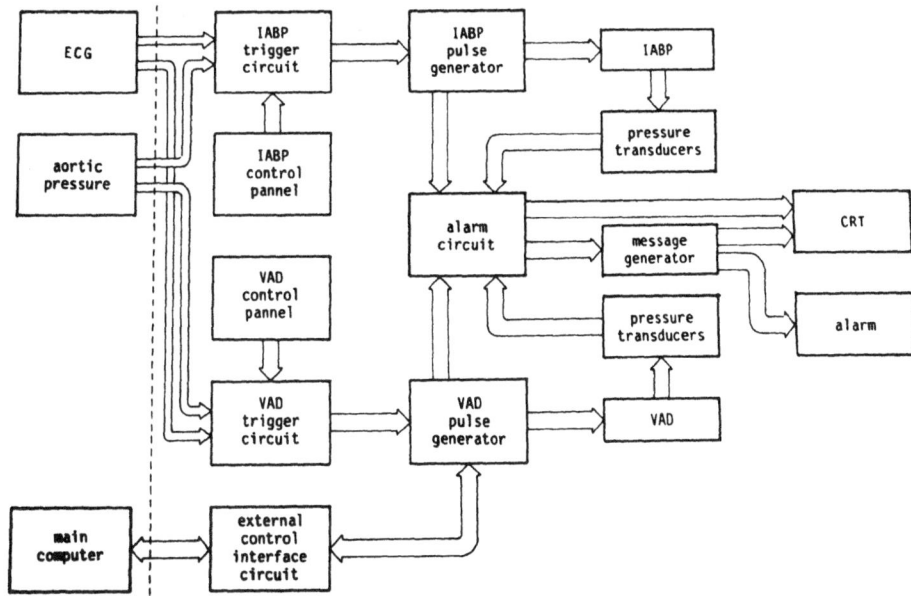

**Fig. 14.8.** Block diagram of IABP and VAD electronic controller and monitor system. The pulse generator of the VAD is shown connected to an externally placed main computer

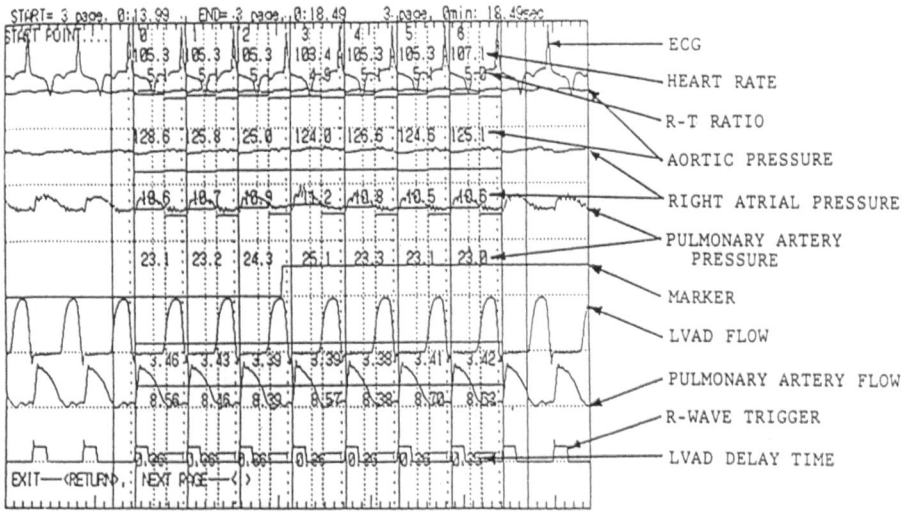

**Fig. 14.9.** An example tracing of hemodynamic data during left atrium-aorta bypass using synchronous VAD pumping. The *numbers* indicate the integrated systolic and diastolic mean values

## Animal experiments

Using this system, left ventricular assist devices were tested in adult goats. After the animal was anesthetized intravenously, respiration was maintained with a Harvard respirator via an orotracheal tube. The left chest was entered through a posterolateral thoracotomy in the fifth intercostal space. An inflow cannula was inserted into the left atrium through the left atrial appendage and an outflow cannula was anastomosed to the descending thoracic aorta with an end-to-side anastomosis. In all the goat experiments, the pump output was kept at around 2 l/min. No anticoagulant was utilized, except for 500-ml administration of low molecular weight Dextran on the day of operation. After the experiment, the animals recovered from the influences of the operative invasion and were put out to pasture.

**Table 14.2.** Diagnosis, operation, and results of three patients with VAD assistance

| Case no. | Age (years) | Sex | Diangosis | Operation | Ventricular assist | | | |
|---|---|---|---|---|---|---|---|---|
| | | | | | VAD | Duration | Wena-off | Long-term survival |
| 1 | 68 | F | LV rupture after MVR | Closure of LV rupture | LVAD | 18 hrs | No | No |
| 2 | 51 | M | OMI | LV aneurysmectomy | LVAD | 5 days | Yes | Yes |
| | | | LVA | re-ACB (Sec 2, 9) | LVAD | 2 days | No | No |
| 3 | 59 | M | OMI ACB VT | | | | | |

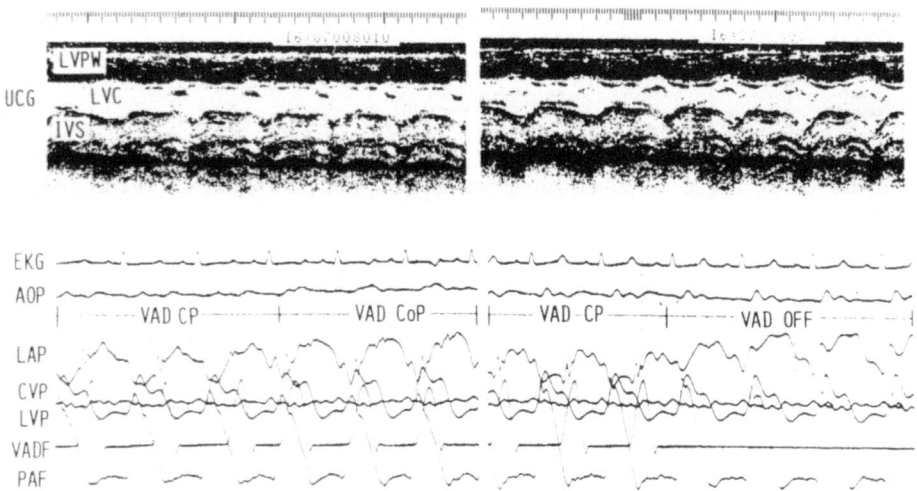

**Fig. 14.10.** Hemodynamic changes during left atrium-aorta bypass in the mode of VAD counter pulsation (*CP*), VAD copulsation (*COP*), and VAD off. *LVC* left ventricular cavity

## Clinical Materials

Based on the results of animal experiments, we recently applied our system in three clinical cases (Table 14.2). Case 1 was a 68-year-old female, who had rupture of the posterior wall of the left ventricle after mitral valve replacement. Case 2 was a 51-year-old male with a huge left ventricular aneurysm following myocardial infarction. Case 3 was a 59-year-old male who underwent two-vessel aortocoronary bypass for an old myocardial infarction and had frequent episodes of ventricular tachycardia. In these three cases, the blood pressure fell below 60 mmHg, when the blood flow from the heart-lung machine was reduced below 70 ml/kg/min, despite the administration of large amounts of catecholamines, adequate volume loading, and the application of IABP. Hemodynamic conditions just prior to the application of VAD fulfilled the criteria for acute profound ventricular failure.

## Results

### Driving system

Figure 14.10 shows an example of automatic control of a left VAD driving with a fixed stroke volume of LVAD. Stroke volume is kept constant even with changes in outflow impedance created by alteration of driving modes from counter pulsation (CP) to copulsation (COP). UCG shows a different left ventricular diameter in the driving modes of CP, COP, and VAD off. These procedures were done with our automatic control system and a programmed menu.

### Animal experiments

Table 14.3 summarizes the results of animal experiments in the most recent 21 cases. Of these 21 cases, two had thrombus formation in the type A (TH-1) and four in the type B (TH-2). However, after design im-

**Table 14.3.** Results of chronic animal experiments using our four types of ventricular assist device

| Experiment no. | Pump type | Survival time | Valve position | Coating material | Thrombus |
|---|---|---|---|---|---|
| 1 | A | 78 days | Nozzle | 610 | + |
| 2 | A | 60 | Nozzle | 610 | + |
| 3 | B | 7 | Cannula | 610 | + |
| 4 | B | 55 | Cannula | 610 | − |
| 850913 | B | 18 | Cannula | 610 | + |
| 851009 | B | 22 | Connector | 51 | − |
| 860107 | C | 33 | Cannula | 51 | − |
| 860131 | C | 16 | Cannula | 51 | − |
| 860314 | C | 38 | Cannula | 51 | − |
| 860404 | C | 34 | Cannula | 51 | − |
| 860606 | D | 27 | Cannula | 51 | − |
| 860723 | D | 17 | Connector | 51 | − |
| 860808 | D | 4 | Connector | 51 | − |
| 860829 | D | 1 | Connector | 51 | − |
| 860905 | D | 34 | Connector | 51 | + |
| 860912 | D | 2 | Cannula | 51 | − |
| 861024 | D | 15 | Connector | 51 | − |
| 861031 | D | 4 | Connector | 51 | − |
| 861114 | D | 32 | Connector | 51 | − |
| 861217 | D | 38 | Connector | 51 | − |
| 870211 | D | 22 | Connector | 51 | − |

*610* Cardiomat 610, *51* Cardiothane 51

**Fig. 14.11.** Model TH-7B in clinical case 2

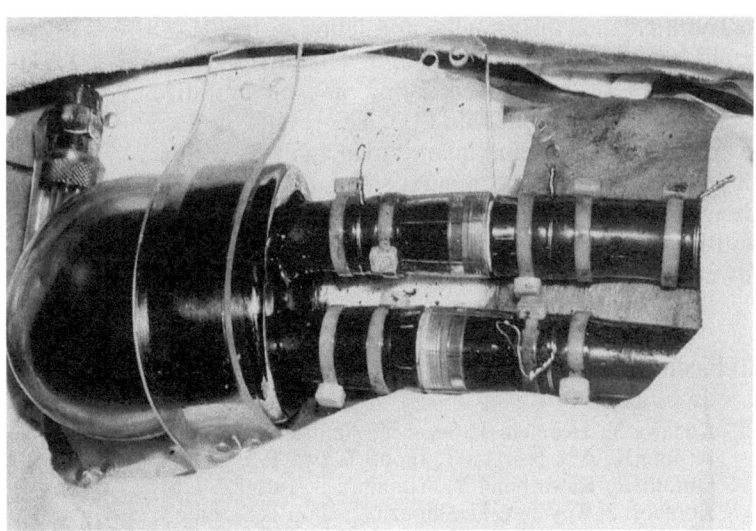

provement of the VAD, only one of fifteen cases (LC: TH-7A, D: TH-7B) showed sudden onset thrombus formation at the apex of the sack after 34 pumping days. We decided to remove the LVAD from the goat; after removal, the animal survived without any complications until it was killed. The blood-contacting surface of coated Cardiothane showed little dip caused by breakage of the coated layer, which was thought to be the origin of sudden thrombus formation in the sack. In the remaining 14 cases, no thrombus formation was observed, either on the surface of the sac or on the prosthetic valves, even without recourse to anticoagulants.

**Clinical materials**

Table 14.2 summarizes the characteristics of three clinical cases of model Th-7B. Left ventricular assists were applied in all cases. Duration of the assistance was 18 h in case 1, 5 days in case 2 (Fig. 14.11) and 2 days in case 3. Cases 1 and 3 did not wean from the VAD because of continued bleeding. Case 2 was weaned on the 5th postoperative day with a stable hemodynamic condition and the patient is still alive. In all cases, there was no thrombus formation in the gross findings, except for a thin circular thrombus at the junction of the connectors and the sack of the blood pump.

## Discussion

We have developed a new VAD and drive system, including an automatic control system. Because there is an urgent need for a practical RVAD and LVAD adequate for use in patients who have major acute myocardiac infarction with deep cardiogenic shock and in patients who have undergone open-heart surgery and cannot be weaned from extracorporeal circulation, even use the best forms of phamacological and IABP installation.

Another indication for the use of this device is the bridge to transplantation. We had a clinical case [2] of 70 days of LVAD pumping with difficulty in weaning, from the LVAD, which was thought to be a case for bridge bypass and heart transplantation. But severe infection beginning 4 weeks after surgery prevented us from performing the transplantation.

The incidence of thrombus formation in the VAD could be reduced by design improvements following the results of flow visualization and quantitative analyses, as shown in Table 14.3. The results of these evaluating methods and quantitative analyses will be of great benefit in the computer simulation of a VAD design. The three clinical applications proved the high antithrombogenecity of the model TH-7B, even at lower flow rates.

## References

1. Kagawa Y, Horiuchi T, Sezai Y, Akutsu T, Akune J, Atsumi K, Abe N, Arai T, Inoue T, Iwa T, Eguchi S, Omoto R, Kawashima Y, Kitamura S, Kusakawa M, Komatus S, Koyanagi H, Shimizu K, Shoji T, Shirabe J, Suzuki A, Seki S, Takeuchi K, Tokunaga K, Nakamura K, Hasegawa T, Fukumatsu H, Fujita T, Furuse A, Hoshono S, Hori M (1987) Current status of clinical application of ventricular assist device in Japan. 15th Jinkoh-Shinzoh to Hojo Konwakai, Rinshou Kyoubugeka, pp 221–261 (in Japanese)
2. Nitta S, Kagawa Y, Hongo T, Horiuchi T, Katahira Y, Fujimasa I, Imachi K, Atsumi K (1986) Clinical experience of left and right ventricular assist devices. Springer, Tokyo, pp 153–158
3. Nitta S, Horiuchi T, Shibouta Y, Ishitoya T, Kagawa Y, Tanaka S, Sato S, Hongo T (1972) Polyurethane-made ventricular assist device with altures cells as an antithrombogenic blood contacting surface. Japan society for Artificial Internal Organs, 1–1, 67 (in Japanese)
4. Nitta S, Sato N, Kagawa Y, Takahashi K, Honda T, Kahata O, Mori H, Horiuchi T, Tanaka M, Meguro T (1976) Noninvasive evaluation of cardiac dynamics during left heart bypass utilizing echo-cardiography. Jpn J Art Org 267–270 (in Japanese)
5. Nitta S, Kagawa Y, Hongo T, Sato N, Katahira Y, Miura M, Akino Y, Yambe T, Nishi K, Tuji T, Yoda R, Tanaka M, Horiuchi T (1987) Preclinical evaluation of an improved and modified ventricular assist device and a driving system. Jpn J Art Org 203–206 (in Japanese)
6. Nitta S, Katahira Y, Yambe T, Tanaka M, Miura M, Sato N, Hongo T, Yoshizawa M, Hu K, Takeda H (1987) Hemodynamic response to an automatic controled ventricular assist device pumping. IEICE Technical Report, pp 1–6 (in Japanese)
7. Nitta S, Katahira Y, Ohkawai H, Tanaka M, Kagawa Y, Hongo T, Miura M, Horiuchi T, Nagase T, Kuwahata H, Miyashita S, Kaneko N, Yora R (1984) Flow visualization study of an artificial heart. Nagare no Kashika 4 (suppl): 21–26 (in Japanese)
8. Katahira Y, Nitta S, Tanaka M, Kagawa Y, Hongo T, Horiuchi T (1985) Flow visualization of artificial heart and its quantitative analysis. Fluid control and measurement. Pergamon, Oxford, pp 165–170
9. Katahira Y, Nitta S, Nanaka M, Hongo T, Kagawa Y (1986) Quantitative analysis of the flow in the artificial heart by the tracer method. Japanese Society of Medical Electronics and Biological Engineering, pp 28–34 (in Japanese)
10. Nitta S, Katahira Y, Yambe T, Tanaka M, Kagawa Y, Hongo T, Sato N, Horiuchi T, Tuji T (1986) A multipurpose driving console for VAD, IABP and PAD. The Japan Society of Medical Electronics and Biological Engineering 25th Conference, p 335 (in Japanese)
11. Nitta S, Katahira Y, Yambe T, Tanaka T, Kagawa Y, Hongo T, Horiuchi T, Uchida N, Miura M, Takahashi A (1986) Development and evaluation of micro sensors for an automatic control system of ventricular assist device. Jpn J Art Org, pp 646–649 (in Japanese)

# Discussion

*Lederman* (ABIOMED): In the two human trials you carried out, were the patients anticoagulated?

*Nitta* (Tohoku University): ACT was kept around 150 without any active heparine administration. In the first case, there was a lot of surgical bleeding.

*Lederman:* I think that a good argument for having the temporary support system outside the body, as we saw in your slides, is that the blood flow in the pumps can be observed and the performances of the system assessed.

# 15. Pulsatile veno-arterial bypass (ECMO) with a pusher-plate pump for profound biventricular failure

Hiroyuki Irie, Taiji Murakami, Hirohumi Izumoto, Koji Takata, Eiji Sugawara, Haruaki Indo, Yuichi Ogoshi, Yoshimasa Senoo, and Shigeru Teramoto[1]

**Summary.** Short-term experiments were undertaken to maintain circulation in goats with profound biventricular failure using of pulsatile veno-arterial (VA) bypass incorporated with a membrane oxygenator.

Our pulsatile VA extracorporeal membrane oxygenation (ECMO) circuit consisted of a 60-ml pneumatic pusher-plate pump and an extracapillary blood flow membrane oxygenator; it had no reservoirs. The right atrium was cannulated and the oxygenated blood was returned to the ascending aorta.

In two goats, pump flows, pressure drops, and aortic pressure waves were measured under various driving conditions. In chronic studies ventricular fibrillation was induced in 13 goats and total circulation was maintained with the circuit driven in the variable rate mode.

The bypass time ranged from 9 to 23 h (mean 12 h 48 min). A pump flow of 60%–120% of native cardiac output was obtained, but each experiment was terminated because of a gradual decrease in pump flow. When the pump flow was 3.0 l/min, the gas flow and pressure drop across the oxygenator was 7.0 l/min and 170 mmHg, and aortic pressure and pulse pressure were 90 and 40 mmHg. The serum free hemoglobin level was elevated but was within an acceptable range.

This pulsatile VA ECMO circuit maintained the total circulation and provided almost the same pulse pressure and aortic dp/dt as native hearts for a short period.

**Key words:** Pulsatile pump—Pusher-plate pump—ECMO—Veno-arterial bypass—Biventricular failure

Left ventricular assist devices (LVAD) have been used for patients with severe cardiac damage and the long-term survival of these patients has been reported [1]. As clinical experience has accumulated, however, associated right ventricular failure has been identified as one of the major limitations of effective circulatory support with LVAD [2, 3], and 20%–30% of patients receiving LVAD have had this problem [4].

When the circulation is assisted by a supportive bypass, pulsatile perfusion is not only useful as a driving force but is also important in maintaining vascular tone, providing good renal blood flow and promoting oxygenation of the tissues [5–7].

Conventional mechanical assisting methods such as intraortic balloon pumping (IABP), veno-arterial (VA) bypass, and LVAD alone are not satisfactory to maintain the circulation in profound biventricular failure.

In this study, a pulsatile VA extracorporeal membrane oxygenation (ECMO) circuit has been designed and tested as a biventricular assist system with pulsatile waves generated by a pneumatically driven pusher-plate pump.

## Materials and methods

Our pulsatile VA ECMO circuit consists of a pusher-plate pump and a membrane oxygenator and has no reservoir (Fig. 15.1). The pusher-plate pump has a stroke volume of 60 ml, two Björk-Shiley valves, and a hall effect sensor, which detects the displacement of

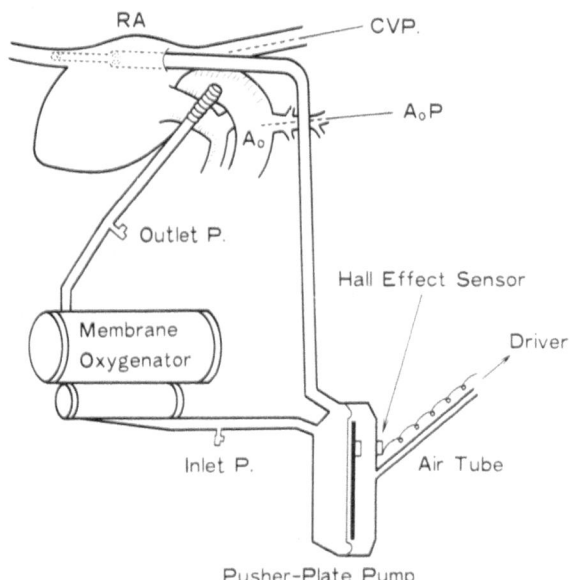

**Fig. 15.1.** Experimental preparation. The pulsatile VA ECMO circuit consists of a pusher-plate pump and a membrane oxygenator, and is primed with a volume of 500 ml. Aortic pressure (*AoP*), central venous pressure (*CVP*) and pressures both at the inlet and outlet of the oxygenator (*Inlet P, Outlet P*) are measured. *RA* right atrium

[1]Department of Surgery, Okayama University Medical School, 2-5-1 Shikata-cho, Okayama, 700 Japan

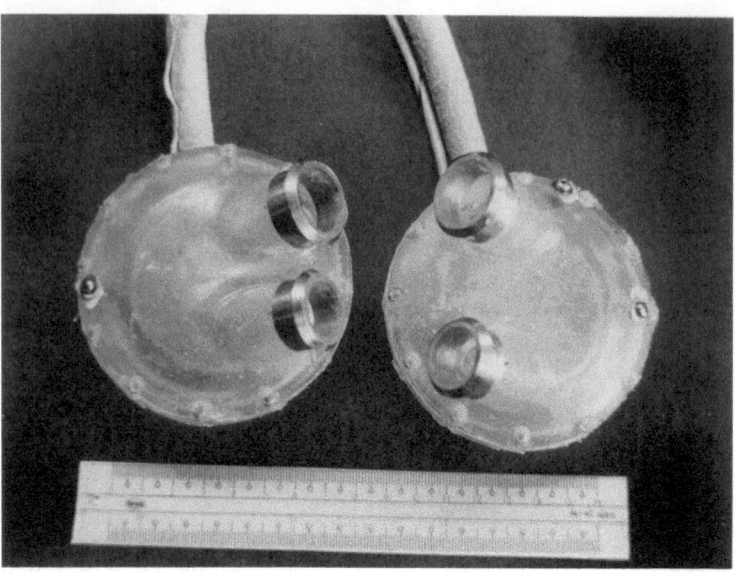

**Fig. 15.2.** A pusher-plate pump. It has a stroke volume of 60 ml and a hall effect sensor to detect displacement of the pusher plate

the pusher plate and calculates pump rate, stroke volume, and pump flow. It is driven pneumatically in three different modes: variable rate mode (VR), fixed rate mode (FX), and synchronized mode (Synchro) (Fig. 15.2). The membrane oxygenator (Sarns 16310) is made of polypropylene, is an extracapillary blood flow type, and is primed with a volume of 320 ml.

Fifteen goats were divided into two groups: two, both weighing 45 kg, were used for acute studies and 13, 26–75 kg, for chronic studies.

After premedication with ketamine (10 mg/kg, intramuscular) and atropine (0.01 mg/kg, intramuscular), each animal was anesthetized with pentobarbital (30 mg/kg, intravenous) and placed on a Harvard animal respirator after tracheal intubation. Anesthesia was maintained with G-O-F ($N_2O$-$O_2$-Fulothane) during the operation and thereafter ketamine was given for sedation. The heart was exposed through a right thoracotomy in which the fourth rib was removed and a vascular graft (10 or 14 mm) was anastomosed to the ascending aorta. The right atrium was cannulated with a two-stage cannula (36–51 F) or venous return cannulas (34 and 36 F). The circuit was primed with 500 ml physiological saline.

Cardiac output was measured by the thermodilution method using a 7-F Swan-Gantz catheter. Catheters were positioned in the aorta and the superior vena cava to measure aortic pressure (AoP), aortic dp/dt, and central venous pressure (CVP). The inlet and outlet of the oxygenator were also connected to transducers to measure pressures (inlet P and outlet P). Arterial blood was drawn to analyze blood gas (Cornig model 158), hematocrit value, activated coagulation time (ACT; Hemocron, International Technidyne Corp., NJ, USA), serum free hemoglobin

(free Hb; tetrametyl benzidin method), and antithrombin III (AT-III; Testzym AT-III kit, KabiVitrum, Sweden). Venous blood was taken to measure blood gas and lactate (lactate test kit, Boehringer Mannheim, Federal Republic of Germany).

The positive driving pressure of the pump was controlled to keep inlet P between 300 and 500 mmHg, and the negative pressure was 10 mmHg. The pump was placed 50 cm below the right atrium and was driven in the variable rate mode to obtain maximal blood flow; subsequently, the heart was induced to ventricular fibrillation (VF) by an electric fibrillator in chronic studies. During bypass, ACT was maintained at three times the preoperative value. Gas flow of the oxygenator was adjusted to keep arterial oxygen and carbon dioxide tension within the normal range, and sodium bicarbonate was injected when necessary. No blood transfusion was carried out during the experiments.

## Results

AoP, CVP, inlet P, outlet P, and pump flow were measured in normal sinus rhythm when the pump was driven by VR, FX, and Synchro modes in acute studies. At 220 mmHg of peak inlet P, pump flows were 1.4, 1.6, and 1.7 l/min in VR, FX, and Synchro 1:1, respectively. At the same time, pressure drops across the oxygenator were 40, 60 and 44 mmHg, respectively. At 360 mmHg of peak inlet P, pump flows were 2.1, 1.7, 1.3, and 1.9 l/min in VR, FX, Synchro 1:1, and Synchro 2:1, respectively; the pressure drops were 130, 140, 100, and 140 mmHg in the same order (Fig. 15.3). At 500 mmHg of peak inlet P, pump flow was 2.3 and 2.0 l/min in VR and FX, respectively. The pressure drops were both 170 mmHg. Pulse pressure of VR, FX, and Synchro 2:1 was 26, 24, and 20 mmHg at 360 mmHg of inlet P, respectively. The pressure waveform of Synchro had its peak in the diastolic phase, but those of the other modes had peaks even in the systolic phase.

In chronic studies, VF was maintained and each experiment was terminated when pump flow decreased to less than 1.5 l/min. The bypass time ranged from 9 to 23 h (mean 12 h 48 min; Table 15.1). Four goats with preoperative hematocrit values of less than 25% did not survive bypasses of more than 12 h.

The time-course changes and waveforms in the animal surviving 23 h 15 min are shown in Figs. 15.4 and 15.5. Pump flow ranged from 2.5 to 3.1 l/min and gradually decreased after 21 h of bypass. Before 21 h had elapsed, total circulation was maintained at an AoP of 70–104 mmHg, an Ao max dp/dt of 600–1800 mmHg/s and a pulse pressure of 20–40 mmHg, whereas these values of the native heart were 110 mmHg, 800 mmHg/s, and 35 mmHg, respectively. Subsequently, AoP decreased as pump flow declined. The hematocrit value decreased from 48% to 35% after the bypass began and then decreased to between 34% and 45% until 21 h had passed. Free Hb level rose from 3.1 to 10.5 mg/dl and the highest value was 25.3 mg/dl. When arterial oxygen saturation was maintained between 98.4% and 100%, venous saturation ranged from 48% to 77%. Venous carbon dioxide tension ranged from 39.5 to 57.0 mmHg when arterial tension was maintained between 27.6 and 46.8 mmHg. This case was terminated when pump flow fell to 1.4 l/min after 23 h of bypass.

Concerning the summarized data (Fig. 15.6), the hematocrit value was 31.0% ± 7.25% (mean ± SD)

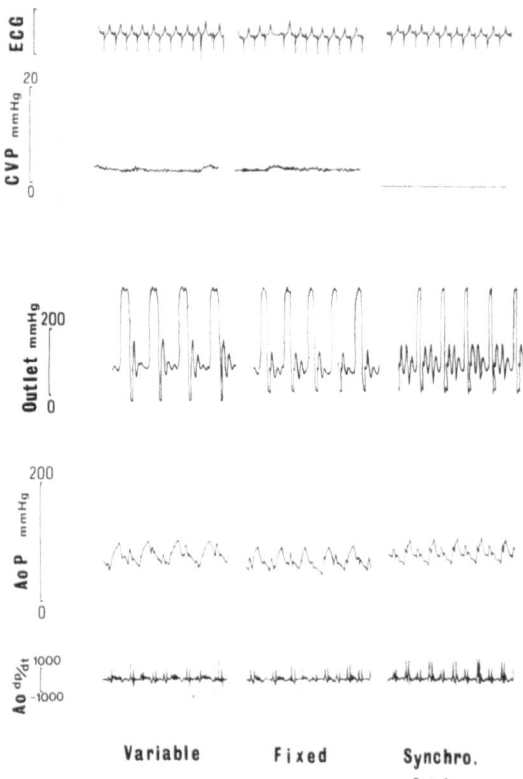

**Fig. 15.3.** Pressure waves in acute study. Peak Inlet P is 360 mmHg. Pump flows are 2.1 (variable), 1.7 (fixed), 1.9 l/min (Synchro 2:1). *CVP* central venous pressure, *AoP* aortic pressure, *Ao* aortic

before bypass, decreasing to 22.6% ± 8.28% after 6 h and 21.3% ± 8.04% after 12 h. Free Hb level was 2.59 ± 1.02 mg/dl before bypass, increasing to 11.22 ± 6.47 after 6 h and 14.93 ± 6.31 mg/dl after 12 h.

**Table 15.1.** Summary of chronic experiments

| Goat no. | Body weight (kg) | Graft (mm) | Venous cannula | ECG | Drive mode | Bypass time (h, min) |
|---|---|---|---|---|---|---|
| 1 | 75 | 10 | Two stage | Vent. fib. | VR | 23, 15 |
| 2 | 26 | 10 | Two stage | Vent. fib. | VR | 11, 15 |
| 3 | 45 | 10 | SVC + IVC | Vent. fib. | VR | 12, 00 |
| 4 | 37 | 10 | SVC + IVC | Vent. fib. | VR | 12, 00 |
| 5 | 38 | 10 | SVC + IVC | Vent. fib. | VR | 9, 00 |
| 6 | 75 | 10 | SVC + IVC | Vent. fib. | VR | 13, 00 |
| 7 | 60 | 10 | SVC + IVC | Vent. fib. | FX | 12, 00 |
| 8 | 60 | 10 | SVC + IVC | Vent. fib. | VR | 10, 00 |
| 9 | 35 | 10 | SVC + IVC | Vent. fib. | VR | 12, 00 |
| 10 | 55 | 10 | SVC + IVC | Vent. fib. | VR | 13, 30 |
| 11 | 70 | 14 | Two stage | Vent. fib. | VR | 15, 45 |
| 12 | 55 | 14 | Two stage | Vent. fib. | VR | 14, 00 |
| 13 | 45 | 14 | Two stage | Vent. fib. | VR | 9, 00 |
| Total | | | | | | 12, 48 |

*VR* variable rate mode, *FX* fixed rate mode

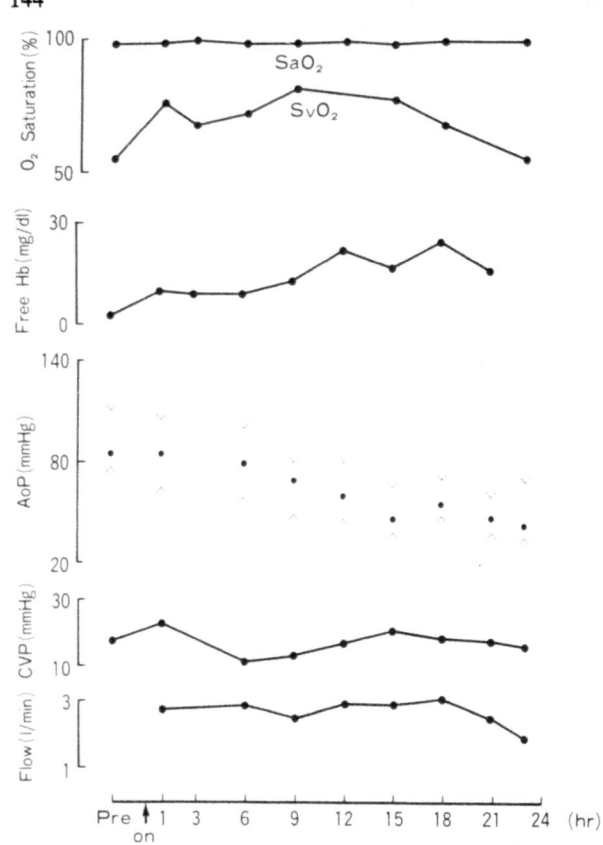

**Fig. 15.5.** Waveforms of goat no. 1 (body weight 75 kg). The heart is in ventricular fibrillation

**Fig. 15.4.** Time-course of goat no. 1 (body weight 75 kg)

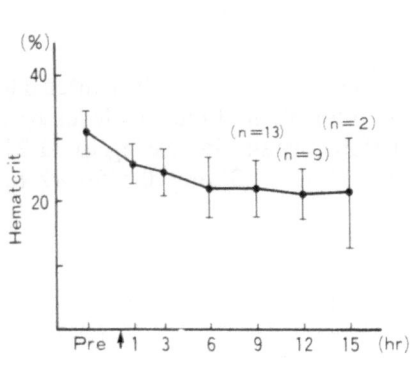

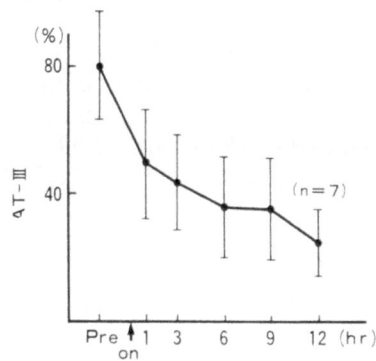

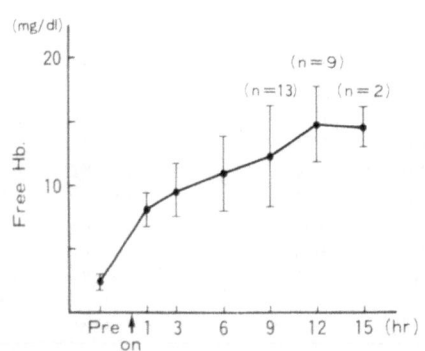

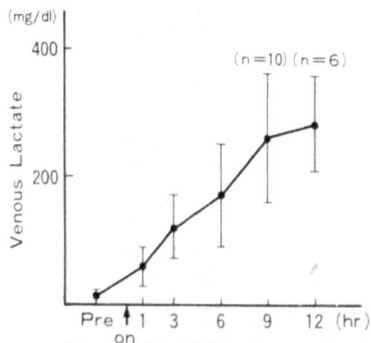

**Fig. 15.6.** Hematocrit value, free hemoglobin (*Hb*), antithrombin III (*AT-III*), and venous lactate in chronic study

Lactate level was $12.9 \pm 4.9$ mg/dl before bypass, increasing remarkably to $177.1 \pm 78.2$ and $264.0 \pm 75.7$ mg/dl after 6 and 12 h, respectively. AT-III value was $79.8\% + 7.4\%$ before bypass and decreased to $36.6\% \pm 16.0\%$ after 6 h and $25.0\% \pm 10.1\%$ after 12 h. The membrane oxygenator needed a flow of gas 2.5 times that of blood, and arterial oxygen saturation was maintained at between 98% and 100% throughout the experiments. When pump flow was maintained at 60%–120% of preoperative cardiac output, AoP stayed over 60 mmHg. Aortic dp/dt was employed for the evaluation of pulsatility. Aortic max dp/dt produced by this device in VF ranged from 800 to 3000 mmHg/s (mean 1391) at 6 h, whereas that of native hearts ranged from 800 to 2100 (mean 1250). CVP was maintained at 7–16 mmHg.

## Discussion

LVAD is a powerful circulatory assisting method when IABP or nonpulsatile VA bypass are not effective. It has been applied to patients with severe cardiac damage after cardiac operations or myocardial infarctions and has enabled such patients to live a long time after discharge [1]. Recent studies, however, indicate that associated or covered right ventricular failures reduce pulmonary blood flow and cause venous congestion, limiting the effectiveness of LVAD [2, 3]. A right ventricular assist device (RVAD) is sometimes combined with the LVAD and is used as a biventricular assist device (BVAD). Attachment of a BVAD is more invasive to the heart and coordinating a BVAD and the beating heart is far more difficult than is the case with an LVAD. To support total circulation with a single pump, an interesting trial has been reported by Sugita et al., in which a failed left ventricle is used as a functional right ventricle with an LVAD [8]. Moreover, Takano et al. reported that the total circulation was maintained with a single ventricle when pulmonary vascular resistance was within the normal range and right atrial pressure was kept at 10–18 mmHg [9, 10]. Pennington et al., however, found that there were no survivors among 16 patients treated with an LVAD who had associated right ventricular failure treated with isoproterenol rather than an RVAD [3]. And Gaines et al. reported that passive pulmonary flow alone provided inadequate pulmonary circulation support when compared with three other mechanical support methods [11].

Concerning recovery of the right ventricle and release of venous congestion, VA bypass with an oxygenator seems to be more effective. Clinical studies of VA bypass show that cases with AoP of less than 60 mmHg were all lost [12]. Thus, we have designed a pulsatile VA ECMO circuit, which provides pulse pressure by a pusher-plate pump. This pump is driven in three different driving modes—VR, FX, and Synchro. Based on the results of acute studies, VR was selected for chronic studies. VR is a stroke volume constant mode which needs no excessive vacuum, prevents atrial wall collapse, and washes out blood to avoid thrombosis [13, 14]. Although there are reports that nonpulsatile flow maintains the total circulation, allowing survival for more than a month [14], and that there are no significant differences between pulsatile and nonpulsatile flow in connection with renal blood flow [16], there are conflicting reports that renal blood flow or urinary output is increased by pulsatile perfusion [5–7]. Discussion regarding these two perfusion methods continues, but pulsatile flow is definitely superior to nonpulsatile flow because its waveform is much closer to that of the natural heart.

In our chronic studies, hematocrit values and free Hb levels were within the acceptable range. This meant that with powerful pulsatile flow propelled into the oxygenator there was not the problem of red blood cell destruction. The reason why pump flow gradually declined was that intravascular fluid escaped into a third space—the pleural and peritoneal cavities. Infusion of blood or albumin might be helpful in maintaining the osmotic pressure and total circulation.

Our circuit has the following advantages: It is driven by a single pump, has no reservoir, is simple and primed without blood, provides pulsatile waves and flow like that of the native hearts, and is useful in respiratory assistance. It has, on the other hand, some disadvantages: It needs an oxygenator and anticoagulation and it is expensive. These points considered, this pulsatile VA ECMO circuit is thought to be effective for circulatory assistance in profound biventricular failure.

## Conclusions

This circuit produced almost the same pulse pressure and AoP dp/dt as a native heart.

This circuit provided a blood flow of 60%–120% that of the preoperative cardiac output.

The free Hb level was elevated but within an acceptable range.

The bypass time ranged from 9 to 23 h.

**Acknowledgments.** The authors thank Dr. Setsuo Takatani (Japan National Cardiovascular Center) and Miss Masako Hata for their technical assistance, and also 3M Health Care Limited and Koshin Medical Company for providing membrane oxygenators.

# References

1. Pae WE, Pierce WS, Pennoch JL, Campbell DB, Waldhausen JA (1987) Long term results of ventricular assist pumping in postcardiotomy cardiogenic shock. J Thorac Cardiovasc Surg 93: 434–441
2. Turina M, Bosio R, Senning A (1978) Clinical application of paracorporeal uni- and biventricular artificial heart. Trans Am Soc Artif Int Organs 24: 625–631
3. Pennington DG, Merjavy JP, Swartz MT, Codd JE, Barner HB, Lagunoff D, Bashiti H, Kaiser GC, Willman VL (1985) The importance of biventricular failure in patients with postoperative cardiogenic shock. Ann Thorac Surg 39: 16–26
4. Farrar DJ, Compton PG, Hershon JJ, Fonger JD, Hill JD (1985) Right heart interaction with the mechanically assisted left heart. World J Surg 9: 89–102
5. Sezai Y, Hasegawa T, Miyamoto A, Kitamura S, Nakaoka Y, Kawano K, Shiono M (1986) Advantages and disadvantages of left ventricular assist device with nonpulsatile flow. Comparison of pulsatile and nonpulsatile perfusion devices. In: Akutsu T (ed) Artificial heart 1. Springer, Tokyo, pp 115–121
6. Mukhenjee ND, Beran AV, Hirai J, Wakabayashi A, Sperling DR, Taylor WF, Connolly JE (1973) In vivo determination of renal tissue oxygenation during pulsatile and nonpulsatile left heart bypass. Ann Thorac Surg 15: 354–363
7. Sink JD, Chitwood WR, Hill RC, Wachsler AS (1980) Comparison of nonpulsatile and pulsatile extracorporeal circulation on renal cortical blood flow. Ann Thorac Surg 29: 57–62
8. Sugita Y, Smith WA, Harasaki H, Jacobs G, Yozu R, Morimoto T, Olsen E, Nose Y (1985) Surgical approaches to applying an LVAD in a "one pump TAH" configuration. Trans Am Soc Artif Intern Organs 26: 235–239
9. Takano H, Taenaka Y, Nakatani T, Umezu M, Matsuda T, Iwata H, Tanaka T, Noda H, Hayashi K, Takatani S, Nakamura T, Seki J, Akutsu T, Manabe H (1984) Circulatory maintenance with a single artificial heart. Trans Am Soc Artif Intern Organs 15: 550–555
10. Takano H, Nakatani T, Fukuda S, Umezu M, Noda H, Adachi S, Matsuda T, Iwata H, Taenaka Y, Tanaka T, Takatani S, Hayashi K, Nakamura T, Seki J, Akutsu T, Manabe H (1986) Prolonged circulatory maintenance with a single artificial heart. Jpn J Artif Organs 15: 592–595
11. Gains WE, Pierce WS, Prophet GA, Holtzman K (1984) Pulmonary circulatory support. A quantative comparison of four methods. J Thorac Cardiovasc Surg 88: 958–964
12. Nawa S, Kioka Y, Komoda T, Shimizu A, Miyachi Y, Ebara K, Tsuji H, Nakayama Y, Murakami T, Uchida H, Senoo Y, Teramota S (1986) Evaluation of the results and causes of unsuccessful cases after assist circulation (IABP), V-A bypass, ECMO and the combination maneuver). Jpn J Artif Organs 15: 549–553
13. Murakami T, Shiotsu K, Kioka Y, Shimizu A, Nakao T, Irie H, Bando K, Senoo Y, Teramoto S (1987) An experimental study of left heart bypass. J Jpn Asso Thorac Surg 35: 297–301
14. Takatani S, Harasaki H, Koike S, Yada I, Yozu R, Fujimoto L, Murabuyashi S, Jacobs G, Kiraly R, Nose Y (1982) Optimum control mode for a total artificial heart. Trans Am Soc Artif Intern Organs 28: 148–153
15. Murakami T, Golding LR, Jacobs GB, Takatani S, Sukalac R, Harasaki H, Nose Y (1979), Nonpulsatile biventricular bypass using centrifugal blood pumps. Jpn J Artif Organs 8: 636–639
16. Dunn J, Kirsh MM, Harness J, Carroll M, Straker J, Sloan H (1974) Hemodynamic, metabolic and hematologic effects of pulsatile cardiopulmonary bypass. J Thorac Cardiovasc Surg 68: 138–147

# Discussion

*Adachi* (Saitama medical School): We use VA bypass for patients suffering from cardiogenic shock after cardiac surgery and we are usually able to maintain the circulation for about 24 h, but after 24 h it is difficult to do so because a lot of plasma is required to maintain the circulatory volume. Do you see any advantage in using the pulsatile rather than the nonpulsatile system?

*Irie* (Okayama University): In this study, we did not make a comparison with the nonpulsatile system, so I cannot give you a definite answer. However, I think that the pulsatile system is advantageous for the peripheral tissues. We measured the osmotic pressure and levels of plasma protein and found the decrease in these parameters to be less with the pulsatile than with the nonpulsatile system in another study.

*Adachi:* About 5 years ago VA bypass appeared to be a very effective treatment for the cardiogenic shock patient. Our recent experience though would suggest that the results from this treatment are not so good and that left ventricular assist is superior.

*Imamura* (Tokyo Women's Medical College): I think there is a problem associated with the VAD, which increases the left ventricular afterload. We usually use IABP along with VAB, otherwise the left ventricular function may deteriorate.

*Irie:* If the failure is only on the left side, IABP is very effective. But if both ventricles are injured, IABP alone is not so effective. In most cases, biventricular failure is encountered after cardiac surgery, so the function of both ventricles has to be assisted. It is easy to change from ordinary cardiac bypass to this kind of circuit.

*Imamura:* With VAB alone, it is necessary to have flow of about 75% or more to support the left ventricle effectively. However, with this amount of flow support, other problems appear, for example, the mitral valve does not open; the VAB flow is limited. Adequate flow is estimated to be about 20% or 30%.

*Irie:* With our circuit, bypass flow is obtained at 60% to 120% of preoperative cardiac output. Sufficient pump flow can thus be obtained with this circuit.

# 16. Ventricular assist device with built-in trileaflet polyurethane valves

Mitsuo Umezu*, Hiroyuki Noda, Yoshiyuki Taenaka, Masayuki Kinoshita, Takehisa Matsuda, Hiroo Iwata, Junji Seki, Kozaburo Hayashi, Takao Nakamura, Eisuke Tatsumi, Akihiko Yagura, Setsuo Takatani, Hisateru Takano, and Tetsuzo Akutsu[1]

**Summary.** A diaphragm-type ventricular assist device (VAD) with one-piece conduit valves made of polyurethane (PU) was developed and its hydrodynamic function, durability, and antithrombogenicity were evaluated.

The mock-loop test indicated that as a result of rapid closure of the leaflet, a pump with the PU valves yielded equivalent output to that of ordinary Björk-Shiley (BS) valves, although a pressure gradient across the PU valves was higher than with BS valves. A durability test, using an accelerated fatigue tester of disk-rotating type, proved that failure occurred in 5% of cases after 2.6 million cycles, corresponding to 1 month's pumping. Fourteen PU valves with the leaflet thickness of 0.30 mm were used for four animal experiments. The animals were divided into two groups: a high-bypass flow group (3.5–4.5 l/min) and a low-flow group (1.8–2.5 l/min). When a thrombus was detected, the pump was changed. In the high-flow group, thrombi on the pump inlet side appeared on the 8th, 16th, and 17th pumping days, while there was no thrombus on the pump outlet side over the same period. Conversely, at the low-flow rate, thrombus formation was found almost simultaneously at the pump inlet and outlet in three of four pairs of valves, on the 5th, 13th, and 25th pumping days. In conclusion, a pump with our prototype PU valves has adequate hydrodynamic performance and acceptable durability for 1 month. Although the antithrombogenicity of the present model was not satisfactory, improvement of the design should upgrade the in vivo performance.

**Key words:** Accelerated fatigue test—Polyurethane valve—Conduit valve—Ventricular assist device—Thrombus formation

Many clinical results with the ventricular assist device (VAD) have shown it to be one of the most effective treatments for patients with severe heart disease, and the quality of the VAD system has been improving. However, the problem of the great expense of the VAD system, especially on pumps where permanent commercial valves are incorporated, still remains. To reduce the cost of the pumps, polyurethane (PU) valves for temporary VAD have been developed, focusing on the simplification of the fabrication technique. This approach is different from previous efforts [1, 2]. This paper deals with in vitro as well as in vivo evaluation of the VAD pump with our prototype PU valves.

## Materials and methods

### Fabrication of pump and valves

Both pump and valves were fabricated with segmented PU (Toyobo TM series) [3]. The pump is a pneumatically driven, diaphragm type, the design of which is the same as that of a commercially available one made by Toyobo Company. In this study, PU valves, developed in our laboratory, were mounted in the VAD pump instead of ordinary tilting disk [Björk-Shiley (BS)] valves, as shown in Fig. 16.1. The PU valves were fabricated by a dipping method. An aluminium mold, the configuration of which was similar to that of the Ionescu-Shiley valve, was dipped into TM-5 solution at a concentration of 10%. Between each dip, the mold was stored in an oven to evaporate the solvent. After the above procedure was repeated five times, the mold was inserted into a polyvinyl chloride (PVC) tube with the same diameter as the mold. Then, this assembly was dipped again three times in TM-5 solution at a concentration of 5%. After the final overnight drying procedure, the one-piece conduit-type PU valve was easily removed from the mold. The leaflet thickness in each valve could be controlled to around 0.30 mm. Since these procedures were simple and reproducible, the current rejection rate of our PU valves is less than 1%, as shown in Fig. 16.2.

### Hydrodynamic evaluation

The PU valves were mounted into a straight pipe and the pressure drop across the valve was measured by changing the steady flow rate. The test for dynamic pump function was performed by using our pulse duplicator system and the relations between pump

---

[1]Department of Artificial Organs, National Cardiovascular Center Research Institute, 5-7-1 Fujishiro-dai, Suita, Osaka, 565 Japan
*Present address: St. Vincent Hospital, Victoria St., Darlinghurst, NSW 2010, Australia

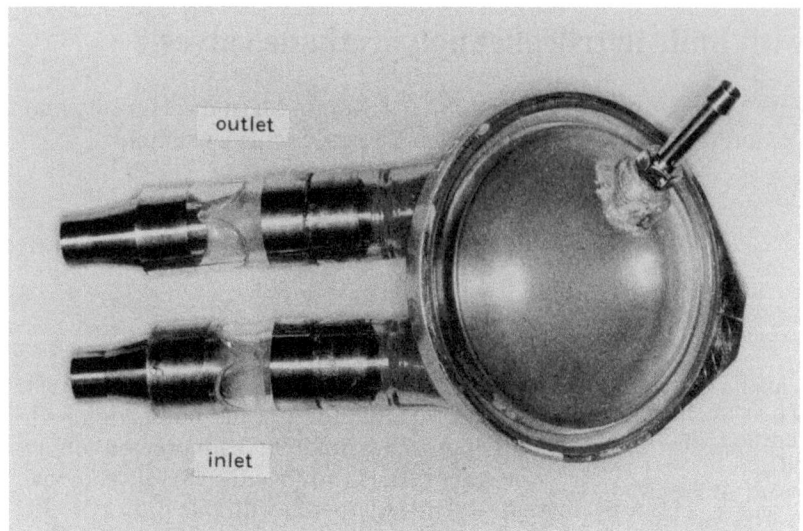

**Fig. 16.1.** Diaphragm type ventricular assist pump with polyurethane valves

flow and percentage systole—systolic fraction in one cardiac cycle (Fs)—were obtained under various pumping conditions.

### Durability test

Since adequate durability of the VAD pump with BS valves had already been certified through chronic animal experiments, the durability test of the PU valves alone was carried out using the Helmholtz-type accelerated fatigue tester [4]. A schematic drawing and basic hydrodynamic waveforms at the valve inlet and outlet under standard drive conditions are given in Fig. 16.3.

### In vitro hemolysis test

Prior to the animal experiments, an in vitro hemolysis test was carried out using a closed-loop mock circulatory system, which consisted of a VAD pump, inlet and outlet compliance tanks, and a variable resistance element (clamp screw) [5]. This simple circuit was filled with bovine fresh blood with a hematcrit of 40%. Two circuits with the same design with different heart valves (PU and BS) were prepared for this test. The blood was circulated for 24 h and the changes in plasma free hemoglobin in each circuit were measured while the pump flow was maintained at a constant level.

### Chronic animal experiments

In vivo evaluation of PU valves was carried out on goats weighting 30–50 kg. The LVAD with the PU valves was implanted in the same way as in normal surgical procedures (Fig. 16.4). The pulse rate was

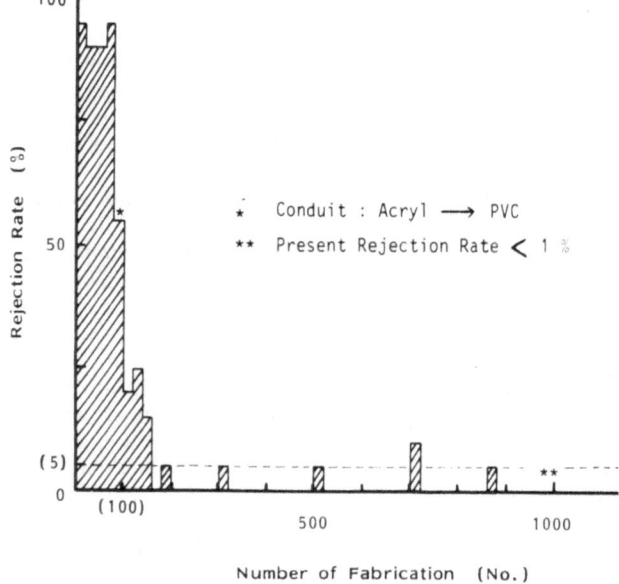

**Fig. 16.2.** Improvement of fabrication technique of conduit-type polyurethane valves

fixed at 70 beats/min throughout the time of LVAD pumping. The experiments were divided into two groups; high-bypass flow group (3.5–4.5 l/min) and low-bypass flow group (1.8—2.5 l/min). Anticoagulation therapy was not used except for the time of LVAD implantation. When a thrombus was detected, the valves were removed together with the pump by cutting the conduits in the vicinity of the reduce connectors. Then, the pump was changed. When the bypass flow could not be maintained within the range given above, the experiments were terminated.

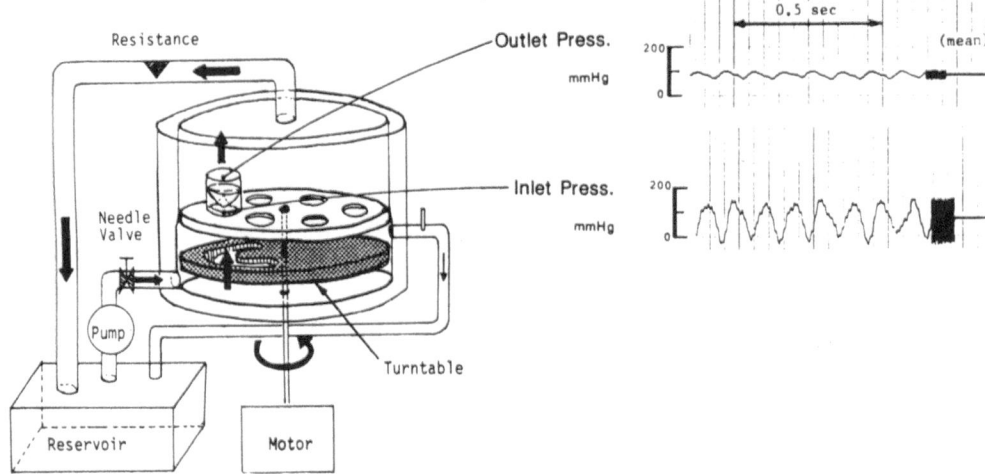

**Fig. 16.3.** PU valve fatigue tester (Helmholtz type). Standard drive condition: rotational speed 1000/min, pump flow 24 L/min, afterload 80 mmHg, six valves tested

## Result

### Hydrodynamics of pump with PU valves

Figure 16.5 shows the pressure gradient across the PU valves and dynamic function of the VAD pump. The pressure gradient curves were not uniform with the increase in flow because of a different opening resistance among the three leaflets due to a slight difference in the leaflet thickness. Although the resistance of the PU valves with a leaflet thickness of 0.30 mm was higher than that of BS valves, a pump with the PU valves yielded an equivalent output because the reflux volume of the PU valves was much less than that of the BS valves owing to the rapid closure of the valve leaflets.

### Durability tests

The results of the durability test are summarized in Table 16.1 [4]. The present valve failure rate after 2.6 million cycles, which corresponds to about 1 month's pumping, was less than 5% under standard drive conditions (flow rate 26.0/6 = 4.3 l/min; afterload 80 mmHg). Most of the valve failure due to the leaflet tear occurred in the vicinity of the conduit-leaflet junction.

### Hemolysis test

Figure 16.6 shows the relations between the level of plasma free hemoglobin and pumping duration [5]. In this figure, the pump inlet and outlet pressure and inflow waveforms are also indicated. The data indi-

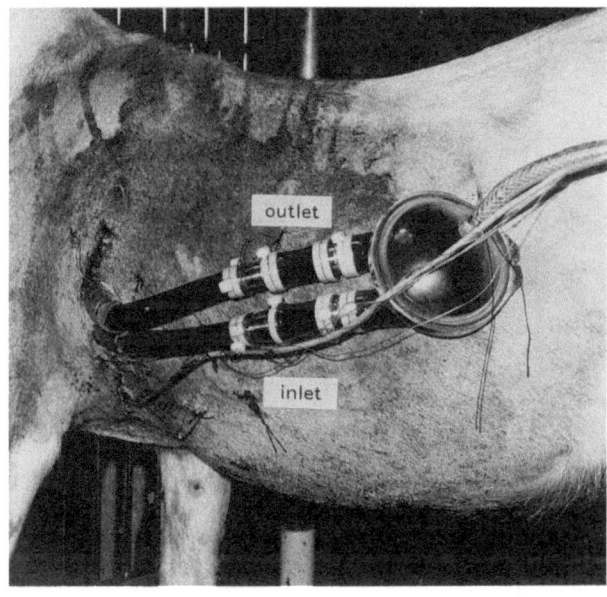

**Fig. 16.4.** In vivo evaluation of PU valves in the goat

cate that the extraordinary high amplitude spike, which is known as the water hammer (WH) phenomenon, was significantly observed at both sides of the disk (BS valves). The amount of plasma free hemoglobin in the circuit with BS valves was 150 mg/dl after 24-h pumping, whereas that with the PU valves was 75 mg/dl. In the case of the PU valves, the drive pressure was maintained higher than in the BS valves. These two facts suggest that the level of hemolysis is closely related to the level of WH.

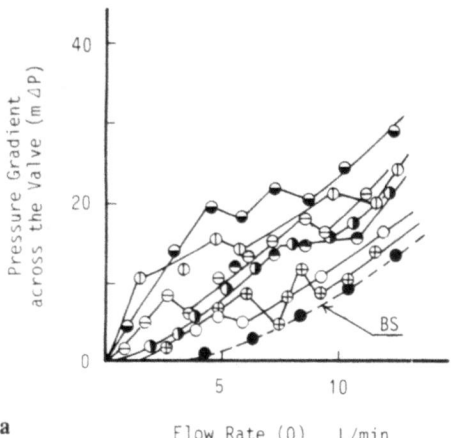

a

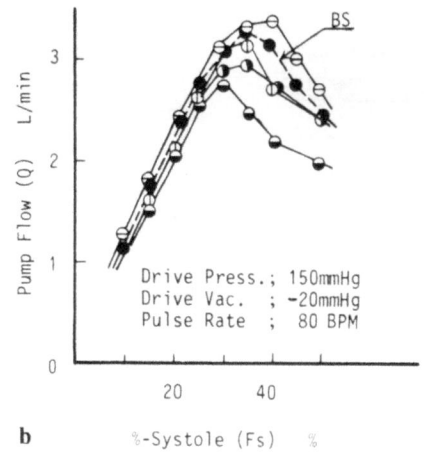

b

**Fig. 16.5a, b.** Basic hydrodynamics of polyurethane valves (PU valves; material—TM-5, coating times—five). **a** Steady flow; **b** pulsatile flow

**Table 16.1.** Durability test results of polyurethane valves by accerelated fatigue tester

| Exp. no. | Rotational speed (rpm) | Testing duration (days) | Cyclic number (cycles) | Number of valves (N) | Number of valves failed (F) |
|---|---|---|---|---|---|
| 1 | 180 | 10 | $2.6 \times 10^6$ | 7 | 1 |
| 2 | 600 | 3 | $2.6 \times 10^6$ | 34 | 0 |
| 3 | 1000 | 1.8 | $2.6 \times 10^6$ | 21 | 2 |
| Total | | | | 62 | 3 |

Present failure ratio $(F/N) < 4.8\%$

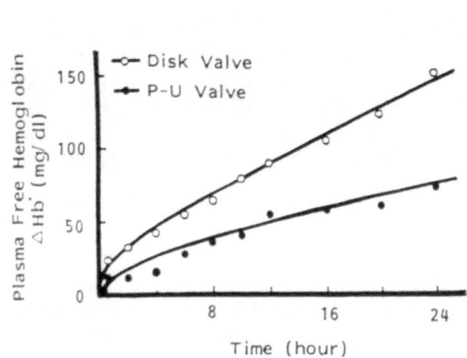

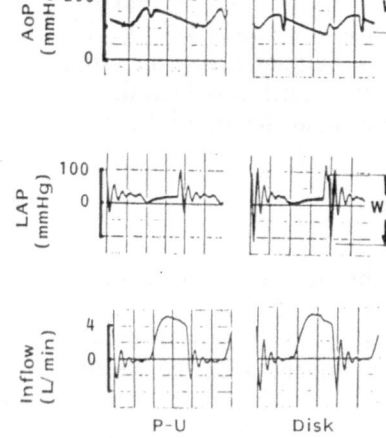

**Fig. 16.6.** Relations of plasma free hemoglobin to pumping time in different types of valves

## In vivo evaluation

Fourteen PU valves were used in four chronic goat experiments. The time-course of the bypass flow in all experiments is plotted in Fig. 16.7. The bypass flow in each case was maintained within the above setting range. In three cases (P8713, P8701, P8622), the

experiments were terminated due to the inflow obstruction. At the time of autopsy, overgrowth of an infected thrombus at the side holes of the inlet cannula was noted. In the other experiment (P8711), the animal accidentally bled to death due to a disconnection between the inflow cannula and inlet valve. Thrombus formation in the chronic experiments is

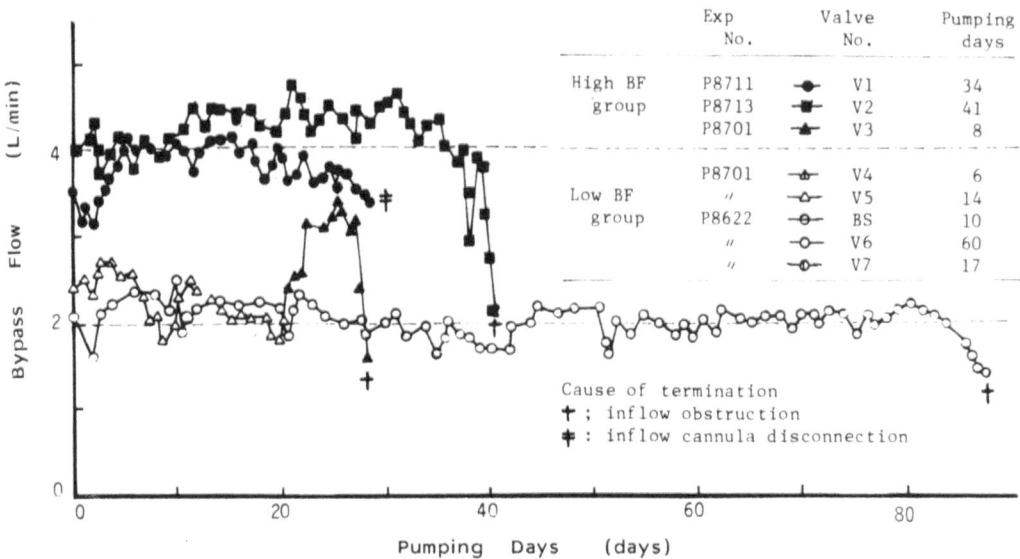

**Fig. 16.7.** Time-course of bypass flow in chronic animal experiments for the evaluation of polyurethane valves

**Table 16.2.** In vivo evaluation of polyurethane valves

| | Exp. no. | Valve no. | Pumping days | Day of thrombus formation | |
|---|---|---|---|---|---|
| | | | | Inlet | Outlet |
| High BF group (3.5–4.5 l/min) | P8711 | V1 | 34 | 17 | — |
| | P8713 | V2 | 41 | 16[a], 40 | — |
| | P8701 | V3 | 8 | 8 | — |
| Low BF group (1.8–2.5 l/min) | P8701 | V4 | 6 | 5 | 5 |
| | P8701 | V5 | 14 | 14 | 8[a], 13 |
| | P8622 | V6 | 60 | 25[a], 60 | 25 |
| | P8622 | V7 | 17 | 17 | — |

[a] Thrombus disappeared after detection
*BF* blood flow, — no thrombus formation

summarized in Table 16.2. In the high-flow rate group, thrombi on the pump inlet side appeared on the 8th, 16th, and 17th pumping days, while there was no thrombus formation at the outlet valves for the same pumping duration. In the group with low flow rate, thrombi formed more frequently than in the high-flow rate group. In three of four pairs of valves, thrombi on both sides were detected almost simultaneously. They appeared on the 5th, 13th, and 25th pumping days. In the case of P8622, the valves (V6 in Fig. 16.7) were evaluated over 2 months, which was the longest period of usage. In this case, thrombi were detected once on both sides on the 25th pumping day and disappeared on the 27th. Subsequently, a small thrombus ($0.5 \times 3$ mm) was detected on the inlet side on the 60th pumping day, while there was no thrombus formation at the outlet valve during the same period. These valves are shown in Fig. 16.8.

Every thrombus in these experiments was detected at the bottom of one of the sinuses, as shown in Fig. 16.9. In all cases, this sinus was located at the lower part of the valve. There was no significant difference in the size of the thrombus between the high and low flow rates at the inlet valve. The size of the biggest thrombus was $3 \times 12$ mm, as shown in Fig 16.10.

## Discussion

### Polyurethane valve design

Most PU valves of a single piece conduit type currently under development have pockets similar to the aortic sinus, aiming to reduce thrombus formation by a good washout effect [6]. Different to this type, our prototype PU valve was built in a conduit with concave

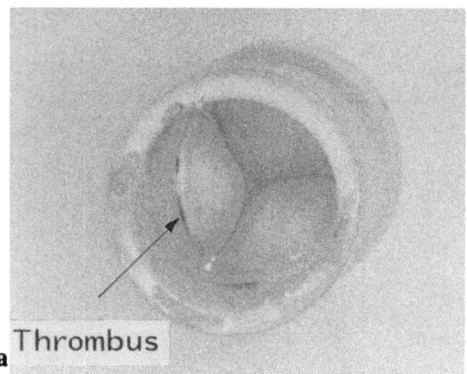
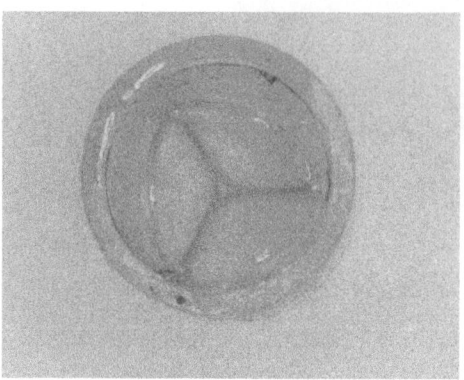

**Fig. 16.8. a** Inlet and **b** outlet PU valves after 2 months, pumping (P8622)

| Exp. No.<br>Pumping days | P8711<br>34 | P8713<br>41 | P8701<br>8 |
|---|---|---|---|
| INLET | (3x12) | (1x8) | (0.5x2) |
| OUTLET | (−) | (−) | (−) |

**a**

**Fig. 16.9a, b.** In vivo evaluation of the PU valves; location and size of the thrombus formed at the bottom of the sinus. **a** High-flow rate group; **b** low-flow rate group. Figures in parentheses indicate size of thrombus (width × length in mm)

| Exp.No.<br>Pumping days | P8701<br>6 | P8701<br>14 | P8622<br>60 | P8622<br>17 |
|---|---|---|---|---|
| INLET | (3x12) | (1x3) | (0.5x3) | (0.5x2) |
| OUTLET | (2x10) | (2x5) | (−) | (−) |

**b**  ( ) ; Size of thrombus (width x length in mm )

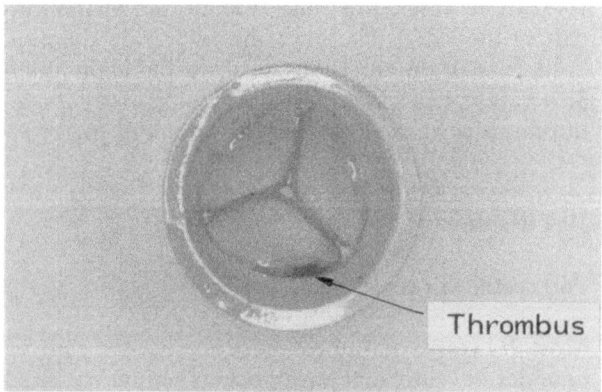

**Fig. 16.10.** The biggest thrombus appeared in the PU valves tested

sinuses, because simplification of the fabrication technique was considered to be the most important factor. Following flow visualization studies using the hydrogen bubble method, the design with the aortic sinus was the most effective for trileaflet valves to achieve an adequate washout on the inner surface of the conduit. These data also suggested that PU valves with a concave sinus, like our prototype, ranked next, and the straight tube was the worst design [7]. The optimum shape of the conduit should be discussed after a higher quality valve has been manufactured, because different mechanical characteristics among the three leaflets of the present PU valves were observed in vitro tests owing to small differences in the leaflet thickness.

## Hydrodynamics of PU valves

As shown in Fig 16.5, the pressure gradient across PU valves was higher than that across BS valves. It is easy to reduce the pressure gradien by decreasing the leaflet thickness. However, from the hydrodynamic point of view, the present PU valves would be suitable for temporary VAD, even if a somewhat higher drive pressure were necessary.

## Valve durability

Even though the VAD pumps were driven under high flow in animal experiments, the leaflet of the PU valves was not torn after a period of 1 month. As expressed in Table 16.1, the PU valves were durable for 1 month's pumping under the accelerated condition [4]. The conditions of the simulation with the valve durability tester were rather more severe than in the actual experiment. Consequently, the guaranteed pumping duration of the VAD with the prototype PU valves was considered to be more than 1 month from the data of durability tests as well as animal experiments.

## Stress-induced thrombus formation.

The following two results were obtained from the animal experiments: (a) The thrombus at the outlet only formed in the low-bypass flow group; (b) the thrombus at the inlet appeared even if the bypass flow was kept at a high flow level. It is commonly accepted that thrombi and calcification might be reduced if the stress on the leaflets could be decreased [2]. The stress under VAD pumping may be very much higher than the pumping of the natural heart, judging from the data on WH measured in the vicinity of the valves [5]. These data also indicate that WH levels at the high-flow rate were remarkably high at both the inlet and outlet of the VAD, whereas the WH level on the pump outlet side was greater than that of the inlet at the low-flow rate. The data can partly explain the two experimental results mentioned above. As a result, stress may be one of the main causes of thrombus formation in addition to the washout effect [3].

## Cause of termination of experiments

The experiments in three cases were terminated by inflow obstruction. Since the forward flow resistance of the PU valve was higher than that of the BS valve, the increase in diastolic vacuum pressure was necessary to obtain adequate inflow filling. This was considered to be one of the reasons for the inflow obstruction; however, similar findings were observed when disk valves were employed for the VAD. The relation between pump-driving condition and thrombus formation must be clarified after the accumulation of further data.

## Conclusion

The VAD pump with the prototype PU valves was evaluated in in vitro and in vivo experiments. The results may be summarized as follows.

—A fabrication technique for PU valves for temporary VAD has been established.

—The VAD pump with the PU valves had equivalent hydrodynamic characteristics to that of BS valves.

—The PU valves were durable under VAD pumping for more than a month.

—Thrombi formed more frequently on the inlet side than on the outlet.

—When the bypass flow was decreased, the incidence of thrombus formation became high.

—Although the causes of thrombus formation have not been clarified yet, improvement of the design promises upgrading of the in vivo performances.

**Acknowledgments.** This study was supported financially in part by a Grant-in-Aid for Scientific Research from the Ministry of Education (No. 62870056) and a Research Grant for Cardiovascular Disease (60A-1) from the Ministry of Health and Welfare.

## References

1. Herold M, Lo HB, Reul H, Mückter H, Taguchi K, Giersiepen M, Birkle G, Hollweg G, Rau G, Messer BJ (1987) The Helmholtz-Institute-tri-leaflet polyurethane heart valve prosthesis: Design, manufacturing and first in-vitro and in-vivo results. In: Planck H (ed) Polyurethane in Biomedical engineering II. Elsevier, Amsterdam, pp 231–256
2. Wisman CB, Pierce WS, Donachy JH, Pae We, Myers JL, Prophet GA (1982) A polyurethane trileaflet cardiac valve prosthesis: in-vitro and in-vivo studies, Trans Am Soc Artif Intern Organs 28: 164–168
3. Umezu M, Noda H, Nogawa A, Nakatani T, Yoshiwara T, Yamadera Y, Taenaka Y, Fukuda S, Iwata H, Matsuda T, Adachi S, Tsuchiya K, Takano H, Akutsu T (1985) Development of built-in polyurethane valves for ventricular assist device. Jpn J Artif Organs 14: 1120–1123
4. Umezu M, Tanaka T, Hayashi K, Iwata H, Seki J, Matsuda T, Takano H, Akutsu T, Ueki Y, Inada K, Tsuchiya K (1987) Accelerated fatigue testing of polyurethane valves for ventricular assist device. Jpn J Artif Organs 16: 362–365
5. Umezu M, Tanaka T, Tsuchiya K (1986) Water hammer phenomenon observed in the artificial heart. Papers on the 1st Symposium on Fluid Control, The Society of Instrument and Control Engineers, Japan, pp 163–168
6. Jansen J, Grevelink JMJ, Kim SW, Kolf WJ, Reul H (1986) New polyurethane trileaflet valves: performance and blood compatibility, Life Support Systems, Proceedings 8th ISAO, pp 130–132
7. Inada K, Ueki Y, Miyakawa A, Tsuchiya K, Umezu M, Tanaka T, Takano H, Akutsu T (1987) Flow visualization in the vicinity of the valve built in the conduit for ventricular assist device, Jpn J Artif Organs 16: 358–361

## Discussion

*Imachi* (University of Tokyo): How do you decide the leaflet thickness; is this just based on experience? Why does the thrombus form inside the valve? Thirdly, how would you compare anti-thrombogenicity and durability of your valve with that of Dr. Lederman?

*Umezu* (National Cardiovascular Center): The valve thickness is determined based on in vitro hydrodynamic tests. The leaflet thickness of the valve is now around 0.3 mm. With regard to the second question, all of the thrombus was observed at the bottom of one leaflet pocket; gravity appears to have played a role here

*Imachi:* Might it not be related to valve thickness? If the leaflet is very thick, there is perhaps inadequate washout when the valve opens.

*Umezu:* I do not think that leaflet thickness plays a major role here.

*Lederman* (ABIOMED, Inc.): I think that the dierence in results between our valve and that of Dr. Umezu is largely attributable to design rather than to material. I noticed in your pressure versus flow curves that the relationship is not continuous. The zigzag pattern of the curve suggests that the leaflets are opening one at a time. If the situation occurs in low-flow conditions, one leaflet will open and remain open, while the other two will not open at all. It is likely that blood will become trapped behind the open leaflet and a clot will develop. We have observed this phenomenon with our valves. The thickness distribution of the leaflets and the similarity in thickness profile of all three leaflets play a very important role in their opening gradually. Your curves clearly show that they are not doing that but instead they are opening one at a time. From your data, I would infer that you have two memory positions, one closed and one open with severe snapping or buckling.

The valves that you showed did not have sinuses and you indicated that you intend to introduce these in future. I think this will help a good deal by insuring that there is good washout behind the leaflets.

# 17. Right ventricular function during left ventricular assistance evaluated by two-dimensional echocardiography

Isao Yada, Chi-Ming Wei, Ryoji Hattori, Manabu Okabe, Tamotsu Morimoto, Tetsuo Mizutani, and Minoru Kusagawa[1]

**Summary.** Right ventricular (RV) function during left heart bypass (LHB) using centrifugal blood pumps was studied in 20 mongrel dogs, which were divided into normal and failing heart groups. RV function was evaluated hemodynamically and by a 2D echocardiography method. Incremental changes in LHB flow ratio from control, 25%, 50%, 75% to the maximum of 85%–100% resulted in decrements of the interventricular septum (IVS) segmental shortening fraction (SSF) from 54% $\pm$ 12%, 43% $\pm$ 5%, 42% $\pm$ 2%, 35% $\pm$ 7% to 1%, respectively. When the LHB ratio was increased from 75% to the maximum level, significant reduction in the RV ejection fraction and a completely depressed left ventricle (LV) were observed. The cross-sectional echo image also revealed profoundly depressed SSF of the IVS and of the nearby RV wall. The LV decompression with the maximum LHB seemed to decrease the contraction capability of the LV wall, including the IVS subsequently causing reduction of the RV wall. This finding was more pronounced in the failing heart group. The excessive LHB for a prolonged duration not only reduces the RV wall contraction capability but may lead to right heart failure.

Our result, therefore, suggests that the LHB ratio of about 75% is optimum for maintenance of normal cardiac function, particularly that of the right heart.

**Key words:** Left heart bypass—Left ventricular assist—Right ventricular function

Circulatory support using a left ventricular assist device (LVAD) is an effective means of treating patients with profound heart failure when drug therapy or intra-aortic balloon pumping (IABP) assistance has no effect. However, with increased usage of the LVAD, the concomitant occurrence of right ventricular failure has also been reported, and this requires extensive medical treatment with catecholamines and sometimes biventricular support with two assist devices [1, 2].

The causes of such right heart failures have been investigated in various experimental studies, but a thorough understanding is lacking. In this study [3–7], changes in right heart function during LVAD assistance were studied in experimental animals using an echocardiography method to elucidate the possible mechanisms related to right heart failure during left heart bypass.

## Materials and methods

### Animal model and experimental method

Left heart bypass, from the left atrium to the descending aorta, was performed in 20 mongrel dogs (mean body weight $24 \pm 4$ kg) using a Bio-pump (Biomedicus, MN, USA). Dogs were anesthetized with an intramuscular injection of ketamine (15 mg/kg), followed by an intravenous injection of pentobarbital (20 mg/kg). After intubation, anesthesia was maintained with a continuous infusion of pentobarbital at the rate of 3 mg/kg/h, and respiration was controlled using a respirator. To prevent the development of atelectasis, end expiratory pressure was set in the positive range of 5–8 cm $H_2O$. Blood gases were frequently checked to correct any evidence of acidosis.

The chest was opened through the left fifth intercostal space. A Sarns 36-F drainage cannula was inserted into the left atrium through its appendage, while a T-shaped return cannula, fabricated in our laboratory, was positioned inside the descending aorta, as shown in Fig. 17.1.

The LVAD circuit was primed with a fluid mixture of blood (10 ml/kg), mannitol (5 ml/kg), and Hespander (5 ml/kg). During the left heart bypass, blood activated coagulation time (ACT) levels were maintained at twice the normal level by continuous intravenous infusion of heparin to prevent blood coagulation.

Monitoring included right (RAP) and left atrial pressures (LAP), left ventricular pressure (LVP), and pulmonary arterial (PAP) and aortic pressures (AoP). A Swan-Ganz catheter was inserted into the pulmonary artery for measurement of the right cardiac output, while the left heart output was determined by implanting an electromagnetic flow probe (Nihon Koden, Tokyo Japan) on the ascending aorta. The bypass flow through the LVAD was monitored using a cannulating-type flow probe connected in the outflow port of the device.

[1]Department of Thoracic Surgery, Mie University School of Medicine, 2-174 Edobashi, Tsu, Mie, 514 Japan

The experimental animals were divided into two groups: one had normal heart function, while in the other group left heart failure was induced by ligating the left anterior descending coronary artery. In both groups, LVAD bypass flow ratio, defined as bypass flow divided by the sum of the bypass flow and aortic flow, was varied from 25%, 50%, 75%, to the maximum of about 85%–100%, where at each bypass flow ratio, cardiac function was studied from the hemodynamic parameters and also using an echocardiographic system (YHP Co. Boston, MA, USA). With regard to infarction size in the left ventricle, the nitroblue tetrazolium (NBT) staining method indicated that it extended to about 30%–40% of the total left ventricle.

### Echocardiographic measurement

The echocardiography probe was placed directly against the posterolateral wall of the left ventricle. After calibrating the measurement at the annular level of the tricuspid valve, cross-sectional views of both ventricles were recorded by short-axis echocardiography. In addition, the movement of the interventricular septum and right ventricular (RV) free wall was quantitatively determined following the procedure described below.

As shown in the upper part of Fig. 17.2, the segmental lengths of both the IVS and RV wall measured along their internal surfaces were obtained during the end-diastolic and end-systolic periods. From these data, the segmental shortening fraction of the IVS, defined as (EDSL–ESSL)/EDSL, that of the RV free wall, and the total segmental shortening of the RV (sum of the IVS SSF and the RV free wall SSF) were determined. The middle part of Fig. 17.2 shows the method of calculating the thickness of the IVS and RV free wall. The IVS wall was divided into four equal sections and measurements were made along the lines originating from the RV internal surface and

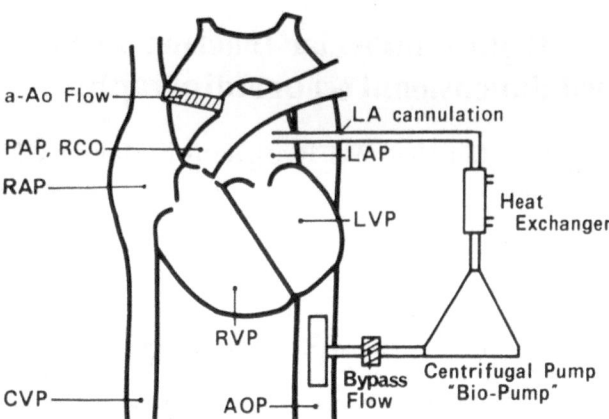

**Fig. 17.1.** Experimental setup of left ventricular assist device. *a-Ao Flow* ascending aortic flow, *LAP* left atrial pressure, *RCO* right cardiac output, *LVP* left ventricular pressure, *PAP* pulmonary arterial pressure, *RVP* right ventricular pressure, *RAP* right atrial pressure, *AOP* aortic pressure, *CVP* central venous pressure

perpendicular to the external surface points denoted by A, B, B', C, and C'. From these data, the percentage wall thickening, defined as (EDT–EST)/EDT, was calculated for each segment. In addition, the internal surface area of the RV was calculated from the computer trace; from this, changes in the RV area from the end-diastolic to end-systolic phase (RVEDA–RVESA = RV area) and the RV ejection fraction (RVEF = RVEDA–RVESA/RVEDA) were obtained. The lower part of Fig. 17.2 shows the relation between the RV volume and RV area obtained from the 2D echocardiography. In this case, the RV volume change was induced by injecting normal saline. The correlation coefficient between the injected saline volume and the RV area obtained from the echocardiographic method was 0.98 with a regression equation of $Y = 0.49X - 2.98$.

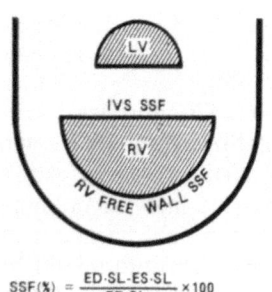
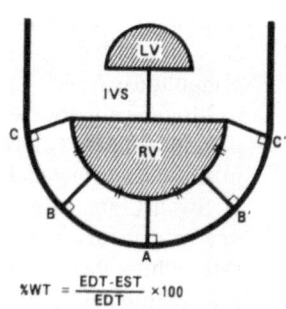
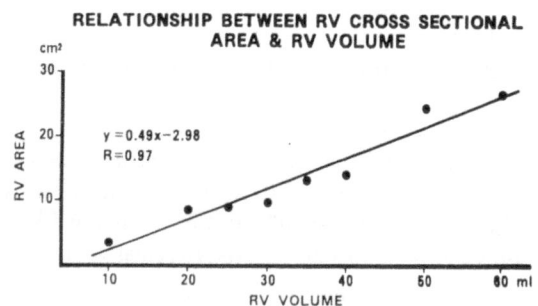

**Fig. 17.2.** Method of measuring segmental shortening fraction (*SSF*) and percentage wall thickening (*%WT*) based on echocardiography. *LV* left ventricle, *RV* right ventricle, *IVS* interventricular septum, *SL* segmental length, *ED* end diastole, *ES* end systole, *T* wall thickness

## Results

The entire series of measurements was completed for each of the 20 dogs. The changes in the RV output are shown in Fig. 17.3. In both the normal and failing heart models, there was a tendency for RV output to increase with an increase in bypass ratio, but the failing heart exhibited a higher rate of increase.

Echocardiograms of both ventricles during 75% bypass (left side) and maximum bypass (right side) are shown for both end-diastolic and end-systolic periods in Fig. 17.4. It was clear from these pictures that the left ventricular cavity was completely decompressed, while that of the RV was significantly distended. At that time, ascending aortic flow decreased approximately to zero, there was almost no pulse in the aortic pressure patterns, and, based on the 2D echocardiogram, aortic and mitral valves remained in the closed position and no leaflet movement was evident.

Segmental shortening of the IVS and RV free wall was examined. The SSF of the IVS in both normal and failing hearts was 35% ± 7% during 75% bypass, but it became almost 0%, indicating no IVS shortening, during the maximum bypass time. On the other hand, the SSF of the RV free wall ranged from 44% to 49% during 75% bypass, and although it decreased to 25% ± 2.5% and 15% ± 1.1% in the normal and failing hearts, respectively, appreciable reduction in the SSF of the RV free wall was recognized during the

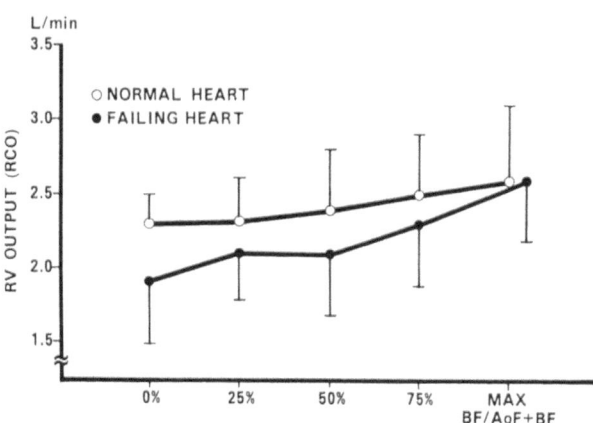

**Fig. 17.3.** Changes in right ventricular output at each bypass flow rate. *BF* bypass flow; *AoF* ascending aortic flow

maximum bypass time. Also, the RV total shortening fraction exhibited a considerably larger reduction when the bypass ratio was changed from 75% to the maximum ($P < 0.005$), as shown in Fig. 17.5.

Percentage changes in the wall thickening, as obtained from the echocardiographic method, are shown in Fig. 17.6. In both normal and failing hearts, the percentage wall thickening of the IVS was 24%–25% and 22%–23% during the control and 75% bypass ratio, respectively; during the maximum bypass ratio it became 0% and no IVS shortening was

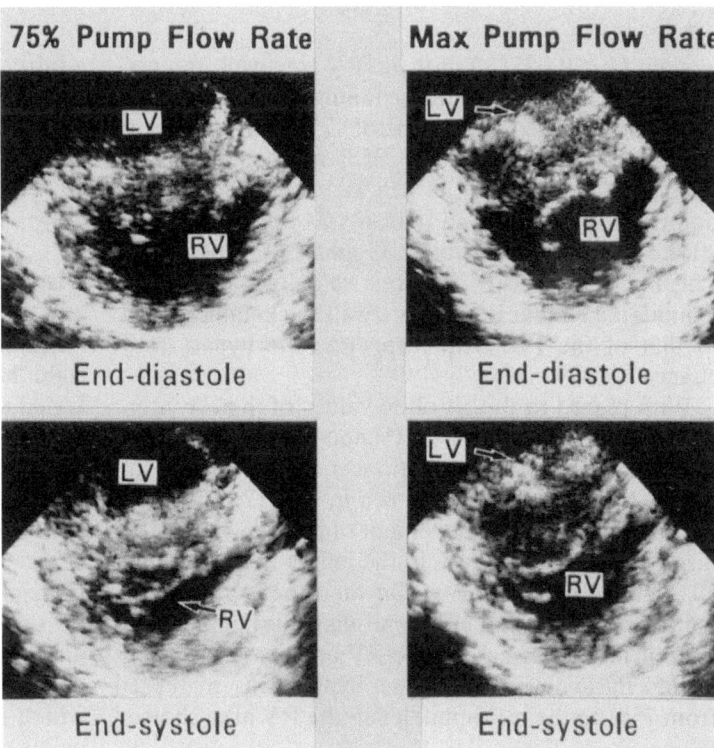

**Fig. 17.4.** Echocardiogram during left heart bypass at 75% and maximum bypass flow rate. *LV* left ventricle, *RV* right ventricle

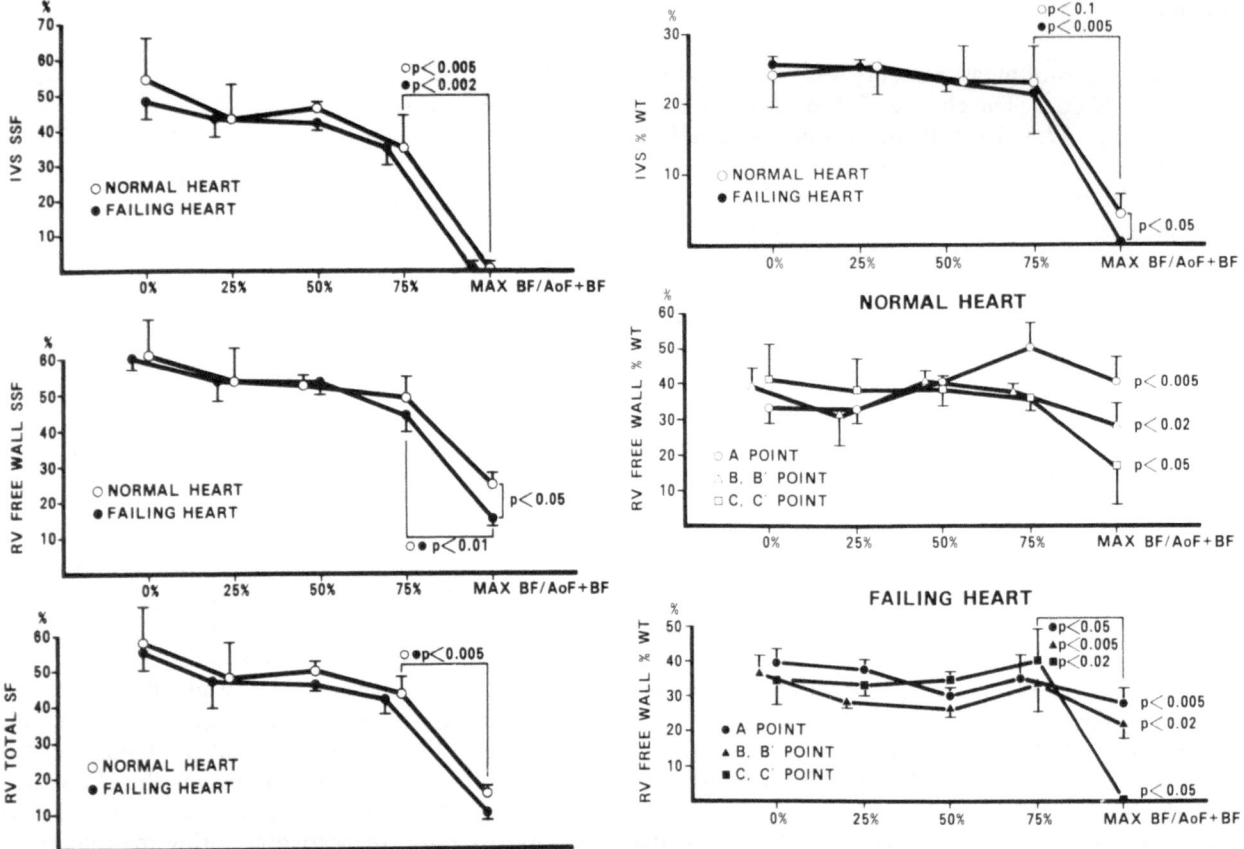

**Fig. 17.5.** Changes in segmental shortening fraction (*SSF*) at each bypass flow rate

**Fig. 17.6.** Changes in percentage wall thickening (%*WT*) at each bypass flow rate

evident ($P < 0.005$). As for the RV free wall, the percentage wall thickening of the failing heart showed the following changes from control, 75%, to maximum bypass: from 39% ± 4% to 35% ± 7% at point A, from 36% ± 5% and 34% ± 9% to 22% ± 4% at points B and B′, and from 34.5% ± 7%, and 40% ± 9% to 0% at points C and C′, respectively. This indicates that the RV free wall closer to the IVS exhibited a similar percentage wall thickening change to that of the IVS with respect to the bypass ratio change.

With regard to the absolute values of the RV area, both RV end-diastolic and RV end-systolic areas during the maximum bypass ratio were much larger than the 75% bypass ratio, as shown in Fig. 17.7. In addition, the paradoxical movement of the IVS was recognized at over 25% bypass in the failing heart and over 50% in the normal heart. On the other hand, along with the increase in the RV end-diastolic and RV end-systolic areas, increase in the RV area was also recognized. Particularly when the bypass was increased from 75% to the maximum level, the RV area showed

a fairly significant increase in both normal and failing hearts. However, RV ejection fraction changes of both groups showed a notable decrease when the bypass ratio was varied from 75% to the maximum ($P < 0.002$).

## Discussion

Although there have been several reports concerning right heart failure during left heart bypass using a LVAD, the mechanism leading to right heart failure is not clear. When such situations arise, catecholamine and/or biventricular support utilizing two assist devices may be used. According to Pierce [8], right heart failure occurred in 6 of 22 patients who had had left ventricular assists after cardiac surgery. Minor deviations in RV function occur as a result of left ventricular decompression associated with LVAD. Farrar et al. [9] suggested that RV function depends on the contractile state of the undecompressed left ventricle, which is mediated through the IVS. Watanabe et al.

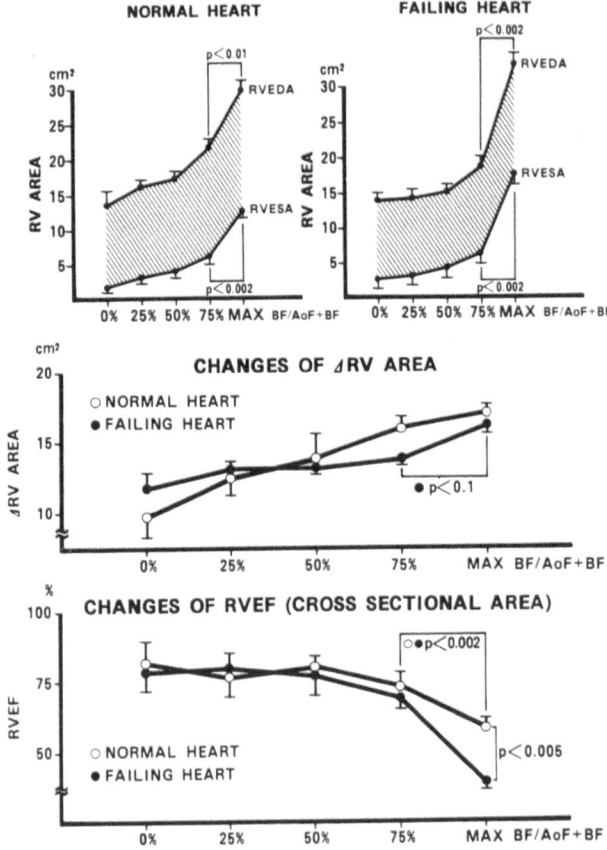

**Fig. 17.7.** Changes in right ventricular ejection fraction (*RVEF*) at each bypass flow rate

to Harada et al. [11], when the IVS function is impaired, left heart bypass may not contribute to RV functional improvement. Moreover, Miyamoto et al. [7] recognized appreciable reduction in dp/dt of the RV during left ventricular decompression; they also found that the systolic SSF of the IVS became almost 0% as evaluated by 2D echocardiography, which is directly related to the impaired function. From these facts, it is apparent that the left heart bypass flow rate should be set at an optimum level, but not at the maximum level, so as to reflect appropriately the body's basal requirements.

Also, in our experiment, left ventricular decompression and concomitant development of RV distension with the start of left heart bypass were observed where these were more prominent in the failing heart animal. With the increase in the left heart bypass ratio, an increase in RV end-diastolic area and left ventricular end-diastolic area/RV end-diastolic area as obtained from the 2D echocardiography were observed. Particularly, when the bypass ratio was increased from 75% to the maximum level, RV ejection fraction area determined from echocardiography decreased significantly, SSF and percentage wall thickening of the IVS became almost zero, and the RV free wall close to the IVS became nearly immobile, thus leaving only the central portion of the RV to be contractile. The suppressed left ventricular wall movement during left ventricular decompression, mediated through the IVS to the RV free wall, seems to restrict the movement of the wall near the IVS. If this condition is sustained for a prolonged period, it is likely to produce right heart failure. Excessively prolonged left heart bypass, therefore, not only reduces the right wall contraction capability but also impairs right heart function, possibly leading to its failure. Hence, an appropriate amount of left heart bypass is important from the standpoint of effectively reducing left heart work load as well as maintaining normal cardiac function, particularly that of the right heart.

[4], Matsuda et al. [5], and Nishigaki et al. [6], who studied the distension of the RV and paradoxical movement of the IVS during left heart bypass using echocardiography, report that the effects of left ventricular decompression upon RV ventricular function can be fairly significant when the bypass ratio approaches 100%.

Rushmer [10] defined the following four mechanisms for the maintenance of RV function: (a) the RV fiber shortens along its longer axis as the papillary muscles inside the RV pull the tricuspid valve down. (b) The distance between the free wall and IVS decreases. (c) The IVS extends into the RV cavity due to an increase in its bending flexibility during left ventricular contraction. (d) Left ventricular contraction pulls the RV free wall attachments toward the left ventricle, thus helping the RV free wall become closer to the IVS.

Of these four factors, (b) to (d) involve the IVS, and hence when its movement is restricted in some way, RV function may be impaired. This shows the important role of the IVS to RV function. According

## Conclusion

During left heart bypass, when the bypass ratio is increased to a maximum level, left ventricular decompression occurs, which in return reduces the IVS contractility. This leads to a significant reduction in the contraction efficiency of the RV. When left heart bypass is continued under this state for a prolonged period, right heart failure may result.

The left heart bypass ratio should be kept at an optimum value of about 75% in order to maintain normal cardiac function, particularly to minimize effects on RV function.

## References

1. Pae We, Rosenberg G, Donachy JH, Landis DL, Phillips WM, Parr GVS, Prophet GA, Piierce WS (1980) Mechanical circulatory assistance for postoperative cardiogenic shock. A three year experience. Trans Am Soc Artif Intern Organs 26: 256–261

2. Olsen EK, Shaffer LJ, Pae WE, Parr GVS, Rosenberg G, Pierce WS (1980) Biventricular mechanical assistance in the postcardiotomy patient. Trans Am Soc Artif Intern Organs 26: 26–33

3. Miyamoto AT, Tanaka S, Matloff JM (1982) Effects of left heart bypass on right ventricular function. Trans Am Soc Artif Intern Organs 28: 543–546

4. Watanabe T, Kagawa Y, Hongo T, Yokoyama K, Shoji Y, Nitta S, Sato N, Tanaka S, Horiuchi T (1982) Effects of left heart bypass evaluated by left ventricular pressure-volume curve. Jpn J Artif Organs 11: 139–142

5. Matsuda H, Hirose H, Nakano S, MaedaSS, Kaneco M, Kato M, Nishigaki K, Otake S, Kawashima Y (1983) Experimental studies of left heart bypass using a centrifugal pump. Heart 15: 1285–1289

6. Nishigaki K, Hirose H, Matsuda H, Nakano S, Maeda S, Kaneko M, Otake S, Hatta T, Nomura F, Kawashima Y (1984) Two-dimensional echocardiograms and right ventricular functional changes during left heart bypass. Jpn J Artif Organs 13: 104–107

7. Miyamoto AT, Tanaka S, Matloff JM (1983) Right ventricular function during left heart bypass. J Thorac Cardiovasc Surg 85: 49–53

8. Pierce WS (1979) Clinical left ventricular bypass: Problems of pump inflow obstruction and right ventricular failure. ASAIO J 2: 1–10

9. Farrar DJ, Compton RG, DajeeH, Fonger JD, Hill JD (1984) Right heart function during left heart assist and the effects of volume loading in a canine preparation. Circulation 70: 708–716

10. Rushmer RF (1982) Cardiovascular dynamics, 4th edn. Saunders, Philadelphia

11. Harada A, Yamate N, Tanaka S, Gomibuchi M, Ikeshita M, Tamauchi S, Shoji T, Takano J, Tanaka K (1984) Right ventricular performance on afterload reduction or pressure overload to left ventricle. Jpn J Artif Organs 13: 165–168

## Discussion

*Nitta* (Tohoku University): You measured right ventricular volume. The wall of the right ventricle has some degree of elasticity, allowing a large amount of saline to be introduced. What is your stopping point in administering saline into the right ventricle?

*Yada* (Mie University): We measure the pressure in the right ventricle.

*Imachi* (University of Tokyo): In your experiments, you used a centrifugal pump. Do you think your results would be very different from the results obtained by a pulsatile pump?

*Yada:* We tried using a pulsatile pump and obtained similar data.

# 18. Reduction of myocardial infarct size by left ventricular assist with revascularization

Hideo Adachi[1], Ryozo Omoto[1], William A. Baumgartner[2], and Bruce A. Reitz[2]

**Summary.** Adequate circulatory support and early revascularization may be a possible therapy for evolving myocardial infarction to salvage the jeopardized myocardium and preserve cardiac function. Optimal support combined with revascularization in this setting, however, remains unknown. The effects of intra-aortic balloon pumping (IABP) and left ventricular assist (LVA), both combined with revascularization for reducing myocardial injury, were studied using a canine model of regional ischemia and reperfusion. Each dog underwent 90 min of ischemia, created by an atraumatic vascular clip on the left anterior descending coronary artery (LAD), followed by 180 min of reperfusion. Circulatory assistance was activated 15 min after occlusion of the LAD. Regional myocardial function was evaluated by a sonomicrometry technique. The hypothermic ischemic myocardium was estimated by an infrared imaging system. The region at risk in the left ventricle and infarcted myocardium was measured by pathological staining methods. A combination of IABP and revascularization showed a smaller infarct size than revascularization alone ($25.2\% \pm 5.1\%$ versus $57.8\% \pm 9.2\%$). A combination of the LVA and revascularization demonstrated the best functional recovery ($9.7\% \pm 2.9\%$ versus $-6.6\% \pm 1.9\%$), the smallest hypothermic area ($14.9\% \pm 1.8\%$ versus $31.6\% \pm 5.2\%$), and the smallest infarct size ($13.0\% \pm 4.1\%$ versus $57.8\% \pm 9.2\%$) compared with controls. These data indicate that emergency coronary revascularization combined with the early use of an LVA may be a possible treatment for evolving myocardial infarction for the effective reduction of the myocardial infarct.

**Key words**: Myocardial infarction—Intra-aortic balloon pump—Left ventricular assist—Sonomicrometry—Infrared imaging

The currently emerging therapy of reperfusion, including intracoronary administration of streptokinase, emergency percutaneous transluminal coronary angioplasty, and emergency surgical revascularization, has been employed for acute coronary occlusion to reduce the size of the infarct and to preserve cardiac function [1–3]. Adequate circulatory support, such as the administration of vasodilators, inotropic agents, and control of circulatory volume, is helpful and necessary for the failing heart. Mechanical assistance is also necessary to maintain the systemic circulation in cases of cardiogenic shock or in preshock patients after acute coronary occlusion. What has not been established is the relative value of the currently available techniques for mechanical support in patients with acute coronary occlusion and revascularization. Mechanical support may increase coronary flow and decrease the ventricular load during ischemia [4]. Mechanical support may attenuate "reperfusion injury" upon reperfusion because of the unloading effect [5]. Optimal mechanical support combined with revascularization for evolving myocardial infarction has not as yet been developed.

This study was designed to evaluate the effects of intra-aortic balloon pumping (IABP) and left ventricular assist (LVA) in reducing the extent of ischemic myocardial injury in a canine model of acute coronary occlusion and subsequent reperfusion. Myocardial injury was estimated by three different means. Myocardial functional recovery in the ischemic area was assessed by a sonomicrometry technique [6]. The hypothermic zone in the left ventricle (LV), which may reflect myocardial injury, was evaluated using an infrared imaging system [7]. The size of myocardial necrosis in the region at risk was measured by standard pathological staining techniques [8].

## Materials and methods

Eighteen mongrel dogs weighing 20–28 kg were anesthetized with intravenous administration of pentobarbital sodium and succinylcholine chloride, intubated, and ventilated with a respirator supplying a mixture of room air and oxygen. After performing a left thoracotomy through the fifth intercostal space, the heart was exposed in a pericardial cradle. Epicardial pacing electrodes were placed on the right atrium and the animals were paced at 150 beats/min. The left anterior descending coronary artery (LAD) distal to the first diagonal branch was exposed in preparation for temporary occlusion by an atraumatic vascular clip. A

[1]First Department of Surgery, Saitama Medical School, Moroyama-machi, Saitama, 350-04 Japan
[2]Division of Cardiac Surgery, The Johns Hopkins Hospital, Baltimore, USA

pair of sonomicrometer crystals was implanted in the LAD distribution to evaluate regional myocardial function. The crystals were positioned 15 mm apart and were oriented perpendicular to the major axis of the LV. LV pressure was measured by a high-fidelity pressure transducer tipped catheter (Millar Instrument, Houston, TX, USA) inserted into the LV through the left atrium (Fig. 18.1).

Each dog underwent 90 min of ischemia created by placing the vascular clip on the LAD. After 90 min of ischemia, the clip was removed and the ischemic region was reperfused for 180 min. The 18 dogs were divided into three groups (Fig. 18.2). In group I (controls, $n = 6$), no further interventions were carried out during ischemia and reperfusion. Central venous pressure and carotid blood pressure were monitored and maintained within 10% of baseline values by the administration of fluids. Blood gases were checked and acidosis was corrected. In group II ($n = 6$), an intra-aortic balloon (12 ml) was inserted through the femoral artery and an IABP (System 90, Datascope, Paramus, NJ, USA) was activated 15 min after occlusion of the LAD. The animals were placed on the IABP during the remainder of the ischemic and reperfusion period. In group III ($n = 6$), the animals were heparinized (300 units/kg), and a 28-F cannula was placed in the left atrium. Blood was removed from this cannula by a centrifugal pump (Centrimed, Hopkins, MN, USA) and returned to the animal via an 18-F cannula placed in the thoracic aorta. The animals were placed on an LAV 15 min after occlusion of the LAD. The extracorporeal circuit was primed with crystalloid solution and Hespan, and a mean aortic pressure of 80–100 mmHg was maintained. LVA provided 80% (mean) of the total systemic flow during ischemia and reperfusion.

In groups II and III, mechanical support terminated 10 min before the end of the reperfusion period for evaluating myocardial injury. LV end-diastolic pressure was adjusted to a baseline value by the administration of fluid, and myocardial function and hypothermic area in the LV were assessed.

Regional myocardial function was measured using sonomicrometry and micromanometry techniques. Pressure-dimension loops were generated by a computer (IBM PC-XA), and the area within the loop was used as an index of the regional stroke work. Myocardial function was reported as percentage recovery of the loop area based on a preischemic value of 100%. Myocardial surface temperature was mapped by a real-time infrared imaging system (Hughes Thermal Video System, Hughes Aircraft, Carlsbad, CA, USA). This system converts invisible infrared radiation to a voltage signal, which cn be imaged on a television display. The camera head was fixed 70 cm from the exposed heart and scanned the heart at 20 fames/s

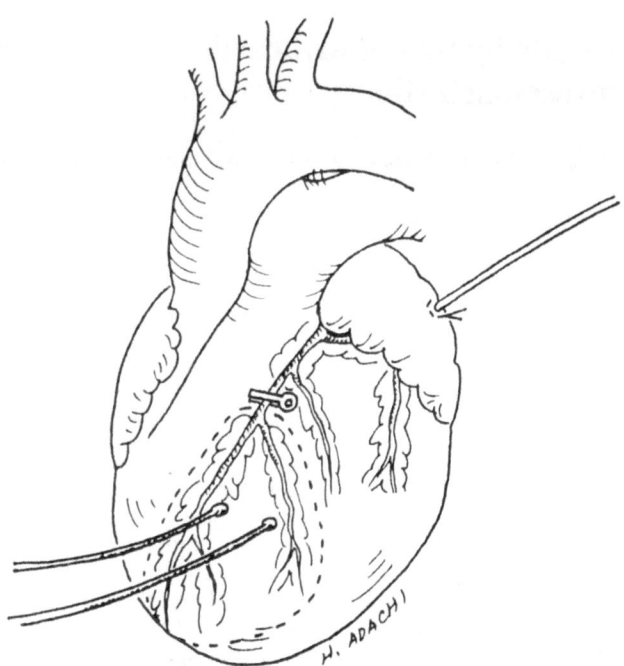

**Fig. 18.1.** Experimental preparation with left anterior descending coronary artery exposure, sonocrystals, and left ventricular micromanometer

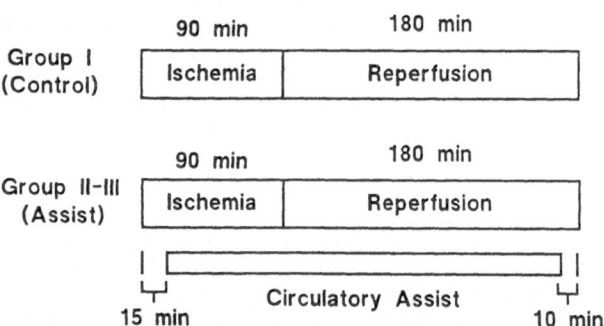

**Fig. 18.2.** Experimental design. Each dog underwent a 90-min period of regional ischemia followed by 180 min of reperfusion. Mechanical support was activated 15 min after occlusion of the artery

with a thermal resolution power of 0.1°C. In the normal dog heart, the anterior wall of the LV showed a homogeneous temprature distribution, reflecting normal perfusion. In the area ofischemia or injured myocardium, surface temperature decreased [7]. The hypothermic area where the temperature decrement was morethan 1.0°C was measured and reported as a percentage of the LV anterior wall area.

Following the experiment, the LAD occluder was replaced and monastryl blue dye was injected into the left atrium to outline the region at risk (RR) for infarction. After removing the right ventricle and atria, the LV was sectioned and incubated in nitro blue

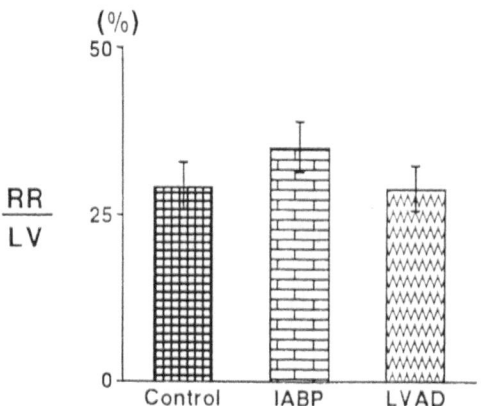

**Fig. 18.3.** The region at risk was measured as percentage of the left ventricular weight. No significant difference was observed among the three groups

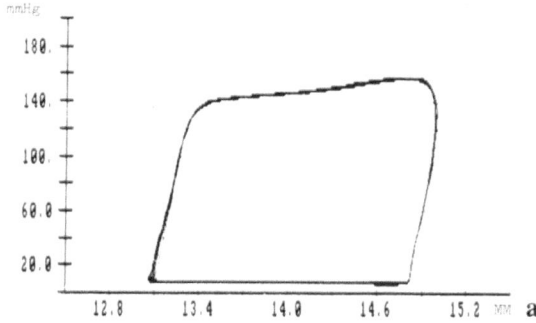

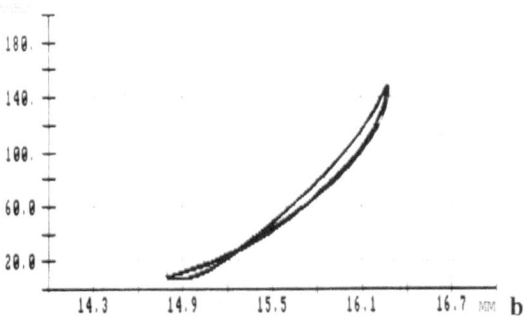

**Fig. 18.4a, b.** Pressure-dimension loops with **a** positive wide area reflecting normal function and **b** negative narrow area reflecting ischemic bulging

tetrazolium chloride solution for 20 min to stain the infarcted myocardium (IM). Pathological myocardial injury was evaluated by calculating the percentage infarction of the LV in the region at risk by a planimetric method.

Statistical significance was examined by Student's $t$-test, analysis of variance (ANOVA) and Duncan's multiple range test provided by CLINFO. All values are expressed as means ± SEM. Results were considered to be significant at a level of $P < 0.05$.

## Results

The region at risk measured as a percentage of the LV did not differ significantly between the groups (group I 29.4% ± 3.6%, group II 35.3% ± 3.8%, group III 29.0% ± 3.4%; Fig. 18.3).

Before ischemia, pressure-dimension loops showed a large positive area, reflecting normal myocardial function. After occlusion of the LAD, the area became small and negative, reflecting lack of myocardial function (Fig. 18.4). Significant decrease from the baseline in myocardial function were observed in all three groups at the end of reperfusion; however, a significant difference was observed in functional recovery between groups I and III. At the end of reperfusion, functional recovery in group I was negative (−6.6% ± 1.9%), reflecting dyskinetic regional wall motion. In group II, functional recovery was slightly positive (1.3% ± 3.3%); however, no significant difference was observed between group II and controls. In group III, regional functional recovery was significantly better than controls (9.7% ± 2.9% versus −6.6% ± 1.9%; $P < 0.001$; Fig. 18.5).

In the infrared images, a sharp outline of the exposed heart was obtained and the anterior wall of the

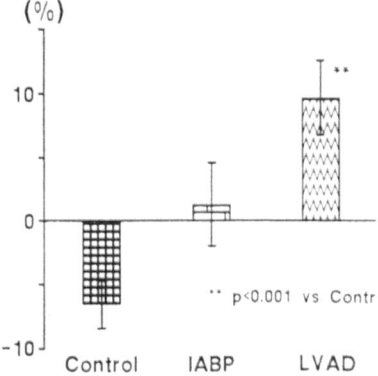

**Fig. 18.5.** Functional recovery was reported as percentage recovery based on a preischemic value of 100%

LV demonstrated an even temperature distribution. After occlusion of the LAD, the surface temperature in the LAD distribution decreased rapidly and the ischemic hypothermic area was clearly differentiated from normal myocardium. After reperfusion, the hypothermic area decreased; however, hypothermia still remained in the region at risk, which may reflect the existence of myocardial injury [7]. In controls, the hypothermic area in the anterior wall of the LV was 31% ± 5.2% at the end of reperfusion. In group II, the hypothermic area (19.6% ± 4.0%) appeared

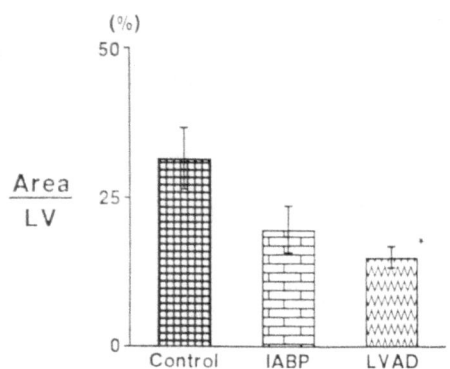

**Fig 18.6.** The hypothermic area where the temperature decrement was more than 1°C reported as a percentage of the anterior wall of the left ventricle. *$P < 0.05$ vs. control

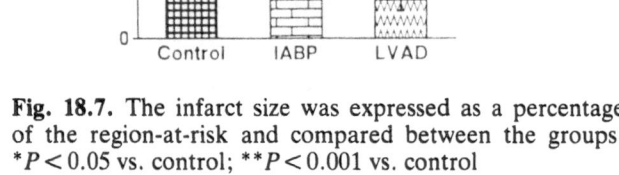

**Fig. 18.7.** The infarct size was expressed as a percentage of the region-at-risk and compared between the groups. *$P < 0.05$ vs. control; **$P < 0.001$ vs. control

smaller than in controls; however, this difference was not significant. Group III animals showed the smallest hypothermic area ($14.9\% \pm 1.9\%$), and there was a significant difference between group III and controls in the size of the hypothermic area ($P < 0.05$; Fig. 18.6).

Although there were no significant differences in the size of the region at risk, the size of myocardial infarction was quite different between the groups. Controls animals demonstrated large infarcts in the region at risk ($57.8\% \pm 9.2\%$). In group II, a significant reduction in the infarct size ($25.1\% \pm 5.1\%$) was observed in the region at risk compared with controls ($P < 0.05$). Group III animals showed the smallest size of infarct in the region at risk ($13.0\% \pm 4.1\%$), and this marked reduction is highly significant compared with controls ($P < 0.001$; Fig. 18.7).

## Discussion

Our results demonstrate that a combination of mechanical support and revascularization is superior to revascularization alone for reducing the size of the infarct in this canine model. The addition of mechanical support to emergent revascularization is a potential therapy for severe acute coronary occlusion [9]. During ischemia, adequate circulatory support is necessary not only to maintain systemic circulation but also to help the failing heart. Early reperfusion is essential to ultimate myocardial viability; however, "reperfusion injury" may occur on reperfusion [10].

IABP is widely accepted for the failing heart because of its relative simplicity, accessibility, and the reduction effect of afterload with augumentation of coronary flow [11]. In our present study, IABP was effective in reducing the myocardial necrosis in the region at risk as expected; however, it could not sustain

the circulation when the cardiac output was very low. A simple, effective, and reliable means of mechanical circulatory support is necessary for patients with cardiogenic shock after acute coronary occlusion (prior to revascularization).

From many experimental and clinical studies using various forms of LVA, LV decompression, reduction of ventricular workload, and decrease of myocardial oxygen consumption may be achieved satisfactory by the use of LVA [12, 13]. Several investigators have reported that LVA effectively reduces myocardial ischemic injury following acute coronary occlusion (without revascularization) and thus may reduce the mortality associated with cardiogenic shock [14]. Open-Chest LVA has been found to be effective in improving cardiac function in patients who could not be weaned from cardiopulmonary bypass after cardiac surgery [15].

Early revascularization is important to salvage the ischemic myocardium, though simple reperfusion may result in "reperfusion injury" [10]. LVA has been demonstrated to be helpful in reducing "reperfusion injury" following coronary artery occlusion [5]. Some investigators have reported the effectiveness of the pulsatile LVA in preventing "reperfusion injury" in a canine model [16]. They used LVA during the initial reperfusion period and showed a significant reduction in the infarct size compared with simple reperfusion. In the present study, LVA was started prior to reperfusion, simulating the clinical case of acute coronary occlusion with cardiogenic shock and subsequent reperfusion. A combination of LVA and revascularization demonstrated significant improvement of regional myocardial function, a significant decrease in the size of the hypothermic area, and a marked reduction in the size of the infarct compared with simple reperfusion. A combination of IABP and revascularization also showed significant reduction in the size of the infarct; however, differences in other measurements between IABP animals and controls were not significant. LVA allows better decompression of the left side of the heart than IABP [17]. We conclude that the combination of LVA and revascularization may be an optimal therapy for evolving myocardial infarction in reducing the size of the infarct. This treatment may be effective in patients with cardiogenic shock who do not respond to IABP support.

Several methods of LVA without thoracotomy have been reported since 1962 [18–19]; however, no standard method has been established. We need to develop a simple, effective, and safe cannulation method for LVA that would allow it to become a primary acceptable means for patients with evolving myocardial infarction and cardiogenic shock.

In summary, the effects of IABP and LVA in the reduction of myocardial injury were studied in the canine model of acute coronary occlusion and reperfusion. LVA combined with revascularization demonstrated the best functional recovery, the smallest hypothermic injured area, and the smallest area of the infarct. Emergency coronary revascularization and the early use of LVA appear to be the optimal means for the reduction of myocardial injury in evolving myocardial infarction.

**Acknowledgments.** Computational assistance was provided by CLINFO, sponsored by NIH Grant RR-00035.

# References

1. Ganz W, Buchbinder N, Marcus H, Mondkar A, Maddahi J, Charuzi Y, O'Connor L, Shell W, Fishbein MC, Kass R, Miyamoto A, Swan HJC (1981) Intracoronary thrombolysis in evolving myocardial infarction. Am Heart J 101: 4–13
2. Meyer J, Merx W, Schmitz H, Erbel R, Kiesslich T, Dorr R, Lambertz H, Bethge C, Krebs W, Bardos P, Minale C, Messmer BJ, Effert S (1982) Percutaneous transluminal coronary angioplasty immediately after intracoronary streptolysis of transmural myocardial infarction. Circulation 66: 905–913
3. Berg R, Selinger SL, Leonard JJ, Grunwald RB, O'Grady WP (1981) Immediate coronary artery bypass for acute myocardial infarction. J Thorac Cardiovasc Surg 81: 493–497
4. Laks HL, Ott RA, Standeven JW, Hahn JW, Blair OM, William VL (1977) The effect of left atrial-aortic assistance on infarct size. Circulation 56 (Suppl 2): 38–43
5. Uretzky G, Franco KK, Paolini D, Cohn LH (1983) Cardiopulmonary bypass during reperfusion after coronary occlusion attenuates the "no reflow" phe-

nomenon in ischemic myocardium. J Thorac Cardiovasc Surg 85: 870–876
6. Forrester JS, Wyatt HL, Luz PL, Tyberg JV, Diamond GA, Swan HJC (1976) Functional significance of regional ischemic contraction abnormalities. Circulation 54: 64–70
7. Adachi H, Johnson DL, Baumgartner WA, Borkon MA, Reitz BA (1986) Real-time infrared imaging for perfusion assessment in heart surgery: An experimental model. Thermology 2: 7–12
8. Lie JR, Pairolero PC, Holley KE, Titus JL (1975) Macroscopic enzyme mapping verification of large homogeneous experimental myocardial infarcts of predictable size and location in dogs. J Thorac Cardiovasc Surg 69: 593–600
9. Mundth ED (1976) Mechanical and surgical interventions for the reduction of myocardial ischemia. Circulation 53 (Suppl 1): 176–183
10. Jennings RB, Reimer KA (1983) Factors involved in salvaging ischemic myocardium: Effects of reperfusion of arterial blood. Circulation 68 (Suppl 1): 25–36
11. Kantrowitz A, Tjonneland S, Freed PS (1968) Initial clinical experience with intra-aortic balloon pumping in cardiogenic shock. JAMA 203: 113–118
12. Wakabayashi A, Kubo T, Gliman P, Zuber WF, Connolly JE (1975) Oxygen consumption of the normal and failing heart during left heart bypass. J Thorac Cardiovasc Surg. 70: 9–18
13. McDonnell MA, Kralios AC, Tagaris TJ, Kuida H (1979) Comparative effect of counterpulsation and left ventricular bypass on myocardial oxygen consumption and dynamics before and after coronary occlusion. Am Heart J 97: 78–88
14. Delaria GA, Johansen KH, Levine ID, Bernstein EF (1974) Reduction in myocardial ischemia by left ventricular bypass after acute coronary artery occlusion. J Thorac Cardiovasc Surg 67: 826–837
15. Spencer FC, Eiseman NG, Trinkel JK (1965) Assisted circulation for cardiac failure following intracardiac surgery with cardiopulmonary bypass. J Thoracic Cardiovasc Surg 49: 56–73
16. Laschinger JC, Grossi EA, Cunningham JN, Krieger KH, Baumann FG, Colvin SB, Spencer FC (1985) Adjunctive left ventricular unloading during myocardial reperfusion plays a major role in minimizing myocardial infarct size. J Thorac Cardiovasc Surg 90: 80–85
17. Mickleborough LL, Rebeyka I, Wilson GJ, Gray G, Desrosiers A (1987) Comparison of left ventricular assist and intra-aortic balloon counterpulsation during early reperfusion after ischemic arrest of the heart. J Thorac Cardiovasc Surg 93: 597–608
18. Dennis C, Carlens E, Senning A (1962) Clinical use of a cannula for left heart bypass without thoracotomy. Ann Surg 156: 623–637
19. Glassman E, Engelman RM, Boyd AD, Lipson D, Ackerman B, Spencer F (1975) A method of closed-chest cannulation of the left atrium for atrial-femoral artery bypass. J Thorac Cardiovasc Surg 69: 283–287

# Part III
# Ventricular Assist Device: Clinical Use

# 19. Clinical experience with ventricular

Yuzuru Kagawa[1], Shinichi Nitta[2], Tadayoshi Hongo[3], Naoshi Sato[1], Takashi Watanabe[1], Naoki Uchida[1], Makoto Miura[1], Yoshiaki Katahira[2], Tomoyuki Yambe[2], Masahiro Ouchi[3], and Takahisa Shibazaki[3]

**Summary.** Since November 1984, eight postcardiotomy patients with ages ranging from 13 to 65 years, have received ventricular assist devices (VADs) at our institute. All the cases fulfilled the criteria for acute profound ventricular failure despite the administration of a large amount of catecholamines and application of intra-aortic balloon pumping (IABP). The original diseases were acute myocardial infarction (AMI) in two, left ventricular (LV) aneurysm in one, severe acquired valvular disease in three, and congenital cardiac anomaly in two cases. Of the eight cases, three with critical preoperative hemodynamic conditions underwent surgery with VAD on standby. The reasons for applying the VAD were difficulty in weaning from extracorporeal circulation (ECC) in five and low cardiac output syndrome after weaning from ECC in three cases. Two types of VAD system were used in this series. VAD systems developed at the University of Tokyo were used in the initial six cases and a blood pump (TH-7), and multipurpose driving system, which were newly developed at our institute, in the most recent two cases. The duration of assistance varied from 18 h to 70 days. Three cases were not weaned from VAD—two because of incomplete surgical repair and one because of multiple organ failure (MOF) after prolonged assistance for 70 days. Of the five patients who were weaned from VAD, two are alive. The remaining three patients were weaned from VAD and died on the 21st, 97th, and 123rd postoperative days. The cause of death was mainly MOF, originating from various complications such as acute renal failure, sepsis, respiratory failure, and cerebral embolism.

**Key words**: Acute profound ventricular failure—Left ventricular assist device—Right ventricular assist device—Long-term survivor

Since the first clinical application of the ventricular assist device (VAD) in Japan in 1980 [1, 2], the number of cases has increased with time and the total number of VAD applications was 51 by the end of November 1986 (Fig. 19.l) [3]. The first long-term survival was achieved in 1985 at our institute [4] and the overall incidence of cases weaned from VAD is now 61% and that of long-term survival 22%. At present, the efficacy of VAD in coping with profound acute ventricular failure is widely accepted and it appears that the indications for the application of VAD are almost standardized. However, there still remain several unclear areas in the practical applications of VADs. We have used VADs in eight postcardiotomy cases. Based on this experience, reconsideration of the indications, an evaluation of the control method of VAD driving, and an analysis of VAD-related complications will be presented in this paper.

## Subjects and methods

Since November 1984, eight patients (five females, three males; age range 13–68 years) received VADs for the relief of postcardiotomy acute profound ventricular failure. The incidence of assisted circulation was 7.3% and that of VAD application 1.5% of all cardiac operations done during the same period at our institute. Details of the subjects are presented in

[1]Department of Thoracic and Cardiovascular Surgery, Tohoku University School of Medicine, 1-1 Seiryo-cho, Sendai, 980 Japan,
[2]Department of Medical Engineering and Cardiology, The Research Institute for Chest Disease and Cancer, Tohoku University, 4-1 Seiryo-Cho, Sendai, 980 Japan
[3]Department of Cardiovascular Surgery, Sendar National Hospital, 2-8 Miyagino, Sendai, 980 Japan

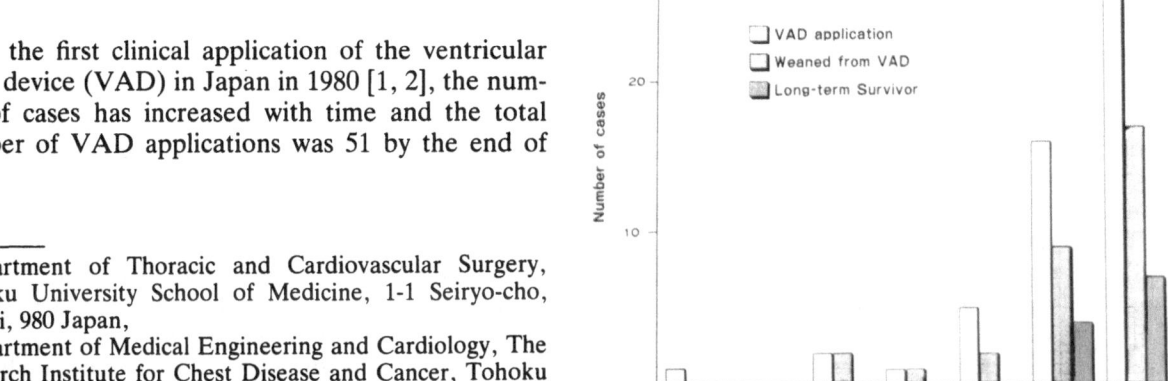

**Fig. 19.1.** Clinical application of VAD in Japan

**Table 19.1.** Subject data

| Case no. | Age (yrs) | Sex | Diagnosis | Operation | VAD standby |
|----------|-----------|-----|-----------|-----------|-------------|
| 1 | 58 | F | Ebstein's anomaly, ASD, CHF (NYHA IV) | TVR, closure of ASD, Plication of atrialized RV | No |
| 2 | 48 | M | ASR, malfunction of mital prosthesis, CHF (NYHA IV) | AVR, Re-MVR | Yes |
| 3 | 49 | F | AMI after PTCA, cardiogenic shock | Emergency ACBG | No |
| 4 | 13 | F | Residual shunt after Fontan's procedure for tricuspid atresia | Closure of residual shunt | No |
| 5 | 55 | M | MR, TR, CHF (NYHA IV) | MVR, TAP | Yes |
| 6 | 65 | F | AMI, VSP, LV aneurysm, cardiogenic shock | Closure of VSP, LV aneurysmectomy | Yes |
| 7 | 68 | F | LV rupture after MVR | Closure of LV rupture | No |
| 8 | 51 | M | OMI, LV aneurysm | LV aneurysmectomy | No |

*ASD* atrial septal defect, *CHF* congestive heart failure, *TVR* tricuspid valve replacement, *RV* right ventricle, *ASR* aortic stenosis and regurgitation, *AVR* aortic valve replacement, *MVR* mitral valve replacement, *PTCA* percutaneous trans-coronary angioplasty, *ACBG* aortocoronary bypass grafting, *MR* mitral regurgitation, *TR* tricuspid valve replacement, *TAP* tricuspid annuloplasty, *OMI* old myocardial infarction

**Table 19.2.** Reasons for application of VAD and types of VAD

| Case no. | Reasons for VA | Hemodynamics just prior to application of VAD | | | | IABP | ECC VA (h) | Assist mode | Type of VAD system | |
|----------|----------------|-----------------------------|---|---|---|------|------------|-------------|--------------------|---|
| | | ECC flow (ml/kg/min) | Blood pressure (mmHg) | Cl (l/min/m²) | LAP [CVP] (mmHg) | | | | Blood pump | Driving system |
| 2 | ECC | 30 | 60 | | | Yes | | LVA | UT | UT |
| 4 | ECC | 70 | 40 | | | Yes (ECMO) | | LVA | UT | UT |
| 6 | ECC | 50 | 70 | | | Yes | | LVA | UT | UT |
| 7 | ECC | 30 | 70 | | | Yes | | LVA | TU | TU |
| 8 | ECC | 60 | 80 | | | Yes | | LVA | TU | TU |
| 1 | LOS | | | | 14 [30] | Yes | 6 | RVA | UT | UT |
| 3 | LOS | | | 1.37 | 31 | Yes | 4 | LVA | UT | UT |
| 5 | LOS | | | 1.5 | 20 | Yes | 2 | LVA | UT | UT |

*ECC* extracorporeal circulation, *LVA* left ventricular assistance, *RVA* ventricular assistance, *UT* University of Tokyo, *TU* Tohoku University

Table 19.1. The original diseases were ischemic heart disease in three, severe acquired valvular disease in three, and congenital cardiac anomaly in two cases. Three of the eight patients, comprising two with severe valvular disease with extremely poor preoperative cardiac functions (cases 2, 5) and one with profound cardiogenic shock due to acute myocardial infarction (AMI) and ventricular septal perforation (VSP; case 6), underwent surgery with the VAD on standby. The reasons for applying the VAD were difficulty in weaning from extracorporeal circulation (ECC) in five cases and low cardiac output syndrome (LOS) after weaning from ECC in the remaining three (Table 19.2).

Two types of VAD system were used in this series. For the initial six cases (cases 1–6), a blood pump (Nihon Zeon Co., Tokyo, Japan) and driving system (Corat, Aishin Seiki Co. Ashiya, Japan), which were developed at the University of Tokyo, were used. For the two most recent cases (cases 7, 8), another type of blood pump (TH-7, Nihon Zeon Co., Tokyo, Japan) (Fig. 19.2) and driving system (Nihon Zeon Co., Tokyo, Japan), which were developed at our institute, were used. The TH-7 blood pump was designed to eliminate thrombus formation within the sac, especially in the low-flow state, through the analysis of flow velocity using a flow visualization technique [5, 6]. The driving system contains two separate drivers, such that simultaneous driving of two pumps or combined driving of the VAD and IABP is possible [7].

Hemodynamic data before and after the application of VAD and VAD-related complications were analyzed.

## Results

### Indication for application of VAD

The Criteria of acute profound ventricular failure, for which the VAD is indicated, are a cardiac index of less than 2.0 1/min/m², blood pressure lower than 80 mmHg, left atrial pressure greater than 20 mmHg, urinary output less than 0.5 ml/kg/min, and so on, despite of the administration of a large amount of catecholamines, adequate volume loading, and application of IABP. The reasons for applying the VAD, hemodynamic conditions just prior to the application, mode of assistance, and type of VAD system for our patients are summarized in Table 19.2. VADs were applied for difficulty in weaning from ECC in five cases (cases 2, 4, 6–8). In these cases, the blood

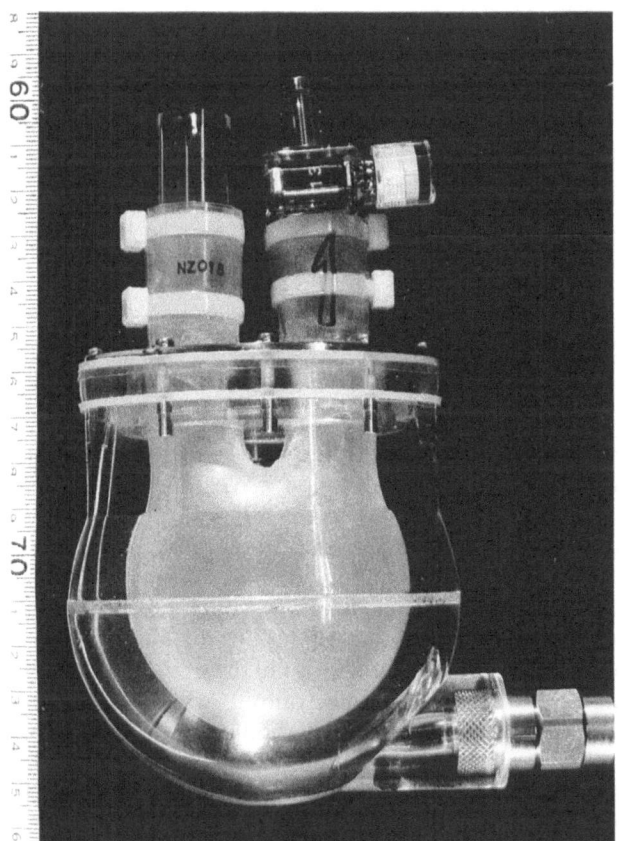

**Fig. 19.2.** TH-7 blood pump

pressure could not be maintained when ECC flow was reduced below 301–70 ml/kg/min. In three cases (cases 1, 3, 5), a gradual fall in blood pressure, decrease in urinary output, bulging and poor contraction of the ventricle, or frequent occurrence of ventricular tachycardia or fibrillation were noted after weaning from ECC. The interval between the termination of ECC and institution of VAD was 2–6 h, which gradually decreased as we accumulated experience. The mode of assistance was left ventricular assist in all cases except case 1, where a surgical intervention was undertaken only for the right side of the heart and the patient appeared to show right ventricular failure after weaning from ECC.

Figure 19.3 shows the pre- and postoperative course of case 6. VSP associated with profound cardiogenic shock following AMI necessitated the administration of a large amount of catecholamines and the application of IABP. Despite intensive treatment, the patient's hemodynamic condition deteriorated and urinary output dropped to zero. Closure of the VSP and left ventricular aneurysmectomy were carried out on an emergency basis with the VAD on standby. After the procedure, the contraction of both ventricles was weak and blood pressure fell to 70 mmHg when ECC flow was reduced to 50 ml/kg/min. Despite a large amount of catecholamines and IABP, weaning from ECC was impossible. Left VAD (LVAD) was applied between the left atrium and the ascending aorta. A left atrial cannula was inserted transatrioseptally. Immediately after going onto LVAD driving, elevation of blood pressure and restoration of urinary output were observed and it was possible to wean the patient from ECC very easily.

Figure 19.4 shows the clinical course of case 3. Following unsuccessful percutaneous transcoronary angioplasty of the left coronary artery, the patient suffered from AMI associated with profound cardiogenic shock. Emergency aortocoronary bypass grafting was carried out. After the patient was weaning from ECC with the assistance of catecholamines and IABP, the hemodynamic situation deteriorated and the frequent occurrence of serious arrhythmias was noted. An LVAD was inserted between the left atrium and ascending aorta. Immediately after going onto left ventricular assistance, the hemodynamic condition stabilized and arrhythmias disappeared.

### Hemodynamics after application of VAD and weaning from VAD

Driving of the VAD was started immediately after connection of the inflow and outflow cannulae to the blood pump was completed. Initially, an asynchronous driving mode was selected and positive and negative pressure, D/S ratio, and pulse rate were

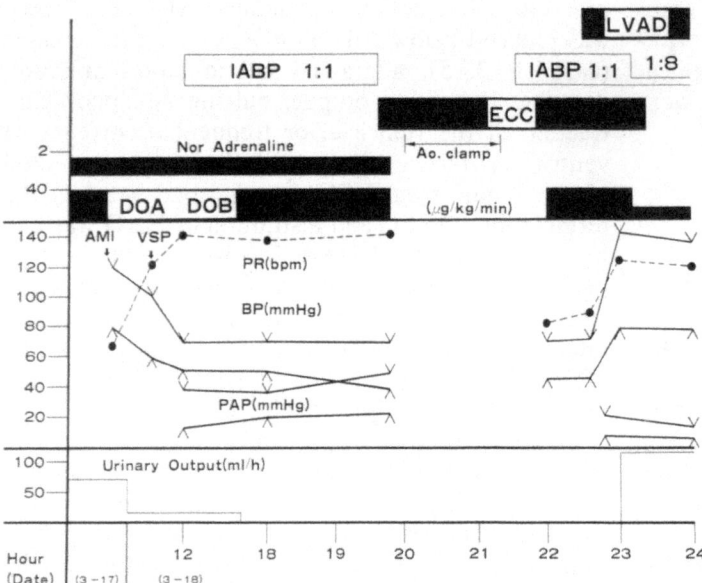

**Fig. 19.3.** Clinical course of case 6 (1). *PR* pulse rate, *BP* blood pressure, *PAP* pulmonary arterial pressure, *DOA* dopamine, *DOB* dobutamine

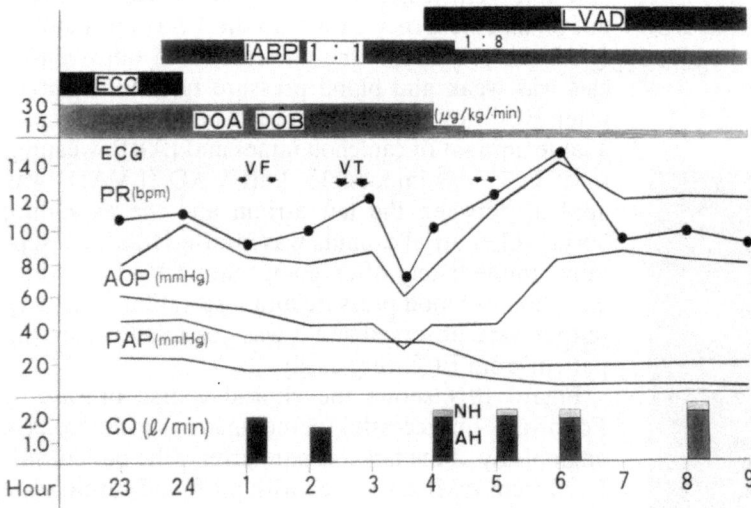

**Fig. 19.4.** Clinical course of case 3 (1). *VF* ventricular fibrillation, *VT* ventricular tachycardia, *NH* natural heart, *AH* artificial heart

settled so as to obtain the largest output from the blood pump. The driving mode as then converted to the synchronous mode as soon as possible, after the hemodynamic condition had stabilized.

Figure 19.5 shows the percentage of VAD flow to the total flow, i.e., the assist ratio of VAD. The assist ratio was 40%–70% and remained almost unchanged throughout the entire period of assistance except in case 3, where there was complication with the cardiac tamponade.

Figure 19.6 shows the clinical course of case 6. Restoration of the cardiac function was achieved on the 14th postoperative day and the patient was weaned from LVAD on the 20th postoperative day.

Figure 19.7 shows the clinical course of case 3.

From the 2nd postoperative day, catecholamine administration was suspended. Weaning from the respirator was achieved on the 4th postoperative day, and from LVAD on the 7th postoperative day.

The timing for weaning from VAD was based on the recovery of cardiac function, which was evaluated by stopping the drive of the VAD for about 15 min after 1 mg/kg heparin was administered. Changes in blood pressure and cardiac output, which was calculated by a thermodilution method using a Swan-Ganz catheter placed in the pulmonary artery, were observed. Figure 19.8 shows the ratio of blood pressure with VAD to that without VAD. This ratio increased daily according to the recovery of cardiac function and exceeded more than 80% prior to weaning from

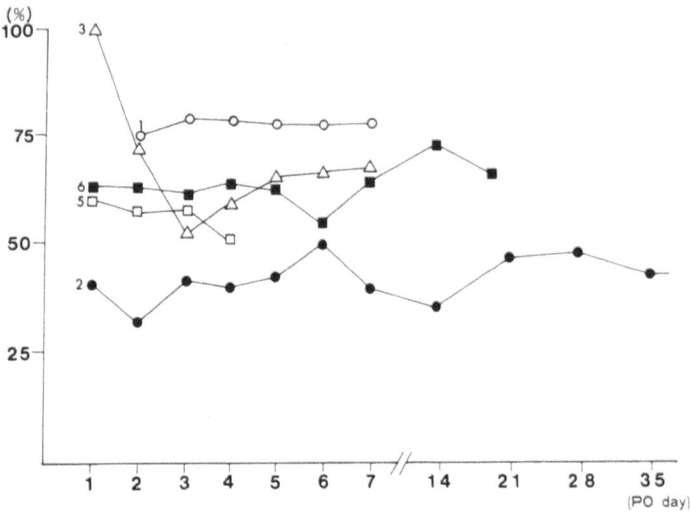

**Fig. 19.5.** Ratios of VAD flow to total flow. Changes in ratios of VAD flow to total flow are shown in percentages. *Numbers* refer to case numbers

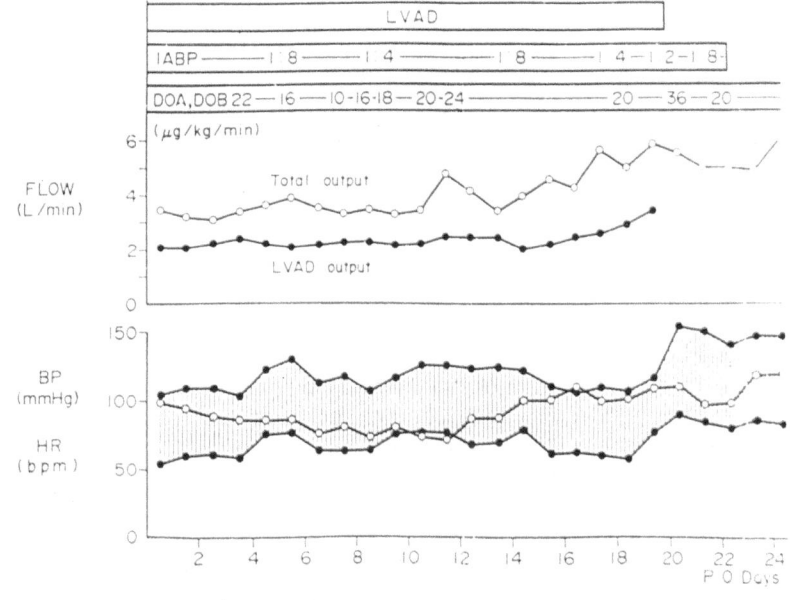

**Fig. 19.6.** Clinical course of case 6 (2). Changes in total flow VAD flow blood pressure and heart rate are shown by postoperative days

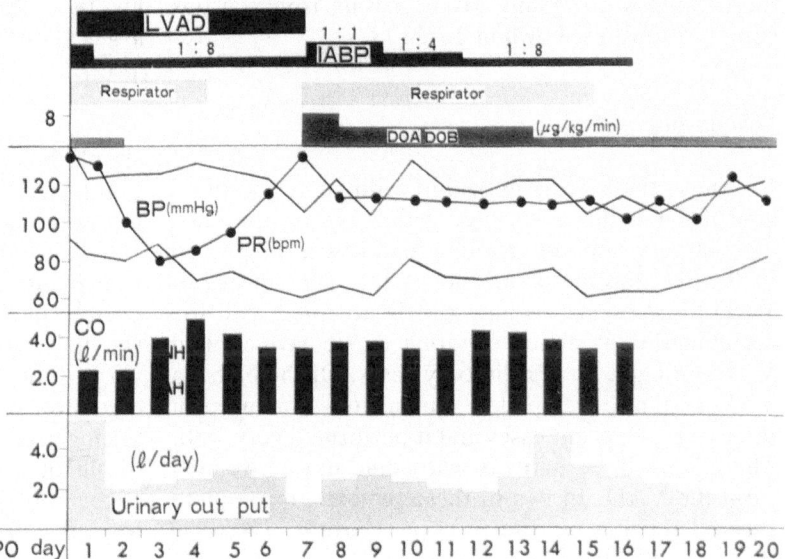

**Fig. 19.7.** Clinical course of case 3 (2)

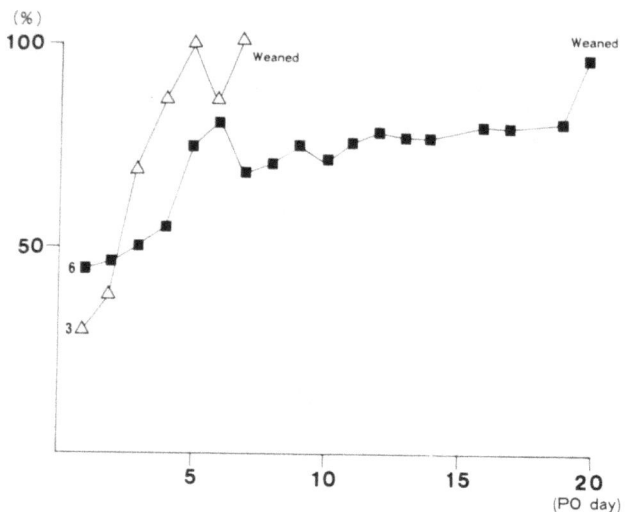

**Fig. 19.8.** Change in ratio of blood pressure with and without VAD. Immediately after institution of VAD, blood pressure fell to less than half when VAD pumping had ceased. Just prior to weaning from VAD, blood pressure did not fall even without VAD pumping. *Numbers* indicate case number

VAD. Figure 19.9 shows changes in left ventricular function in case 6 without the aid of an LVAD. Cardiac function recovered gradually and the cardiac index reached 4.0 l/min/m$^2$ when the pulmonary arterial wedge pressure was 20 mmHg on the 20th postoperative day, which was the day of weaning the patient from the LVAD,

### Summary of results

Table 19.3 shows a summary of the results. The duration of assistance varied from 18 h to 70 days. Of the eight patients, three could not be weaned from VAD. Incomplete surgical repair provoked poor recovery of cardiac function in two cases (cases 4, 7). The remaining case (case 2) became dependent on the LVAD and died of multiple organ failure (MOF) after very prolonged assistance. Three patients died after weaning from the VAD (case 1, 5, 6). The cause of death in these cases were mainly MOF, arising from various complications, as shown in Table 19.3.

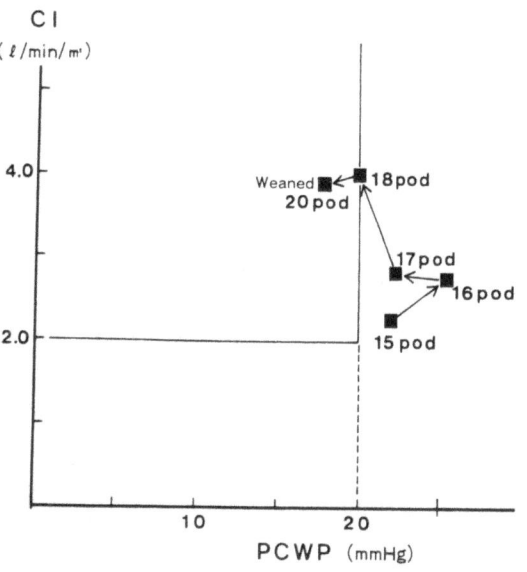

**Fig. 19.9.** Changes in left ventricular function of case 6. *pod* postoperative day

### Discussion

Recently, the success in dealing with acute profound ventricular failure associated with AMI, or after cardiac surgery and convention treatment have proved ineffective, has increased rapidly [8]. The efficacy of VAD in such cases is now widely accepted with the accumulation of clinical experience. We have applied VADs in eight postcardiotomy cases. Of the eight, a VAD system developed at our institute was used in the two most recent cases and it performed very well. There were three patients who could not be weaned from the VAD. In two of these patients, incomplete surgical repair gave rise to poor recovery of cardiac function. In these cases, the indication for VAD

should have been given greater consideration. In the other patient who became dependent on the VAD, measures such as the application of a permanent VAD, total artificial heart implantation, or heart transplantation should have been performed. To decide the timing for weaning, stopping the drive of the VAD for about 15 min after giving heparin was very useful. The cause of death of the patients who died after weaning from the VAD were mainly MOF, arising from various complications. To improve the results of the clinical application of VADs, an analysis of the etiology of MOF, establishing countermeasures to cope with MOF, and preventing complications are indispensable.

**Table 19.3.** Summary of results

| Case no. | Duration of VA | Weaned | Outcome | Time of death | Cause of death |
|---|---|---|---|---|---|
| 2 | 70 days | No | | | Dependency on VAD→ prolonged VA→ infection→ MOF |
| 4 | 28 h | No | | | Incomplete surgical repair→ circulatory failure |
| 7 | 18 h | No | | | Incomplete repair of LV rupture→ bleeding |
| 1 | 7 days | Yes | Died | 21 PO day | ARF, sepsis |
| 5 | 4 days | Yes | Died | 97 PO day | Cerebral embolism→ MOF |
| 6 | 20 days | Yes | Died | 123 PO day | Respiratory failure→ sepsis→ MOF |
| 3 | 7 days | Yes | Alive | | |
| 8 | 5 days | Yes | Alive | | |

*VA* ventricular assist, *VAD* ventricular assist device, *MOF* multiple organ failure, *LV* left ventricular, *PO* postoperative, *ARF* acute renal failure

# References

1. Atsumi K (1981) Clinical application of mechanical assist heart pump. Jpn J Artif Organs 10: 661–664
2. Furuta S, Wanibuchi Y, Inou T, Kyo S, Urushino K, Kaneko K, Koike R, Taketa K, Ono T, Atsumi K, Fujimasa I, Imachi K, Miyake H, Takido N, Nakajima M (1981) The first clinical experience of circulatory assist using partial artificial heart. Jpn J Artif Organs 10: 657–660
3. Kagawa Y, Horiuchi T, Sezai Y, Akune J, Atsumi K, Abe N, Arai T, Inoue T, Iwa T, Eguchi S, Omoto R, Kawashima Y, Kitamura S, Kusakawa M, Komatsu S, Koyanagi H, Shimizu K, Shoji T, Shirabe J, Suzuki A, Seki S, Takeuchi K, Tokunaga K, Nakamura K, Hasegawa T, Fukumasu H, Fujita T, Furuse A, Hoshino S, Hori M (1987) Current status of clinical application of ventricular assist service in Japan. JATS 7: 223–227
4. Kagawa Y, Hongo T, Sato N, Uchida N, Miura M, Nitta S, Horiuchi T, Atsumi K, Fujimasa I, Imachi K, Naka-jima M (1986) Clinical application of partial artificial heart. In: Nose Y, Kjellstrand C, Ivanovich P (ed) Progress in artificial organs—1985. ISAO, Cleveland pp 436–440
5. Nitta S, Kagawa Y, Hongo T, Horiuchi T, Katahira Y, Fujimasa I, Imachi K, Atsumi K (1985) Clinical experience of left and right ventricular assist device. In: Akutsu T (ed) Artificial heart 1. Sringer, Tokyo, pp 153–158
6. Katahira Y, Nitta S, Tanaka M, Kagawa Y, Hongo T, Horiuchi T (1985) Flow visualization of artificial heart and its quantitative analysis. Fluid control and measurement, Pergamon, Oxford pp 165–170
7. Nitta S, Kagawa Y, Sato N, Katahira Y, Miura M, Akino Y, Yambe T, Nishi K, Tsuji K, Yoda R, Tanaka M, Horiuchi T (1987) Preclinical evaluation of an improved and modified ventricular assist device and driving system. Jpn J Artif Organs 1: 203–206
8. Kagawa Y, Abe Y, Hongo T, Sato N, Sato K, Horiuchi T (1985) Current problems in surgical treatment for acquired heart disease. JJSS 86: 31–34

# Discussion

*Hill* (Pacific Presbyterian Medical Center): What was the control mechanism for pumping? Was it synchronized with an EKG?

*Kagawa* (Tohoku University): At first, we drive the VAD, asynchronously to the R waves of EKG until the patient's hemodynamic conditions get stabilized. After that, we drive in the synchronous mode, mainly in the mode of conterpulsation.

# 20. Clinical evaluation of left ventricular assist device in six cases

Motomi Shiono, Takamitsu Hasegawa, Akira Miyamoto, Shinzo Kitamura, Shogo Umeda, Hidetomo Rikukawa, Shoji Shindo, Yukihiko Orime, Hiroaki Hata, and Yukiyasu Sezai[1]

**Summary.** During recent years, ventricular assist devices (VADs) have demonstrated early clinical applications in circulatory support, with the potential of increasing use. VAD systems have been used in more than 50 cases in Japan, although a significant change in survival was achieved in only 15% of the cases. There have been a number of difficulties inherent to both the hardware and techniques of clinical application. Retrospective analysis of six cases where VADs were applied clinically are reviewed. Left ventricular assist devices (LVADs) were indicated in five patients for cardiopulmonary bypass (CPB) weaning and in one patient for postcardiotomy low output syndrome (LOS). Five cases could be weaned from LVAD, however one patient failed and was classified as LVAD dependent. In the group which could be weaned from LVAD, two patients died from multiple organ failure (MOF) and two from heart failure. Long-term survival was significant in only one patient. A clinical evaluation of the LVADs suggests that there was a remarkable hemodynamic improvement in postoperative pump failure in all six cases, and total cardiac output index should be maintained at more than 2.2–2.5 l/min/m² for the prevention of hypoperfusion of vital organs. Antithrombogenicity of the system was satisfactory, though thrombi were observed microscopically. The method and indication for removal of LVAD have not been established; however, these problems may be resolved as the number of clinical cases increase in future.

**Key words**: Ventricular assist device—Left ventricular assist device—Multiple organ failure

At present, progress in cardiovascular surgery has been rapid and remarkable; it has been accompanied by the clinical application of mechanical circulatory assistance devices. As an example, intra-aortic balloon pumping (IABP) has been successful for postcardiotomy pump failure. At the same time, however, limitations of IABP in circulatory assistance have also been recognized. Ventricular assist devices (VADs) have demonstrated early clinical capabilities of far more profound circulatory support with the potential of increasing use during recent years [1–3]. VAD systems have been used in more than 50 cases in Japan, but significant long-term survival was achieved in only

15% of cases. There are a number of problems involved in both the hardware and techniques in the clinical application of VAD systems.

A retrospective analysis was performed in six cases where left ventricular assist devices (LVADs) were applied clinically, and clinical indications and problems are discussed.

## Materials and methods

### LVAD system

#### Blood pump

An air-driven pump is used in this system (Fig. 20.1). Made from vinyl chloride resin, the inner surface of the pump is covered with Cardiothane of polyurethane and silicone copolymer (Nihon Zeon Co., ltd). The pump housing consists of polycarbonate, and several ventricular volumes are available. The standard sizes are 60 and 40 ml. On the inflow and outflow sides, spherical disc-type valves of Björk-Shiley, 18 mm inside diameter, are fixed. On the outflow side, an electromagnetic flow probe can be attached.

#### Cannulae

The design of the cannulae, connecting the blood pump and the body circulation system, can be altered depending on the procedures for the body approach that the surgeon chooses (Fig. 20.2). For the inflow side, the cannula can be inserted into the atrium or atrial appendix. The outflow side consists of a polytetrafluoroethylene (PTFE; Goretex) vascular prosthesis covered with Cardiothane and can be connected to the body circulation system by an end-to-side anastomosis.

#### Driving unit

The air-driven apparatus, Corart type 102 (Aishin Seik Co., ltd.) is an air-pulse generation system originally designed for clinical use with a maximum flow of 18 l/min, a maximum air pressure of 300 mmHg, and a maximum vacuum pressure of 150 mmHg (Fig. 20.3). These values, however, can be altered depending on

[1] 2nd Department of Surgery Nihon University School of Medicine, 30-1 Oyaguchi-kamimachi, Itabashi-ku, Tokyo, 173 Japan

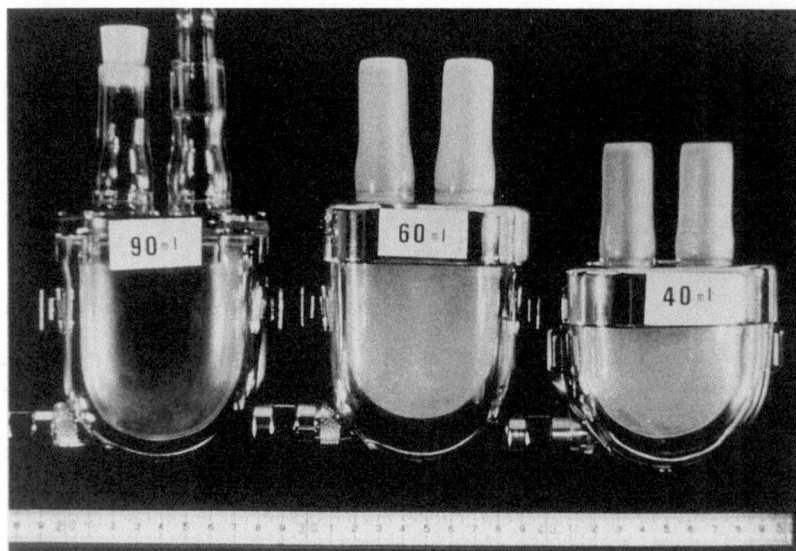

**Fig. 20.1.** Sac-type blood pump; 60 and 40 ml are most commonly used for adults

**Fig. 20.2.** Cannulae for LVAD

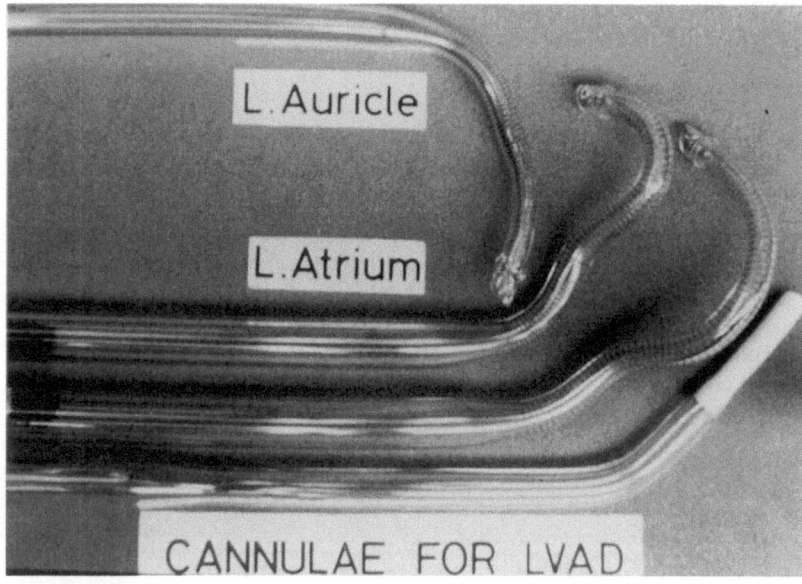

the selection of the original driving power. Adjustment of the system is automatically controlled by three microcomputers mounted inside the system, and the pumping rate, ejection time, and driving pressure can be remote controlled. ECG synchronization facilities are incorporated in the system and the cycle of assistance can be selected to wean the patient. Computerized programming for all other controls is also possible.

In terms of durability and reliability, the device has a built-in power source and a compact, small, compressed air bottle as a pneumatic drive supply, which is effective for 30 min and can be used during the transfer of patients from the operating room to the ICU or during a power shortage.

### VAD system

The pump and circulation system can be connected in three basic ways. The first is a left ventricular assist with a left ventricular bypass between the left atrium and aorta. The second is a right ventricular assist with a right ventricular bypass between the right atrium and pulmonary artery. The third way is by connecting to total heart assist and performing concurrent left and right ventricular bypasses.

### Clinical application of LVAD

The hemodynamic criteria for the indication of the use of ventricular assist devices are those presented by Pierce et al. [12] (Fig. 20.4). Since completion of the system in September 1982, we have had the opportunity to apply the LVAD system clinically. The device was used to assist in six cases (Table 20.1). The assist interval of the LVAD was 3–238 h (mean 114.4 h), and the indication was for CPB weaning in five cases and postcardiotomy LOS in one. In five cases, successful weaning from the LVAD was possible, however in one case there was failure and the patients was classified as LVAD dependent. Of the patients that could be weaned from the LVAD, two died form multiple organ failure (MOF) [4–6] and two form heart failure, and long-term survival was significant in only one patient. Retrospective analysis was performed in six cases that were clinically treated with an LVAD, and the clinical indications and problems encountered in Japan are discussed.

## Clinical cases and results

### Indication and effect of LVAD

Postoperative mechanical circulatory assistance has been done with an IABP and LVAD, however, at the same time the limitations of the IABP [7, 8] for profound pump failure have also been recognized. With these limitations in mind, the criteria for application of the LVAD have been proposed to be a cardiac index of less than 1.8 l/min/m², pulmonary capillary wedge pressure greater than 25 mmHg, and systolic arterial pressure less than 80 mmHg. The overall clinical impression is added to these parameters as an important criterion. After LVAD assistance, hemodynamic improvement was noted in all cases that fell into Forrester grade III or IV before LVAD use [13]. At the time of weaning from the LVAD, all cases fell into grade I, and a remarkable improvement was achieved (Fig. 20.5).

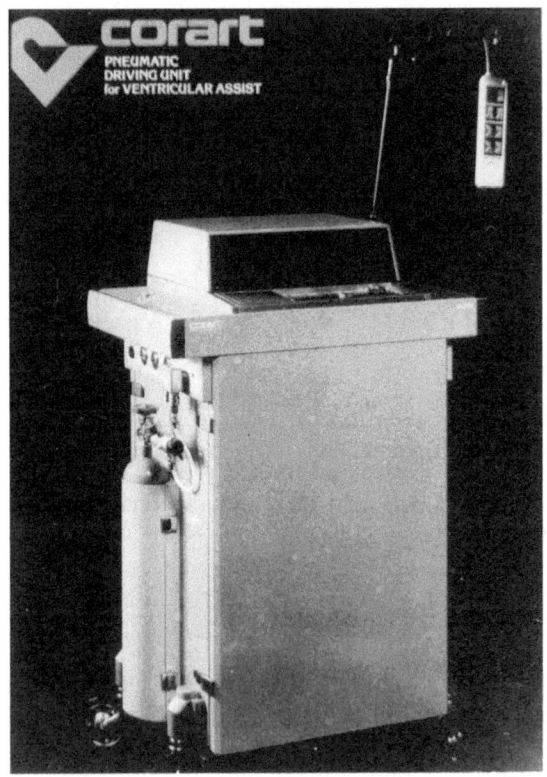

**Fig. 20.3.** Pneumatic driving unit "Corart 102"

### Driving method of LVAD in cases which progressed to MOF

Patients 2, 3, and 4 died from MOF and patients 2 and 4 progressed to oliguria, showing a rapid increase of blood urea nitrogen (BUN) and creatinine after weaning from the LVAD and subsequently needed peritoneal dialysis [9, 10]. In case 2, the total cardiac output index was maintained at approximately 2.0 l/min/m² during LVAD assistance, and hemodynamic improvement was not obtained after weaning from

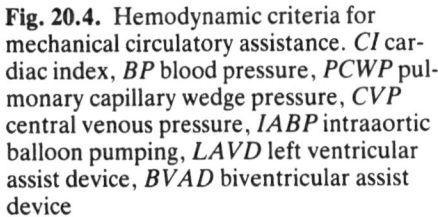

**Fig. 20.4.** Hemodynamic criteria for mechanical circulatory assistance. *CI* cardiac index, *BP* blood pressure, *PCWP* pulmonary capillary wedge pressure, *CVP* central venous pressure, *IABP* intraaortic balloon pumping, *LAVD* left ventricular assist device, *BVAD* biventricular assist device

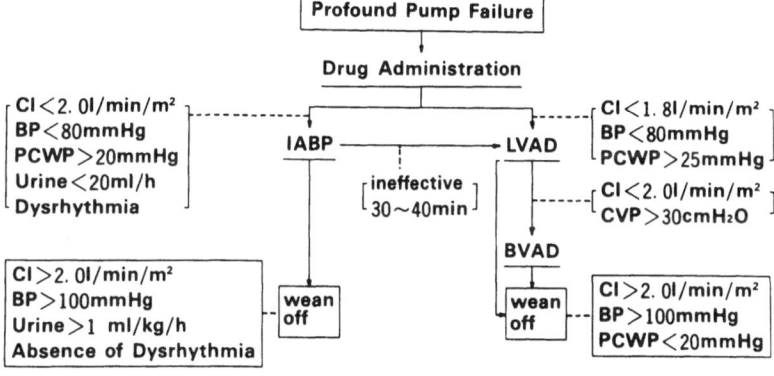

**Table 20.1.** Clinical applications of LVAD

| Case no. | Age (yrs) | Sex | Dx | Procedure | Indication | Assist interval (h) | Weaning | Prognosis |
|---|---|---|---|---|---|---|---|---|
| 1 | 62 | F | AR + MS | AVR + MVR | CPB weaning | 3 | Possible | Died (arrhythmia) |
| 2 | 23 | F | MR + TR | MVR + TAP | LOS | 118 | Possible | Died (MOF) |
| 3 | 55 | F | AMI, VSP | Patch closure | CPB weaning | 238 | Impossible | Died (MOF) |
| 4 | 71 | M | AR + MS OMI, LVA | AVR + MVR, aneurysmectomy, CABG | CPB weaning | 118 | Possible | Died (MOF) |
| 5 | 54 | M | OMI, LVA | Aneurysmectomy, CABG | CPB weaning | 95 | Possible | Survived |
| 6 | 40 | F | Post-MVR AR + TR | AVR + TVR | CPB weaning | 96 | Possible | Died (heart failure) |

*AR* aortic regurgitation, *MS* mitral stenosis, *MR* mitral regurgitation, *TR* tricuspid regurgitation, *AMI* acute myocardial infarction, *VSP* ventricular septal perforation, *OMI* old myocardial infarction, *LVA* left ventricular aneurysm, *AVR* aortic valvular replacement, *MVR* mitral valvular replacement, *TAP* tricuspid annuloplasty, *TVR* tricuspid valvular replacement, *CPB* cardioplumonary bypass, *LOS* low output syndrome

the LVAD. Prolongation of the LOS condition progressed into MOF despite a life-saving attempt (Fig. 20.6). In case 4, double valvular replacement, coronary artery bypass graft, and left ventricular aneurysmectomy were performed simultaneously for severe combined vascular disease. Aortic cross clamping and CPB time were prolonged in both cases, which was attributed to the deterioration. CPB was discontinued under LVAD assistance, however the flow of 2.2 l/min/m² was not sufficient for recovery of the vital organs. Just after weaning from the LVAD, renal insufficiency became apparent and the patient progressively deteriorated into MOF (Fig. 20.7). In case 5, however, the total cardiac output index was consistently maintained at 3 l/min/m² and organ perfusion was still inadequate. In case 3, with an anterior myocardial infarction complicated by VSP, an emergency operation was performed because of the appearance of MOF. The condition improved transiently after the operation, which included CPB and LVAD; however, the patient continued to be LVAD dependent and died of MOF (Fig. 20.8).

### Weaning time and method of LVAD in cases with pump failure

In cases 1 and 6, heart failure appeared clinically soon after weaning from the LVAD, and case 1 showed progression of right ventricular failure, and LOS in which IABP was not effective [11] (Fig. 20.9). In case 6, cardiac output was not measured by the thermodilution technique because of triple valve replacement; however, reduction of cardiac output such as a decrease in glomerular filtration rate (GFR) was recog-

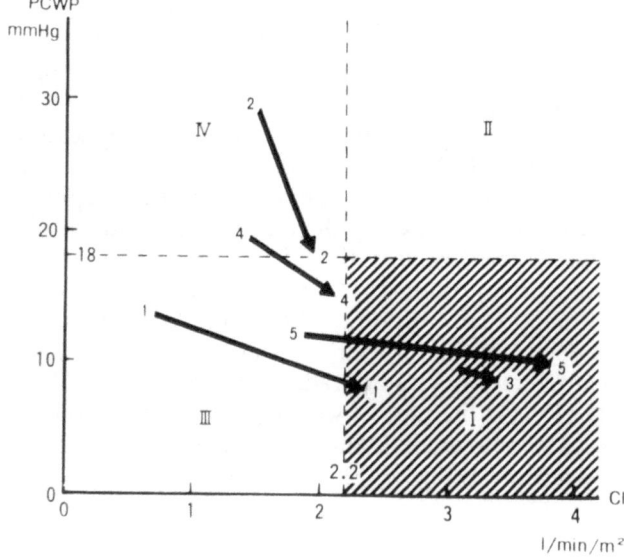

**Fig. 20.5.** Hemodynamic changes after LVAD application

nized clinically, right heart overloading progressed, and the patient expired (Fig. 20.10). These two cases suggest that the assist interval of LVAD should be longer than 3 or 4 days and the weaning technique is confronted with difficulties.

### Antithrombogenicity of system

Thromboembolic complications were not apparent in any cases during and after LVAD assistance. In cases 1, 2, and 3, anticoagulation therapy with

**Fig. 20.6.** Clinical course in case 2

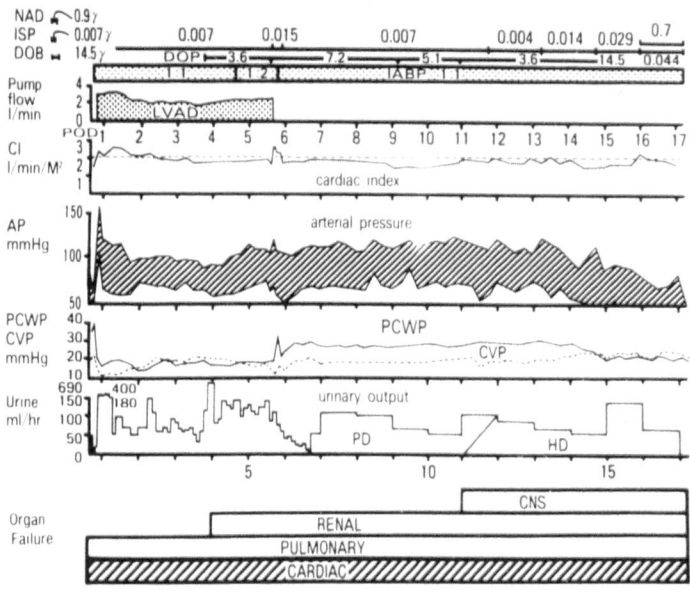

**Fig. 20.7.** Clinical course in case 4

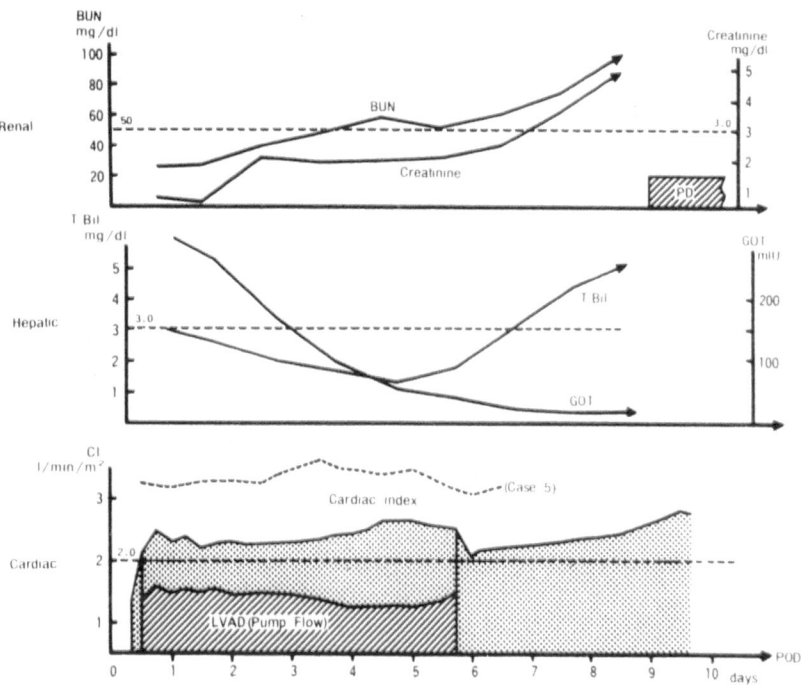

heparin, in which ACT was maintained from 150 to 200 s, was performed and thrombus formation was not apparent either in the blood pump or the cannulae. In the latter three cases, in which anticoagulation therapy was performed only with urokinase, a small number of thrombi were found in the connector portion of the pump and cannulae. Antithrombogenicity was satisfactory is most clinical cases.

## Discussion

In recent years, the VAD system has been demonstrated to be an early, effective clinical application of a profound, increased circulatory support. Since 1982, an LVAD has been clinically applied in six cases at our institute, and each case has provided further knowledge about the system [1–3].

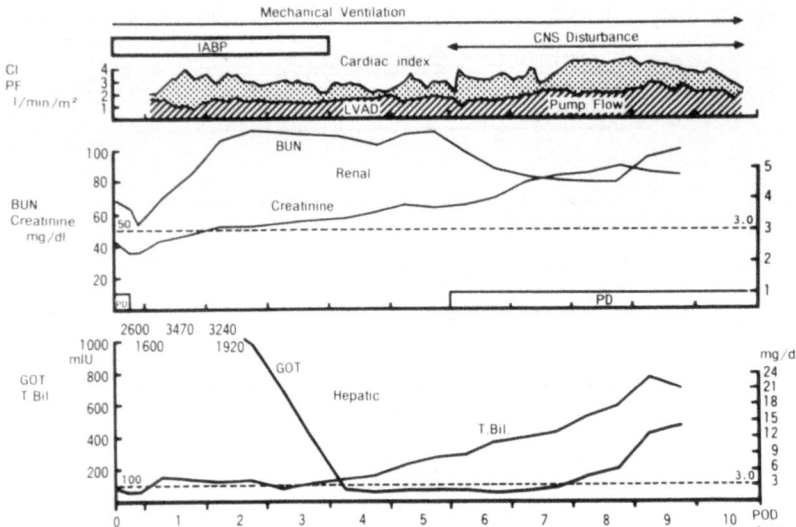

**Fig. 20.8.** Clinical course in case 3

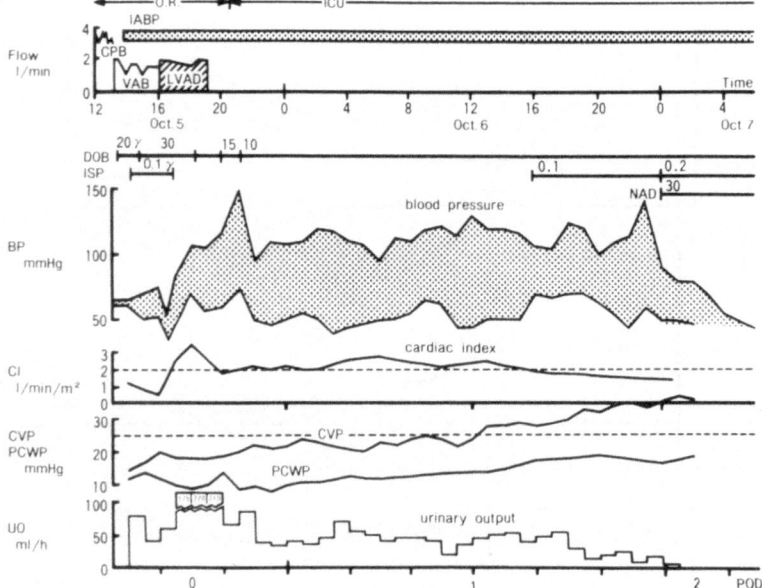

**Fig. 20.9.** Clinical course in case 1

Criteria for the indications for LVAD use have already been established in cases where the IABP has not been found to be effective. It has been reserved as a final alternative following previous poor results. The hemodynamic effects of the LVAD are remarkable, but in many cases there was no significant life-saving effect and the patients ultimately died of MOF. The LVAD is also limited, like the IABP, in cases of LVAD dependence and MOF.

In cases where the LVAD has been applied, low preoperative cardiac functions and latent origin failure progressed to MOF by the additional risks of surgical intervention and CPB. Prolongation of operation time, moreover, and CPB time may result in respiratory or renal insufficiency. Any significant life-saving effect of mechanical circulatory support, in general, has still been poor.

MOF, in this study, has been defined as:
a) Lung—dependency on mechanical ventilation
b) Kidney—BUN > 50 mg/dl, creatinine > 3 mg/dl
c) Liver—total bilirubin > 3 mg/dl, transaminase > 100 mIU
d) Digestive system—bleeding
e) CNS—coma or semicoma

MOF is diagnosed when ever two organ systems meet the above criteria.

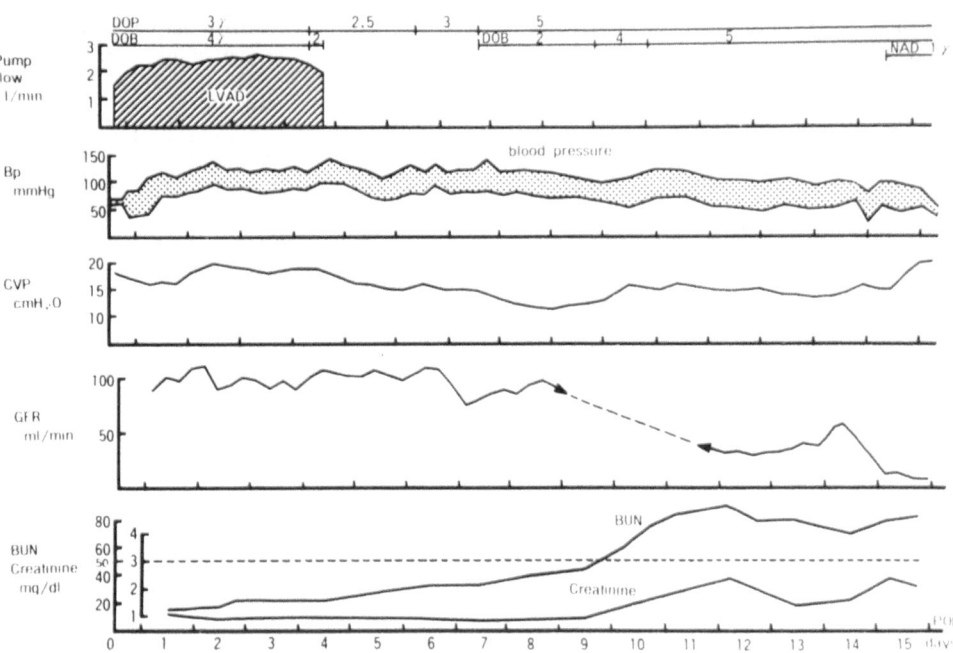

**Fig. 20.10.** Clinical course in case 6

In the cardiac surgical field, LOS or pump failure appears first, then there is a need for mechanical ventilator support, and finally renal insufficiency becomes apparent, which progresses to MOF. During LVAD assistance, therefore, the total cardiac output index is maintained at 2.2–2.5 l/min/m² because a low output state already complicates the recovery from the latent injuries to the vital organs. The pump flow of the VAD should be maintained by volume enhancement and there must be an increase of negative pressure to the pump. With regard to the weaning from LVAD, in many cases it is possible to wean from the LVAD, but long-term survival is still disappointing. At present, the indications and techniques for removal of the LVAD have not been established and current weaning criteria follow those of Pierce [11, 12].

The assist pump is discontinued for 60 s at: (a) LAP $\leq$ 20 mmHg; (b) systolic blood pressure $\geq$ 100 mmHg; (c) cardiac index $\geq$ 2.0 l/min/m²
The above criteria must be applied every 6 h over a period of 24 h prior to assist pump removal. The cardiac index, however, should be maintained for at least 2.2–2.5 l/min/m² after removal of the LVAD. It is also apparent that there is a limitation to the antithrombogenicity in the blood pump when used in a low pump flow state and, therefore, continuous weaning from the LVAD is difficult. Thromboembolic complications, however, were not apparent in any of the six cases during or after VAD support. In cases 4, 5, and 6, in which anticoagulation was performed by a small amount of urokinase, insignificant thrombus formation was noted in the connector. Antithrombogenicity was satisfactory, however considerations

should be given not only to the timely use of anticoagulant but also to the improvement of the pump, cannula, tube connections, prosthetic valve, and selection of the proper size and flow rate of the pump. The method and indications for discontinuation of the LVAD have not been established, though these problems might be resolved as the number of clinical cases increases in the future. Continued efforts are required to improve further the hardware and techniques in accordance with the advances in ventricular assist devices.

### References

1. Sezai Y, Miyamoto A, Tanoi H, Kitamura S, Kawano K, Hagiwara H, Takahashi K, Rikukawa H, Shiono M, Orime Y, Niino S (1983) Ventricular assist device system and clinical experience of 2 canes weaned from left ventricular assist device. JATS 3: 734–740
2. Sezai Y, Hasegawa T, Miyamoto A, Kitamura S, Kawano K, Shiono M, Shindo S, Rikukawa H, Orime Y, Atsumi K, Fujimasa I, Imachi K (1985) Clinical application of ventricular assist device. Medicina Philosophica 4: 708–714
3. Sezai Y, Miyamoto A, Tanoi H, Kitamura S, Kawano K, Hagiwara H, Takahashi K, Rikukawa H, Shiono M, Ogasawara K, Orime Y, Niino S, Atsumi K, Fujimasa I, Imachi K (1983) Clinical experiences of left ventricular assist device. Jpn J Artif Organs 12: 1024–1028
4. Eiseman B, Beart R, Norton L (1977) Multiple organ failure. Surg Gynec Obstet 144: 323–326
5. Fry DE, Pearlstein L, Fulton RL, Polk HC (1980) Multiple system organ failure. Arch Surg 115: 136–140
6. Baue AE, Guthrie D (1983) Multiple systems failure and circulatory support. Jpn J Surg 13: 69–85

7. Shiono M, Hasegawa T, Miyamoto A, Kitamura S, Umeda S, Kawano K, Shindo S, Rikukawa H, Sezai Y, Atsumi K, Fujimasa I, Imachi K (1986) Clinical and hemodynamic evaluation of IABP and LVAD. Jpn J Thorac Surg 39: 208–212

8. Shiono M, Miyamoto A, Kitamura K, Nakamura S, Ogasawara K, Sezai Y, Saito T (1982) Balloon counterpulsation for acute right ventricular failure due to right ventricular infarction in swine. Jpn J Artif Organs 11: 1224–1227

9. Miyamoto A, Tanoi H, Kitamura S, Kawano K, Takido N, Sezai Y, (1984) Multiple organ failure after open heart surgery. JATS 4: 296–300

10. Shiono M, Hasegawa T, Miyamoto A, Kitamura S, Kawano K, Shindo S, Rikukawa H, Orime Y, Namiki Y, Sezai Y, Atsumi K, Fujimasa I, Imachi K (1986) Retrospective analysis of multiple organ failure cases: effectiveness and limitations of mechanical circulatory assistance. Jpn J Artif Organs 15: 521–524

11. Shiono M, Miyamoto A, Kitamura S, Shindo S, Akiyama K, Orime Y, Takido N, Namiki Y, Sezai Y, Atsumi K, Fujimasa I, Imachi K (1985) Clinical application of IABP and LVAD. Jpn J Artif Organs 14: 567–570

12. Myers JL, Pierce WS (1981) The role of the ventricular assist pump for postcardiotomy cardiogenic shock: A four and one-half year experience. Proceedings of ISAO 5 (Suppl): 244

13. Forrester JS, Diamond G, Chatterjee K, Swan HJC (1976) Medical therapy of acute myocardial infarction by application of hemodynamic subsets. N Engl J Med 295: 1356, 1404

## Discussion

*Hill* (Pacific Presbyterian Medical Center): Did you begin by having three different pump sizes?

*Shiono* (Nihon University): No, we began with two sizes; 60 and 80 ml of ventricular volume. In the first three cases, the ventricular volume was 60 ml. In the latter three cases, we used 40 ml of ventricular volume.

*Hill:* Do you have any preference from a hemodynamic point of view?

*Shiono:* The hemodynamic effect is almost same with the two sizes, but the weaning technique was different because of antithrombogenicity. A small pump size of 40 ml needs a high, frequent beat rate when a large output is needed; antithrombogenicity is thought to be better under certain conditions of pump flow.

# 21. Left ventricular assist device: Experimental and clinical study

Masayoshi Okada, Maki Kubota, Masanao Imai, Yoshimi Koyama, and Kazuo Nakamura[1]

**Summary.** Recently, intra-aortic balloon pumping (IABP) has been widely employed clinically as a means of mechanical circulatory assistance. However, there have been a few patients who could not be saved from severe heart failure after a cardiac operation in spite of IABP assistance. An evaluation of the left ventricular assist device (LVAD) was experimentally carried out for profound heart failure after acute myocardial infarction, which was produced by multiple ligations of the coronary arteries. Consequently, the efficacy of the LVAD was clearly confirmed hemodynamically in comparison with another means of mechanical assistance such as VA bypass and IABP + VA bypass.

On the basis of our experimental studies, the LVAD was successfully employed in a 68-year-old female patient who underwent closure of a ventricular septal rupture (VSR) and AC bypass for VSR following acute myocardial infarction (AMI). She was weaned from the LVAD and IABP 7 days after surgery. Our experience concerning the LVAD in mechanical circulatory assistance is reported in detail.

**Key words:** Acute myocardial infarction—Severe heart failure—Mechanical circulatory assistance—Left ventricular assist device—Intra-aortic balloon pumping

Satisfactory results after cardiac surgery in patients with severe ventricular dysfunction have been obtained by improvements in the operative techniques and myocardial protection during cardiopulmonary bypass [1–6]. There are still, however, a few patients whose hemodynamic condition cannot be improved by means of intensive medical treatment. In those cases, it may be considered that mechanical circulatory assistance in addition to conventional medical treatment is the best way to save their lives.

During the past decade, mechanical circulatory assistance was utilized in 155 patients with cardiogenic shock or low cardiac output syndrome after acute myocardial infarction (AMI) and cardiac surgery. The number of cases of mechanical circulatory assistance consisted of 144 cases with intra-aortic balloon pumping (IABP), ten with IABP + VA bypass, and one with left ventricular assist device (LVAD) + IABP (Table 21.1). In general, 70% of the patients could be weaned from the circulatory assistance. Conversely, it appeared that these procedures brought no hemodynamic improvements in the remaining cases [1].

Recently, left ventricular assist devices (LVADs) have been employed in patients with cardiogenic shock after surgery for mechanical complications following AMI. For those patients, the LVAD is now essential to improve the hemodynamics and save lives [7–12]. Here some problems concerning the mechanical circulatory assistance will be discussed from our experience in this field.

## Materials and methods

Sixty-three mongrel dogs weighing between 12 and 18 kg were used in this study. The chest was opened through the fourth intercostal space under general anesthesia and respiration was maintained with a respirator. AMI was produced by multiple ligations of the coronary arteries [13, 14]. Mechanical circulatory assistance such as IABP, left heart bypass (LHB), and LVAD with an air-driven pumping chamber was initiated when cardiogenic shock and severe heart failure developed (Fig. 21.1) [15–17]. A centrifugal pump was also utilized as an LHB between the left atrium and aortic arch.

Table 21.1. Clinical experience with IABP

| Indication | No. of cases | Weaned cases from IABP |
|---|---|---|
| Cardiogenic shock due to AMI | 44 | 21 (47.7) |
| LOS and shock after cardiac surgery | 83[a] | 58 (69.8) |
| Evolving MI | 13 | 13 (100) |
| Unstable angina | 15 | 13 (86.7) |
| Total | 155 | 105 (67.7) |

[a] IABP + VA bypass was done in ten cases and LVAD in one

[1]Department of Surgery, Division II, Kobe University School of Medicine, 7-5-2 Kusunoki-cho, Chuo-ku, Kobe, 650 Japan

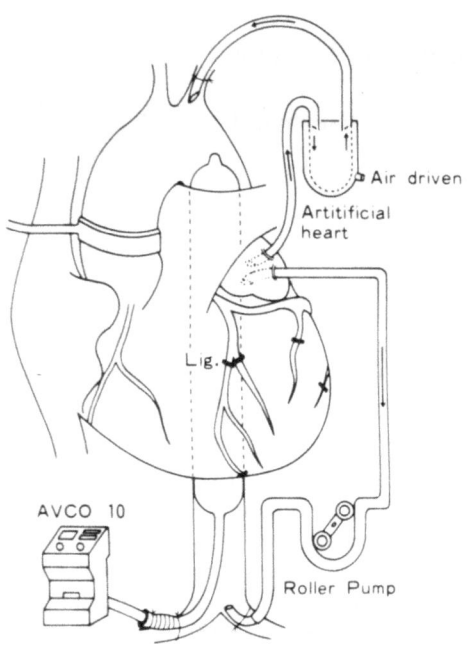

**Fig. 21.1.** Schematic illustrations of mechanical circulatory assistance

**Table 21.2.** Limitations of IABP assistance

Hemodynamic
 Cl < 1.6 l/min/m²
 LVedp > 25 mmHg
 PAWP (mean) > 30 mmHg
 Qp/Qs > 4.5

Angiographic
 Noncontractile area > 40%
 EF < 0.30
 LVEDVI > 150 ml/m²

Infarcted area
 >50% of free wall of LV

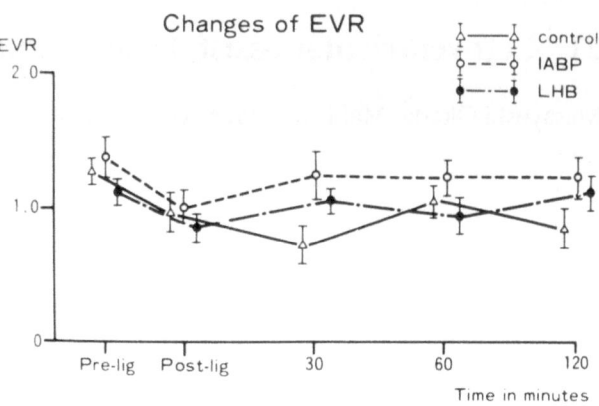

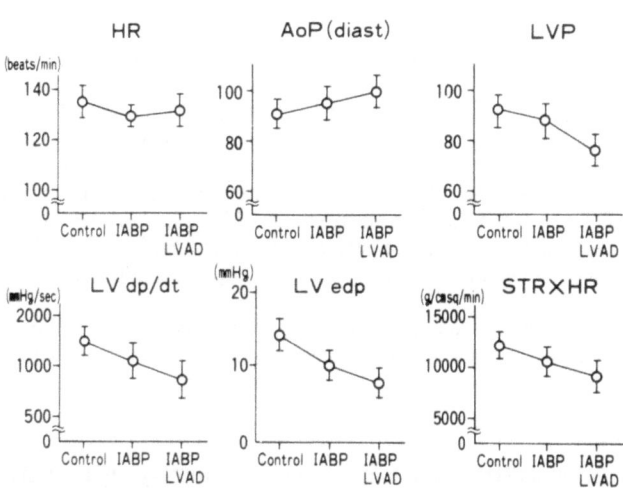

**Fig. 21.3.** Hemodynamic comparisons between IABP and IABP + LVAD

## Results

### Experimental study

By multiple ligations of the coronary arteries, an infarcted area of 25%–65% in the free wall of the left ventricle was obtained. Cardiogenic shock occurred, of which the infarcted area reached more than 45% of the free wall of the left ventricle. Thereafter, three types of circulatory assistance were carried out to compare their effects on the hemodynamics [17].

The IABP did not show any effect when the infarcted area was greater than 50% of the free wall of the left ventricle, which apparently indicates the limitations of IABP in cardiac assistance (Table 21.2) [1].

Comparing the IABP and LHB, where the flow rate was about 30% of the cardiac output, IABP was more effective than LHB in improving the hemodynamics even with changes in the endocardial viability ratio (EVR), cardiac output, and left ventricular end-diastolic pressure (LVedp) (Fig. 21.2) [16]. However, in LHB where the flow rate was more than 50% of the cardiac output, LHB was more effective than IABP.

In hemodynamic changes between IABP and LVAD + IABP, significant improvements in aortic pressure (AoP), left ventricular pressure (LVP), LV max dp/dt, and LVedp were observed especially when IABP and LVAD were combined (Fig. 21.3).

Left cardiac assistance by a centrifugal pump was also experimentally carried out in dogs with heart failure following multiple ligations of the coronary arteries. Mean AoP was maintained at 90 mmHg and mean left atrial pressure (LAP) at 7 mmHg by initiation of the centrifugal pump. In addition, LVP

**Fig. 21.4.** Effects of centrifugal pump on hemodynamics

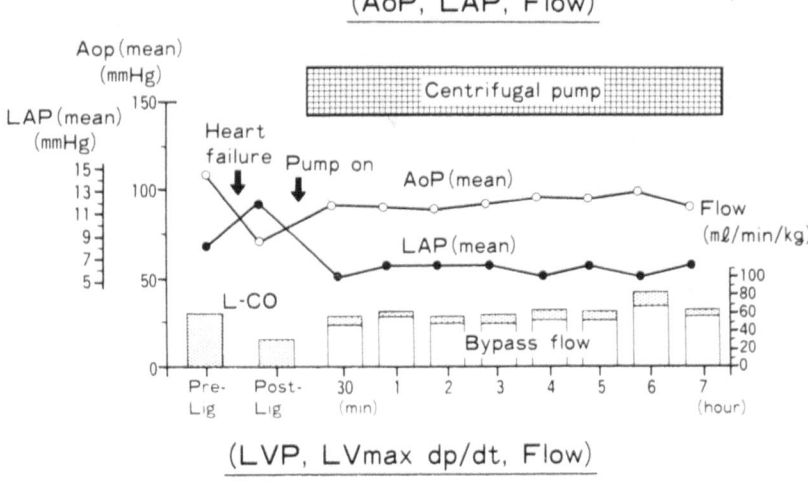

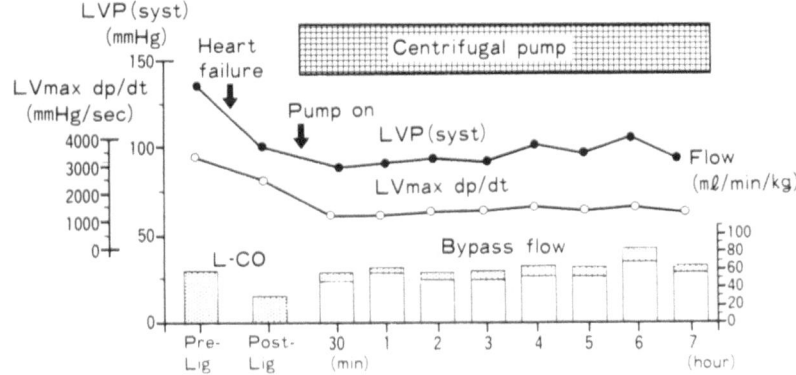

and LV max dp/dt also improved. However, there were no remarkable changes in right ventricular function (Fig. 21.4, 21.10a) [18].

On the basis of our experimental study, the most significant effects on the hemodynamics were obtained by applying the LVAD. Our protocol for indicating the assisted circulation is shown in Fig. 21.5 [19].

### Clinical study

On the basis of favorable experimental results, the LVAD was clinically employed in a 68-year-old female patient. She was admitted to our hospital because of severe chest pain and dyspnea. AMI was confirmed on ECG and holosystolic murmur occurred 2 days after the onset of chest pain. On the color Doppler echocardiogram, ventricular septal rupture (VSR) following AMI was clearly recognized (Fig. 21.6a). On the coronary angiogram, 99% stenosis of the left anterior descending artery (LAD) and 75% stenosis of the circumflex artery were noted (Fig. 21.6b).

Cardiogenic shock occurred after the onset of VSR, and IABP was immediately initiated. Simultaneously,

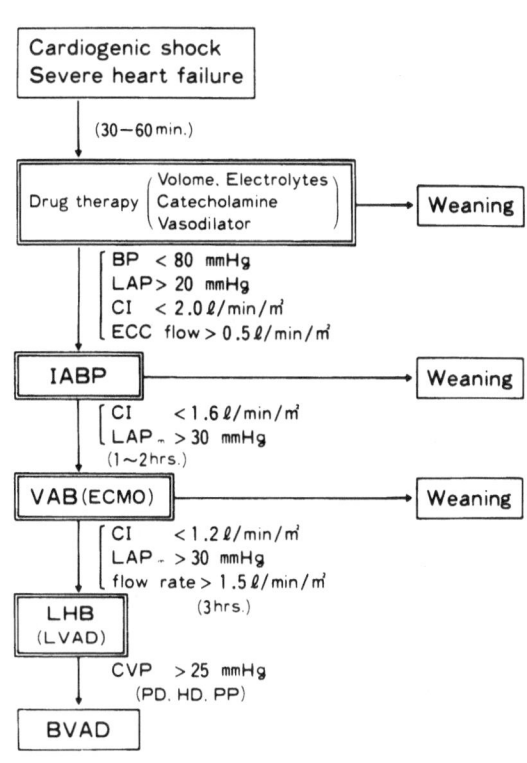

**Fig. 21.5.** Indications of assisted circulation

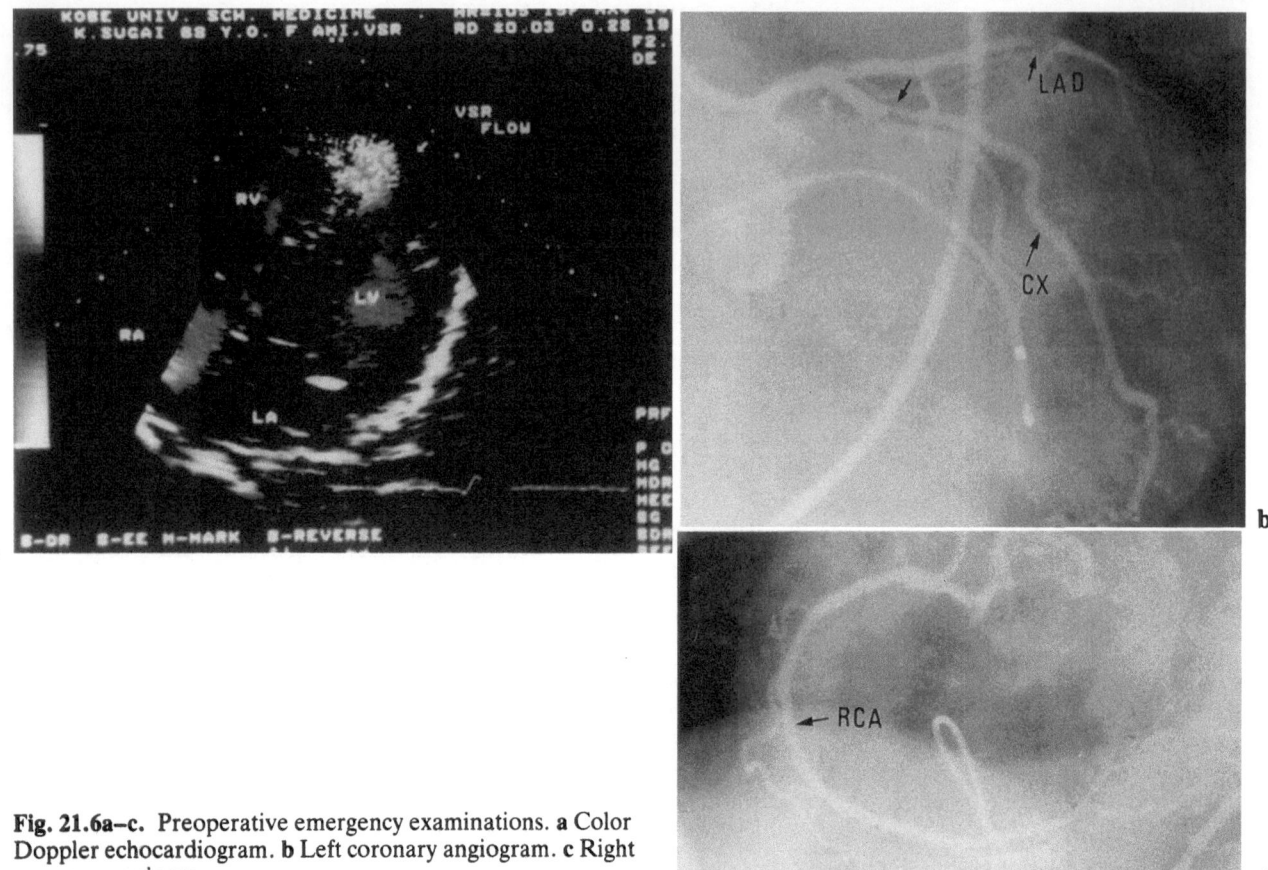

**Fig. 21.6a–c.** Preoperative emergency examinations. **a** Color Doppler echocardiogram. **b** Left coronary angiogram. **c** Right coronary angiogram

Swan-Ganz catheterization was performed. Consequently, high pressure in the right atrium and right ventricle as well as the pulmonary artery was clearly recognized (Table 21.3). The pulmonary to systemic flow ratio (Qp/Qs) was 1.87 and left to right shunt was 48%. Since the cardiac condition was in grade IV of the NYHA, an emergency operation was carried out on the day of admission. The operation was performed with the aid of cardiopulmonary bypass. First, aortocoronary bypass to the Cx using a saphenous vein was performed, and the VSR, $25 \times 15$ mm in size, was closed with a Teflon felt patch through the incision of the left ventricle (Fig. 21.7). The operation was uneventful with no complications. However, the cardiopulmonary bypass could not be removed despite the administration of a large amount of catecholamines. So, LVAD was immediately initiated (Fig. 21.8) [19]. An outflow cannula was sewn to the anterior wall of the ascending aorta and an inflow cannula was sewn to the left atrium.

By initiating the LVAD (air-driven, diaphragm-type system bypass between the left atrium and the ascending aorta), the patient was easily weaned from cardiopulmonary bypass, and good arterial pressure

of over 90 mmHg was obtained [20]. Thereafter, she was carefully managed in the CCU under the control of the LVAD (Fig. 21.9).

Full bypass using the LVAD was safely performed for 3 days after surgery. Good hemodynamics and urination were maintained during the LVAD. Thereafter, reduction of cardiac assistance was gradually performed. Consequently, the LVAD was removed on the 7th pumping day. IABP assistance was changed from 8: 1 to 1: 1. On the day after removal of the LVAD, the patient was also weaned from IABP (Fig. 21.10a) The findings of the chest x-ray film also showed an apparent improvement (Fig. 21.11). However, IABP was restarted because of low cardiac output syndrome (LOS), and hemofiltration was done 2 weeks after surgery due to a marked increase of BUN or creatinine and a decrease in the urine volume. The need to apply the IABP seemed to depend on the procedures used to remove the LVAD or on the recurrence of AMI. But, these values increased abruptly 3 weeks after surgery. On the other hand, in enzyme activities during and after LVAD, GPT was under 100 international units/l, but LDH and total bilirubin were high (Fig. 21.10b, c).

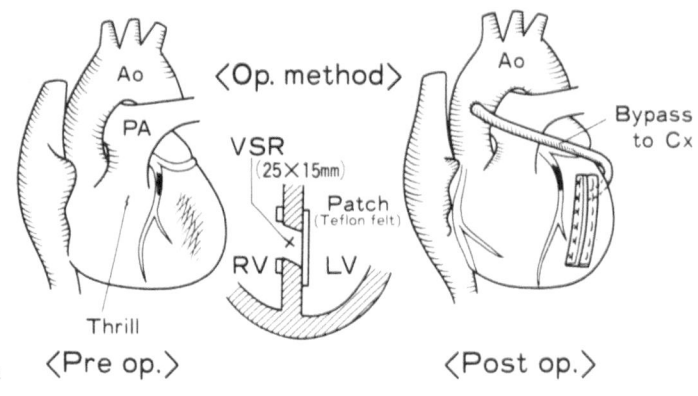

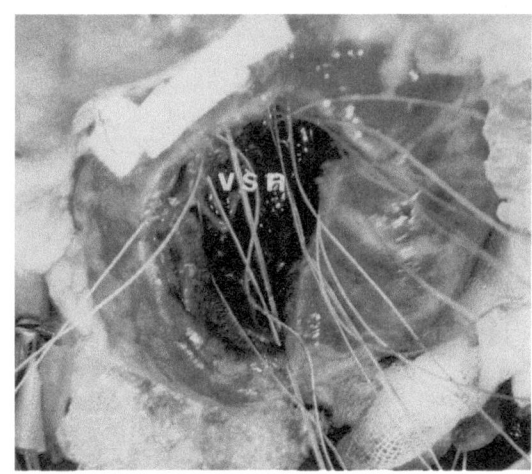

**Fig. 21.7. a** Operative method. **b** Intraoperative view

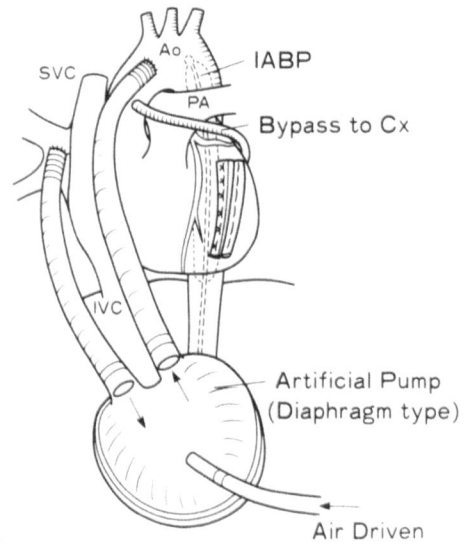

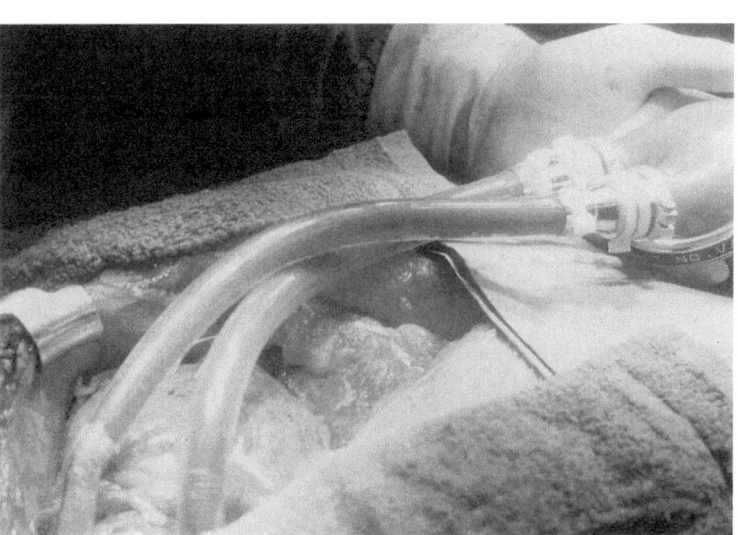

**Fig. 21.8a, b.** Left ventricular assist device. **a** Method. **b** Intraoperative view

**Table 21.3.** Cardiac conditions on admission

| Heart rate | 83/min |
| Blood pressure | 85/45 mmHg |

Swan-Ganz catheterization data

| RA | 20/10 (15) mmHg | I | → 20/4 (11) |
| RV | 44/8 edp-20 | A | → 42/4 − 18 |
| PA | 38/19 (28) | B | → 36/19 (25) |
| PC | 26/15 (20) | P | → 16/7 (13) |

Qp/Qs   1.87
l → r shunt   48%

CAG
  LAD (No 7)   99%  } stenosis
  Cx (No 14) 75%

UCG
  VSR (+)

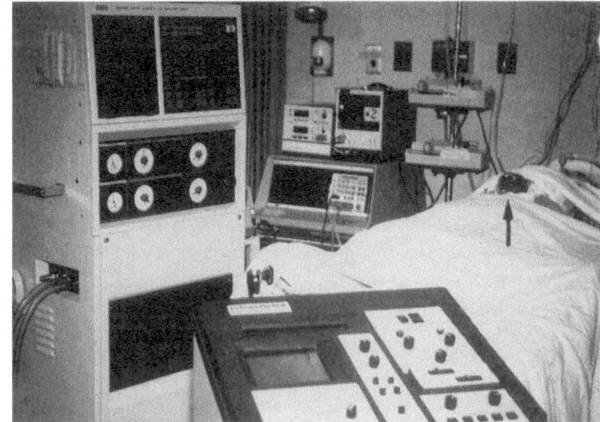

**Fig. 21.9.** LVAD + IABP in CCU

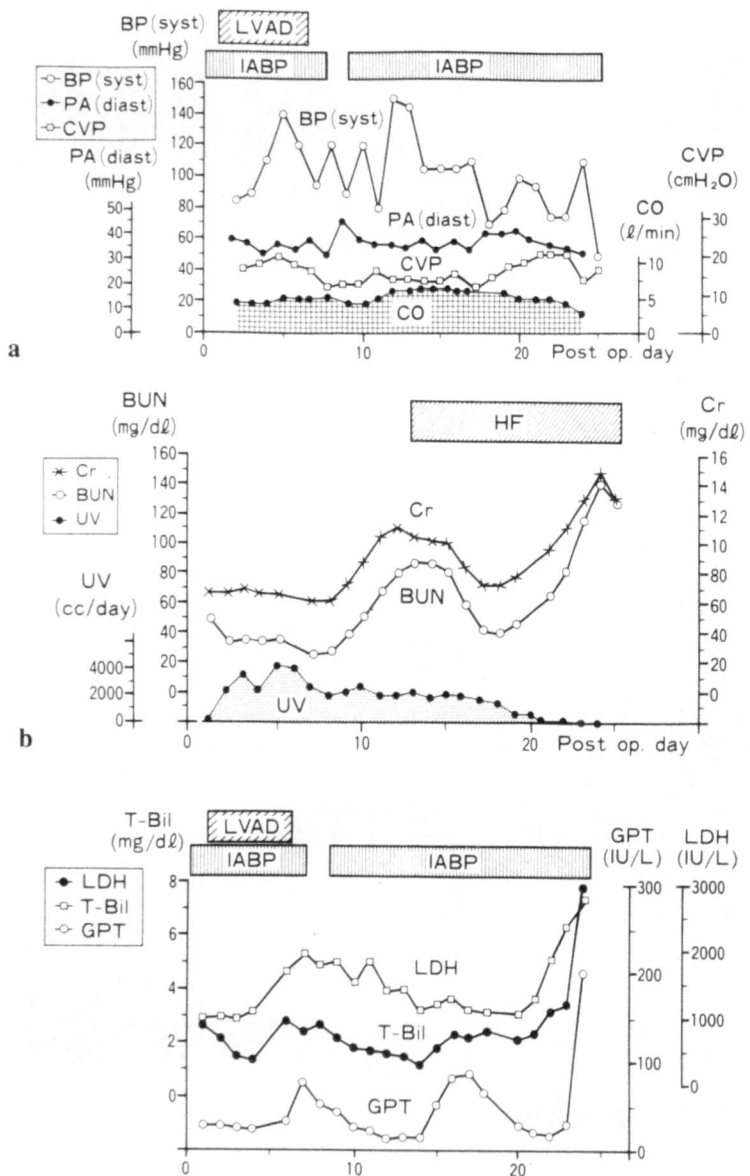

**Fig. 21.10a–c.** Clinical course during LVAD.
**a** Hemodynamic changes. **b** Renal functions.
**c** Enzyme activities

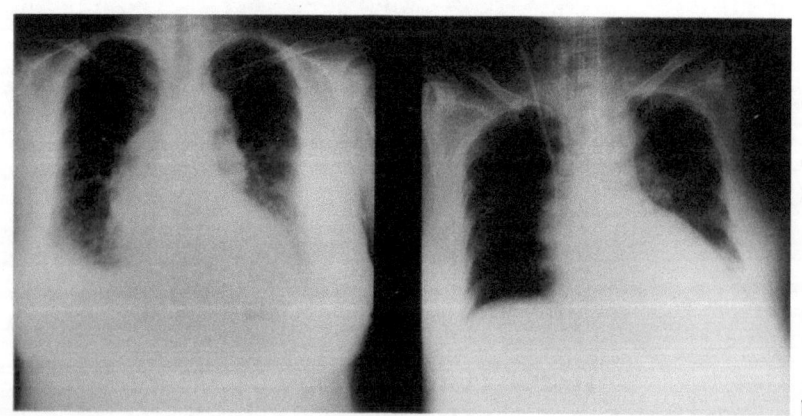

**Fig. 21.11a, b.** Findings of chest X-ray film. **a** Preoperative. **b** Postoperative

Despite hemofiltration, these values increased abnormally 3 weeks after surgery. Unfortunately, the patient died of renal failure 24 days after surgery. AC bypass to the circumflex artery was patent and closure of VSR was found to be perfect at autopsy. An obstructive coronary artery and extensive myocardial necrosis were observed by microscopic examination (Fig. 21.12).

## Discussion

There are many kinds of mechanical circulatory assistance such as IABP, VA bypass, and LHB with a centrifugal pump or a ventricular assist device (VAD). Selection of the type of cardiac assistance should be based on the severity of cardiac failure [21–27].

From our experimental study, LVAD was the most useful and effective procedure for improving the hemodynamics of the failing heart. We have used the LVAD in one clinical case with cardiogenic shock following AMI associated with VSR. Full bypass for 3 days with LVAD was very effective in improving the cardiac function.

The flow rate was gradually reduced from 2.5 to 0.3 l/min/m$^2$ according to the hemodynamics. With the reduction of the cardiac assistance by LVAD, IABP assistance was increased from 8:1 to 1:1 to maintain adequate blood pressure. During initiation of LVAD, the activated coagulation time (ACT) was carefully controlled by the administration of heparin to between 200 and 250 s to prevent blood coagulation in the artificial blood pump. The patient was successfully weaned from the LVAD and then the IABP. Thus, the combined methods were more effective than any other type of mechanical circulatory assistance. There were no complications concerning the LVAD. A great problem at present, however, is avoiding MOF during and after the use of the LVAD. To prevent MOF, intensive management was required for each vital organ, such as the kidney, liver, and lung. In the near future, temporary use of mechanical circulatory assistance or a total artificial heart might also be recommended as a bridge to heart transplantation [28–35].

In conclusion: (a) The LVAD should be used when a bypass flow more than 50% of the cardiac output is required; (b) synchronous utilization and combined procedures with IABP are useful for improving the hemodynamics; (c) IABP is not always necessary if pressure assistance can be obtained by an LVAD; (d) assisted circulation starts from the IABP and ends by itself.

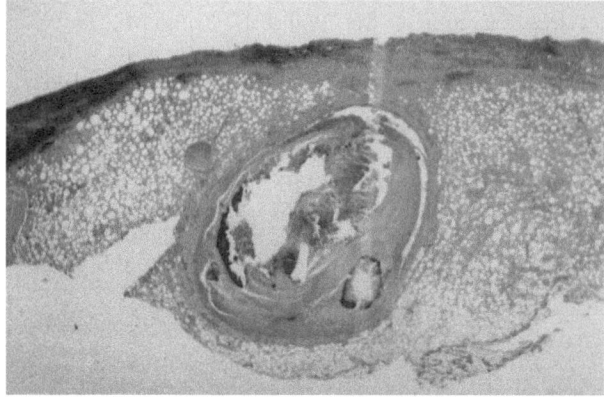

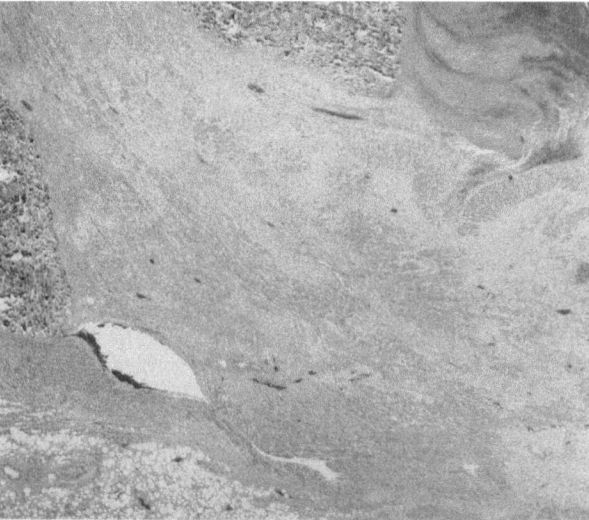

**Fig. 21.12a, b.** Microscopic findings. **a** Coronary artery (LAD). **b** Extensive necrosis of left ventricle

## References

1. Okada M, Nakamura K (1986) Indications and limitations of IABP. Jap J Thorac Surg 39: 172–181
2. Pennington DG, Swartz M, Codd JE, Merjavy JP, Kaiser GC (1983) Intraaortic balloon pumping in cardiac surgical patients: A nine-year experience. Ann Thorac Surg 36: 125–131
3. Goldberger M, Tabak SW, Shak PK (1986) Clinical experience with intraaortic balloon counterpulsation in 112 consecutive patients. Am Heart J 111: 497–502
4. Sanfelippo PM, Baker NH, Ewy HG, Moore PJ, Thomas JW, Brahos GJ, McVicker RF (1986) Experience with intraaortic balloon counterpulsation. Ann Thorac Surg 41: 36–41
5. Heitmiller R, Jacobs ML, Daggett WM (1986) Surgical management of postinfarction ventricular septal rupture. Ann Thorac Surg 41: 683–691

6. Alcan KE, Stertzer SH, Wallsh E, Bruno MS, DePasquale NP (1984) Current status of intra-aortic balloon counterpulsation in critical care cardiology. Critical Care Medicine 12: 489–495

7. Edelman SK (1980) Timing during concomitant abdominal left ventricular assist device (ALVAD) and intra-aortic balloon pumping (IABP) in man. Trans Am Soc Artif Inter Organs 26: 450–454

8. Pae WE, Rosenberg G, Donachy H, Landis DL, Phillips WM, Parr GVS, Prophet GA, Pierce WS (1980) Mechanical assistance for postoperative cardiogenic shock: A three year experience. Trans Am Soc Artif Intern Organ 26: 256–261

9. Atsumi K (1984) Ventricular assistance—Development and clinical application of a new device. In: Unger F (ed) Assisted circulation, 2nd edn. Springer, Berlin pp 100–114

10. Dew PA, Olsen DB, Kessler TR, Coleman DL, Kolff WJ (1984) Mechanical failure in vivo and in vitro studies of pneumatic total artificial hearts. Trans Am Soc Artif Intern Organs 30: 112–116

11. Takano H, Nakatani T, Taenaka Y, Umezu M (1986) Development of the ventricular assist pump system: Experimental and clinical studies. In: Akutsu T (ed) Artificial heart 1 Springer, Tokyo, pp 141–151

12. Nitta S, Kagawa Y, Hongo T, Horiuchi T, Katahira Y, Fujimasa I, Imachi K, Atsumi K (1986) Clinical experience of left and right ventricular assist devices. In: Akutsu T (ed) Artificial heart 1. Springer, Tokyo, pp 153–158

13. Swan HJ, Forrester JS, Diamond G, Chatterjee K, Parmely WW (1972) Hemodynamic spectrum of myocardial infarction and cardiogenic shock. A conceptual model. Circulation 45: 1097–1110

14. Resnekov L (1983) Cardiogenic shock. Chest 83: 893–898

15. Okada M, Asada S (1979) Assisted circulation—especially IABP. Jpn J Thorac Surg 32: 645–657

16. Okada M, Horii H, Ikuta H, Shimizu K, Isaji S, Tsuruta H, Takahashi H, Matsuda S, Yano H, Yoneda K, Kawai M, Iizuka M, Hironaka S, Shiozawa T, Okuno K, Nakamura K (1982) The effects of mechanical circulatory assistances for acute myocardial infarction-IABP and left heart bypass (using roller pump, or artificial heart). Jpn J Artif Organs 11: 114–119

17. Okada M, Shiozawa T, Iizuka M, Okuno K, Hironaka S, Matsuda S, Yoneda K, Yano A, Kawai M, Nakamura K, Asada S (1984) The effect of intraaortic balloon pumping (IABP) on cardiogenic shock due to acute myocardial infarction. Kobe J Med Sci 30: 35–51

18. Kubota M, Okada M, Imai M, Nakamura K (1986) Experimental studies on assisted circulation by centrifugal pump. Presented at the 39 th J Jap Assoc Thorac Surg, Oct. Tokyo

19. Okada M (1987) An evaluation of simultaneous application of IABP during ventricular assist device. Jpn Ann Thorac Surg 7: 230–235

20. Okada M, Kubota M, Imai M, Koyama Y, Koterazawa T, Nakamura K (1987) Left ventricular assist device: Experimental and clinical study. Proceedings of 2nd international symposium on artificial heart and assist device. p 24

21. Okada M, Shiozawa T, Iizuka M, Okuno K, Chen CC, Matsuda S, Yoneda K, Yano A, Kawai M, Asada S (1979) Experimental and clinical studies on the effect of intra-aortic balloon pumping for cardiogenic shock following acute myocardial infarction. Artif Organs 3: 241–246

22. Okada M, Matsuda S, Kusumoto N, Shio K, Ohta T, Shiozawa T, Okuno K, Iizuka M, Kozawa S, Nakamura K (1984) Intraaortic balloon pumping (IABP) in patients with cardiogenic shock and mechanical complication due to acute myocardial infarction. Jpn Ann Thorac Surg 4: 926–932

23. Matsuda S, Okada M, Yamamoto S, Ohta T, Ohyabu H, Kuris S, Shida T, Shio J, Tachibana F, Nakamura K, Tsuruta H, Goto T, Ogawa K (1983) Combined use of ECMO with IABP for cardiogenic shock. Jpn J Artif Organs 12: 362–366

24. Bernhard WF, Clay W, Gernes D, Hougen T, Sherman C, Burke D, Schoen TJ, Poirier VL (1985) Temporary and permanent left ventricular bypass: Laboratory and clinical observations. World J Surg 9: 54–64

25. Pennington DG, Bernhard WF, Golding LR, Berger RL, Watson JT (1985) Long-term follow-up of postcardiotomy patients with profound cardiogenic shock salvaged by ventricular assist device. Circulation 70 (Suppl II): 70–84

26. Kafrouni G (1984) Intraaortic balloon counterpulsation. Am J Surg 147: 731–734

27. Kantrowitz A (1986) The ninth Hastings lecture, Spectrum. Artif Organs 10: 497–510

28. Pierce Ws (1986) The artificial heart—1986: Partial fulfillment of a promise. ASAIO Trans 32: 5–10

29. Kresh JY, Kerkhof PL, Goldman SM, Brockman SK (1986) Heart-mechanical assist device interaction. ASAIO Trans 32: 437–443

30. Cortesini R, Berloco P (1986) Alternatives to heart transplantation. Cardiologia 31: 1065–1968

31. Wolner E (1986) Artificial heart in heart transplantation—A review. Z Kardiol 75: 125–126

32. Firth BG (1987) Replacement of the failing heart. Am J Med Sci 293: 50–65

33. Vasku J (1987) Use of total heart replacement in clinical practice. Importance of experimental preparation in relation to legal, ethical and social aspects. Cas Lek Cesk 126: 33–40

34. Copeland JG, Levinson NM, Smith R, Icenogle TB, Vaughn C, Chung K, Otto R (1986) The total artificial heart as a bridge to transplantation. A report of two cases. JAMA 256: 2991–2995

35. Griffith BP, Hardesty RL, Kormos RL, Trento A, Borovetz HS, Thompson ME, Bahnson HT (1987) Temporary use of the Jarvik-7 total artificial heart before transplantation. N Engl J Med 316: 130–134

## Discussion

*Hill* (Pacific Presbyterian Medical Center): Do you turn the interior balloon off completely at any time?

*Okada* (Kobe University): No, we do not turn off inserted balloon assistance (IABP) completely at any time to prevent thrombus formation during left ventricular assist device (LVAD). IABP assistance, such as 8: 1, is employed if hemodynamic conditions can be adequately maintained by LVAD. We control activated coagulation time (ACT) with heparin for 200–250 s during LVAD. By the way, IABP support of 1: 1 can be utilized at the time of weaning from LVAD

# 22. Clinical considerations of life-saving effect of left ventricular assist device

Hiroyuki Noda, Hisateru Takano, Yoshiyuki Taenaka, Masayuki Kinoshita, Eisuke Tatsumi, Mitsuo Umezu, Akihiko Yagura, Hiroyoshi Sekii, Takeshi Nakatani, Hiroo Iwata, Setsuo Takatani, Takehisa Matsuda, Yoshitsugu Kito, Tsuyoshi Fujita, Tetsuzo Akutsu, and Hisao Manabe[1]

**Summary.** Our left ventricular assist device (LVAD), containing an automatic level control of total systemic flow and left atrial pressure, was clinically applied in 16 patients (aged 3–73 years) with cardiogenic shock following acute myocardial infarction (AMI; nine cases) and cardiac surgery (seven cases). The entire circulation was well maintained at the normal level and the LVAD was successfully removed in nine patients (56%). Three patients (19%) could be discharged with a satisfactory condition. Removal of left ventricular overload with the use of the LVAD prevented overextension of the impaired myocardium, and the gradual increase in left ventricular work promoted the compensatory ability of the residual myocardium. This recovery mechanism was established in chronic animal experiments using goats. However, the clinical problem with the treatment was the preexisting myocardial damage, such as fibrosis caused by rheumatic myocarditis and ischemia in the residual myocardium. In addition, although the natural heart recover, several patients died of multiple organ failure, which had developed during the prolonged low perfusion period prior to left ventricular assistance. In conclusion, the timely use of LVAD proved to be effective in treatment of cardiogenic shock, but preexisting myocardial damage and delayed application will considerably decrease the chance of a favorable recovery in clinical cases.

**Key words:** Left ventricular assist device—Acute cardiogenic shock—Multiple organ failure

The mortality in profound heart failure following acute myocardial infarction (AMI) or after cardiac surgery is still high even though potent medical therapy or intra-aortic balloon pumping (IABP) are used. In our coronary care unit, patients who fell into cardiogenic shock of Killip grade 4 and Forrester grade 4 did not usually survive despite the application of various kinds of conventional therapy. Recently, the left ventricular assist device (LVAD) has been inducted in the treatment of intractable pump failure as an effective method. At our hospital, we have treated 16 patients with cardiogenic shock using the automatic LVAD system which was originally developed at our research institute. The present study was aimed to establish the clinical problems on the recovery mechanism of the failing heart and also the factors affecting the survival rate as compared with the results of animal experiments.

## Materials and method

### Description of LVAD system

The LVAD system utilized in this study was originally developed at our research institute and consists of an air-driven, diaphragm-type blood pump (stroke volume 70 ml for adults and 20 ml for children) made of segmented polyetherpolyurethane (supplied by TOYOBO Co., Ltd., Japan) and driving console which alternately supplies compressed air and a vacuum to drive the blood pump. This driving console has a level control system which can automatically regulate the pump flow in response to changes in the systemic circulatory condition [1]. The unit also has an electrocardiographic synchronization system, which allows the assist pump to be driven in a counterpulsation mode against the heart output. This LVAD system was used in both the clinical and experimental studies.

### Indication and operative method

An outline of the indications for LVAD use is presented in Fig. 22.1. The major indications include: (a) cardiac output below 2.0 l/min/m²; (b) left atrial pressure or pulmonary arterial wedge pressures over 18 mmHg; (c) systemic systolic pressure below 80 mmHg. These indications are used not only for postoperative heart failure but also for AMI with shock. The patient in Killip grade 4 and Forrester's subset 4 is also a candidate for application of the LVAD. All pumps were implanted between the right side of the left atrium and ascending aorta under extracorporeal circulation.

[1]National Cardiovascular Center, 5-7-1 Fujishiro-dai, Suita, Osaka, 565 Japan

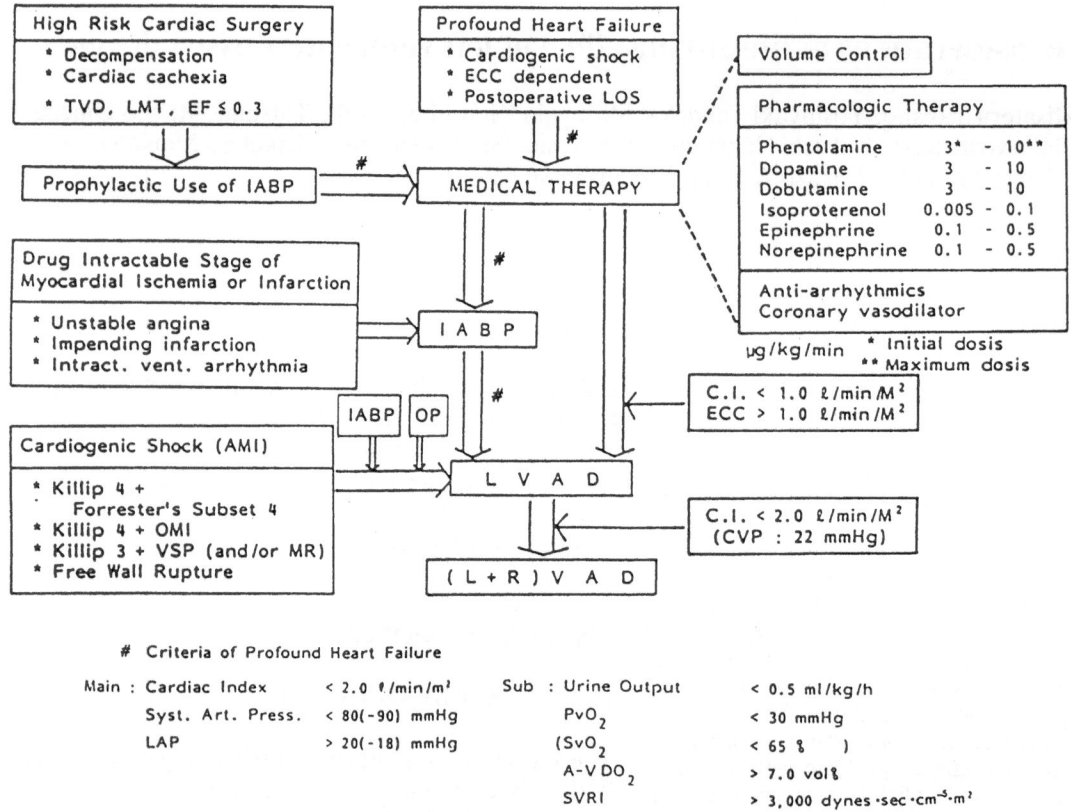

**Fig. 22.1.** Schematic drawing of indication of left ventricular assist device. *TVD* Tri-vessel disease, *LMT* left main trunck disease, *ECC* extracorporeal circulation, *IABP* intra-aortic balloon pumping, *OP* operation, *CI* cardiac index, *CVP* central venous pressure, *LAP* left atrial pressure, *OMI* old myocardial infarction, *VSP* ventricular septal perforation, *MR* mitral regurgitation, *LOS* low output syndrome, *PvO2* mixed venous oxygen pressure, *SvO2* venous oxygen saturation, *A-VDO2* arterial mixed venous oxygen difference, *SVRI* systemic vascular resistance index, *LVAD* left ventricular assist device, *L + R* left and right.

### Outline of patients

From 1982 until July 1987, 16 patients were treated with the LVAD system; their data are summarized in Table 22.1. The age ranged from 3 to 73 years and there were ten males and six females. Ten of the patients suffered from AMI. In three of the AMI cases (no. 2, 4, and 7), ventricular septal perforation occurred within 5–7 days after AMI. Although an emergency patch closure of perforation was performed in these cases, cases 2 and 7 were not weaned from extracorporeal circulation (ECC). Thus, the LVAD was applied to maintain the systemic circulation. In case 4, the LVAD was electively applied in order to prevent overloading of the left ventricle. In five AMI cases, the LVAD was applied following emergency aortocoronary bypass grafting (ACBG). Two AMI patients received no ACBG because the appropriate time for emergency ACBG had already passed.

Case 4, the child, received closure of a ventricular septal defect and could not be weaned from ECC. The small-type LVAD was applied, and this became the world's first case of an LVAD being used in a child. In case 5, there was massive bleeding from the left ventricular rupture after mitral valve replacement. The LVAD was applied in order to decompress the left ventricle. The LVAD was also performed in cases with postoperative heart failure following mitral valve replacement, left ventricular aneurysmectomy, patch enlargement of supraaortic stenosis, and reconstruction of a thoracic aortic aneurysm.

### Results

The clinical results are shown in Table 22.2. In the ventricular septal perforation patients, the LVAD was successfully removed. Although one patient died of cerebral hemorrhage 35 days after removal, two patients were discharged from hospital with a satisfactory condition. Three of the five patients who under-

**Table 22.1.** Patients in whom left ventricular assist was applied in the treatment of cardiogenic shock

| No. | Age (yrs) | Sex | Diagnosis | Operation | Indication | Assist |
|---|---|---|---|---|---|---|
| 1 | 36 | F | MSR, TR, giant LA | MVR, TAP, LA plication | Postop. LOS | LVAD |
| 2[a] | 62 | F | AMI + VSP | Patch closure, resection of LV infarcted area | ECC dependent | LVAD |
| 3[a] | 52 | M | ASR, MSR, AMI & VF during CAG | AVR, ACBG (1) | ECC dependent | LVAD + RVAD |
| 4 | 3 | M | VSD + PH | Patch closure | ECC dependent | LVAD |
| 5 | 66 | F | MS | MVR (LV rupture) | Intractable repair | LVAD |
| 6[a] | 66 | M | OMI, AMI & VT during CAG | ACBG (2) | ECC dependent | LVAD |
| 7[a] | 71 | F | AMI + VSP | Patch closure | Elective use | LVAD |
| 8[a] | 60 | M | AMI + shock | ACBG (1) | Card. shock ECC dependent | LVAD |
| 9 | 26 | M | Supravalvular AS | Aortoplasty (VA bypass) | ECC dependent | LVAD |
| 10[a] | 69 | M | AMI + shock | (−) | Card. shock | LVAD |
| 11[a] | 73 | F | AMI + VSP | Patch closure | ECC dependent | LVAD |
| 12 | 44 | M | OMI, VT, LA aneurysm | Aneurysmectomy, cryosurgery | Postop. LOS | LVAD |
| 13 | 73 | M | AMI + shock | (−) | Card. shock | LVAD |
| 14 | 57 | M | OMI + AP during | ACBG (3) | Postop. LOS | LVAD |
| 15 | 62 | M | AMI, shock during PTCR | ACBG (2) | Card. shock | LVAD |
| 16 | 73 | M | TAA | Reconstruction | Postop. LOS | LVAD |

[a] Emergency operation

*LOS* low output syndrome, *AMI* acute myocardial infarction, *OMI* old myocardial infarction, *VSP* ventricular septal perforation, *ASR* aortic stenosis and regurgitation, *TAA* thoracic aortic aneurysm, *MSR* mitral stenosis and regurgitation, *VF* ventricular fibrillation, *VT* ventricular tachycardia, *AP* angina pectoris, *CAG* coronary angiography, *AVR* aortic valve replacment, *ECC* extra corporeal circulation, *ACBG* aortocoronary bypass grafting, *LVAD* left ventricular assist device

**Table 22.2.** Clinical results of treatment

| No. | Age (yrs) | Sex | Indication | Assist | Duration | Weaned | Results |
|---|---|---|---|---|---|---|---|
| 1 | 36 | F | Postop. LOS | L | 14 days | Yes | Died (MOF, sepsis: 1 day after removal) |
| 2 | 62 | F | ECC dependent | L | 15 days | Yes | Hospital death (cerebral bleeding: 35 days after removal) |
| 3 | 52 | M | ECC dependent | L + R | 4 h | No | Died (peripheral insufficiency) |
| 4 | 3 | M | ECC dependent | L | 3 days | Yes | Died (respiratory failure: 20 days after removal) |
| 5 | 66 | F | Intractable repair | L | 22 h | No | Died (bleeding from repaired LV wall) |
| 6 | 66 | M | ECC dependent | L | 7 days | Yes | Died (MOF, 11 days after removal) |
| 7 | 71 | F | Elective use | L | 7 days | Yes | Alive (discharged and well) |
| 8 | 60 | M | Card. shock ECC dependent | L | 14 days | Yes | Died (MOF, sepsis: 10 days after removal) |
| 9 | 26 | M | ECC dependent | L | 3 h | No | Died (respiratory failure, CVA during VAB) |
| 10 | 69 | M | Card. shock | L | 12 days | No | Died (respiratory failure) |
| 11 | 73 | F | ECC dependent | L | 6 days | Yes | Alive (in general ward) |
| 12 | 44 | M | Postop. LOS | L | 6 days | No | Died (respiratory failure) |
| 13 | 73 | M | Card. shock | L | 12 days | Yes | Hospital death (respiratory failure: 149 days after removal) |
| 14 | 57 | M | Postop. LOS | L | 7 days | Yes | Alive (discharged) |
| 15 | 62 | M | Card. shock | L | 41 days | No | Died (MOF) |
| 16 | 73 | M | Postop. LOS | L | 1 h | No | Died (respiratory failure) |

*MOF* multiple organ failure, *LVAD* left ventricular assist device

went ACBG could be weaned from the LVAD. Two of three weaned patients died of multiple organ failure, which might have been caused by the prolonged low cardiac output condition before LVAD application. Only one survivor (case 14) among the ACBG patients received implantation of the LVAD without delay. The systemic circulation in case 15, where there was a broad left ventricular infarction became dependent in the LVAD during the clinical course, and several trials of weaning failed. The patient died of respiratory failure following 41 days of pumping. Case 3 had cardiac massage for over 1 h and the peripheral vessels completely collapsed when the LVAD was applied. In case 10, weaning from the assistance was not carried out because the general condition became critical due to respiratory failure; however, recovery of the heart was observed enhococcardiographically. Case 13 without ACBG was weaned from the assist pump, and the patient later underwent ACBG because of a prolonged ischemic attack.

In the pediatric case, the LVAD was removed on the 4th postoperative day (POD). The patient died of pulmonary vascular constriction, which occurred suddenly on the 7th POD. In the left ventricular rupture

case, uncontrollable bleeding caused death. In case 1 with mitral valve replacement, the LVAD was successfully removed, but the patient's general condition had become critical because of multiple organ failure and sepsis, and the patient died the day after removal. Both patients with aortic aneurysm and aortic stenosis died soon after application of the LVAD because of respiratory failure.

The weaning ratio from the LVAD in all patients was 56%. Hemodynamic changes in the nine weaned patients are summarized in Fig. 22.2. Total flow (bypass flow + cardiac output) was well maintained at a level of 3.0–3.5 l/min/m$^2$ while the left ventricular function recovered as evidenced by an increase in the heart rate and a left atrial pressure higher than normal. Right ventricular failure gradually recovered during pumping. To estimate heart function clearly, an echocardiographic examination was performed. A gradual increase in left ventricular (LV) capacity, recovery of abnormal LV wall motion, and increase in ejection fraction of the left ventricle were seen as the heart recovered.

Only three patients were discharged from the hospital. The cause of death in the patients weaned from

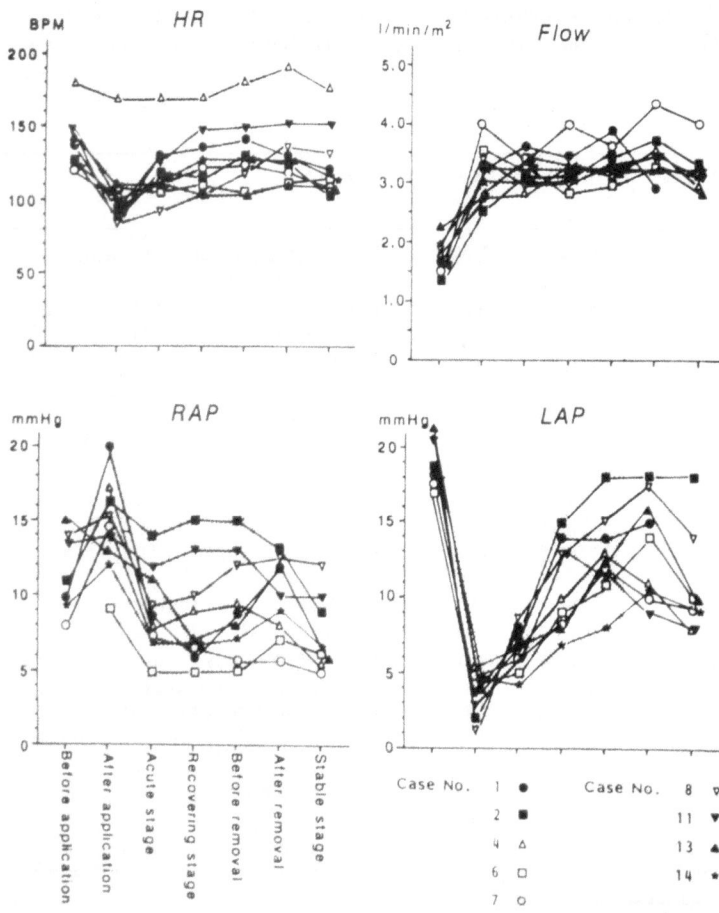

**Fig. 22.2.** Hemodynamic changes in patients who were weaned from assisted circulation before, during, and after LVAD assistance

| | | LUNG | KIDNEY | LIVER | D I C | BRAIN | INFECTION | EMBOLISM | RESULT | CAUSE OF DEATH | EPISODE PRIOR TO APPLICATION |
|---|---|---|---|---|---|---|---|---|---|---|---|
| 36 | female | O | O | O | ● | | ● | MV | death | MOF | delayed application |
| 62 | female | ● | ● | ● | ● | O | | | death | cerebral hemorrhage | delayed application |
| 3 | male | ● | ● | | ● | O | ● | lung | death | respiratory failure | long term ECC |
| 66 | male | ● | ● | ● | ● | | O | | death | MOF | delayed application |
| 71 | female | O | O | O | O | | ● | | alive | | |
| 60 | male | O | ● | O | ● | | ● | LV | death | MOF & infection | delayed application |
| 73 | female | O | O | | O | | O | | alive | | |
| 73 | male | O | ● | | O | O | O | LV | death | cerebral infarction infection | |
| 57 | male | | O | | | | O | | alive | | |

**Fig. 22.3.** Complications and episodes prior to pump application in the patients who were weaned from assisted circulation. A *closed circle* indicates that some special treatment was required, such as high-frequency oscillated ventilation for lung complications, peritoneal dialysis for kidney, plasma pheresis for liver. A *closed circle* in *INFECTION* also indicates that sepsis was ascertained by blood culture

the assist pump was multiple organ failure, which was closely related to the systemic conditions before LVAD application (Fig. 22.3)

## Pathological findings of the heart in clinical cases

Generally, the infarcted myocardium changed either into granulation tissue in the patients who died in the early post-AMI period or was replaced with fibrous tissue and became a solid scar in the patients who survived longer than 1 month after AMI. In addition, the residual myocardium became hypertrophic when compared with normal myocardium. In case 2, AMI with a ventricular septal perforation, the reduced LV capacity following resection of the infarcted wall returned almost to normal. In some cases where emergency ACBG was performed, hemorrhagic necrosis into the bypassed area of myocardium was observed (Fig. 22.4).

## Discussion

Prior to clinical application, we set up two types of experimental model using adult goats to examine the clinical condition; one was the AMI model and the other the postcardiotomy global myocardial ischemia (GMI) model [1, 2]. Of AMI in the LV free wall, 70%–90% was made by ligation of the coronary artery in the ten goats. The GMI model was made by anoxic

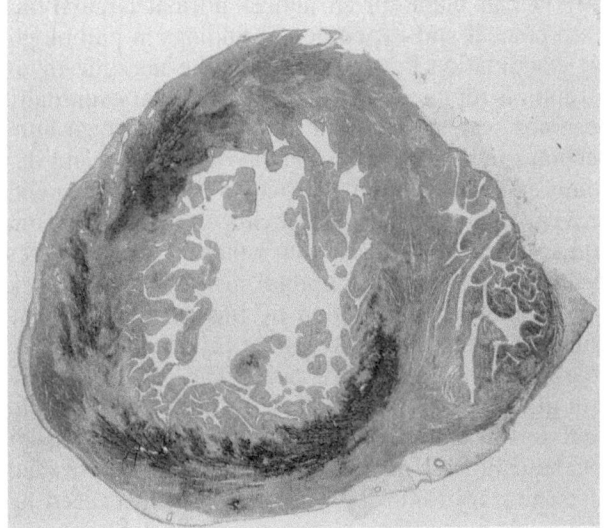

**Fig. 22.4.** Ring slice of the heart in case 8; the patient died of multiple organ failure and sepsis. Hemorrhagic necrosis was seen in the bypassed area of myocardium

arrest at normal temperature for 30 min and 60 min in three animals each. The LVAD was installed between the left atrium and descending aorta. The LVAD was introduced to maintain systemic circulation and its effect on both profound heart failure models was evaluated. In AMI animals with less than 80% LV infarction, systemic circulation was well maintained with the use of the LVAD only, and heart function recovered sufficiently for the LVAD to be removed. Also in GMI models, LVAD was removed successfully in three of six animals. In both models, the failing heart recovered by an increase in the LV capacity, heart rate, and preload to LV. The causes of death were ventricular arrythmia or right ventricular failure, not malfunctions of other organs. Pathological findings showed tight scar formation of the infarcted myocardium, and myocardial cells in the normal region seemed to be hypertrophic in AMI models. In GMI models, patchy necrosis was seen in the myocardium, and islets of normal myocardial cells were surrounded by tight fibrous tissue. No profound organ failure was seen in either model.

In our experimental study, the LVAD was an extremely powerful method for to treating cardiogenic shock as it could substitute for up to 100% of cardiac function. However, our clinical results were not satisfactory. It is important to establish what disturbs the improvement in survival rate.

### Recovery mechanism of the failing heart

The severely impaired heart cannot maintain the normal circulation without an LVAD. However, the heart that has recovered from heart failure with the LVAD can maintain an almost normal circulation. Both clinical and experimental findings in pathological examination have shown that the necrotic myocardium is replaced with fibrous tissue that eventually becomes scar tissue, while the residual myocardium becomes hypertrophic. Removal of overload and decompression of the left ventricle at the beginning will prevent overextension of the impaired myocardium and accelerate scar formation, which no longer causes dyskinetic movement. Gradual increase in LV work will promote compensation by the residual myocardium. However, the preexisting myocardial damage delays recovery in clinical cases. The pumping duration in survivors was 6–7 days, while in patients who died it was either extremely short or long except for the child case and case 12, where the patient died of respiratory failure. Myocardial fibrosis caused by rheumatic myocarditis or broad myocardial ischemia, which developed during the prolonged period of low cardiac output, were obstacles to recovery of the impaired myocardium.

### Multiple organ failure as complications

Although 56% of the patients were weaned from the assist pump, only 19% of the total patients were discharged from the hospital. Omitting the two long-term survivors, patients died of renal, hepatic, respiratory, and/or other organ failure, which originated from a prolonged period of low output before the LVAD application. A close relation was seen between the severity of complication and the period of application. It is important to note that all survivors were treated by LVAD immediately when their circulatory condition deteriorated and there was no delay in its application. If use of the LVAD is delayed, sequelae in the major organs will follow, even though the heart may recover from profound heart failure. Since hemodynamic derangement will promptly progress, it is important to bear in mind that the decision to use the LVAD should not be delayed; it is better to apply it before major organs, including the heart itself, are irreversibly damaged.

### Systematic use of LVAD

Richenbacher et al. reported [3] that early hemodynamic stabilization with the LVAD should minimize the chance of hypoperfusion and its sequelae. We also believe that ventricular assistance should be introduced with greater care to treat acute cardiac failure and improve the survival rate. Our clinical experience suggests two basic concepts for establishing the proper way of LVAD application. The first is that acute cardiogenic shock should be treated, in consideration of possible use of the LVAD. When a trial for weaning from the extracorporeal circulation fails, the LVAD must be applied immediately without any hesitation as in the case of as IABP. Especially in the treatment of AMI with shock, the LVAD should be the first form of management before cardiac catheterization in some cases. The second concept is deciding the concomitant surgery when the LVAD is applied to AMI with shock. The emergency ACBG is still uncertain in its life-saving effect because the patient in shock occasionally cannot tolerate major surgery. In addition, the bypass operation to the infarcted myocardium may not only be ineffective in recovering heart function but also result in acceleration of hemorrhagic necrosis of the ischemic myocardium in patients with shock. We had two clinical cases with a large area of myocardial infarction, but subsequent ACBG was not performed [4]. Although both patients died of complications, their heart function recovered, and in one case the heart recovered enough to be weaned from the assist pump. This result suggests that the LVAD alone can be used to support the patient in cardiogenic shock, and ACBG should be considered after recovery from the shock. Following this experience, a therapeutic concept of acute myocardial infarction has been established, as outlined in Fig. 22.5. In this concept, any patient in shock of Killip grade 4 and Forrester 4, or with mechanical complications such as septal perforation or free wall rupture, is treated as a candidate for LVAD application. In applying this concept, it is important for there to be cooperation work among physicians, surgeons, nurses, and paramedics.

**Fig. 22.5.** Systematic introduction of left ventricular assistance to the treatment of acute myocardial infarction with cardiogenic shock

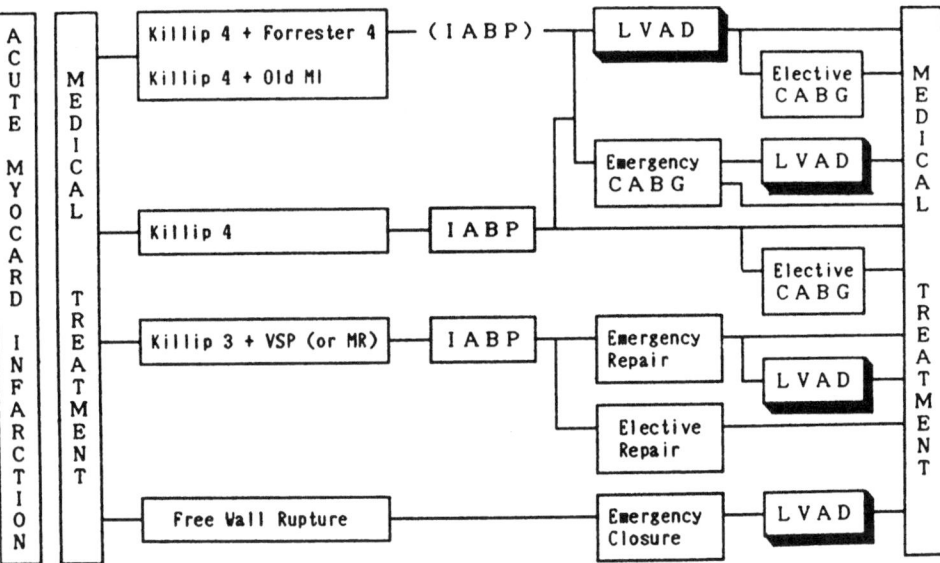

## Conclusions

The LVAD was applied to 16 cardiogenic shock patients including ten cases with AMI. The LVAD was effective in maintenance of the systemic circulation and the pump was removed in 56% of the patients. Preexisting myocardial damage and delayed LVAD application will considerably reduce the change in clinical cases. This clinical experience clearly shows the importance of timely use of the LVAD and the establishment of a therapeutic concept in treating cardiogenic shock using LVAD.

## References

1. Takano H, Nakatani T, Taenaka Y, Umezu M, Matsuda T, Iwata H, Adachi S, Tanaka T, Noda H, Fukuda S, Seki J, Nakamura T, Takatani S, Hayashi K, Akutsu T, Manabe H (1985) Recovery mechanism from postoperative profound heart failure by an automatic left ventricular assist system. Trans Am Soc Intern Organs 31: 198–201

2. Nakatani T, Takano H, Taenaka T, Umezu M, Tanaka T, Yutani C, Matsuda T, Iwata H, Noda H, Nakamura T, Takatani S, Seki J, Hayashi K, Akutsu T, Manabe H (1984) Therapeutic effect of left ventricular assist device on induced profound left ventricular failure—evaluation by left ventriculography. Trans Am Soc Artif Intern Organs 30: 533–538

3. Richenbacher WE, Dash H, Buick MK, Pierce WS (1984) Utilization of left ventricular assistance in patients with acute myocardial infarction and cardiogenic shock. ASAIO J 7: 32–40

4. Takano H, Nakatani T, Noda H, Umezu M, Fukuda S, Tanaka T, Matsuda T, Iwata H, Takatani S, Taenaka Y, Kinoshita M, Kumon K, Kito Y, Yutani C, Fujita T, Manabe H, (1986) Clinical consideration of a left ventricular assist system for acute myocardial infarction with cardiogenic shock. Trans Am Soc Intern Organs 32: 467–473

# Discussion

*Hill* (Pacific Presbyterian Medical Center): his is certainly an area that we must pay a great deal of attention to. It is not enough simply to insert these pumps; there should be clarity as to what can be salvaged, and these multiple organ problems make for a very difficult salvage.

Have you changed your attitude at all with respect to how quickly you insert a pump? Do you tend to insert the pump quickly so as to save the lungs, kidneys, etc?

*Noda* (National Cardiovascular Center): We usually receive the patients a long time after they have gone into cardiogenic shock. So we insert the pump as soon as possible.

*Copeland* (Arizona Health Science Center): In heart transplantation, we use a limit for candidate selection of pulmonary vascular resistance of about 6 Wood units. Some groups will perform transplants at 6–8 Wood units. Very few groups would exceed this. In a group of patients who are candidates for transplantation, a certain number will have slightly elevated to moderately elevated pulmonary vascular resistance. Assuming that this type of device is used to support these patients, how do you decide which patients need univentricular and which biventricular support?

*Takano:* We usually use a left ventricular assist device, but if cardiac output is less than 2.0 l/min/m$^2$ we use a right ventricular assist device in addition to LVAD.

*Copeland:* So you would basically put in the left ventricular assist device and then if the output was sufficient you would leave it; if it was insufficient you would put in a right ventricular assist device.

*Takano:* At that time, we would use a pulmonary vasodilator such as Tolazoline.

*Imamura:* This is an interesting question I think since we have the experience with the Fontan procedure in tricuspid atresia, in which the right ventricle does not work or there is very weak ejection. Nevertheless, a good right heart circulation can be maintained with the Fontan procedure. This procedure is only indicated in patients with less than 4 Wood units, so I think that patients with over 5 Wood units should also receive heart support.

*Copeland:* Yes that has certainly been our experience with the Fontan procedure, where even though patients are selected very carefully some do die.

# Part IV
# Bridge Used to Transplantation

# 23. Early experience with the total artificial heart as a bridge to cardiac transplantation

Jack G. Copeland, Richard G. Smith, Timothy B. Icenogle, and Richard A. Ott[1]

**Summary.** The experience with artificial hearts at the University of Arizona is described and case reports of the five patients who received them are presented. In one patient, it was seen that problems with the fit of the device resulted in fatal complications. Most world experience at present is with the Jarvik heart and the current model of choice is the 70-cm³, since it smaller than the 100-cm³ and there is reduced chance of trouble with the fit. Hemolysis is not a problem if excessive transfusion can be avoided. Bleeding is always a threat in complex cardiac surgery with grafting. Embolism and infection may be inevitable, but the evidence in one patient showed that there is no necessity to perform transplantation immediately. It is recommended that patients who have previously been selected for orthotopic transplantation and begin an accelerated decompensation are the best candidates for temporary orthotopic mechanical support.

**Key words**: Bridge to transplantation—Pneumatic orthotopic device—Biventricular device—Fit problems

In March 1985 when we implanted the "Phoenix heart" in a desperately ill young man [1, 2], who later died after cardiac transplantation, considerable controversy ensued. Critics and supporters were given much attention by the media, and "bioethecists" were called upon to provide some "perspective." It was clear to those of us directly involved in the care of the young man in question that we had observed and documented a definite improvement in his condition during 11 h of support with the orthotopic pneumatic pulsatile biventricular pump. And my greatest regret was that the patient was not supported for a longer period of time, which might have permitted greater recovery prior to his second transplant.

Our use of the device, while unplanned, was not a new idea. Total artificial hearts had previously been implanted by Cooley in bridge-to-transplant attempts in 1969 and 1981 [3]. The technology of 1985 and the success of DeVries and Joyce in "permanent" total heart implants [4] and Pennington, Oyer, and Hill [5] in temporary support with ventricular assist devices of

various kinds set the stage for our next bridge attempt in August, 1985 [5].

This patient, the first to survive total artificial heart implantation followed by cardiac transplantation, remains alive and works full time as assistant manager of a grocery store today. Since then, many bridge-to-transplant procedures with implanted orthotopic biventricular pumps have succeeded and the media and public seem to be less interested in this promising experimental field.

Here, I would like first to summarize briefly the world experience with total artificial hearts [5] and then discuss the five implants in four patients at our institution.

## The world experience with bridge to cardiac transplantation

From 4 April 1969 until March 1987, there were 61 implants of orthotopic biventricular pneumatic pulsatile artificial hearts. Five of these were "permanent implants" as shown in Table 23.1.

Fifty-six hearts were implanted with the intent to bridge critically ill patients until the time of transplantation. At this writing, 39 patients have had heart transplants, 25 of these (64%) are alive and 18 (46%) have been discharged. Table 23.2 lists the first ten bridge-to-transplant patients.

Etiologies for end-stage cardiac disease have been ischemic heart disease (24), cardiomyopathy (22), viral (four), congenital (two), post partum (two) and valvular (two). The mean age has been 40 years (range 18–58 years). Since the first use of the Jarvik 7–70, which has a theoretical stroke volume of 70 cm³ as opposed to the Jarvik 7 with a 100-cm³ stroke volume, by Joyce et al. [6] more than twice as many smaller devices have been used. Only a few other devices have been tried: Penn State (two), Unger (two), Berlin (one), and Phoenix (one). There has been only one mechanical device failure, a strut fracture of the Shiley disc valve in DeVries's first patient (Clark). The implant time for bridge patients has, in most cases, been less than 2 weeks, ranging from 0.5 to 244

[1]Arizona Health Sciences Center, 1501 North Campbell Avenue, Tucson, AZ 85724, USA

**Table 23.1.** "Permanent" implants

| Implant date | Patient | Age | Surgeon/location | Device | Days | Status |
|---|---|---|---|---|---|---|
| 12/02/82 | Clark | 61 | DeVries/Salt Lake | Jarvik 7 | 112 | Died |
| 11/25/84 | Schroeder | 52 | DeVries/Louisville | Jarvik 7 | 622 | Died |
| 02/17/85 | Haydon | 58 | DeVries/Louisville | Jarvik 7 | 488 | Died |
| 04/07/85 | Stenberg | 53 | Semb/Stockholm | Jarvik 7 | 227 | Died |
| 04/14/85 | Burcham | 62 | DeVries/Louisville | Jarvik 7 | 10 | Died |

**Table 23.2.** Bridge to cardiac transplant with total artificial heart

| Implant date | Patient | Age | Surgeon/location | Device | Days | Status |
|---|---|---|---|---|---|---|
| 04/04/69 | Karp | 47 | Cooley/Houston | Liotta | 2.5 | Died |
| 07/23/81 | Meuffels | 36 | Cooley/Houston | Akutsu | 2.2 | Died |
| 03/06/85 | Creighton | 33 | Copeland/Tucson | Phoenix | 0.5 | Died |
| 08/28/85 | Drummond | 25 | Copeland/Tucson | Jarvik 7 | 9.5 | Alive |
| 10/18/85 | Mandia | 44 | Pierce/Hershey | Penn St. | 12 | Died |
| 10/24/85 | Gaidosh | 47 | Griffith/Pittsburgh | Jarvik 7 | 4 | Alive |
| 12/18/85 | Lund (F) | 40 | Joyce/Mpls | Jarvik 7-70 | 45 | Died |
| 02/03/86 | Chayrez (F) | 40 | Copeland/Tucson | Jarvik 7-70 | 4 | |
| 02/09/86 | Chayrez | | Copeland/Tucson | Jarvik 7-70 | 244 | Died |
| 02/03/86 | Buvello | 39 | Griffith/Pittsuburgh | Jarvik 7 | 12 | Alive |
| 02/03/86 | Kent | 41 | Frazier/Houston | Jarvik 7 | 31 | Alive |

days. Most patients have been treated with heparin and dipyridamole, with some centers using aspirin as well. There have been four strokes, two with residual sequelae and five transient ischemic attacks. Among 59 implants, there were 14 reoperations for hemorrhage, and among 35 cases reported [6] the average blood replacement was 14 units. Hemolysis has not been a problem with the Jarvik system since the Utah driver dp/dt was lowered in May 1985 to the range of 3500–4500 mmHg/s [7]. Finally, infections have been noted on transcutaneous pneumatic drive lines in six cases, involving the total artificial heart in four cases.

## Total artificial heart as bridge to heart transplantation—Our experience

At the University of Arizona in Tucson we have implanted five artificial hearts in four patients (Table 23.3).

### Case 1

Our first case was a 33-year-old man with ischemic cardiomyopathy, an ejection fraction of 5%, and frequent runs of ventricular tachycardia. He received a cardiac transplant on 5 March 1985 (ischemic time 105 min). Graft function was sluggish, immediately requiring 4 $\mu$g/kg/min isoproterenol and 1 $\mu$g/min epinephrine. Several days later, we found the cardiac donor had six blood cultures postive for *Pseudomonas*

*aeruginosa*, which may have accounted for depression of the heart and subsequent cardiac arrest 24 h after the transplant.

The patient was resuscitated with open-chest massage ($1\frac{1}{2}$ h) and placed on cardiopulmonary bypass (bubble oxygenator) for $7\frac{1}{2}$ h, while we initially attempted to find a second donor heart and, when that search failed, until we completed the implantation of the Phoenix heart. This heart, which was designed by K. Cheng and had been implanted 12 times in calves, was previously untried in humans.

We experienced some technical difficulties [2] in implantation of the device, but found the function to be adequate to support the patient with normal blood pressure (110–120/40 mmHg) near normal central venous pressure (10–13 mmHg), and a urine output of at least 100 cm³/h.

Because of pressures from outside (news media, FDA, peers) [2] and from internal pressures resulting from our lack of experience, we proceeded to a second transplant as soon as a heart became available. After 11 h of adequate physiological support with the Phoenix heart, it was removed and replaced with a donor heart which sustained for 2 h 12 min of ischemic time. Very poor function characterized by right and left ventricular failure, large amounts of inotropic support, immediate rise in central venous pressure to 25–30 mmHg, and immediate fall off in pO₂ and urine output were noted. The patient died after 33 h of pulmonary edema, pseudomonas pneumonia with multiple abcesses, and low cardiac output.

**Table 23.3.**

| | Patient | | | | |
|---|---|---|---|---|---|
| | TC | MD | BC | BC | BS |
| Date implantation | 03/06/85 | 08/29/85 | 02/03/86 | 02/09/86 | 11/25/86 |
| Age | 33 | 25 | 40 | 40 | 43 |
| Sex | M | M | F | F | F |
| Heart disease | Ischemic | Myopathy | Viral | Rejection | Congenital |
| Weight (kg) | 65.5 | 103 | 65 | 65 | 84 |
| Height (cm) | | | | | 157 |
| Sternum-spine (cm) | | | | | |
| Device | Phoenix | Jarvik 7 | Jarvik 7-70 | Jarvik 7-70 | Jarvik 7-70 |
| Transplant | Yes | Yes | Yes | Yes | No |
| Outcome | Died | Alive | Rejection | Died | Died |

We learned from this case that support and resuscitation of a critically ill patient was possible with an orthotopic pneumatic device. Introspect, we regretted that support had not been for a long enough period to return the patient to a more stable condition or to determine that he could not be improve.

**Case 2**

A 25-year-old man with a chronic cardiomyopathy presumed to be viral in origin was admitted in late August 1985 with an ejection fraction of 10%, acidosis, hypothesion, and delirium [2]. Continued deterioration led us on 29 August 1985 (in the absence of a suitable doner) to implant a Jarvik-7 heart.

We had no difficulty implanting the heart into this patient using the techniques described by DeVries and Joyce [4]. Time on cardiopulmonary bypass was 117 min. His large pericardial space easily accepted the Jarvik-7 and neither pleural space was opened. Bleeding was not a problem, the 24-h total for chest tube drainage was 690 cm$^3$.

We were initially cautious in our support running cardiac outputs in the range of 5–6 l/min. The patient was not acidotic and had an excellent urine output, but had poor peripheral pulses and a high core temperature (38°–38.5°C) until we increased the output by using vacuum in diastole and higher drive pressures, raising his cardiac output to 7–8 l/min. At this point, excellent pulses were palpable in all extremities and his core temperature dropped while his skin temperature rose (measured by great toe surface probe). For us, this was a dramatic demonstration not only of life support but also of excellent control of the cardiac output (Fig. 23.1)

In addition to initial timidity regarding cardiac output control, we focused on our patient's fluid balance and were delighted that within 4 days it could be dropped by 18 l and the lungs completely cleared of pulmonary edema (Fig. 23.2). This rapid drop in total body water, however, had two adverse effects. First, it forced us to cut back on cardiac output because of the drop in preload. Second, it led to a concentration of clotting factors and platelets. We felt, in retrospect, that the combination of decreased flow through the device plus recovery of the patient's coagulation factors and platelet count to normal and/or high levels (Fig. 23.3) led to platelet and fibrin deposition in crevices located at the inflow and outflow valve mounts (Fig. 23.4). One of these on the left side may have led to a stroke on day 7 diagnosed by the presence of right-sided weakness and expressive aphasia. Serial computed tomgographic brain scans failed to reveal infarction or homorrhage and the weakness disappeared within several days. The expressive aphasia was progressively less detectable and disappeared about 3 weeks posttransplantation.

Heparin therapy (Fig. 23.3) was progressively increased. The thrombin time, which is a sensitive test for the presence of heparin, was maintained at $1\frac{1}{2}$ times the normal level. Unfortunately, we did not use the partial thromboplastin time to monitor heparin therapy, but as seen in Fig. 23.4 it remained normal most of the time.

Retrospective evaluation of this case led us to adopt two approaches to prevent thromboembolism. The first is to maintain a high normal cardiac output by maintaining adequate hydration (CVP 8–10 mmHg) and vasadilation if necessary and by adjusting the drive system to deliver a high heart rate (120/min) and high cardiac output while maintaining pressures high enough the eject each ventricle fully on every beat and modifying the percentage systole (usually 45%–55%) and vacuum (usually around −5 cmH$_2$O) to optimize ventricular filling at reasonable CVP levels. The data from Levinson et al. [7] support the concept of a high heart rate associated with a lower stroke incidence.

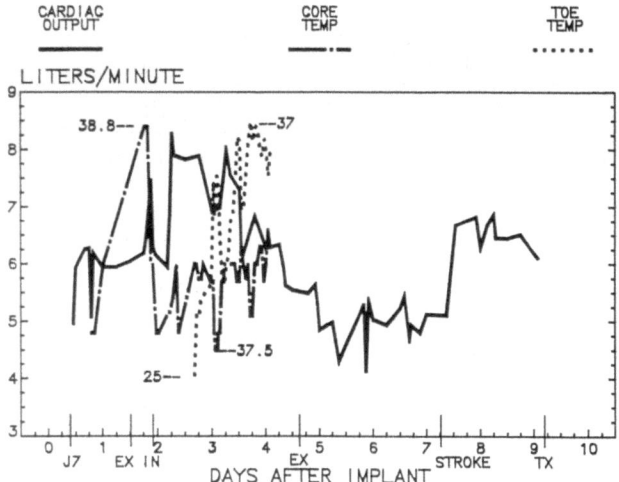

**Fig. 23.1.** Cardiac output, core temperature, and toe temperature in patient 2

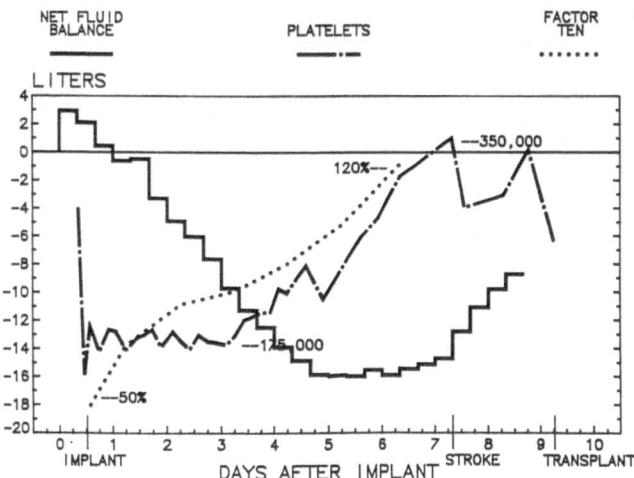

**Fig. 23.2.** Net fluid balance, platelet count, and factor 10% of normal in patient 2

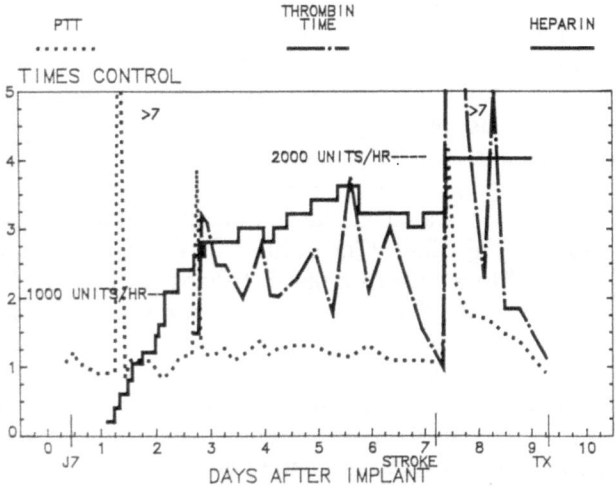

**Fig. 23.3.** Partial thromboplastin time (*PTT*), thrombin time, and heparin dosage in units per hour plotted versus time for patient 2

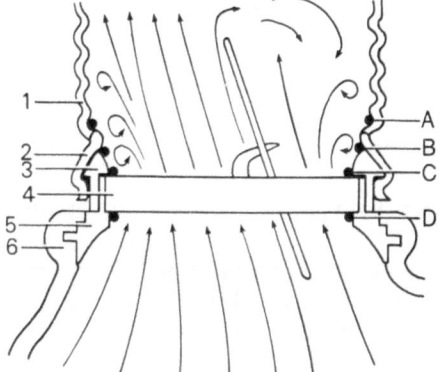

**Fig. 23.4.** A cut-away view of the outflow tract from the Jarvik-7 device with possible sites of eddy currents and sites at which tiny fibrin and platelet deposits found in case 2

Nine and a half days after the initial implant, a heart was transplanted from 19-year-old male with a 102-min ischemia time. We experienced no problems with removal of the Jarvik 7 heart or with the technical features of the transplant. In retrospect, we believe it is extremely important to remove the patient's heart distal to the atrioventricular groove when implanting the Jarvik 7 in order to have excellent artial compliance and in anticipation of adequate remaining atrial cuffs at the time of transplantation.

Posttransplantation, this patient had two rejection episodes and disseminated toxoplasmosis apparently acquired from his donor Intracellar forms were seen on numerous biopsy specimens for approximately 1 month into his therapy (sulfadiazine, pyrimethamine) and have not been seen since.

The patient has been working for nearly 1 year and is over 18 months posttransplantation.

**Case 3**

A 40-year-old famale, mother of three, presented with acute cardiac decompensation 1 week following the onset of a viral syndrome. Initial cardiac biopsy demonstrating myocyte necrosis led us to treat with high-dose steroids, azathioprine, and amantadine and to attempt to stabilize her with maximal inotropic therapy until the myopathic condition improved. The blood pressure was 80–85 mmHg systolic, left ventricular pressure 25 mmHg, and she developed severe pulmonary edema and acute renal failure.

In the face of hemodynamic deterioration, an acute postviral setting with the presence of influenza A detected by immunofluorescent stain, staining of nasopharyngeal material, and in the presence of what might have been a lupus-like syndrome, all of which were relative contraindications to transplantation, we proceeded to implantation of a Jarvik-7-70 total artificial heart. The procedure was accomplished without difficulty. At pathological examination of the patient's heart we found 50%–60% of the patient's ventricular myocardium destroyed apparently by direct viral damage (viral particles were found in the dead myocytes on immunofluorescent staining).

Postimplantation, the hemodynamics were stable, but the coagulation system was abnormal. A platelet defect identified by prolonged bleeding time and in vitro decreased platelet aggregation was present. We, nevertheless, felt early (2nd day) that heparinization was essential and proceeded as planned with a heparin bolus (5000 units) followed by continuous infusion. In retrospect, this was probably unncessary in the light of her poor platelet function. Unfortunately, each time we attempted heparinization the patient bled through her chest tubes and developed signs suggestive of atrial cuff tamponade with rising filling pressure and falling cardiac output. This was relieved with vigorous stripping of the chest tubes, but precipitated her first cardiac transplant on 7 February 1986.

Hyperacute rejection by according to histological evidence (interstitial hemorrhage and polymorphonuclear infiltration, plugged capillaries, appearance of antiheart antibodies on immunofluorescent stain) and time course (1 1/2 days) led to acute decompensation and cardiac arrest, requiring closed then open cardiac massage.

The patient was rapidly returned to the operating room and had a second Jarvik 7–70 implant on 9 February 1986. This time, there was little atrial tissue available to aid in the atrial quick concect cuff anastomoses or in the leftward positioning of the heart in such a small woman. An anatomical probrem created by this situation, inferior vena caval compression, went unnoticed for 8 days until the development of ascites led to bedside catheterization, showing a 10-mmHg gradient at the caval-atrial junction. Reoperation on post implant day 9 to correct this consisted of: (a) umbilical tape sling around the right ventricle of the device and a lateral rib (about r-7) which was tightened enough to move the heart several centimenters leftward (before reoperation simply pulling on the drive lines had been of no value), and (b) turning the edge of the aterial quick connect cuff, which seemed to be pressing on the inferior vena cava into an everted position with the use of a horizontal mattress stitch, which was then passed around the tricuspid valve mount (Figs. 23.5, 6).

Many other problems plagued this unfortunate patient, as shown in Table 23.4.

For approximately 2 1/2 months (9 February to 1 May 1986), numerous complications (Table 23.4) were treated. By 1 May, however, the patient was stable, able to walk ride an exercise cycle, go out of the building, take baths in a tub, interact with her family, and behave as a "normal" person tethered to a drive console. Attempts were made to personalize her environment: room decoration, a portable bed for her

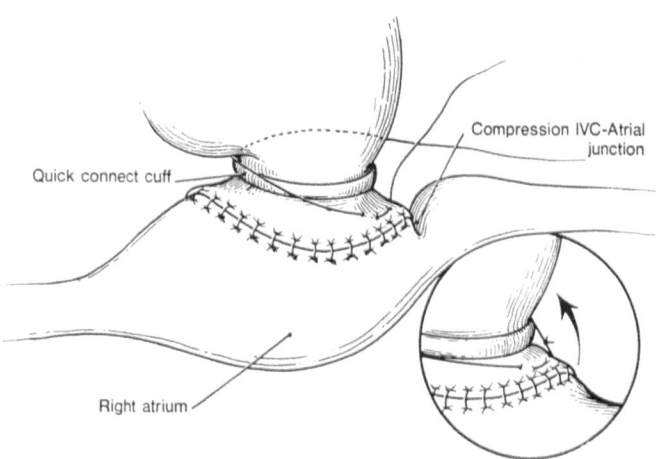

**Fig. 23.5.** In case 3 at reoperation, the first maneuver was to unkink the superior vena cava using the suture material to evert the quick connect cuff near the inferior vena cava

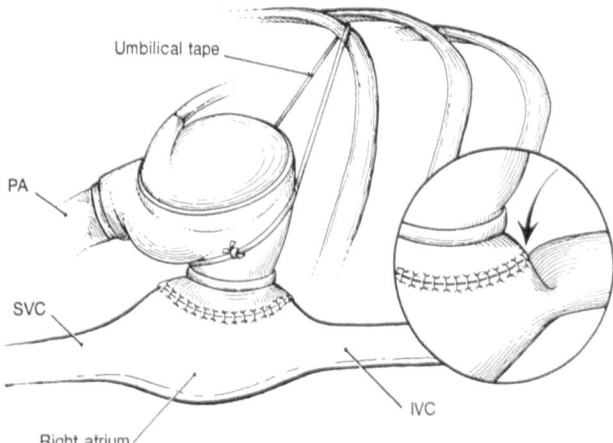

**Fig. 23.6.** Also in case 3, in order to eliminate further the kink in the inferior vena cava, an umbilical tape was passed laterally around the seventh rib and used to sling the right ventricle. This enabled us to eliminate entirely the inferior vena cava to right atrial gradient which initially was greater than 10 mm Hg

**Table 23.4.** Complications of patient B.C.

| Infections | Days after 2nd implant | Treatment |
|---|---|---|
| Influenza A sepsis | 0–12 | Intravenous ribavirin |
| Candida sepsis | 12–21 | Intravenous amphotericin B |
| Enterobacter sepsis | 18–31 | Intravenous imipenum |
| Herpes simplex sepsis, intermisttent urinary tract infections | 43–52 | Intravenous acyclovir |
| Drive line infection | 30–244 | Local treatment |
| Mediastinal infection | 220–244 | Debridement drainage 9/16/86 |
| Surgical complications | | |
| Inferior vena cava compression | 0–9 | Decompression (date) |
| Delayed splenic rupture | 23 | Splenectomy 3/4/86 |
| Other complications | | |
| Renal failure | 0–78 | Dialysis and continuous hemofiltration |
| Prolonged intubation | 0–41 | Extubation (date) |
| Pancreatitis | 0–8 | Nasogastric drainage |
| Ileus | 0–60 | Intravenous alimentation |
| Persistent cytotoxic antibodies | 0–244 | Plasmaphresis, total nodal irradiation (2000 rad) |
| Autoantibodies | 0–244 | Irradiation (2000 rad) |
| TIA | 212 | 36-h left facial nerve and left upper extremity palsy |

mother, television, home cooked meals, and family social events. In fact, her family, including mother, father, and three children spent much of their time with her. Remote total artificial heart monitoring by computer interfacing removed engineers and monitoring devices from the room. Limited nursing and medical personnel contact except for two daily visits were enforced. All of this was felt to have given her a "reasonable" quality of life until mid-September.

During this time, she was free of any evidence of thromboembolism on a continuous infusion of heparin (to maintain PTT at 1 1/2 to 2 times normal) and dipyridamole (100 mg, four times per day). The cardiac output was maintained at 6.5–7 l/min and heart rate at 125/min. Positive cytotoxic antibodies remained against 70%–100% of a random panel of lymphocytes. The patient was crossmatched against 80 possible donors throughout the United States with only one negative crossmatch in a reasonable donor. That donor was used for a stable (class III) recipient.

Eventually, the drive line infections led to mediastinitis and a partial drainage and debridement was done on 16 September 1986. The patient had had a TIA (Table 23.4) of 36-h duration on 8 September. There was no trend toward decreasing titers of cytotoxic antibodies. It was, therefore, decided in consultation with the patient and family to proceed with a transplant once the infection was controlled. Accordingly, the patient was treated with total nodal irradiation (2000 rad) and four plasmaphreses, which dropped her autoantibody levels to titers of less than 1:20.

On 11 October 1986, a transplant with an excellent donor heart (ischemic time 40 min) was performed.

Initial excellent cardiac function degeneration to poor function over a 2-h period and the patient died. Once more, the time course and histology were compatible with hyperacute rejection.

**Case 4**

A 43-year-old, 84-kg (157 cm) woman with Ebstein's anomaly and a tiny left ventricle decompensated after implantation of an automatic internal defibrillator. Her course was marked by persistent acidosis, hypotension, pulmonary edema, intubation, and acute renal failure.

A Jarvik 7–70 was implanted on 25 November 1986 at the time of implantation; the device was allowed to slide over her left pericardium (which had been mobilized as a flap to just above phrenic nerve) into the left chest. The fit seemed to be adequate, though slighly tight prior to chest closure. As soon as the chest was closed, there was a prolongation of the ventricular fill time and flattening of the filling curve compatible with either inflow obstruction or hypovolemia. We observed her for 72 h, then reopened the chest, and in an effort to enlarge the thorax placed metallic struts across the sternum, which were wired in place maintaining a 2.5- to 3-cm-cleft between the sternal edges. Because of her moderate obesity, we were able to close subcutaneous tissue and skin over the defect. Unfortunately, this proved inadequate and persistence of her pulmonary edema finally led us, with spousal consent, to turn off the device on the 9th postimplantation day. At the postmortem examination, there was severe compression of both atria. This was most striking on the left, where the pulmonary veins were flattened and the upper and lower pulmonary veins were nearly occluded by white thrombi.

Even though this patient weighed 84 kg she had a small skeleton. Retrospective radiological sizing with films made from Jarvik 7–70 phantoms suggested that the heart should have fit better. We have hypothesized that her small native left heart compared with a huge right heart may have predisposed her to have a "medial" total artificial heart position and that this in combination with preimplantation stiff lungs, which left little room for the Jarvik 7–70, may have led to the unfortunate outcome.

## Conclusions

There is no doubt that currently available biventricular pneumatic pulsatile devices placed orthotopically with transcutaneous drive lines can support life in patients who may then be successfully transplanted. For the most part, the world experience is with Jarvik hearts. The current model of choice is the 70-cm$^3$ device because it is smaller and may be implanted with less fear of "fit problems" than the 100-cm$^3$ model. As our case 4 illustrates, a fit problem may be a fatal disaster.

The fears of excessive bleeding, hemolysis, embolism, and infection with the use of these devices are not as prohibitive as we suspected. Bleeding is always a threat in complex cardiac surgery with grafting. Hemolysis is not a problem if excessive transfusion can be avoided. Embolism and infection may be inevitable, but as seen with our patient B.C. there is no need to rush immediately to transplantation. And if the implanted patient does not meet local transplant selection criteria, we have enough information now to recommend that they not be accepted for tranplantation.

We would recommend patients who have previously been selected for orthotopic transplantation and begin an accelerated decompensation (our case 2) as the best candidates for temporary orthotopic mechanical support. In these patients, there is no question about whether recovery of the native heart is possible or whether a reversible myocardial insult is present. The plan to do an orthotopic transplant indicates that a cardiectomy is necesssary.

This type of device when suitably placed provides excellent control of the circulation. There is no requirement for intensive care of the native heart since it is gone along with toxic antiarrythmic medications, risk of embolizing a mural thrombus, and the constant balancing of a univentricular device vis-à-vis the native heart. Further, if pulmonary edema is present with accompanying elevation in pulmonary vascular resistance, the biventricular device requires only an upward adjustment in right drive pressure. With a univentricular device, one must worry not only about the pulmonary vascular resistance but also the right heart capacity to pump at a normal output.

These patients can be returned to normal hemodynamic function immediately and with time many types of organ failure heretofore felt irreversible may be reversed to normal.

Only time and more experience along with improved technology will provide us with a family of devices to support and replace the heart. Until more definitive developments, the pneumatic orthotopic devices can be recommended as life-saving in selected patients.

## References

1. Vaughn CC, Copeland JG, Cheng K, Austin J, Levinson MM Interim heart replacement with a mechanical device: An adjunct to management of allograft rejection. Heart Transpl 4 (5): 502–505
2. Copeland JG, Levinson MM, Smith R, Icenogle TB, Vaughn C, Cheng K, Ott RA, Emery RW (1986) The total artificial heart as a bridge to transplantation: A report of two cases. JAMA 256 (21): 2991– 2995
3. Cooley DA (1982) Staged cardiac transplantation: Report of 3 cases. Heart Transpl 1: 145–153
4. DeVries WC, Joyce LD (1983) The artificial heart. CIBA Clin Symposia 35: 4–32
5. Joyce LD et al. (1987) JACC 9: 28A
6. Joyce LD, Johnson KE, Pierce WS, DeVries WC, Semb BKH, Copeland JG, Griffith BP, Cooley DA, Franzier OH, Cabrol C, Keon WJ, Unger F, Bucherl ES, Wolner E (1986) Summary of the world experience with clinical use of total artificial hearts as heart support devices. Heart Transpl 5 (3): 229–235
7. Levinson MM, Copeland JG, Smith RG, Cork RC, DeVries WC, Mays JB, Griffith B, Kormos R, Joyce LD, Pritzker MR, Semb BKH, Koul B, Menkis AH, Keon WJ (1986) Indexes of hemolysis in human recipients of the Jarvik-7 total artificial heart. J Heart Transpl 5: 236–248
8. Levinson MM, Smith RG, Cork R, Gallo J, Icenogle TB, Emery RW, Copeland JG (1986) Three recent cases of the total artificial heart before transplantation. J Heart Transpl 5: 215–228

# Discussion

*Taenaka* (National Cardiovascular Center): With regard to selection of the device, I think that availability is one of the most important factors. Generally speaking, each device, left ventricular assist device and total artificial heart, has its own merits and demerits. For patients who are candidates for heterotopic cardiac transplantation and patients with an extremely small chest, a left ventricular assist device should be used. In cases of rejection after transplantation, the total artificial heart should be applied. I think it is desirable to have both devices at hand. How do you feel about this?

*Copeland* (Arizona Health Sciences Center): I agree with you completely. If the surgeon is not tied down to any particular approach, this gives the patient the best possible chance for survival. As you say, there are a great many factors to be taken into account with respect to selection of the device. Any one device is not necessarily the best for every patient. I agree with you that a very small patient is best treated with an external left ventricular assist device. The larger patient may be a candidate for an internal left ventricular assist device or a total artificial heart. A patient with global failure of the heart, such as one who is rejecting the heart, is obviously a candidate for replacement of both ventricles. I think as we learn more and more we will come to realize that there is a place for different types of devices.

*Geselowitz* (Pennsylvania State University): Would you please comment on the use of a total artificial heart rather than an assist device?

*Copeland:* The major advantage with the total artificial heart is that it gives complete control over the circulation provided there is an adequate fit and normal mechanical function of the device. It is very easy to use. However, at present it is not so good for long-term use because of infection, the risk of thromboembolism, and severe scar tissue formation around the device, making the eventual transplantation almost impossible. In the last patient I showed, the very small patient who was not really an optimal candidate for tranplantation, if he had had a total arti-

ficial heart that would have been the best choice for him. I think that total implantability will be an important factor when it is developed. It will provide us with another way to approach these critically ill patients.

*Gaselowitz:* Don't you think that you can obtain as much control with a biventricular assist? There also seems to be for some reason a lower incidence of thromboembolism and strokes with the assist device than with the total artificial heart.

*Copeland:* The total artificial heart seems to have a bad reputation with respect to thromboembolism from the so-called permanent experience where all the patients suffered from stroke. However, if all the data on the bridge to transplantation are examined there are only two cases of stroke out of over 60 patients. This is not a bad record for thromboembolism.

I agree that biventricular support is possible. It is only possible with those ventricular assist devices that are external. There are basically two or three pneumatic devices that can be used right now in that situation. For surgeons who are skilled in their use they may be just as good, but it is difficult for me to imagine anything as simple as a biventricular, pneumatic, implantable, orthotopic device being able to control the hemodynamics. In some institutions, there is often no nurse or engineer present in the room. I am not sure that this can be done with the patient's own heart in place. The total artificial heart eliminates the need for cardiac drugs, many of which are very depressive in their effects on the rhythm, etc.

In our own limited experience with a univentricular assist using an external device, we found that proper atrial drainage is a key point; if this is not precisely managed, the patient may do very badly or even die as a result of hemodynamic problems and renal problems from hemolysis. Perhaps with experience, surgeons can become very skilled with the techniques involved here, but not all patients have large atria or the correct anatomy for good function of this type of device.

I believe it is much better for there to be a full variety of devices available to meet all situations.

*Copeland:* Now Japanese surgeons are doing LVAD without any possibility of following heart transplantation. I hope someday soon that heart transplantation will become available in Japan. There are a number of teams in Japan who have the capability and capacity to be successful with heart transplantation.

*Imamura* (Tokyo Women's Medical College): You have emphasized the importance of a high heart rate and high cardiac output. I wonder if the heart rate should be reduced during sleep?

*Copeland:* Our reason for using a high heart rate and cardiac output is to discourage thromboembolism, which can of course occur at any time. We only adjust the heart rate and drive-line pressures in response to hemodynamic changes in the patient, such as significant bleeding or reduction in volume from diuresis. If the patient becomes hypertensive during the day, as a result, say, of stimulation from seeing his friends or riding a bicycle, we modify drive-line pressures, the percentage of systole, or the time when ejection occurs. These are very minimal. With the current device, I feel it is best to run high output through the device, thereby washing the device as much as possible.

*Imamura:* When do you start the anticoagulation? Do you start with heparin?

*Copeland:* We start with dipyridamol down nasogastric tube within the first 6 hr after implantation. We do not believe it is necessary to start heparin for at least 2 days. We feel that it is important to obtain good coagulation at all of the suture lines, needle holes, etc. in the patient before heparin is initiated. Further, we are not aware of any embolic events that have occurred within the 1st week after these types of implants. Looking at De Vries' data with permanent implants, all the emboli occurred after 100–120 days. So we feel very comfortable about waiting for at least 48 h, and if there is more bleeding we would wait longer before starting heparin.

*Imamura:* What about streptokinase or urokinase?

*Copeland:* No, we have not used any of the clot-dissolving agents, such as streptokinase, urokinase, or tissue plasminogen activator, since we feel that these would probably cause more bleeding. However, in the long-term situation after some healing has occurred I think there is a case for using something like a tissue plasminogen activator to be given intravenously. This should have the effect of cleaning out the entire inside of the device. This would make an interesting subject for experimental work which would have to be done in humans.

*Yozu* (Keio University): Yesterday I asked the same question of Dr. Hill. Let me ask the same question to you. Does a patient with an artificial heart go to the top of the waiting list for transplantation? Do you wait at all to obtain better function of other organs or do you put the new heart in as soon as you find a donor heart?

*Copeland:* What we have done in the past has not been optimal and we have learned from this experience. Our current policy, which we applied in our last three cases with the device is that we do not consider a patient a candidate for transplantation until he meets all the criteria that we set for other patients: if the urine output is down, if we suspect there is an infection, if the patient is comatose, etc. If any of those numerous contraindications are present, the patient is not considered for transplantation. Only if the patient met all the criteria would he go on the list and then he would go to the top.

The other aspect that your question raises is the very delicate subject that we try to discuss now with the patient and his family before we perform an implant: What do we do if a contraindication to implantation arises, e.g., the patient suffers a stroke or goes into renal failure, do we turn the machine off or not? Generally, our feeling is that if a patient reaches a point of noncandidacy for transplantation then we should have a plan ahead of time. I cannot say what the plan is for every patient, but I think that in certain cases one should turn the machine off.

# 24. Prolonged circulatory maintenance with a left ventricular assist device during cardiac arrest

Hisateru Takano, Yoshiyuki Taenaka, Takeshi Nakatani, Hiroyuki Noda, Masayuki Kinoshita, Sachito Fukuda, Eisuke Tatsumi, Akihiko Yagura, Hiroyoshi Sekii, Setsuo Takatani, Tetsuzo Akutsu, and Hisao Manabe[1]

**Summary.** The occurrence of an intractable severe biventricular failure, ventricular fibrillation, or cardiac arrest during the use of a left ventricular assist device (LVAD) is a serious problem. The purpose of this study is to examine the feasibility of prolonged circulatory maintenance with an LVAD alone during cardiac arrest until heart transplantation is performed. After an LVAD was inplanted between the left atrium and aorta in 12 goats, ventricular fibrillation was induced. When pulmonary vascular resistance was in the normal range (less than 15 000 $dynes.s.cm^{-5}.kg$), the circulation was well maintained with an LVAD alone as long as right atrial pressure was kept at 14–16 mmHg. Under such conditions, the flow fluctuated between 80 and 140 ml/kg/min depending on the animal's demand, and the mean arterial pressure was kept above 80 mmHg. The goats behaved quite normally. However, pooling of pleural effusion was a serious problem in maintaining normal circulation for a prolonged duration. Maintenance of the total protein level above 6.0 g/dl could delay or prevent pooling of effusion. The longest survival period to date has been 38 days. When pulmonary vascular resistance is in the normal range, an LVAD alone during cardiac arrest will provide sufficient time to try a further treatment such as heart transplantation or total artificial heart replacement.

**Key words**: Left ventricular assist device—Cardiac arrest—Ventricular fibrillation—Pulmonary vascular resistance

Recently, clinical trails with a left ventricular assist device (LVAD) for patients with profound heart failure which is beyond the limit of intra-aortic balloon pumping (IABP) have been undertaken worldwide [1–4]. The purpose of using an LVAD for heart failure is to maintain normal circulation and to help the failing heart recover. However, the occurrence of an intractable severe biventricular failure, ventricular fibrillation, or cardiac arrest during LVAD assistance is a serious problem because pulmonary venous return decreases and thus the LVAD cannot maintain sufficient flow. The authors previously reported feasibility study of circulatory maintenance with only an LVAD in acute experiments [5]. The purpose of the present study was to examine the feasibility of circulatory maintenance with only an LVAD during cardiac arrest for a prolonged duration.

## Materials and methods

The LVAD system consists of a blood pump and an automatic control drive unit (CDU), both of which were originally developed at our institute. The blood pump is an air-driven, diaphragm-type pump with an effective stroke volume of 70 ml and a maximum output of 7.0 l/min. The inlet and outlet conduits are connected to the left atrium (LA) and the descending aorta, respectively, through the chest wall, and the pump is placed paracorporeally on the chest wall. The main system of the CDU was designed to include features of an automatic level control system for left atrial pressure (LAP) and the flow. A detailed description of this system can be found elsewhere [6, 7].

Twelve young goats weighing between 13 and 40 kg were used in the chronic experiments. A sterile technique was adopted throughout the surgery. Thoracotomy was performed through the left fifth costal bed. After the blood pump was installed between the left atrium and descending aorta, left heart bypass was started. Preset LAP levels of the automatic level control system were set at 0–5 mmHg, where for these values, the flow through the LVAD was usually maintained at 80–140 ml/kg/min. After the chest was closed, the goat was placed in a cage and extubated after waking. The circulating blood volume was increased by blood or plasma transfusion to keep the right atrial pressure (RAP) above 10 mmHg. Ventricular fibrillation was then induced by an electric fibrillator (Fig. 24.1).

Blood flow through the pump (the flow), RAP, LAP, pulmonary arterial pressure (PAP), and aortic pressure (AoP) were continuously monitored. Analyses of blood gas, blood cell count, and blood chemistry were periodically performed. Pulmonary vascular resistance (PVR), PVR index (PVRI), and systemic vascular resistance (SVR) were calculated from the following equations:

[1]Department of Artificial Organs, National Cardiovascular Center Research Institute, 5-7-1 Fujishiro-dai, Suita, Osaka, 565 Japan

$$PVR = \frac{PAP - LAP \text{ (mmHg)}}{\text{Flow (l/min)}} \times 79.92 \text{ (dynes.s.cm}^{-5})$$

$$PVRI = PVR \times \text{body weight (kg) (dynes.s.cm}^{-5}.\text{kg)}$$

$$SVR = \frac{AoP - RAP \text{ (mmHg)}}{\text{Flow (l/min)}} \times 79.92 \text{ (dynes.s.cm}^{-5})$$

Autopsies were performed after the termination of each experiment.

## Results

### Overall results

One goat (case 1) with a patent foramen ovale had high flows of above 130 ml/kg/min due to right to left

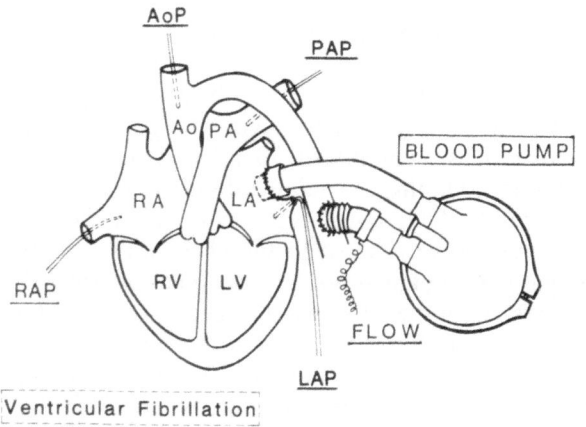

**Fig. 24.1.** Schematic illustration of experimental model. *RA* right atrium, *RAP* RA pressure, *Ao* aorta, *AoP* aortic pressure, *PA* pulmonary artery, *PAP* PA pressure, *LA* left atrium, *LAP* LA pressure, *RV* right ventricle, *LV* left ventricle

shunt at the atrial level. As the goat was uneasy with a PaO$_2$ of less than 40 mmHg, defibrillation was performed on the 2nd day. In two of the twelve goats (cases 2 and 6), PVR increased by initial blood transfusion, preventing the flow from increasing more than 50–60 ml/kg/min even when RAP was kept above 25 mmHg. These goats died of low output syndrome. The other nine goats behaved quite normally until the flow decreased. Pleural effusion and ascites were observed in most goats, but their onset was different in each case. The longest survival period was 38 days. The causes of death were bleeding after thoracentesis, gastric bleeding, inflow obstruction due to pannus formation, disconnection of drive airline, hepatic failure, and compression of both atria by pleural effusion. Overall results are shown in Table 24.1.

### Representative cases

#### Case 9

Case 9 was a goat weighing 40 kg (Fig. 24.2). Ventricular fibrillation was induced after blood and plasma transfusion. Mean AoP and flow dropped temporarily to 44 mmHg and 60 ml/kg/min, respectively, but they returned to a permissible range by elevation of RAP to 15–20 mmHg following immediate increase in SVR and plasma infusion. From the 2nd day, all hemodynamic parameters became stable, and the goat behaved quite normally. Neither notable pleural effusion nor ascites were noticed by ultrasonic method until the 21st day.

Total protein level was maintained above 6.0 g/dl, PaO$_2$ was above 70 mmHg, and PVR was within the normal range until pleural effusion appeared. From the 21st day, the goat had diarrhea, and total protein level decreased. Simultaneously, pleural effusion increased, PaO$_2$ decreased, the PVR was elevated, and the flow decreased in spite of high RAP and LAP.

**Table 24.1.** Overall results of circulatory maintenance with LVAD during cardiac arrest

| No. | Body weight (kg) | Flow (ml/kg/min) | Duration (days) | Cause of termination |
|-----|------------------|------------------|-----------------|----------------------|
| 1.  | 27 | 130–163 | 2  | Hypoxia (RA to LA shunt due to FO) |
| 2.  | 22 | 106–58  | 1  | High PVR after blood transfusion |
| 3.  | 23 | 109–117 | 5  | Bleeding after thoracentesis |
| 4.  | 23 | 75–88   | 5  | Gastric bleeding |
| 5.  | 22 | 91–114  | 17 | Bleeding after thoracentesis |
| 6.  | 21 | 67–57   | 1  | High PVR after blood transfusion |
| 7.  | 13 | 102–120 | 4  | Bleeding after thoracentesis |
| 8.  | 30 | 83–94   | 16 | Inflow obstruction |
| 9.  | 40 | 78–105  | 32 | Compression of both atria by effusion |
| 10. | 28 | 64–93   | 13 | Accident (escape from cage) |
| 11. | 31 | 119–164 | 22 | Hepatic failure |
| 12. | 30 | 113–143 | 38 | High PVR after blood transfusion |

*RA* right atrium, *LA* left atrium, *FO* foramen ovale, *PVR* pulmonary vascular resistance

**Fig. 24.2.** Case no. 9. Hemodynamic changes, profiles of total protein, blood gas, blood chemistry, and hematology. *RAP* right atrial pressure, *LAP* left atrial pressure, *mAoP* mean aortic pressure, *SVR.I* systemic vascular resistance index, *PVR.I* pulmonary vascular resistance index, *T.P* total protein, *T.Bil* total bilirubin

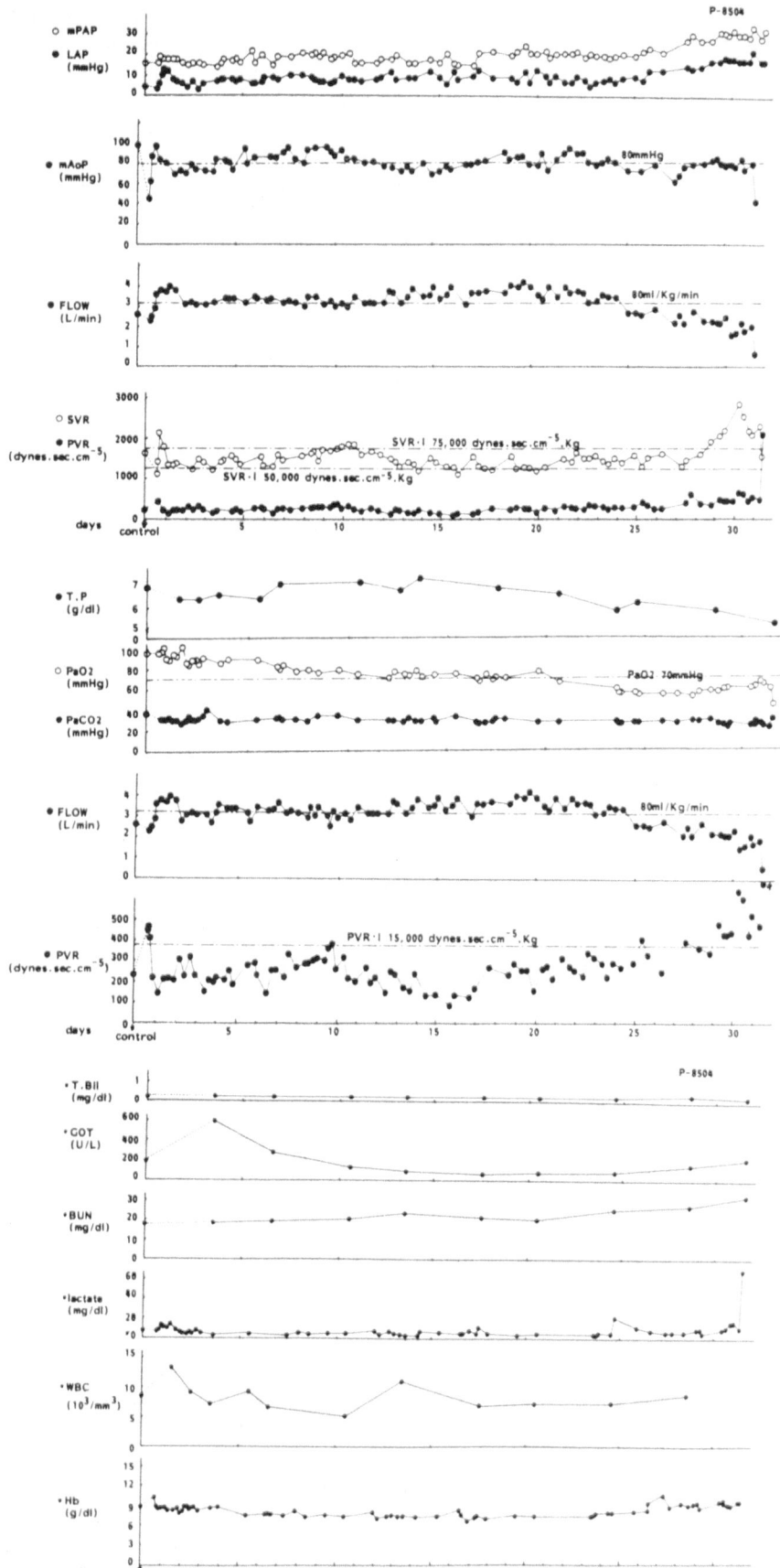

Low flow and high RAP caused a further increase in pleural effusion.

Glutamic-oxaloacetic-transaminase (GOT) and total bilirubin levels, which indicate liver function, blood urea nitrogen level, which indicates renal function, and lactate level, which indicates peripheral circulation, stayed within the normal ranges until the terminal stage. An early increase in GOT may be due to myocardial atrophy or degeneration. The goat died on the 32nd day. Autopsy revealed pleural effusion compressing both atria. Thus, high RAP and LAP were due to the pressure developed by pleural effusion. Venous congestion was very remarkable in the major visceral organs.

### Case 12

Case 12 was the longest survival case (Fig. 24.3). This goat had an adequate mean AoP of above 70 mmHg; the flow was above 100 ml/kg/min. RAP was maintained below 16 mmHg and PVR was within the normal range.

The hemoglobin level was above the control and total protein level was above 6.0 g/dl throughout the entire course. However, the $PaO_2$ level decreased slightly but was above 70 mmHg.

Glutamic-pyruvic-transaminase (GPT), total bilirubin, creatinine, and lactate levels of this goat stayed almost within normal ranges until 7th week. Elevation of GPT, total bilirubin, and lactate levels on the 8th day may have been due to the reaction following the second blood transfusion. The cause of the increase in lactate level at the terminal stage is unknown.

This goat died on the 38th day due to acute severe low pump output and hypoxia following blood transfusion. Pleural effusion and ascites were much less than in the other goats.

### Hemodynamic changes

When ventricular fibrillation was induced, the flow decreased and mean AoP and SVR dropped. However, SVR immediately increased, and RAP and LAP were elevated. Subsequently, AoP and the flow returned to a permissible range. Since RAP tended to decrease with time in the early stages, blood or plasma transfusion was performed to increase RAP in order to keep the flow above 80 ml/kg/min. However, the PVR of two goats markedly increased, resulting in low LAP in spite of high RAP and low flow of less than 60 ml/kg/min, and the experiments were terminated. When the PVR was in the normal range, the pressure gradient between the RA and LA was 7–10 mmHg. LAP increased as RAP increased; hence, the flow increased in proportion to RAP. Collapse of the LA, produced by strong suction by the LVAD, increased PVR and decreased the flow. One goat with a patent foramen ovale had high flows of above 130 ml/kg/min due to right to left shunt at the atrial level. As the goat was uneasy with $PaO_2$ of less than 40 mmHg, defibrillation was performed. The other nine goats had an adequate mean AoP of above 70 mmHg and a flow of between 80 and 140 ml/kg/min, but RAP was usually maintained at 14–16 mmHg. The goats behaved quite normally in the cage and also during exercise. When pleural effusion increased, venous return to the heart was suppressed and PVR increased, resulting in a decrease of the flow. Low flow caused a further increase of pleural effusion. This vicious cycle accelerated, deteriorating the goat's general condition.

### Changes in RAP, $PaO_2$, total protein levels and appearance of pleural effusion

Figure 24.4 shows the time-course of changes in RAP, $PaO_2$, and total protein levels in six animals which survived longer than 10 days. The circulatory condition maintained with an LVAD alone during cardiac arrest is similar to a severe right heart failure. High RAP produces pooling of pleural and visceral effusion. The RAP level ranged from 10 to 19 mmHg. However, in our early experiments with case 5, pooling of effusion appeared on the 4th day. When pleural effusion increased, venous return to the heart was suppressed and PVR increased, resulting in a decrease of the flow and exerting pressure upon the atria and lungs. This vicious cycle accelerated, deteriorating the goat's general condition. In this case, the total protein level was low, so an attempt was made to keep it higher than 6.0 g/dl. Consequently, appearance of effusion was delayed or prevented in the animals after case 5. Since in case 9 the total protein level was maintained above 6.0 g/dl, even the RAP level was around 19 mmHg, pleural effusion did not appear until the 4th week, when total protein level decreased below 6.0 g/dl. Maintaining high total protein as well as low RAP is important to prevent pooling of pleural and visceral effusion. $PaO_2$ was maintained well until pleural effusion became significant.

### Changes in blood and blood chemistry

The hemoglobin level was usually high, because of blood transfusions, but in some cases it was within the normal level. The white blood cell count was usually within the normal range provided that infection did not occur. GOT and total bilirubin levels, blood urea nitrogen level, and lactate level stayed within normal ranges until the terminal stage. At the terminal stage these parameters became elevated.

**Fig. 24.3.** Case no. 12. Hemodynamic changes, profiles of total
protein, blood gas, blood chemistry, and hematology. *RAP* right
atrial pressure, *LAP* left atrial
pressure, *mAoP* mean aortic
pressure, *PVR.I* pulmonary
vascular resistance index,
*T.P* total protein

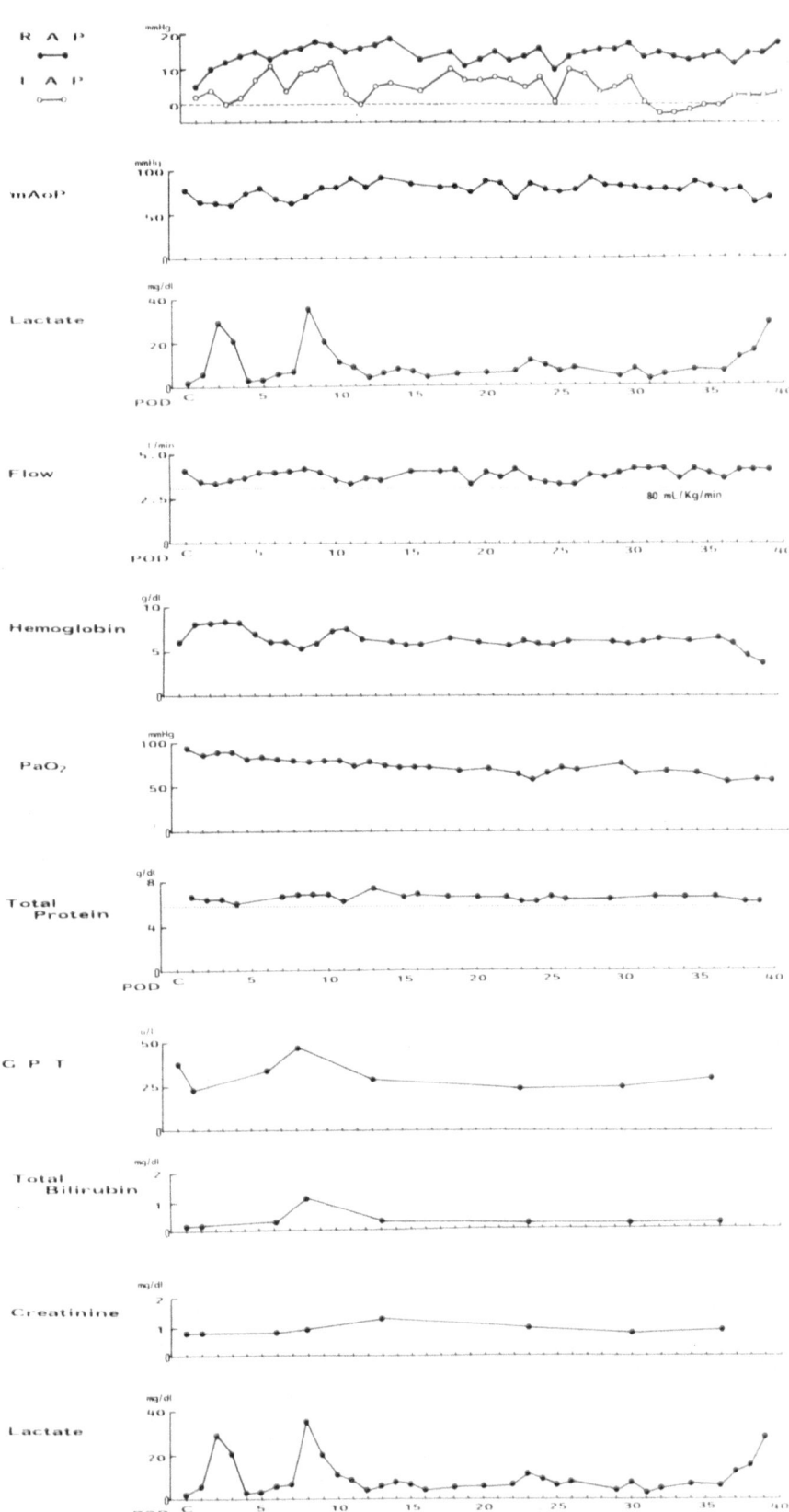

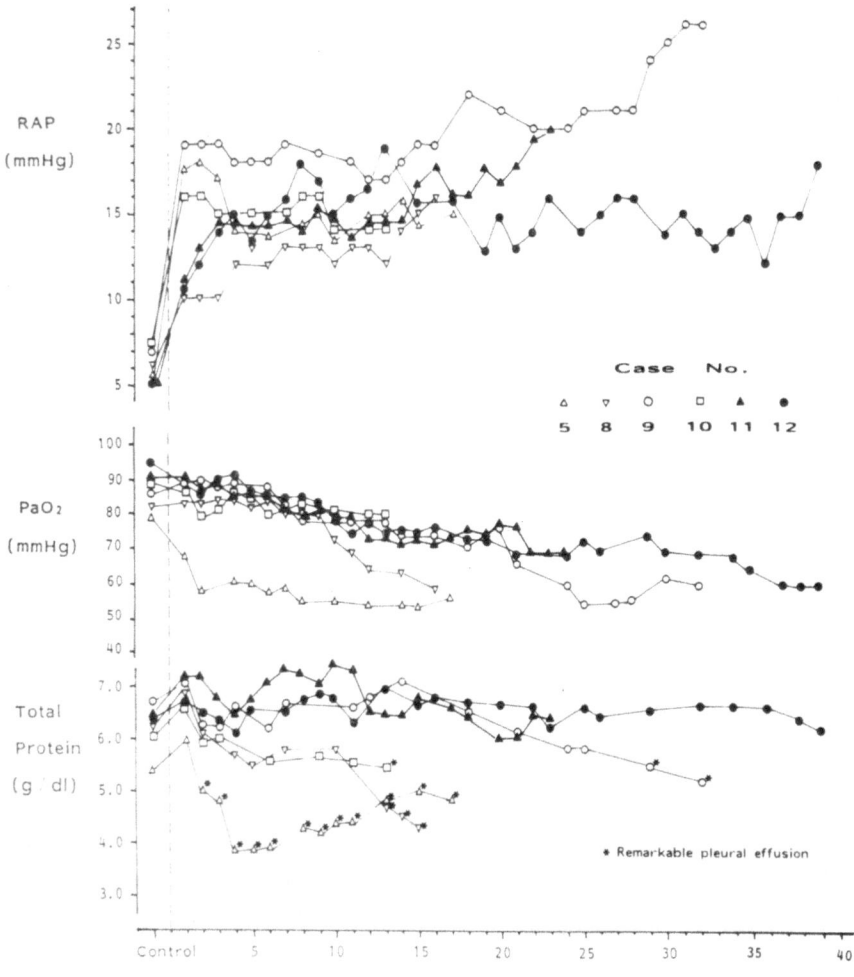

**Fig. 24.4.** Time-course of changes in right atrial pressure (*RAP*), PaO₂, and total protein levels in six goats which survived longer than 10 days. *Asterisks* indicate remarkable pooling of pleural effusion

## Discussion

As a means of salvaging an unrecoverable ventricular fibrillation or cardiac arrest during LVAD assistance, biventricular bypass, implantation of a total artificial heart (TAH), or heart transplantation have been carried out [8, 9]. On the other hand, a right heart bypass operation, sacrificing the right ventricle (Fontan's procedure) [10, 11], has been widely performed, and many patients have been able to return to work. Also, Hennig et al. [12] reported a TAH experiment in which complete right pump failure occurred, but the animal's circulation was successfully maintained for a period of 49 days with the left-side pump alone. These facts suggest that the left-side pump alone can maintain both systemic and pulmonary circulation during cardiac arrest.

We have previously reported a feasibility study of circulatory maintenance with an LVAD alone in an acute experiment [5]. The purpose of the present study was to examine the feasibility of circulatory maintenance for a prolonged duration.

### Principle of circulatory maintenance with an LVAD alone during cardiac arrest

An LVAD sucks or pumps up blood from the LA, therefore LAP decreases during pump diastole. At the same time, RAP decreases as shown in Fig. 24.5. This phenomenon was clearly seen at high RAP and LAP (Fig. 24.5, left), and even at RAP levels of 12–16 mmHg this pump-up effect was also noted (Fig. 24.5, right). At low RAP levels, however, RAP waveform lagged behind that of LAP. This lag may have developed due to the increased transport time of blood across the narrowed pulmonary vasculature, which is caused by diminished blood volume. These facts support the point that circulatory maintenance with an LVAD alone during cardiac arrest is based on the pressure gradient between RAP and LAP and pump-up effect through the lung.

**Fig. 24.5.** Principle of circulatory maintenance with a left ventricular assist device along during cardiac arrest. Left atrial pressure (*LAP*) and also right atrial pressure (*LAP*) decrease during pump diastole. *AoP* aortic pressure

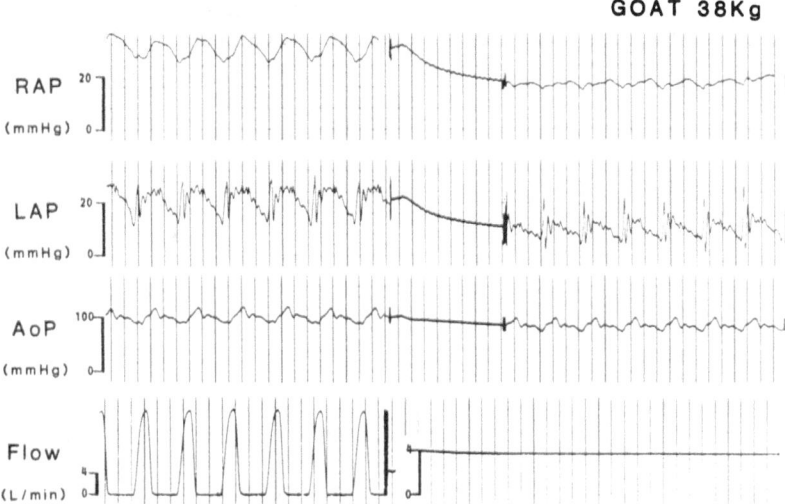

GOAT 38Kg

### Factors contributing to circulatory maintenance for prolonged duration

The PVR level is a major factor related to successful circulatory maintenance. Because of the capillaries in the pulmonary system, a certain grade of resistance from the RA to LA cannot be avoided. Provided that PVR was in the normal range, the pressure gradient from the RA to LA was 7–10 mmHg. If PVR is high, the pressure gradient across the lungs becomes higher, thus requiring RAP to be kept at a higher level in order to yield a sufficient flow. However, there is a limit for the upper level of the RAP, because high RAP usually causes venous congestion, resulting in pleural effusion and ascites. Therefore, PVR should be kept in the normal range. Factors affecting high PVR are blood transfusion, certain types of drugs, pleural effusion, etc. In the authors' experience with goats, blood transfusion increased PVR even when the cross-match test was negative. When PVR was high, a vasodilator, especially tolazoline and isoproterenol, decreased PVR. This study in goats suggests that for successful circulatory maintenance with only an LVAD, PVRI values should be less than 15 000 dynes.s.cm$^{-5}$.kg or preoperative PAP values should be less than 15 mmHg. The PVR level tended to decrease with time even if pleural effusion did not accumulate. The pulmonary vasculature may adapt itself to a new situation.

The RAP level is the second factor related to circulatory maintenance. High RAP produces pooling of pleural and visceral effusion. With regard to the pressure gradient between the RA and LA, when the PVR is normal, the RAP should be 14–16 mmHg.

Movement or exercise caused the flow to change. RAP increased during exercise, and LAP increased as RAP increased. Because the CDU in our LVAD sys-

tem has an automatic level control system for LAP that can maintain the LAP at a constant level, the flow increases in proportion to RAP. A flow of 80–140 ml/kg/min is sufficient for the goat to behave normally in the cage and also during exercise.

### Prevention of pleural and visceral effusion

Because the circulatory situation maintained with an LVAD alone during cardiac arrest is similar to a kind of severe right heart failure, pleural effusion and ascites tend to pool. In our early experiments, pooling of effusion appeared approximately on the 4th day. In these cases, the total protein level was below 5.5 g/dl, so an attempt was made to keep it higher than 6.0 g/dl. Consequently, the appearance of effusion was delayed in cases after case 5. Low RAP also delayed the appearance of effusion. Maintaining high total protein as well as low RAP is important to prevent pooling of pleural and visceral effusion.

### Conclusion

When PVR was in the normal range (less than 15 000 dynes.s.cm$^{-5}$.kg), circulation was well maintained with only an LVAD as long as RAP was kept between 12 and 16 mmHg. Under such conditions, the flow fluctuated between 80 and 140 ml/kg/min, depending on the animal's demand, and the mean AoP was kept above 80 mmHg; the goats behaved normally. However, pooling of pleural effusion and ascites was a serious problem in maintaining the circulation for a prolonged period. Maintenance of the protein level above 6.0 g/dl would delay or prevent pooling of effusion. The longest survival time to date has been 38 days. In consideration of the results of the Fontan's procedure, an LVAD alone during cardiac arrest may maintain the circulation much longer in the clinical situation than in goat experiments. When PVR is in the normal range, an LVAD alone during cardiac arrest will allow enough time for a further treatment such as heart transplantation or total artificial heart replacement.

## References

1. Pierce WS, Donachy JH, Landis DL, Brighton JA, Rosenberg G, Migliore JJ, Prophet GA, White WJ, Waldhausen JA: Prolonged mechanical support of the left ventricle. Circulation 58 (Suppl): 133–146, 1978
2. Pae WE, Jr, Pierce WS: Mechanical left ventricular assistance: Current devices, future prospects. In: Surgery for the complications of myocardial infarction. Moran JW, Michaelis LL (eds.), Grune & Stratton, New York, 1980, pp. 411
3. Pennington DG, Samuels LD, Williams CB, Palmer D, Swartz MT, Codd JE, Merjavy JP, Lagunoff D, Joist JH: Experience with the Pierce-Donachy ventricular assist device in postcardiotomy patients with cardiogenic shock. World J Surg 9: 37–46, 1985
4. Takano H, Nakatani T, Noda H, Umezu M, Fukuda S, Tanaka T, Matsuda T, Iwata H, Takatani S, Taenaka Y, Kinoshita M, Kumon K, Kito Y, Yutani C, Fujita T, Akutsu T, Manabe H: Clinical consideration of left ventricular assist system for acute myocarcial infarction with cardiogenic shock. Trans Am Soc Artif Intern Organs 32: 467–473, 1986
5. Takano H, Taenaka Y, Nakatani T, Umezu M, Matsuda T, Iwata H, Tanaka T, Noda H, Hayashi K, Takatani S, Nakamura T, Seki J, Akutsu T, Manabe H: Circulatory maintenance with a single artificial heart. Trans Am Soc Artif Intern Organs 30: 550–05, 1984
6. Takano H, Taenaka Y, Nakatani T, Akutsu T, Manabe H: Successful treatment of profound left ventricular failure by automatic left ventricular assist system. World J Surg 9: 78–88, 1985
7. Takano H, Nakatani T, Taenaka Y, Umezu M: Development of the ventricular assist pump system: Experimental and clinical studies. In: Artificial Heart-1, Akutsu T (ed.), Tokyo, 1986, Springer-Verlag, p. 141–151
8. Hill JD, Farrar DJ, Hershon JJ, Compton PG, Averg GJ, Litwak P, Foran WS, Dunlap TE, Levin BS: Bridge to cardiac transplantation: Successful use of prosthetic biventricular support in a patient awaiting a donor heart. Trans Am Soc Artif Intern Organs 32: 233–236, 1986
9. Pennock JR, Pierce WS, Campbell DB, Pae WE, Davis D, Hensley FA, Richenbacher WE, Waldhausen JA: Mechanical support of the circulation followed by cardiac transplantation. J Thorac Cardiovasc Surg 92: 994–1004, 1986
10. Fontan F, Baudet E: Surgical repair of tricuspid atresia. Thorax 26: 240–248, 1971
11. Girod DA, Fontan F, Deville C, Ottenkamp J, Choussat A: Longterm results after the Fontan operation for tricuspid atresia. Circulation 75: 605–610, 1987
12. Henning E, Weidermann H, Keilbach H, Schessler A, Stelter U, Baer P, Bucherl ES: Maintaining the circulation with only left pump after total artificial heart replacement. Life Support system (Proc 10th Ann Mtg European Society of Artificial Organs) 2: 1–4, 1983

# Discussion

*Imamura* (Tokyo Women's Medical College): I am particularly impressed with your results concerning the case where a patient is supported by a temporary device and cardiac arrest suddenly occurs but the medical staff do not notice the cardiac ventricular fibrillation. Your experiments have demonstrated that good circulation can be maintained for a certain period of time. How long is it possible to wait before making a countershock without inducing right ventricular failure?

*Takano* (National Cardiovascular Center): It is a difficult question. As you know, our experiments were carried out on goats. Dr. Fontan has developed his right atriopulmonary shunt operation at the sacrifice of right ventricular function. In his experiments on dogs, all the animals died. However, when he tried this procedure in a clinical case, the patient was able to survive and return to work. From this fact, if pulmonary vascular resistance is not high, our procedure can perhaps maintain circulation much longer in humans than in animals.

*Portner* (Novacor Medical Corporation): Much of our own experience would support your data. In animal experiments, there have been many occasions when with a single left ventricular assist system we have been able to support the entire circulation. The key factor of course as you pointed out is essentially normal pulmonary vascular resistance. There have been many occasions when we have had ventricular fibrillation, sometimes for as long as days, though none were as long as in your experience.

In our experience with patients in the bridge to transplant, we have again observed ventricular fibrillation, normally for very short periods and generally with spontaneous reversion back to sinus rhythm. Here we used, of course, only a single left ventricular assist. In one particular patient, there were sustained ventricular tachycardia rates of as high as 200 beats/min for days at a time with maintenance of normal output and pressure. In some patients who have presented with what appeared to be severe biventricular failure at the time of implant, we have found over a period of time that the initial pulmonary hypertension and severe right ventricular failure correct themselves. This was particularly true in the patient I described yesterday who was supported for a period of 3 months. There is a change in pulmonary capillary wedge pressure from preoperative values of 40 mmHg to a normal level of 23 mmHg after about 3 weeks. We feel that in many of these patients, the elevated pulmonary vascular resistance is reactive in nature and once the systemic side of the hemodynamics is corrected the right-sided situation will correct itself. So, we feel that in many cases a single left ventricular assist device will satisfactorily support the circulation.

*Akutsu* (National Cardiovascular Center): I was at the Texas Heart Institute when there was the first clinical use of a ventricular assist device as a bridge to transplantation by Dr. Cooley and his associates. This first use was not intentional. When the postcardiotomy patient had ischemic contracture of the left ventricule which developed into a stone heart, only one ventricular assist device was available and they put it in. They maintained the entire circulation of the patient for a week. I think that Dr. Takano's design is an attempt to improve this idea by experimental means.

*Copeland:* In heart transplantation, we use a limit for candidate selection of pulmonary vascular resistance of about 6 Wood units. Some groups will perform transplants at 6–8 Wood units. Very few groups would exceed this. In a group of patients who are candidates for transplantation, a certain number will have slightly elevated to moderately elevated pulmonary vascular resistance. Assuming that this type of device is used to support these patients, how do you decide which patients need univentricular and which biventricular support?

*Takano:* We usually use a left ventricular assist device, but if cardiac output is less than 2 liters/m² we use a right ventricular assist device in addition to LVAD.

*Copeland:* So you would basically put in the left ventricular assist device and then if the output was sufficient you would leave it; if it was insufficient you would put in a right ventricular assist device.

*Takano:* At that time, we use a pulmonary vasodilator such as Tolazoline.

*Imamura:* This is an interesting question I think since we have the experience with Fontan procedure in tricuspid atresia, in which the right ventricle does not work or there is very weak ejection. Nevertheless, a good right heart circulation can be maintained with the Fontan procedure. This procedure is only indicated in patients with less than 4 Wood units, so I think that patients with over 5 Wood units should also receive heart support.

*Copeland:* Yes that has certainly been our experience with the Fontan procedure, where even though patients are selected very carefully some do die.

# 25. Potential candidates for bridge bypass

Eisaburo Imamura, Kiyoyuki Eishi, Hiroshi Nishida, Masahiro Endo, Akimasa Hashimoto, and Hitoshi Koyanagi[1]

**Summary.** Among the 3143 patients undergoing open heart operations at the Heart Institute of Japan, 34 patients were treated with assisted circulation for longer than 60 min in addition to balloon pumping. A total of 21 patients (62%) were lost due to failure of weaning. Of the 13 patients in whom weaning was possible, three died due to fatal arrhythmias and two died of device-related complications. The remaining eight patients (25%) survived and did well for up to 5 years postoperation. It is concluded that choice of an appropriate ventricular assist mode is of the utmost importance and that four patients in this series might have been potential candidates for bridge bypass to heart transplantation and one for heart-lung transplantation.

**Key words**: Bridge bypass—Heart transplantation—Venoarterial bypass—Left ventricular assist device

Adequate use of intra-aortic balloon pumping (IABP) in addition to dopamine and other types of cardiovascular drug therapy has contributed greatly to the improved operative results in recent years [1, 2]. However, a number of patients still die of intractable low cardiac output syndrome. Some of these patients cannot be taken from cardiopulmonary bypass despite intensive drug therapy and IABP. In addition, a few patients develop sudden cardiac arrest in the immediate postoperative period. For these moribund patients, more aggressive therapeutic approaches are essential to save life. These include temporary assisted circulation [3, 4], permanent cardiac substitute, and bridge bypass to heart transplantation.

We review here our past with assisted circulation. The purpose of this paper is to document the practical efficacy of each mode of mechanical assist device and to increase our understanding with regard to future application of bridge bypass or permanent cardiac substitute.

[1] Department of Cardiovascular Surgery, The Heart Institute of Japan, Tokyo Women's Medical College, 8-1 Kawada-cho, Shinjuku-ku, Tokyo, 162 Japan

## Subjects and methods

During the 6½ years from January 1981 until June 1987, we performed 3755 total cardiovascular operations at the Heart Institute of Japan, Tokyo Women's Medical College. Of the 3143 patients (83.7%) undergoing open heart surgery, 554 were treated postoperatively with IAPB, and 45 of them required additional circulatory support for longer than 60 min. Eleven patients who were either younger than 20 years or who died as a result of technical problems such as uncontrollable bleeding were excluded, and the remaining 34 patients form the basis of this study.

They were 21 men and 13 women, ranging in age from 22 to 69 (mean 46.7) years. Twenty-two patients had cardiac valve disease, ten had ischemic heart disease, and two had a congenital anomaly. Assist duration ranged from 1 to 169 h (mean 29.6 h).

All but one patient were treated with assisted circulation in combination with IABP. The later received extracorporeal membrane oxygenator therapy to manage the lung bleeding, which had been caused by ascending aortic aneurysm prior to Bentall's procedure.

The decision to apply the assisted circulation was made when ventricular fibrillation occurred frequently or peak arterial (mostly augmented diastolic) pressure was below 90 mmHg and mean left atrial pressure above 20 mmHg constantly under IABP treatment. Cardiac output measurement using a Swan-Ganz catheter was not made in most of these cases to avoid unnecessary artificial stimulation, which might have induced fatal arrhythmias.

Table 25.1 illustrates the hemodynamic effects of each method of assisted circulation employed in this series: venoarterial bypass with oxygenation (VAB), isolated left ventricular bypass without oxygenation (ILB), and biventricular bypass with oxgenation (BAB). A single unit was designed to convert from one mode to another in order to manage the varying hemodynamics properly.

**Table 25.1.** Hemodynamic effects of assisted circulation

| | Preload | | Afterload | | Arti-ficial lung |
|---|---|---|---|---|---|
| | LV | RV | LV | RV | |
| IABP | → | → | ↓ | → | No |
| Venoarterial bypass (VAB) | ↓ | ↓↓ | ↑ | ↓ | Yes |
| Isolated LV bypass (ILB) | ↓↓ | ↑ | ↓ or →[a] | → | No |
| Biventricular bypass (BVB) | ↓↓ | ↓↓ | ↓ or →[a] | ↓ or →[a] | Yes |

*LV* left ventricle, *RV* right ventricle, *IABP* intra-aortic ballon pumping
[a] Depending on whether ECG-synchronized or not

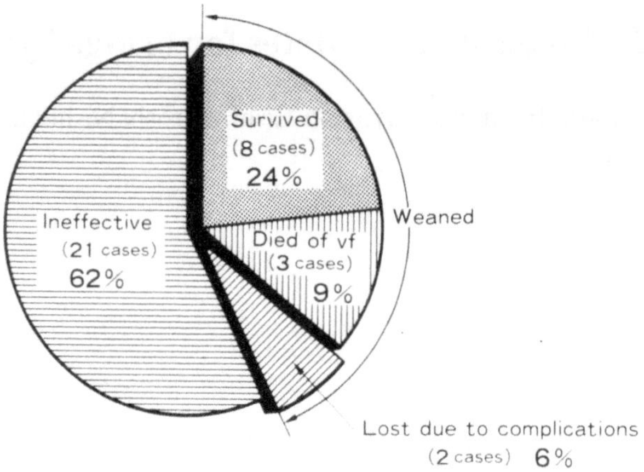

**Fig. 25.1.** Results of assisted circulation (34 patients)

**Table 25.2.** Results of assisted circulation by year

| Venoarterial bypass | Year | Isolated LV bypass biventricular bypass |
|---|---|---|
| ■■●●● | 1981 | |
| ■□□□□ | 1982 | |
| ●●●● | | |
| ■●● | 1983 | ●■ |
| ■● | 1984 | ■▲ |
| | 1985 | ○□●● |
| ● | 1986 | ○●●● |
| △ | 1987.6 | ○ |

○ valve, □ coronary, △ congenital, ● died, ■ survived

**Table 25.3.** Results of assisted circulation by duration

| Venoarterial bypass | Duration | Isolated LV-bypass biventricular bypass |
|---|---|---|
| ●●●●● | 1–3 h | ○ |
| ■■■□□□ | | |
| ●●●●●● | 4–24 h | ○● |
| ▲■ | | |
| | 1–3 days | △ |
| | 4 days | ○ |
| | or | ■■ |
| ● | longer | ●● |
| | | □ |

○ valve, □ coronary, △ congenital, ● died, ○ survived

## Results

Figure 25.1 shows the results of assisted circulation (AC). There were 21 patients (62%) in whome weaning failed. Of the 13 patients where weaning could be carried out, three died due to recurrent ventricular fibrillation while in the intensive care unit, and two patients were lost as a result of AC-related complications. The remaining eight patients, one-fourth of the series, survived and did well for up to 5 years postoperatively.

Among the 22 patients who underwent valve replacement, there were only three survivors. Four of the ten patients with coronary surgery and one of the two patients with a congenital defect repair were successfully treated with assisted circulation.

Early in this series, we employed venoarterial bypass in 20 cases (Table 25.2). It was effective in three of the seven patients with coronary bypass graft-ing in one with congenital defect repair, but it was unsuccessful in all of the 12 patients after valve replacement. Later, we used either isolated left ventricular bypass, biventricular bypass, or a combination of both in 14 patients. It was effective in three of the ten patients with valve replacement and in one of the three patients who underwent ischemic heart surgery, but unsuccessful in one with congenital defect repair.

No significant correlation was found between the duration of circulatory support and survival rate in the present series (Table 25.3). Table 25.4 summarizes the morbidity and mortality associated with assisted circulation. Premature weaning resulted in death in three cases. Two patients were lost due to fatal complications (DIC and sepsis, respectively). Four patients might have been the potential candidates for bridge bypass to heart tranplantation and one for heart-lung transplantation.

**Table 25.4.** Morbidity and mortality associated with assisted circulation

| Patient | Age (yrs) | Sex | Procedure | Assist circulation | | Outcome |
|---|---|---|---|---|---|---|
| **Premature weaning** | | | | | | |
| 1 S.N. | 63 | M | LV-aneurysmectomy | BVB | 1.0 h | vf, 3 h |
| 2 A.U. | 34 | M | MVR | BVB | 44.3 h | vf, 16 h |
| 3 Y.T. | 33 | M | MVR | BVB | 16.2 h | vf, 32 h |
| **Fatal complications** | | | | | | |
| 1 S.K. | 57 | M | AVR | VAB | 6.5 h | DIC, 3 days |
| 2 I.Y. | 38 | F | AVR | BVB | 95 h | Sepsis, 27 days |
| **Potential candidates for bridge bypass** | | | | | | |
| 1 M.I. | 50 | F | MVR | ILB | 109 h | Irreversible myocard. damage |
| 2 M.O. | 22 | F | MVR | BVB | 96 h | Irreversible myocard. damage |
| 3 H.S. | 42 | F | Bentall | BVB | 16 h | Irreversible myocard. damage |
| 4 K.A. | 42 | M | CABG | BVB | 43 h | Irreversible myocard. damage |
| 5 Y.T. | 38 | F | Bentall | ECMO | 120 h | Lung bleeding |

## Discussion

The principal aim of temporary circulatory assist is to reduce the energy consumption until the myocardial cells regain normal energy production [5]. Energy production and consumption in the damaged myocardium must be normally balanced, otherwise low output syndrome or severe arrhythmias may ensue [6]. In this series, we employed three different modes of extracorporeal assisted circulation in addition to IABP. All but one were designed to be able to convert from one mode to another in a single unit. The latter, which was the left ventricular assist device of Tokyo University (Atsumi model), was also found to be useful at the practical level.

The venoarterial bypass was most commonly used, but a drawback with this is an increase in left ventricular afterload. Isolated left ventricular bypass does not need an oxygenator and allows prolonged circulatory support, but it tends to increase preload of the right ventricle. Biventricular bypass predominantly diminishes preload of both ventricles [7]. However, the afterload of this setting is dependent on whether the arterial return is ECG-synchronized or not.

The role of the temporary assisted circulation leaves a few questions unanswered. The first concerns the timing of weaning.

In three cases, we ecountered apparent premature weaning. All three patients developed ventricular fibrillation after the assist device was removed and died. To avoid this, assist of a sufficient duration seems necessary. On the other hand, there is the problem that prolonged circulatory support is apt to increase the incidence of complications. We had two such cases.

It is possible that temporary assisted circulation is no longer effective after myocardial damage has

crossed the point of irreversibility. Pennington et al. [8], Zumbro et al. [9], Hill et al. [10], and Pennock et al. [11] successfully established the concept of bridge bypass where a mechanical heart device is temporarily used until an appropriate donor heart becomes available. We had five such cases among the 34 patients undergoing extended mechanical support following cardiac operation.

In summary, choice of an adequate ventricular assist mode is of the utmost importance. A switch system in one unit from biventricular to univentricular assist is useful for properly managing the unstable hemodynamics. Some of the 16 patients who were unsuccessfully treated with venoarterial bypass could have been saved by ECG-synchronized left ventricular assist device. Four of the ten patients in whom biventricular assist had failed might have been potential candidates for bridge bypass to heart transplantation and one for heart-lung transplantation.

## References

1. Pierce WS, Parr GVS, Myers JL, Pae WE Jr, Bull AP, Waldhausen JA (1981) Ventricular-assist pumping in patients with cardiogenic shock after cardiac operations. N Engl J Med 305: 1606–1610
2. Pennock JL, Pierce WS, Wisman CB, Bull AP, Waldhausen JA (1983) Survival and complications following ventricular pumping for cardiogenic shock. Ann Surg 198: 469–478
3. Levinson MM, Copeland JG (1987) Technical aspects of total artificial heart implantation for temporary applications. J Cardiac Surg 2: 3–19
4. Schoen FJ, Palmer DC, Bernhard WF, Pennington DG, Haudenschild CC, Ratliff NB, Berger RL, Golding LR, Watson JT (1986) Clinical temporary ventricular assist; Pathologic findings and their implications in a multi-institutional study of 41 patients. J Thorac Car-

diovasc Surg 92: 1071–1081

5. Ban T, Fukumasu H, Soneda J, Iways F, Hoshino S, Yuasa S (1987) Clinical application of left ventricular assist devices. J Cardiac Surg 2: 21–36

6. Takano H, Nakatani T, Taenaka Y, Umezu M, Matsuda T, Iwata H, Adachi S, Tanaka T, Noda H, Fukuda S, Seki J, Nakamura T, Takatani S, Hayashi K, Akutsu T, Manabe H (1985) Recovery mechanism from postoperative profound heart failure by an automatic left ventricular assist system. ASAIO 31: 196–201

7. Pennington DG, Merjavy JP, Swartz MT, Codd JE, Barner HB, Lagunoff D, Bashiti H, Kaiser G, Willman VL (1985) The importance of biventricular failure in patients with postoperative cardiogenic shock. Ann Thorac Surg 39: 16–26

8. Pennington DG, Codd JE, Merjavy JP, Swartz MT, Kaiser G, Barner HB, Willman VL (1984) The ex-
panded use of ventricular bypass systems for severe cardiac failure and as a bridge to cardiac transplantation. Heart Transplant 3: 170–175

9. Zumbro GL Jr, Shearer G, Kitchens WR, Galloway RF (1985) Mechanical assistance for biventricular failure following coronary bypass operation and heart transplantation. Heart transplant 4: 348–352

10. Hill JD, Farrar DJ, Hershon JJ, Compton PG, Avery GJ, Levin BS, Brent BN (1986) Use of a prosthetic ventricle as a bridge to cardiac transplantation for postinfarction cardiogenic shock. New Engl J Med 314: 626–628

11. Pennock JL, Pierce WS, Campbell DB, Pae WE Jr, Davis D, Hensley FA, Richenbacher WE, Waldhausen JA (1986) Mechanical support of the circulation followed by cardiac transplantation. J Thorac Cardiovasc Surg 92: 994–1004

# Discussion

*Copeland* (Arizona Health Science Center): Do you always implant right and left atrial cannulae and do you always include a "y" in your arterial limb so that you can go through the oxygenator or bypass the oxygenator?

*Imamura* (Tokyo Women's Medical College): Recently yes. It does depend on the hemodynamic condition of the patient, but in extremely severe cases two cannulae should be placed–one in the right atrium and the other in left. When the hemodynamics improve, biventricular assist is changed to univentricular assist.

# Part V
# Electrical Energy System and Its Transmission

# 26. Energy systems for chronic circulatory support

John C. Moise[1]

**Summary.** The ventricular assist energy system being developed by Nimbus to drive and control the Cleveland Clinic intrathoracic blood pump is described. In the longest in vivo test in the calf, the ventricular assist system was implanted for a period of 6 1/2 months when the experiment was electively terminated. For most of the experimental period, an implanted variable volume device and transcutaneous transmission energy system was utilized. The efficiency of the energy converter in the test was within 2% of the pretest value. Energy converter endurance testing showed that with the exception of gear pump bearings, which exhibited 4 $\mu$m of wear after 5 years, none of the components showed significant wear. Details of clinical trials currently underway are described.

**Key words:** Energy system—Clinical trials—Ventricular assist

A variety of energy systems for driving and controlling blood pumps have been under development. The term "energy system" as used in this paper includes energy source, storage, transmission, and conversion devices as well as control elements. In the material below, there is a brief discussion of the approaches which have been taken to provide energy systems which drive and control blood pumps used for chronic ventricular assist and total heart replacement. This is followed by a more detailed discussion of the ventricular assist energy system being developed by Nimbus under NHLBI sponsor-ship to drive and control the Cleveland Clinic intrathoracic blood pump.

## Energy systems—general considerations

### Energy sources

A wide variety of energy sources have been considered and evaluated for powering implantable circulatory support systems. Table 26.1 summarizes both intracorporeal and extracorporeal sources and their corresponding energy transmission approaches.

Two approaches to utilizing biological energy sources have been evaluated. Significant work is being done on utilizing muscle power to drive circulatory assist devices [1, 2]. The work discussed indicates that the transformed muscle is limited in its ability to provide circulatory support. Another approach which has been investigated and abandoned is the biological fuel cell. The chance of such a process producing the many watts of energy needed to drive an implanted criculatory support device is remote.

Extensive development work has been done utilizing thermal energy sources powering heat engines. The two principle energy sources which have been evaluated are the plutonium 238 radioisotope, which has a sufficiently long half-life to power a circulatory support device for 10 years without a significant loss of power and heat of fusion salts, which are periodically heated and melted. Although from a patient viewpoint the radioisotope heat source is by far the least invasive of all energy sources, the political aspects of using the relatively large radioisotope source are daunting and work utilizing such a source has been de-emphasized.

Thermal energy system development in the United States has concentrated on the use of mixed fluoride heat of fusion salts. The University of Washington [3] and Nimbus [4] are developing left ventricular assist systems based on this technology. The University of Washington approach utilizes a Stirling hydraulic engine, where the power output of the Stirling engine appears in the form of hydraulic power. The hydraulic fluid is then used to power a linear actuator and also to control synchronization with the heart. The Nimbus approach utilizes a Stirling thermocompressor whose direct output is pressurized helium. The helium gas is then used to drive and control the blood pump. Eight hours of freedom from external energy sources can be provided within a charging time of approximately 1 h.

The primary emphasis in circulatory support energy system development has been on approaches which utilize extracorporeal energy sources and transmit energy either percutaneously or transcutaneously to an implanted device. Magnetic couplings have been proposed [5] to transmit rotary motion from an exter-

---
[1]Nimbus, Inc., 2945 Kilgore Rd., Rancho Cordova, CA 95670, USA

**Table 26.1.** Energy sources for chronic circulatory support systems

| Source | Characteristics | Status |
| --- | --- | --- |
| Intracoporeal | | |
| Noncardiac muscle | Transformed skeletal muscle, appears limited to IABP type application | Investigating basic characteristics |
| Biological fuel cell | Impractical at multiwatt power levels required | No known activity |
| $P_U$ 238 radioisotope | Reliable energy source, severe political problems | No kown active development—USSR? |
| Extracorporeal to intracorporeal | | |
| Magnetic coupling | Secondary of coupling equivalent mechanically to electric motor rotor, anatomically constrains location of circulatory support system, eliminates percutaneous penetrations | Was proposed for driving centrifugal blood pump |
| Pneumatic | Requires air compressor and large percutaneous penetrations, limited potential for chronic systems, concern for infection | Used with Jarvik-7 TAH patients |
| Hydraulic | Requires hydraulic pump, low pressure requires large percutaneous penetrations, high pressure smaller penetrations, concern for infection | Limited investigation of low pressure, no known high-pressure development |
| Electrical-percutaneous | Small percutaneous access required (larger if vent tube incorporated), somewhat less concern for infection if vent tube not used | Novacor has used in bridge patients |
| Electrical transcutaneous | Utilizes transcutaneous transformer and rectifier, eliminates percutaneous penetration | Thermedics and Novacor have developed systems, has not yet been used clinically |
| Electrical transcutaneous and thermal energy storage | Transformer periodically transfers energy to heat of fusion thermal salt allows ~ 8 h freedom from extra-corporeal energy source | Thermal systems being developed by Nimbus and University of Washington |

nal motor to an implanted coupling secondary. These devices have been evaluated for driving centrifugal blood pumps. Percutaneous pneumatic and hydraulic energy transmission have also been evaluated with emphasis on the pneumatic approach. An extracorporeal pneumatic source has been used in the Jarvik total heart replacement device. Chronic circulatory support devices can be developed based on pneumatic sources and percutaneous access although the problem of infection of the large percutaneous penetrations remains to be of concern. In addition, the electropneumatic conversion device that would be required for patient mobility is relatively bulky.

These considerations have led to a major development emphasis on devices which can be powered electrically utilizing either transcutaneous energy transmission by means of a transformer or percutaneous access. For conventional cyclic delivery blood pumps, percutaneous access can involve either a vent tube, which results in an access site approximately the same size as one of the pneumatic lines required for a pneumatically powered device, or a small percutaneous access utilized only for electrical energy transmission can be employed. In this case, an internal variable volume device or some double blood pump arrangement is needed. In the case of continuous delivery centrifugal pumps, a small percutaneous access device can be utilized. Transcutaneous energy transmission resolves the skin penertration issue but involves a more bulky system and efficiency degradation associated with the transformer and implanted rectifier [6]. (This paper by Altieri and Watson also has a good recent summary of NHLBI sponsored work on energy transmission and electrical LVASs.)

## Energy conversion approach

Table 26.2 lists thermal energy conversion approaches which have received development attention in the USA. The thermoelectric approach has the advantage of simplicity and reliability but when coupled to re-

**Table 26.2.** Thermal energy conversion approaches

| Approach | Characteristic | Status |
|---|---|---|
| Thermoelectric | Reliable but low efficiency | No known activity |
| Rankine cyclic steam engine | Low efficiency | No known current activity |
| Tidal regenerator engine | Relatively low efficiency | No known current activity |
| Organic Rankine cycle | Relatively low efficiency | No known current activity |
| Stirling mechanical | High efficiency but complex and bulky | No known current activity |
| Stirling hydraulic | High efficiency, hydraulic actuation and control | Being developed by University of Washington for use with thermal energy storage |
| Stirling thermocompressor | High efficiency, Pneumatic actuation and control | Being developed by Nimbus for use with thermal energy storage |

**Table 26.3.** Electrical energy conversion approaches

| Approach | Characteristic | Status |
|---|---|---|
| Piezoelectric | Inefficient—requires major motion amplification | No known current development work |
| Direct linear electrical actuator | Simple—relatively inefficient due to high force required with large magnetic gap | Feasibility investigations |
| Solenoid with spring and linkage | Permits high solenoid efficiency, requires high power ($\sim 1$ kw) pulse for a few milliseconds, high force dry lube bearings | Being developed by Novacor, 14 bridge patients as of May 1987, in device readiness testing |
| Rotary motor with cam or roller screw | Relatively high efficiency by eliminating intermediate energy conversion, high force, dry lube bearings | Gould/THI—Development on system with gear train, no known current activity<br>Thermedics—1 revolution per beat, in device readiness testing<br>Penn State—roller screw system being developed<br>Takatani—cylindrical cam being developed<br>Mitamura—ball screw being developed |
| Low-pressure electrohydraulic | Direct actuation of sac-type pump with hydraulic fluid supplied by axial or centrifugal flow pump, moving parts in hydraulic fluid, relatively low efficiency | University of Utah continues development<br>Abiomed LVAS in device readiness testing<br>Fujimasa in development |
| High-pressure electrohydraulic | Hydraulic pump supplies fluid to magnetically coupled actuator, moving parts in hydraulic fluid | Nimbus LVAS in device readiness testing |

quired additional energy conversion steps, the resulting low efficiency requires an unacceptably large thermal source. Three Rankine cycle approaches received development attention. The conventional "steam" engine [7] had very low efficiency under the constraints of artificial heart application. An organic Rankine cycle engine [8], which theoretically had higher efficiency, received some development attention but was not pursued. The Tidal Regenerator engine [9] had a high degree of regeneration and higher efficiency but was still not fully competitive with Stirling type engines in this application. A mechanical Stirling engine [10] was partially developed which utilized a flexible cable and scotch yoke drive for a total heart blood pump. Thermal system development in the United States today is concentrated on the Stirling hydraulic and Stirling thermocompressor approaches, which were discussed in the previous section.

In the 1980s, most energy conversion development resources have been concentrated on electrical energy converters (Table 26.3). A piezoelectric approach [11] received some attention but the bulky lever systems needed for motion amplification was a serious drawback. Some development work continues on the simplest approach to driving a pusher plate blood pump—direct linear electromagnetic actuation [12]. However, the large force of approximately 5 kg and the large magnetic gap of over 1 cm suggest that this approach will be bulky and inefficient. A more efficient approach [6] involves utilizing a solenoid to cock a spring, which then drives the blood pump. This approach is in an advanced state of development and has been used as a temporary VAS with percutaneous access in 14 patients. The nature of this device requires dry lubrication of bearings, which carry the actuation load.

Mechanical actuation utilizing a rotary electric motor has been under development by a number of investigators. In the Thermedics approach [6], a cam is directly actuated by a motor which has one revolution per beat. Takatani [13] utilizes a cylindrical cam to actuate the pusher plate. Somewhat higher rotational speeds and lower torques are achieved by Pierce [14] utilizing a roller screw and Mitamura et al. [15] utilizing a ball screw. The approach developed by Gould [6] utilized a gear train to achieve much higher motor speeds. All of these approaches require dry lubricated bearings, which must react the full blood pump load.

An approach that is attractive in its basic simplicity is the low-pressure electrohydraulic energy converter. An axial or centrifugal flow hydraulic pump provides fluid for actuating a sac-type blood pump. In various versions, the pump is reversed [16], a valve is utilized [6], or two hydraulic pumps [17] are employed to accommodate systolic and diastolic requirements. A long endurance life can be projected due to hydraulic lubrication of moving parts. However, demonstrated efficiencies are very low, pressure-sensing transducers are required, and long-term diffusion of saline or hydraulic fluid across the blood pump diaphragm remains as an issue.

The "high"-pressure electrohydraulic approach utilized in the Nimbus/Cleveland Clinic LVAS has certain unique characteristics. Driving a blood pump by means of high-pressure hydraulic or pneumatic actuation has a number of advantageous features including: (a) Configurational flexibility, only the relatively compact actuator must be placed along the axis of the blood pump; the fluid source and control components can be packaged for best anatomical compatibility. (b) Low bearing loads, the direct blood pump actuation load of approximately 5 kg is reacted by fluid $\Delta P$ with only secondary loads requiring accommodation by dry lubricated bearings. (c) Synchronization without transducers or electronic elements, the information required for synchronization with the heart can be derived from actuator flow. (d) Fluid actuation allows the use of a small, high-speed power source to drive the inherently low-speed high force blood pump; the same result as can be obtained from a gear train. (e) By operating all moving elements except the bearings which react secondary actuator loads in hydraulic fluid, a very long life energy system can be realized.

Careful design is required to avoid prolems associated with the use of fluid actuation. These include fluid contamination, leakage, and the requirement to seal hermetically the actuation fluid. Contamination issues must be addressed by thorough cleaning of all parts before assembly, clean assembly, and filtration to remove any residual contamination and the small amount of debris generated by operation of the system. In the Nimbus high-pressure hydraulic and pneumatic actuators, hermetic sealing is facilitated by the use of a linear magnetic coupling to transmit driving force from the actuator piston to the blood pump. Laser-welder closures are utilized to complete hermetic sealing of the system.

## Electrohydraulic intrathoracic lvas

### System

The Nimbus electrohydraulic energy system will be described in some detail to highlight circulatory support energy system considerations. The energy system is required to drive and control the Cleveland Clinic Foundation intrathoracic blood pump. To minimize intrathoracic volume, the energy system is located in space made available by rib excision. By taking advantage of the configurational flexibility charactersitic of hydraulic actuation, the energy system components are arranged in the rectangular configuration shown in Fig. 26.1.

The resulting ventricular assist system (Fig. 26.2), which has been developed jointly by Nimbus and the Cleveland Clinic Foundation, consists of: an intrathoracic blood pump, an electrohydraulic parathoracically located energy converter, an intrathoracic varible volume device, a subcutaneous internal battery, a transcutaneous energy transmission system, a diagnostic data transmission and monitoring system, and an external battery assembly.

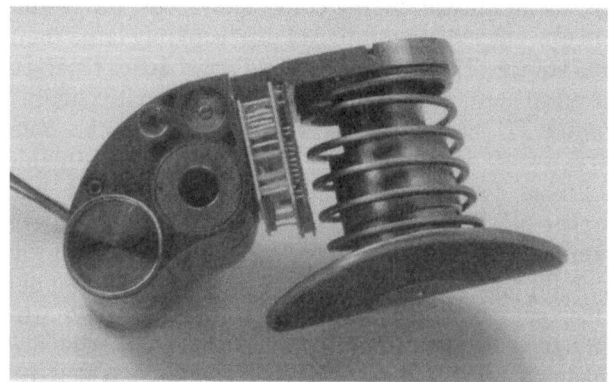

**Fig. 26.1.** Electrohydraulic energy converter

**Fig. 26.2.** Electrical ventricular assist system

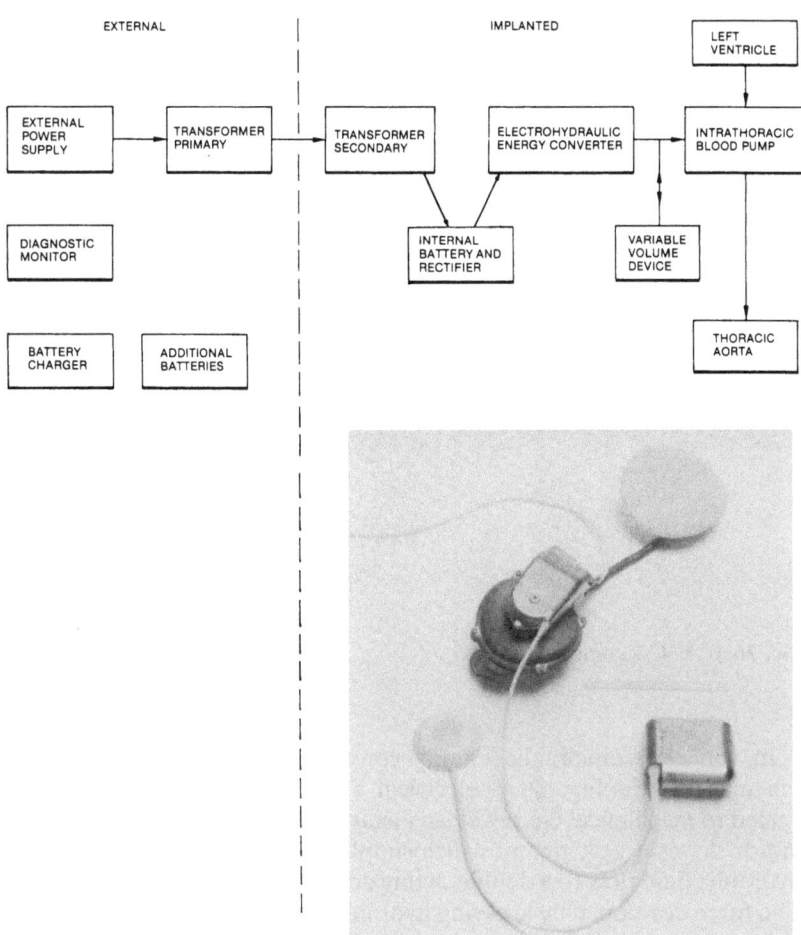

The blood pump is located in the left thorax with the inlet close coupled to the ventricular apex. A tissue valve is integrated with the apical tube. Blood is returned from the pump to the descending thoracic aorta. The energy converter is located in an approximately rectangular enclosure integral with the blood pump outer housing. The parathoracic enclosure is accommodated by removal of a segment of the sixth or seventh rib. The surrounding rib cage provides firm fixation of the blood pump/energy converter module. Of the total blood pump/energy converter volume of 400 cm$^3$, less than half lies within the thorax. The variable volume device, located superior to the pump at the level of the third or fourth rib, is connected to the variable volume space by a subcutaneous tube. Twelve volts dc power is supplied to the energy converter from a internal battery assembly, which is located subcutaneously in the abdomen. The internal battery assembly contains the battery and a rectifier which accepts ac power from the secondary coil of the energy transmission transformer. This secondary coil is positioned subcutaneously over the left second or third rib. The primary coil is supplied by a power oscillator located in the battery belt.

The pusher plate type blood pump utilizes investment cast titanium housings and a compression molded high flex life Hexsyn (Goodyear) rubber diaphragm. The blood-contacting surfaces of the pump are covered with a thin seamless layer of glutaraldehyde cross-linked gelatin. Adhesion of the gelatin layer is promoted by salt impregnation "texturing" of the rubber diaphragm surface and a plasma-sprayed deposition of fine titanium particles on the inner pump housing. The blood pump housing has been refined to fit the maximum number of potential patients.

**Electrohydraulic energy system**

All of the energy converter hydraulic components are integrated into a titanium housing. The housing and components are shown in Fig. 26.3. The compact and light-weight housing is fabricated by laser cutting a series of 20-ml miniplates with appropriate patterns, placing in a stack, and diffusion-bonding them. This fabrication process is a very compact approach to interconnecting the various fluid components of the actuation and control system within the housing.

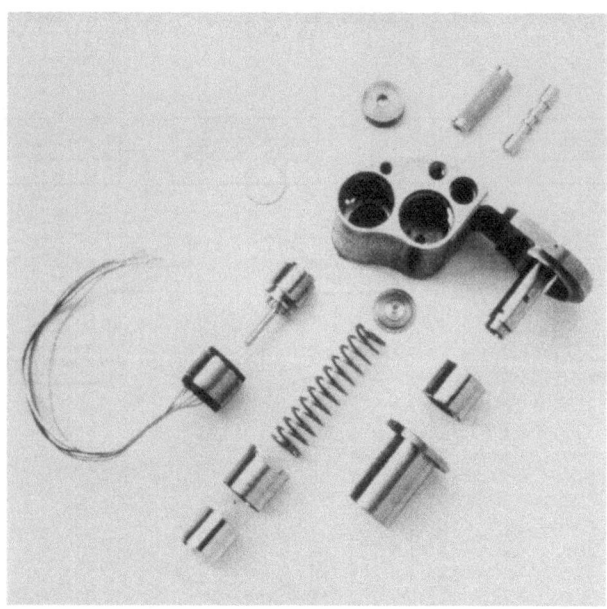

**Fig. 26.3.** E3C-2 components

In the electrohydraulic energy converter, shown schematically in Fig. 26.4, electrical energy is converted to mechanical energy by an electric motor. The motor drives a gear pump, which supplies controlled hydraulic fluid flow to a double-acting actuator piston. The force developed by applying hydraulic pressure to either side of the piston is transmitted to the blood pump pusher plate through the magnetic coupling, resulting in controlled displacement of the blood pump pusher plate/diaphragm.

A compression spring is located between the energy converter housing and the pusher plate to store alternately energy during blood pump filling and contribute energy during ejection. The use of a spring reduces peak hydraulic power demand and the forces on the magnetic coupling. The force supplied by the actuator main spring is a primary factor in establishing the left ventricular pressure required to move the pusher plate—the lower the spring force, the lower the ventricular pressure during heart systole.

The three-phase synchronous motor utilizes rare earth permanent magnets in the rotor to supply the magnetic field. The electrical power is supplied to the stator through circuitry which contains an inverter and a frequency varying circuit. The frequency, which determines electric motor speed, is derived from a microprocessor controller.

High-pressure fluid is alternately supplied to the top of the actuator piston during blood pump ejection and to the bottom of the piston during pump filling. The control logic and valving providing this function make up the hydraulic control circuit. This circuit consists of a two-position spool valve, check and diaphragm valves, a hydraulic switch, and an accumulator. The use of the force balance-based sensing approach provides for reliable synchronous counter-pulsation without the use of ECG signals or pusher plate position sensing and associated complex electronic signal processing. The actuator force balance is such that a blood flow of approximately 4 l/min is maintained if the heart were to fibrillate. Under these conditions, the system runs at a high beat rate with a short stroke.

A gear pump, shown in Fig. 26.5, is the source of pressurized hydraulic fluid. The pump incorporates

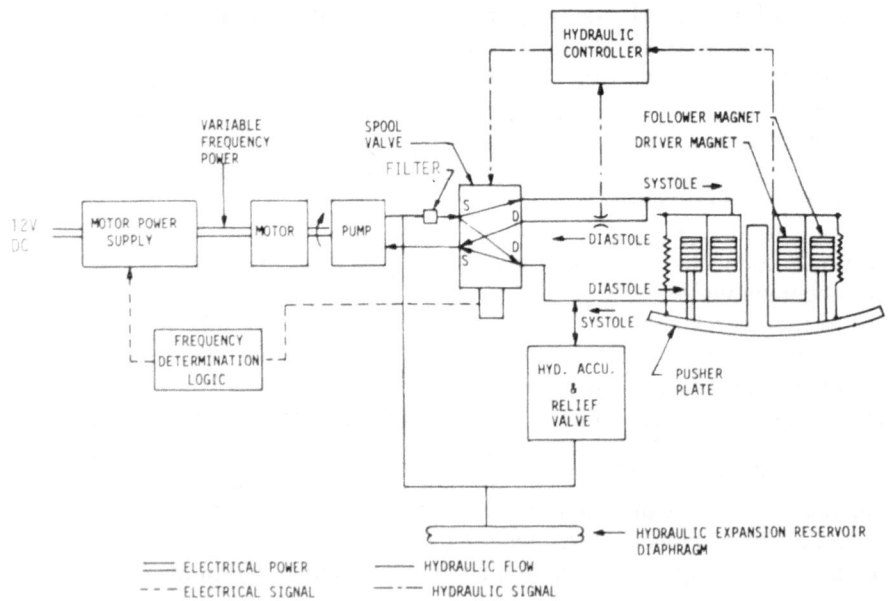

**Fig. 26.4.** Electrohydraulic energy converter schematic

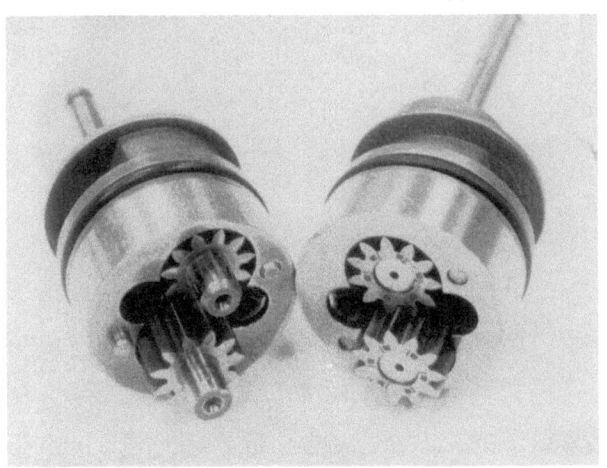

**Fig. 26.5.** E3C gear pumps, −1 and −2 configurations

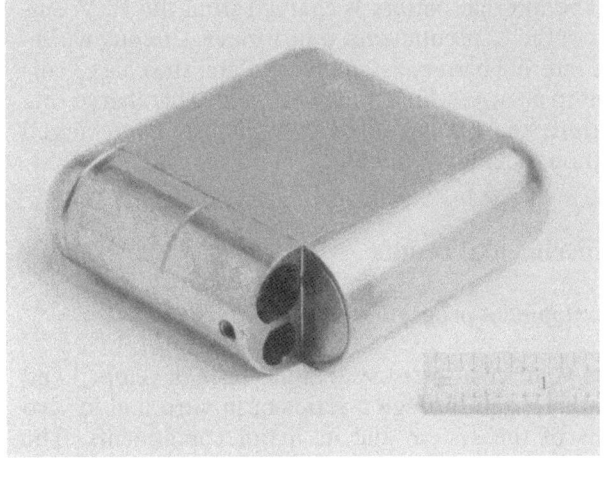

**Fig. 26.6.** Hermetically sealed internal battery

two spur gears, which are mounted on shafts supported by hydrodynamic journal bearings. Axial centering is provided by the hydrodynamic wedge action associated with the slightly rounded gear leading edge. The pump runs free of any mechanical contact between moving parts. The nominal speed range for the gear pump is 5000–10000 RPM, corresponding to a flow rate range of 0.5–1.0 in³. s. The differential pressure required during blood pump fill is approximately 40 psi. During ejection, the systemic blood flow resistance determines the pressure. The positive displacement gear pump must develop the hydraulic pressure required to displace the blood. Pressure ranges from 20 to 100 psi for an aortic pressure range of 70–200 mmHg.

Electrical elements of the energy converter consist of the motor, a motor power and control circuit, a hydraulic interface circuit, and an output signal conditioning circuit. Electronic elements are contained in the hybrid circuit package, which is mounted to the energy converter housing to facilitate heat removal (Fig. 26.1).

The motor consists of a six-pole permanent magnet rotor and a three-phase stator wound in a "delta" configuration. The rotor is mounted directly to the shaft of the hydraulic pump and runs submerged in the hydraulic oil. The motor output torque ranges from 0.5 to 1.5 oz in.

The power circuit converts 10–18 V dc into three-phase ac power pulses. The circuit monitors motor rotor position and modulates phase voltages to maintain the motor at the optimum torque angle. The circuit's control logic is provided by a CMOS microprocessor. A pulse width-modulated signal indicating spool valve position is generated by a Hall sensor to provide input to the microprocessor. This signal con-

tains the information from which the required motor speed is derived.

The motor speed varies in a controlled manner depending on patient activity level. The speed is adjusted so that the hydraulic flow is optimized for any particular physiological condition. This means that at low beat rate or stroke volumes the VAS has a longer period available to eject its blood volume. The motor speed is reduced slowing the ejection velocity of the blood pump. The ejection duration is regulated to provide the minimum speed required for system synchronization, thus increasing efficiency.

### Internal battery

The internal battery (Fig. 26.6) is designed to accommodate temporary interruptions of external power and to provide a nominal once a day period of operation for 30 min with an output of 7 l/min at an average aortic pressure of 100 mmHg. The battery is comprised of nine nickel-cadmium (NiCd) individual cells, which produce a nominal 10.8 V output, housed in a hermetically sealed 6Al-4V titanium case; it is implanted subcutaneously in the lower left hand side of the abdomen. The case is contoured to provide anatomical compatibility. Charging current is limited to the C/10 rate by a current limiter. A connector is housed on one end of the battery to allow for internal battery removal if required. A hermetic seal is maintained through the use of brazed-in glass to metal feedthroughs. A 20-ml copper sheet located between the internal components and the housing is used to distribute heat generated by the power transmission rectifier more uniformly over the internal battery surface.

The internal battery is charged from the 12-V output of the transcutaneous transformer. Circuity within the internal battery assembly regulates the charge current to 60 mA, which is the C/10 rate. This charge rate permits the battery to be continuously overcharged without degrading cell life.

## Experimental results

### Development program

The ventricular assist system has been developed and characterized through a series of in vitro and in vivo tests of the system and its major components. The longest calf in vivo test of implanted system elements was electively killed after $6\frac{1}{2}$ months. This experiment utilized an implanted variable volume device and a transcutaneous energy transmission system for most of the experimental period. The pertinent energy system results of in vitro and in vivo development to date are discussed below.

In vitro testing has been utilized for energy converter development, performance testing, and endurance testing. Development testing has utilized the standard NHLBI mock loop and modifications to the loop to simulate better left ventricular failure. In vitro characterization is also utilized to evaluate changes in energy converter performance as a result of chronic in vivo testing. The efficiency of the energy converter utilized in a 6 1/2-month in vivo test was within 2% of the pretest value.

Energy converter endurance testing has been conducted to evaluate wear characteristics. With the exception of gear pump bearings, which exhibited 4 $\mu$m of wear after 5 years of endurance testing, none of the components showed significant wear. The above data puls a gear pump modification which reduces bearing loads indicate that the energy converter has an endurance life well in excess of 5 years.

Energy converter electronics have been developed in parallel with the hydromechanical components. Standard printed circuit board electronics were utilized during the development phase. These have been replaced by two hybrid microcircuits which are compact enough to be integrated with the energy converter mechanical components. The electronics development was relatively straightforward since synchronization is accomplished hydraulically.

A positive result of the energy converter development program was repeated demonstration that performance of the unit would degrade slowly rather than fail abruptly. Ample warning is available to remove the energy converter cover and take corrective action.

Internal batteries have been tested in conjunction with VAS in vivo tests. However, the majority of bat-

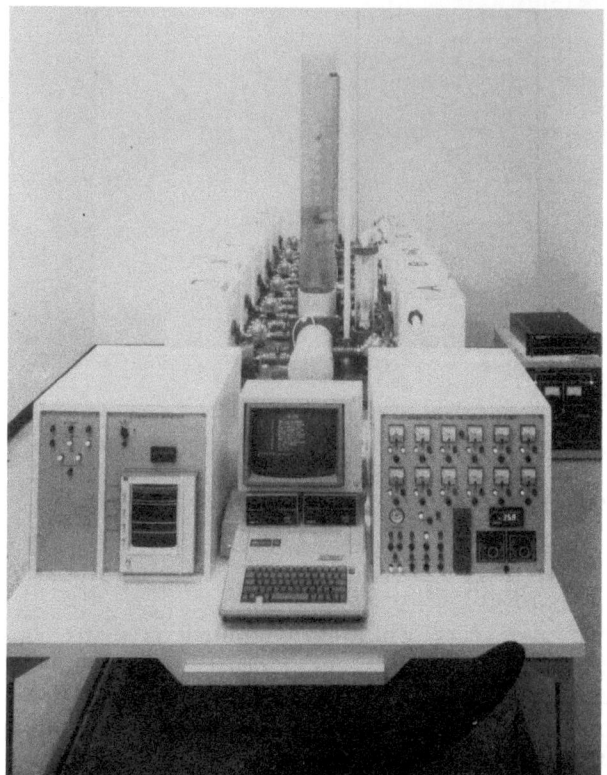

**Fig. 26.7.** Nimbus VAS reliability test facility

tery life data have been generated by means of in vitro tests at body temperature. These tests are conducted with a current requirement profile which matches that of the energy converter during operation. Battery capacity initially decreases but after approximately 20 cycles a steady state capacity is reached.

### Device readiness testing

#### Reliability test facility

The electrohydraulic intrathoracic LVAS described above is currently undergoing device readiness testing in preparation for clinical trials. Device readiness testing involves one in vitro and two in vivo test phases. In vitro reliability testing involves running 12 systems on the test device shown in Fig. 26.7. This device is designed to accommodate 12 systems running simultaneously and provide for automatic control of flow and pressures handled by the test systems as well as automated data recording. The implanted components of each VAS are immersed in saline baths, and the systems are operated, pumping water in a closed flow loop. A centralized heating and sterilization system is used for the loop's water supply. Similarly, a central heating and sterilization circuit is used to supply and circulate flow to the saline baths. Flow to each VAS is controlled through a two-way valve that is cycled on-off at a prescribed beat rate. This valve action causes the VAS to operate in synchronization with the on-off sequence. An on-line, dedicated computer system is used to sample automatically and record test data from each VAS. A master sequencer is used to control flow valve timing and data logging cycles for all systems. The entire test facility essentially fits on and under a 9-ft long, 4-ft wide, by 3-ft high table.

## Performance in vivo studies

Studies will be carried out in animals to demonstrate and document the in vivo performance of the VAS. The major objectives of acute in vivo experiments are as follows:

a) To demonstrate the consistent response of the VAS to various physiological and transiently unphysiological states
b) To establish the range of responses
c) To demonstrate the consistency of the response among systems

A total of four experiments will be conducted with a nominal duration of 2 weeks each. The duration of the experiment may be altered depending on the course of the hemodynamic variables.

## Chronic in vivo studies

Studies will be carried out in animals to demonstrate and document the in vivo performance of the VAS. The two major objectives of chronic in vivo experiments are as follows:

a) To demonstrate operation of the VAS in its final prototype configuration
b) To demonstrate operation of the system with minimal adverse effects on the animal

These objectives are to be achieved in five animals for periods of 5 months (on average), resulting in at least 25 animal-months of testing. Each experiment is expected to last a minimum of 4 months. Other experiments may be terminated before the 4 months are up in the case of failures unrelated to the LVAS and one experiment will deal with LVAS-related failure.

## References

1. Chachques J, Grandjean P, Vasseur B, Hero M, Perier P, Bourgeois I, Fardeau M, Carpentier A (1985) Electrophysiological conditioning of latissimus dorsi muscle flap for myocardial assistance. In: Nose' Y, Kjellstrand C, Ivanovich P (eds) Progress in artificial organs. ISAO, Cleveland, pp 409–412
2. Bitto T, Mannion J, Hammond R, Cox J, Yamashita J, Duckett S, Salmons S, Stephenson L (1985) Preparation of fatigue-resistant diaphragmatic muscle grafts for myocardial replacement. In: Nose' Y, Kjellstrand C, Ivanovich P (eds) Progress in artificial organs. ISAO, Cleveland, pp 441–446
3. White MA (1985) Implantable energy source for artificial hearts. In: Akutsu T (ed) Proceedings of the 1st international sysmposium on current problems for further development of artificial heart and assist device. Springer, Tokyo, pp 33–48
4. Blubaugh AL, Bulter KC, Schneider JA, Moise JC, Fujimoto L, Kiraly R, Smith WA, Nose' Y (1983) Thermally and electrically powered left ventricular assist devices. Progress in artificial organs. ISAO, Cleveland, pp 91–97
5. Bernstein EF, Cosentino LC, Reich S, Stasz P, Scott DR, Dorman FD, Blackshear PL A compact low hemolysis, non-thrombogenic system for non-thoracotomy prolonged left ventricular bypass. Trans Am Soc Artif Intern Organs 20B: 643
6. Altieri FD, Watson JT (1987) Implantable ventricular assist systems. Artificial organs II, 3: 237–246
7. Radioisotope Powered Artificial Heart Program (1974) NHLBI Annual Report, Contract NO1-HV-2-2900T, (PB 236 21/AS)
8. Energy Converter for Cardiac Devices (1975) NHLBI Annual Report, Contract NO1-HV-3-2925, (PB 251 257/AS)
9. Hagen KG (1975) Vapor cycle energy system for implanted circulatory assist devices. NHLBI Annual Report NO1-HV-4-2909-2
10. Westinghouse Astronuclear Laboratory, Evaluation of Practicability of a Radioisotope Thermal Converter for an Artificial Heart Device (1973) AEC Phase I Final Report, WANL-3043-1
11. Development of an Implantable Piezoelectric Driving System for a Circulatory Assist Device (1975) Annual Report, Contract NIH-9-2253, (PB 243 436/AS)
12. Kovachs SG, Weber DO, Yarnoz MD (1982) Ventricular kinetics of a magnetically actuated artificial heart. Proceedings of fourth annual conference IEEE engineering in medicine and biology society, pp 139–144
13. Takatani S (1985) Toward a completely Implantable total artificial heart system. In: Akutsu T (ed) Proceedings of the 1st international symposium on current problems for further development of artificial heart and assist device. Springer, Tokyo, pp 51–57
14. Rosenberg G, Snyder AJ, Weiss W, Landis DL, Pierce WS, Greathous SL, Ostroff AH, Geselowitz DB (1982) An electric motor driven total artificial heart. Proceedings of fourth annual conference IEEE engineering in medicine and biology society. Philadelphia, pp 111–116
15. Mitamura Y, Okamoto E, Mikami T (1985) Motor-driven artificial pump. In: Akutsu T (ed) Proceedings of the 1st international symposium on current problems for further development of artificial heart and assist device. Springer, Tokyo, pp 71–75
16. Jarvik PK, Lioi AP, Isaacson MS, Orth J, Nielsen SD, Kessler TR, Olsen DB, Kolff WJ (1982) Development of a reversing electrohydraulic energy converter for left ventricular assist devices. NHLBI Final Report NO1-HV-72975-3
17. Fujimasa I, Imachi K, Nakajima M, Mabuchi K, Chinzei T, Abe Y, Atsumi K (1985) Practical energy source and energy transmission for the total artificial heart. In: Akutsu T (ed) Proceedings of the 1st international symposium on current problems for further development of artificial heart and assist device. Springer, Tokyo, pp 59–62

## Discussion

*Yamada* (Shinsyu University): Of the four kinds of linear motor that are available, which do you think is the best for the artificial heart?

*Mosie* (Nimbus Inc.): Well I am looking forward to hearing your own answers to this at the end of this session. I was merely pointing out that with a linear motor or direct-drive blood pump, the device has high load and low speed. I certainly do not have a favorite among linear motors.

# 27. Development of transcutaneous energy transmission system for totally implantable artificial heart

Yuusuke Abe[1], Tsuneo Chinzei[2], Iwao Fujimasa[2], Kou Imachi[1], Kunihiko Mabuchi[1], Kiyoshi Maeda[1], Masahiko Asano[1], Akimasa Kouno[1], Toshiya Ono[1], and Kazuhiko Atsumi[1]

**Summary.** A transcutaneous energy transmission system (TETS) was composed of a couple of coils, which formed a transformer across the skin, a driving circuit, and a rectifying circuit. By using coreless coils and a high driving frequency (100–160 kHz), more than 25 W of electric power could be transmitted with 78.5% of maximum efficiency (dc to dc). In animal experiments, the primary coil temperature during operation was under 39°C on thermograms. After 10 months of implantation of a secondary coil coated with epoxy resin, it was wrapped by a thin capsule of connecting tissue. No obvious tissue reaction was recognized.

**Key words:** Transcutaneus energy transmission—Artificial heart

The possibility of long-term survival with the artificial heart (AH) has been demonstrated in animal experiments, and its clincial application has already begun. Following this, the development of a totally implantable AH, where both the AH driver and blood pumps are implanted inside the body, is highly required.

One of the difficulties in realizing the totally implantable AH is the energy source, because the use of atomic energy is not possible due to social and technical limitations. Therefore, secondary battery implantation and its charging from a primary source placed outside the body is generally considered to be the best solution in many laboratories. The object of this study is to develop a noninfectious energy transmission method with high transmission efficiency for a totally implantable AH.

## Method

The transcutaneous energy transmission system (TETS) is a wireless energy transmission method. TETS was designed under the following specifications and considerations: (a) It is composed of a couple of coils which form a transformer across the skin (Fig. 27.1). (b) The primary coil rests on the skin; the secondary coil is implanted under the skin. These two coils make a concentric coupling (Fig. 27.2). (c) With regard to size, the outer diameter of the secondary coil, inner diameter of the primary coil, and the turns of both coils are 6 cm, 8 cm, and less than 30 turns. (d) The transmission power is more than 20 W and transmission efficiency is more than 70%. (e) The temperature rise of the coils should be low to prevent thermal damage. (f) the configuration of the coils should fit well into the body. (g) The secondary coil should have tissue compatibility.

The following points were examined in in vitro and in vivo experiments:
a) The optimal structure of coils
   1) Cored or coreless
   2) Concentric or modified concentric type (Fig. 27.3) in order to obtain a good fit in the body
   3) Kind of coil wire
   4) Number of turns of the coils
b) Optimal oscillating frequency
c) Heat generation measurement of coils
d) In vivo stability and tissue compatibility of the coil

[1] Institute of Medical Electronics, Faculty of Medicine, University of Tokyo, 7-3-1 Hongo, Bunkyo-ku, Tokyo, 113 Japan
[2] Research Center of Advanced Science and Technology, University of Tokyo, 4-6-1 Komaba, Meguro-ku, Tokyo, 153 Japan

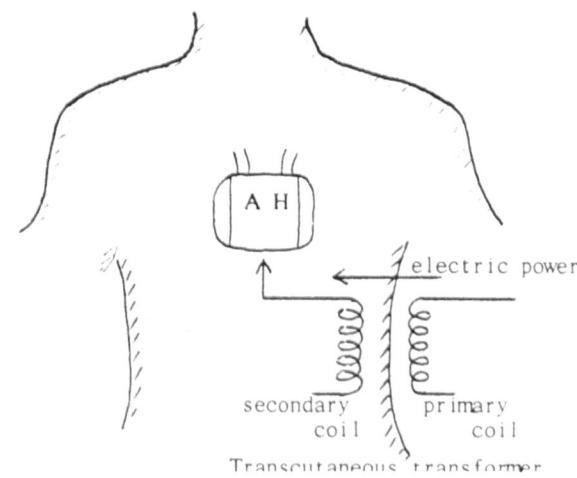

**Fig. 27.1.** Transcutaneous energy transmission system

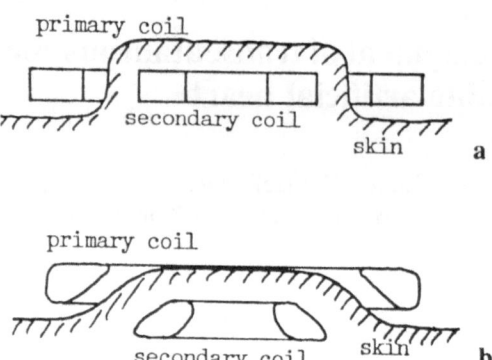

**Fig. 27.3a, b.** Cross sections of **a** concentric type and **b** modified concentric type

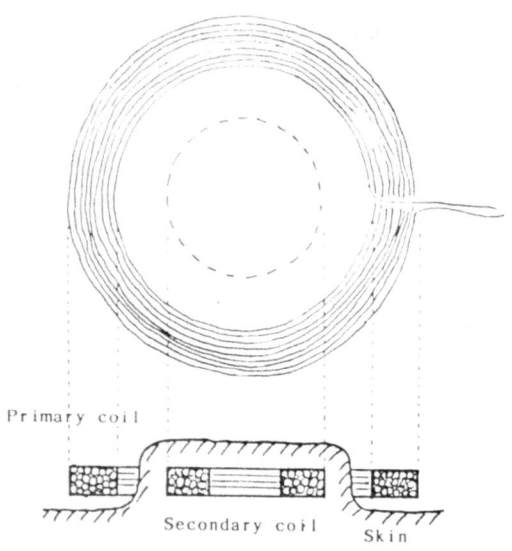

**Fig. 27.2.** Coupling method

**Fig. 27.4.** Block diagram of the circuit

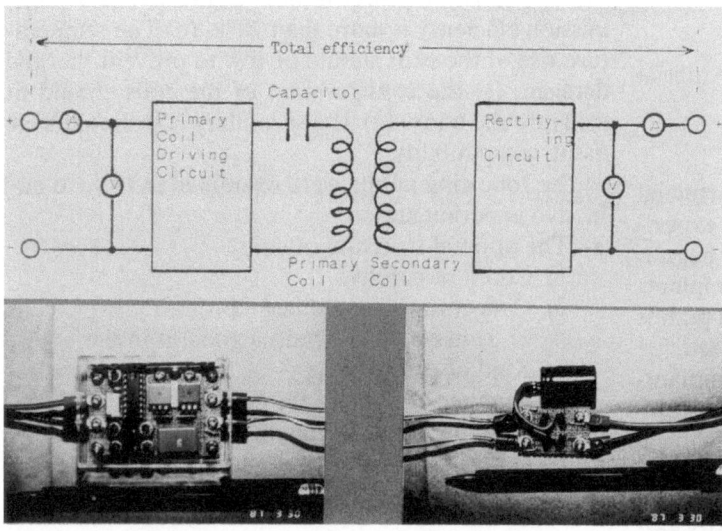

## Results

### System

A block diagram of this TETS is shown in Fig. 27.4, and Fig. 27.5 is a whole view of this system. In the primary coil driving circuit, the capacitor and coil forms an oscillating circuit to supply high voltage and a high-frequency sine wave current to the primary coil. The source voltage was controlled at 20–40 V as required by the secondary power supply. The driving frequency of this circuit could be changed from 75 to 450 kHz. The induced current of the secondary coil was corrected to dc by the rectifying circuit.

The primary and secondary coils were made of Litz wire with a cross section of 0.5 mm² or 0.75 mm² for expecting skin effect. Twenty and thirty turns of the

concentric and modified concentric types of coils were made (Fig. 27.6).

### In vitro experiment

The microcompressors used in the air-driven AH driver were used for the standard load of required power (Fig. 27.5). To drive two microcompressors, 18 W of electrical power was required.

The relation between the turns of the coil, configuration of the coil, and transmission efficiency is shown in Fig. 27.6. The optimum frequency was 100–160 kHz, which depended on the gap of the coils, turns of the coils, and whole circuit impedance. The transmission efficiency was measured at the best gap of the coils. More than 70% of transmission efficiency was obtained with both 20 and 30 turns and the con-

**Fig. 27.5.** Whole view of TETS

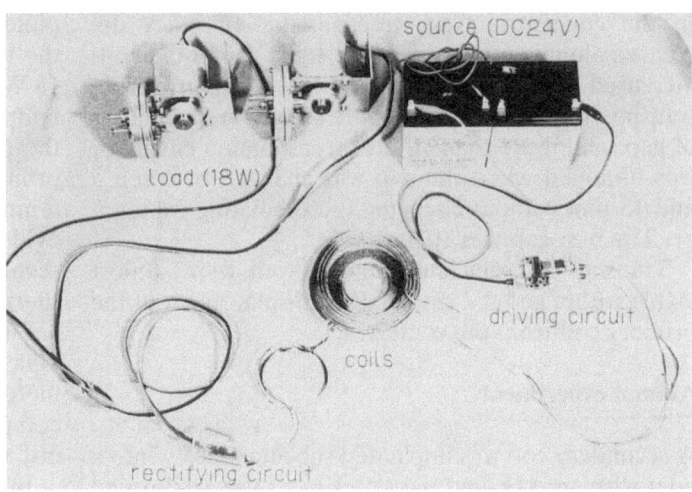

**Fig. 27.6.** Relations between efficiency, frequency, turns of coil, and coupling method

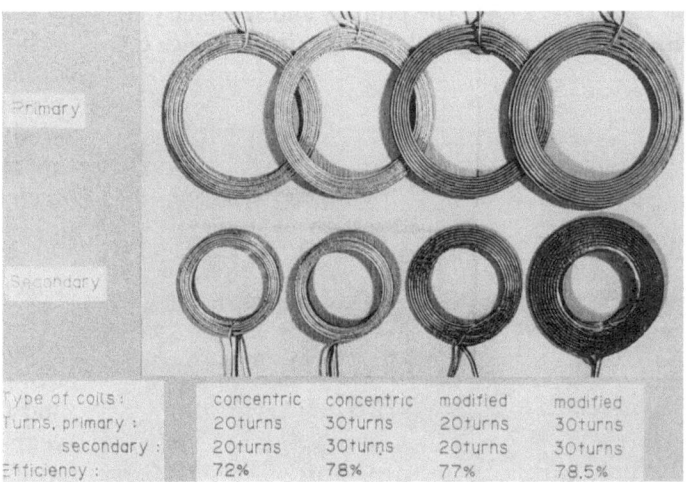

**Fig. 27.7.** Relations among efficiency, gap of coils, and coupling method

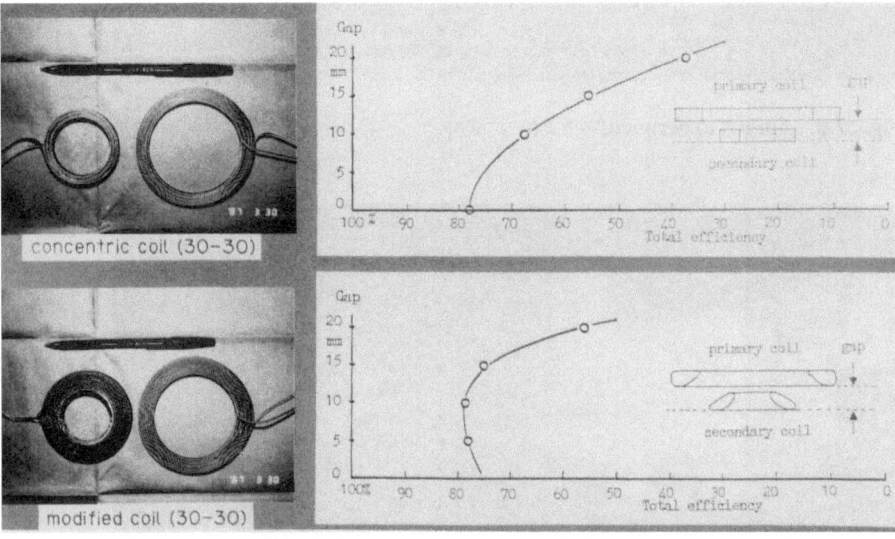

centric and modified concentric types. The modified concentric type was better than the concentric type, and the best efficiency was 78.5% at 30 turns. The maximum transmission energy was more than 25 W, which was measured by giving overdriving voltages to these compressors. The change of transmission efficiency was less than 1% when the transmission energy was changed between 10 and 25 W.

The relation between the type of coil, gap of the coils, and transmission efficiency is shown in Fig. 27.7.

In the concentric type, transmission efficiency decreased along a quadratic curve as the gap of the coils increased. However, in the modified concentric type, transmission efficiency was more stable for the change of gap, and more than 70% of transmission efficiency was obtained when the gap was changed between 5 and 15 mm without changing the oscillating frequency. The best gap was 10 mm wide.

Transmission efficiency and power were almost stable within about 2 cm of lateral displacement of the primary coil from the center.

### Animal experiment

A secondary coil was implanted subcutaneously into a goat with an AH, and the experiment was performed for 5.5 h (Fig. 27.8). The primary and secondary coils with 20 turns were used in this experiment. Since complete coupling was obtained between the two coils, the transmission efficiency and power were 72% and 18 W, which were the same as in the in vitro test. The temperature rise of the coils was measured by infrared thermography (Fig. 27.9). The temperature of the primary coil was 39.0°C on the thermogram at room temperature, and no thermal damage to the skin was evident. No temperature rise of the skin where the secondary coil was implanted was observed on the thermogram.

During this experiment, no influence on the measuring instruments, such as electromagnetic flow meters, transducers, and on the operating microcomputer were evident, and all the systems ran without any disorders.

In the experiment investigating the stability of the coil in the body, a secondary coil coated with epoxy resin was still able to transmit the power with the same transmission efficiency after 10 months of implantation in a rabbit (Fig. 27.10). The coil was covered with a thin capsule of connecting tissue; neither an obvious tissue reaction nor tissue necrosis were seen (Fig. 27.11).

### Discussion

Among the many kinds of TETS, those of Thermedics Co. [1] and Novacor Medical Co. [2] are best known and they have been under research for more than 10 years. Both systems use a transcutaneous transformer with coreless coils and high frequency. In the former, a small secondary coil cast in a convex shape and a ring-shaped primary coil form a concentric coupling across the skin. The primary coil has three turns and the secondary coil 28. The frequency is 160 kHz, and

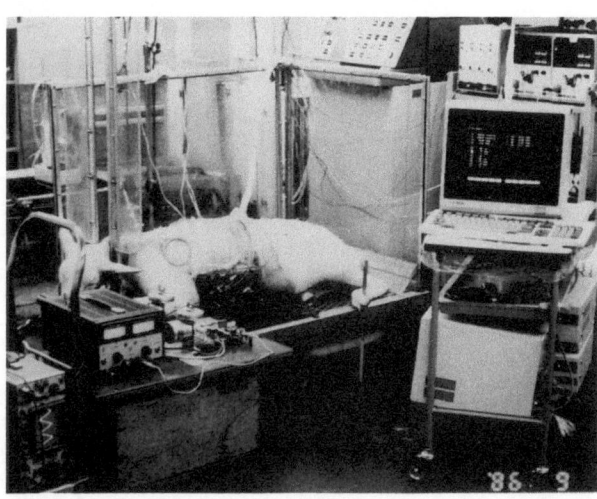

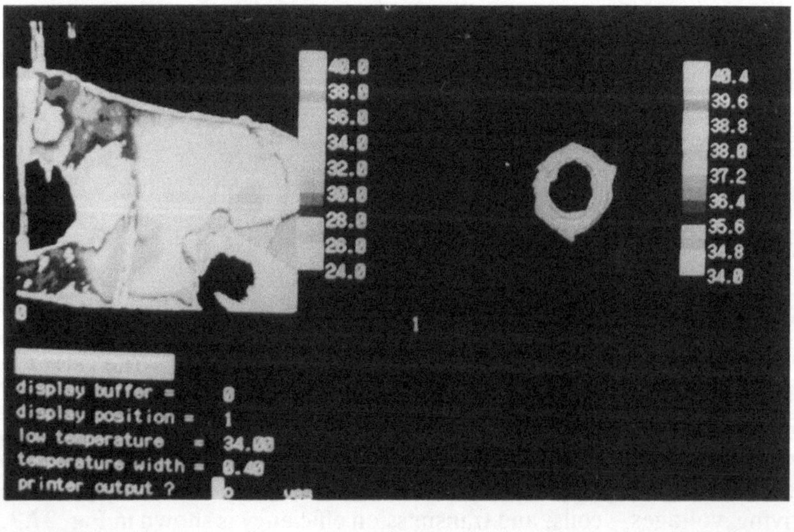

**Fig. 27.8.** Animal experiment—5.5 h

**Fig. 27.9.** Thermogram of coils after 5.5 h of operation. Primary coil temperature was 39.0°C

**Fig. 27.10.** Secondary coil implanted for 10 months in rabbit. Power could be still transmitted

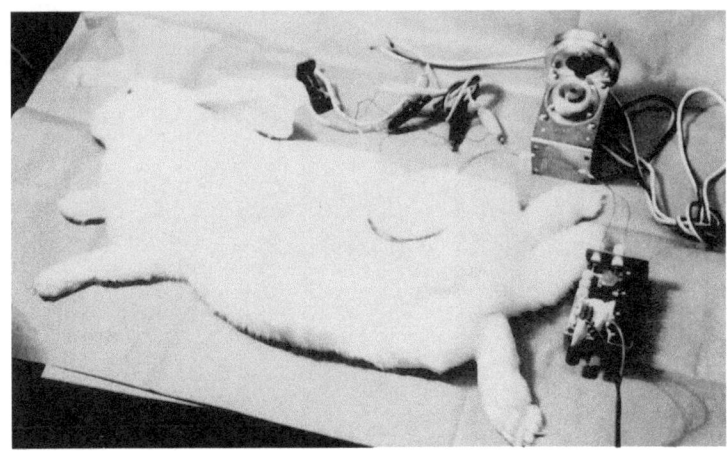

the efficiency is 75%–80%. The Novocor model has a belt-skin transformer. In this type of TETS, the secondary coil is implanted under the skin around the abdomen and the primary one is set in belt like concentric coupling. The maximum efficiency is 84%. But the details of the construction and the circuits have not been reported. Therefore, we had to devise our own method of construction.

The practicability of our type of TETS was demonstrated by using a couple of cored coils and a high-frequency driving current. But the low transmission efficiency and thermal damage to the skin as a result of the high temperature increase in the primary coil were a problem. By using coreless coils, those problems were eliminated. It was demonstrated that high performance could also be obtained with our system. The best efficiency was obtained at 30 turns of the modified concentric type of coil, but the number of turns had to be modified according to different conditions, such as whole circuit, required voltage, source voltage. The configuration of the coils turned out to be important not only in the fitting to the body but also in the stability of virtual deviation of primary coil.

Good compatibility of the secondary coil to the living tissue was obtained by an epoxy resin coating, but a further comparitive study with other tissue-compatible materials, e.g., silicone rubber, is required. Further study in a long-term experiment is also necessary.

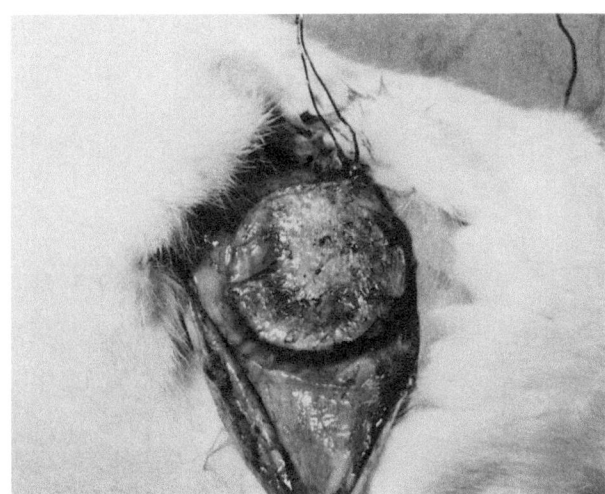

**Fig. 27.11.** Coil wrapped by a thin capsule of connecting tissue

## References

1. Sherman C, Clay W, Dasse K, Daly B (1981) Energy transmission across intact skin for powering artificial internal organs. Trans Am Soc Artif Intern Organs 27: 137
2. Miller PJ, Green GF, Chen H, Ramasmy N, Laforge DH, Jassawalla JS, Ream AK, Oyer PE, Portner PM (1983) In vitro evaluation of a compact implantable left ventricular assist system (LVAS). Trans Am Soc Artif Intern Organs 29: 55.

# Discussion

*Portner* (Novacor Medical Corporation): Have you done any measurements on the change in coupling coefficient or change in efficiency with a lateral displacement of the primary relative to the secondary? It seems to me that the major potential problem with this type of transmission system when used practically in a clinical setting is the alignment of the primary relative to the secondary.

*Abe* (University of Tokyo): We measured the stability against the sliding direction. With 2-cm displacement, more than 70% efficiency could be obtained.

*Portner:* As I understand it from the diagram you showed, there is an attempt to provide self-alignment by the shape of the internal and external coils. Have you had any long-term experience in animals of pressure necrosis in the overlying tissues? Have you observed any pathological effects on the tissues because of the transmitted magnetic field?

*Abe:* At first, the problem was not the pressure necrosis but the temperature rise due to the change in frequency.

*Portner:* What about the potential for pressure necrosis—damage to the tissue because of the placement of the primary over the secondary? As you know in the USA, Thermedics developed a similar kind of design to the one you presented. They had severe problems with pressure necrosis which necessitated elimination of the cone shape. Do you have any data with respect to the tissue?

*Abe:* In experiments with a 10-month implantation, pressure necrosis and damage due to the influence of the magnetic field were not observed.

*Portner:* Do you perform any histological studies of the tissues?

*Abe:* Yes, but I do not have the slides with me today.

*Portner:* Do you have any thoughts as to how you would use this device in a patient, i.e., how would you maintain the coupling physically over a long period of time with a high degree of reliability such that the patient does not feel any concern?

*Abe:* That is an important point and one which will require a good deal of consideration in the future.

*Moise* (Nimbus Inc.): We have used the Thermedics transformer for 4 months in vivo and we did not observe any of these problems. Victor Poirier of Thermedics presented a paper at this symposium 2 years ago and discussed some configuration modifications that they made which I understand do not make the device flat. They achieved good results with this in the tissue area. We were planning to use a bra-type system to hold the primary over the secondary.

*Geselowitz* (Pensylvania State University): Our in vivo experience in this area has also been good, although this is an area that requires more work. With your 78% efficiency, where do the losses occur?

*Abe:* I think the losses occur mainly in the wire of the coils, the driving transistor, and the coupling of the coils.

*Geselowitz:* Do you have more precise data as to how much energy is dissipated into the coils, how much into body tissue, etc?

*Abe:* No, I am not sure exactly.

*Moise:* I would think that most of the internal losses occur in the rectifier, which is one of the reasons why we had to add a thin copper sheet. The secondary coil does not show significant losses as far as we have been able to determine.

# 28. Development of transcutaneous energy transmission system

Yoshinori Mitamura[1], Atsushi Hirano[1], Eiji Okamoto[1], and Tomohisa Mikami[2]

**Summary.** The transcutaneous energy transmission system has been developed for use with electric artificial hearts. The system is composed of a transcutaneous transformer, power oscillator, and output power conditioning system. The transcutaneous transformer is formed from two ferrite cores. The external core is concave at the base and the internal core convex at the top. Since the internal core causes a bulge in the skin, the projections on the external portions can engage the internal portion of the primary core and prevent lateral motion of the primary core. The number of turns of the coils is determined in order to satisfy minimum power loss conditions. The power oscillator converts the power drawn from an external 12-V dc source into a 50-kHz square wave to excite the primary coil. Both the primary and secondary coils are series-tuned at the operating frequency using capacitors. Output voltage is regulated by controlling the duty ratio of the square pulse supplied to the primary coil. Information on output voltage is transmitted through the skin by infrared pulses.

Efficiency of the energy transmission system was measured, when 20 W was transmitted at a core separation of 5 mm. Overall efficiency was 74%. The temperature rise was measured in a chronic experiment by implanting the device in a dog. The temperature rise in the tissue was less than 1°C when 30 W was transmitted.

**Key words:** Transcutaneous energy transmission—Artificial heart

The next generation of artificial hearts and permanent cardiac assist systems will be actuated electrically rather than by compressed gases. Electrical actuation permits the design of systems free of tubes through the skin. Electric systems promise dramatic improvements in the quality of life of pump-dependent patients.

Electric artificial hearts require significant power levels which cannot be met by implanted battery systems. Although there are a variety of possible methods for transporting energy into the body, schemes involving electromagnetic coupling are currently receiving the most attention. Coupling types essentially fall into two broad categories: (a) audio frequency transmission using a magnetic ferrite material [1–3]; (b) radio frequency transmission by means of pancake air-core coils [4–7]; and (c) radio frequency transmission using the belt skin transformer [8, 9].

Air core transformers have some potential disadvantages, such as large size and less coupling between the external and internal coils. To solve these problems, a new transformer was formed from a pair of concave and convex ferrite cores. The external device is concave at the base; the upper surface of the internal device is convex. Since the internal device causes a bulge in the skin, the projections on the external portions can engage the internal portion of the primary core and prevent lateral motion. The external device is taped in place under the light tension of an elastic band. The developed transcutaneous energy transmission system includes output voltage regulation and an implanted rechargeable backup battery. These functions are effective for keeping a constant power supply to the load in the event of dislocation of the coils, drop in primary battery voltage, and so on. It is the purpose of this study to demonstrate the feasibility of the developed transcutaneous energy transmission system for delivering the power of 22 W necessary for driving electric artificial hearts.

## Materials and methods

The transcutaneous energy transmission system is composed of a transcutaneous transformer, power oscillator, output power conditioning system, rechargeable back-up battery, and alarm system (Fig. 28.1).

### Transcutaneous transformer

Three types of transcutaneous transformer have been developed: concave/convex core type, pot core type, and air core type (Fig. 28.2). The concave/convex core-type transformer is formed from two ferrite cores

[1]Department of Medical Electronics, Research Institute of Applied Electricity, Hokkaido University, Kita 12, Nishi 6, Kita-ku, Sapporo, 060 Japan
[2]Department of Biomedical Systems Engineering, Graduate School of Engineering, Hokkaido University, Kita 13, Nishi 8, Kita-ku, Sapporo, 060 Japan

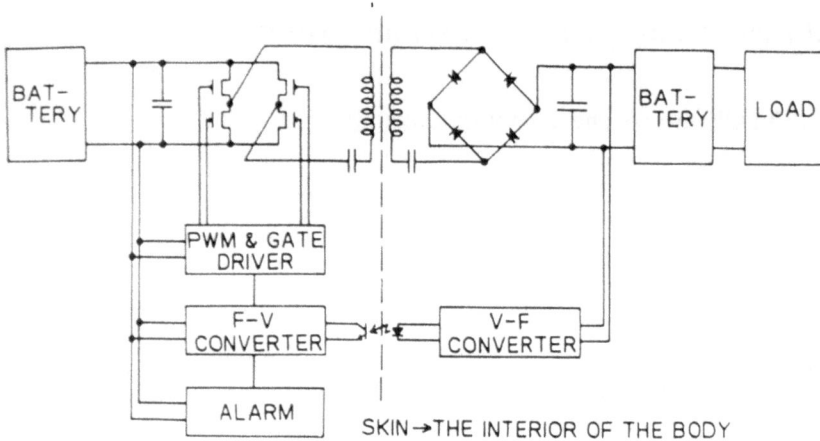

**Fig. 28.1.** Block diagram of transcutaneous energy transmission system

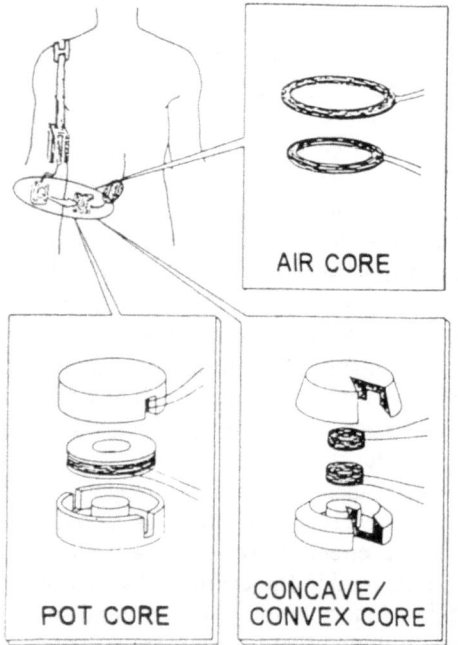

**Fig. 28.2.** Three types of transcutaneous transformer: air core type, pot core type, and concave/convex core type

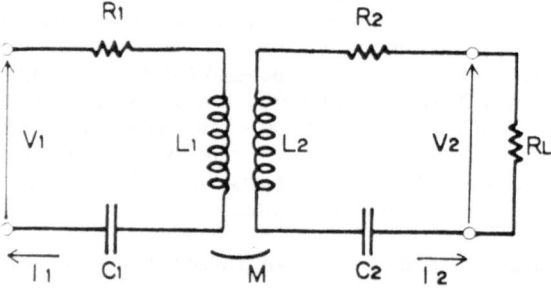

**Fig. 28.3.** Equivalent circuit of transcutaneous transformer

(TDK, specific permeability of 3300). the implanted secondary device is a convex ferrite core measuring 5.6 cm in diameter at the base, 4.0 cm in diameter at the upper surface, 1.3 cm high, and weighing 96 g. The windings have 20 turns of Litz wire (0.12/45). The superficial primary coil has 15 turns of the same wire wound inside a concave ferrite core with a diameter of 6.2 cm at the base, a diameter of 4.4 cm at the top surface, and a weight of 97 g.

Each half of the pot core-type transformer is a ferrite core (TDK, P59/36 Z-52S, specific permeability of 3300), 5.9 cm in diameter, and 1.6 cm thick. The windings have 15 turns of Litz wire. The weight of each unit is 150 g.

The secondary coil of an air core-type transformer contains 25 turns of Litz wire wound in a tight spiral with an inner diameter of 5.0 cm and a weight of 20 g.

The superficial primary coil contains 20 turns of the same wire wound in a tight spiral with an inner diameter of 7.0 cm and a weight of 25 g.

### Theoretical consiserations

In the transcutaneous energy transmission system, both the primary and secondary coils are series-tuned at the operating frequency using capacitors (Fig. 28.1). To find the conditions for minimizing the losses in the coils, we shall first consider the equivalent circuit of Fig. 28.3. The equations at the resonant frequency are:

$$V_1 = R_1 I_1 + jwMI_2 \tag{1}$$

$$V_2 = jwMI_1 + R_1 I_2 \tag{2}$$

and

$$V_2 = -R_L I_2 \tag{3}$$

where $M$ is the mutual inductance of the two coils, $V_1$ the voltage applied to the transcutaneous transformer, $V_2$ the output voltage of the transformer, $I_1$ the current supplied by the source, $I_2$ the current in the load, $R_1$ the loss in the primary coil, and $R_2$ the loss in the secondary coil.

The power loss is given by:

$$P_{loss} = (R_1|I_1|^2 + R_2|I_2|^2)/2 \tag{4}$$

The received load power $P_{load}$ is given by:

$$P_{load} = (R_L|I_2|^2)/2 \tag{5}$$

Equations (1) to (5) yield:

$$P_{loss} = P_{load}(R_1((R_L + R_2)^2/w^2M^2 + R_2)/R_L \tag{6}$$

At this point, it is convenient to introduce a set of dimensionless quantities to eliminate $R_1$ and $R_2$. These parameters are defined by:

$$D_1 = R_1/wL_1; \quad D_2 = R_2/wL_2 \tag{7}$$

Using (7), (6) becomes:

$$P_{loss} = P_{load}(D_1(R_L + wL_2D_2)^2/k^2\,wL_2 + wL_2D_2)/R_L \tag{8}$$

where $k$ is the coefficient of coupling ($M = k\sqrt{L_1L_2}$). By differentiating $P_{loss}$ with respect to $L_2$ and setting the result as equal to zero, one finds that the load condition for minimum power loss under the power supply of $P_{load}$ to the load $R_L$ is:

$$L_2 = R_L/(w\sqrt{D_2^2 + D_2k^2/D_1}) = N_2^2 L_{2S} \tag{9}$$

where $N_2$ is the number of turns of the secondary coil and $L_{2S}$ the self inductance for $N_2 = 1$.

When the resistance $R_1$ is sufficiently small, Eq. (1) can be approximated by:

$$|V_1| = wM|I_2| = wN_1N_2M_S|I_2| \tag{10}$$

where $N_1$ is the number of turns of the primary coil and $M_S$ the mutual inductance for $N_1 = N_2 = 1$.

Equation (5) gives the unique current $I_2$ which provides the load $R_L$ with the power of $P_{load}$. Therefore, for a given $V_1$, Eq. (10) becomes:

$$wN_1N_2M_S = |V_1/I_2| = \text{const.} \tag{11}$$

Equations (9) and (11) yield the optimum number of turns which provides the load with the given power.

### Power oscillator and output power conditioning system

The power MOS-FETs (Hitachi, 2SJ122 and 2SK428) convert the power drawn from an external 12-V dc source into a 10- to 100-kHz square wave to excite the transformer primary coil. The implanted portion of the system contains the secondary coil and series

capacitor followed by a full-wave rectifier (Schottky barrier diodes, Toshiba 5FWJ2S41) and filter.

The output power conditioning is a variation on the switching regulator. The output voltage is converted into its proportional pulse frequency by a V-F converter. The information on pulse frequency is transcutaneously transmitted by a photo-coupler (Sharp, GL513F and PT550F). The infrared emitter used (GL-513F) has a peak emission wavelength of 950 nm and the phototransistor (PT-550F) has a peak spectral sensitivity of 800 nm. Absorption coefficient ($\mu$) of the skin is about 12 cm$^{-1}$ at 950 mm and 14 cm$^{-1}$ at 700 nm, where I (intensity) is $I_0e^{-\mu x}$ (x: distance). Therefore, the infrared signal can be transmitted through the skin for up to several centimeters. The pulse frequency is proportionally changed into voltage by an F-V converter. This voltage is compared with the nominal value for the output voltage and, according to the error signal, the duty cycle of the primary pulse is varied by switching the regulator control circuit.

### Rechargeable backup battery and alarm system

A sealed rechargeable lead storage battery (Matsushita, LCT-812 0.8 A h, 12 V dc), measuring $61 \times 25 \times 95$ mm and weighing 320 g, is connected in parallel to the load. Electric energy can be supplied by the backup battery for at least 10 min.

The alarm system always monitors the transmitted infrared signal. If the amplitude decreases below the threshold level due to dislocation of the transformers or the pulse frequency drops below the threshold level due to a decrease in output voltage, the alarm system makes a warning signal.

### Experimental studies

The efficiency of the energy transmission system was measured, when 20 W was transmitted at a core separation of 5 mm. Three types of transformer were tested at frequencies of 20, 50, and 100 kHz. The optimal number of windings and the method of power measurement are summarized in Fig. 28.4. The overall efficiency is summarized in Fig. 28.5. The efficiency decreased with increased frequency in the core-type transformers, while it increased in the air core-type transformer. Maximum overall efficiency was 73% in the air core-type transformer at 100 kHz, 73% in the concave/convex core-type transformer at 50 kHz, and 74% in the pot core-type transformer at 50 kHz. Energy losses in each subsystem are shown in Fig. 28.6. The loss in the transformer accounted for 6% of the transmitted total energy, the loss in the inverter, rectifier, and filter 16%, and the loss in the control circuit 4%.

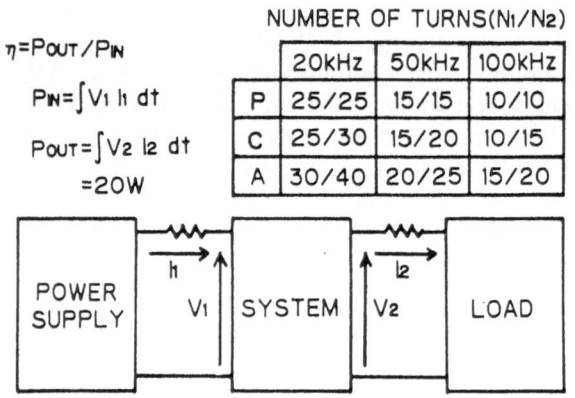

NUMBER OF TURNS($N_1$/$N_2$)

$\eta = P_{OUT}/P_{IN}$

$P_{IN} = \int V_1 I_1 \, dt$

$P_{OUT} = \int V_2 I_2 \, dt$

$= 20W$

| | 20kHz | 50kHz | 100kHz |
|---|---|---|---|
| P | 25/25 | 15/15 | 10/10 |
| C | 25/30 | 15/20 | 10/15 |
| A | 30/40 | 20/25 | 15/20 |

**Fig. 28.4.** Optimum number of windings in three types of transformer and method of measurement of power transmission efficiency. *P* pot core type, *C* concave/convex core type, and *A* air core type

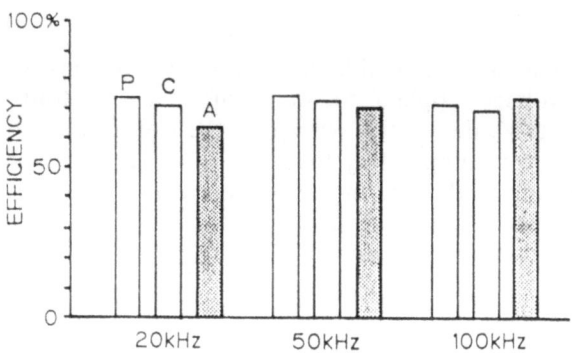

**Fig. 28.5.** Total efficiency of transcutaneous energy transmission system when 20 W was transmitted. *P* pot core, *C* concave/convex core, *A* air core

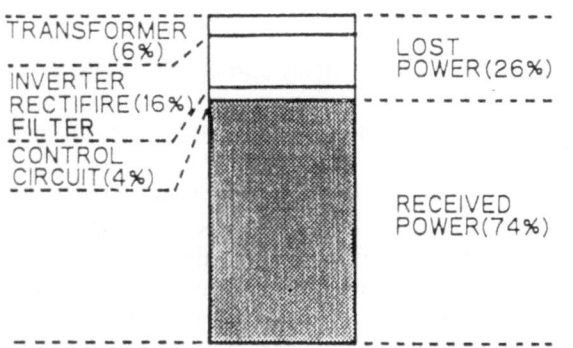

**Fig. 28.6.** Losses in each subsystem of transcutaneous energy transmission system employing the pot core-type transformer when 20 W was transmitted at 50 kHz

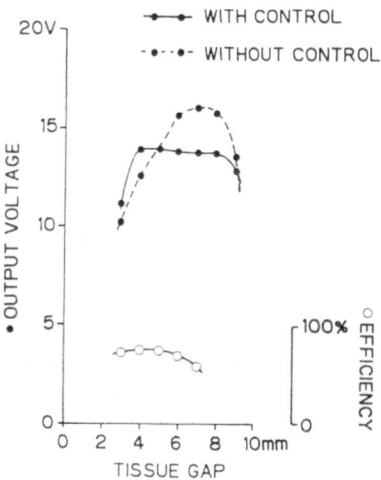

**Fig. 28.7.** Voltage control for the changes in tissue gap when 20 W was transmitted using the pot core-type transformer at 50 kHz

The output voltage control for the changes in tissue gap and radial misalignment are shown in Figs. 28.7 and 28.8 respectively. The output voltage is kept almost constant for changes in the tissue gap of 4–8 mm. The output voltage is also maintained almost constant for changes in the radial displacement of 0–10 mm. Control of the output voltage for changes in the load is demonstrated in Fig. 28.9. Fluctuation of the output voltage is less than 7% for changes in the load from 10 ohms to infinity.

The temperature rise was tested in a chronic experiment by implanting the device (pot core type) in a dog and measuring the temperature rises with implanted thermisters. Three thermisters were used: one on the outside of the internal core, one in the tissue, and one on the outside of the external core. The temperature was monitored by changing the power delivered to the load from 10 to 30 W. The temperature rise in the tissue was less than 1°C when 30 W was transmitted.

## Discussion

Various types of transcutaneous energy transmission system have been developed to power the implanted electric artificial hearts [1–9]. However, several problems still remain to be solved such as high transmission efficiency, permissible temperature rise, easy fitting, regulated output voltage, and safety.

High energy transmission efficiency is essential for a battery-powered biomedical system, because it prolongs the life of the external battery and minimizes the possibility of burns due to high heating loss. High transmission efficiency was attained in our system by employing an optimum number of winding turns and through the use of MOS-FETs and Schottky barrier diodes, which have low on-resistance and excellent high switching charactersitics. The total efficiency of 74% and transmission efficiency of the transformer of

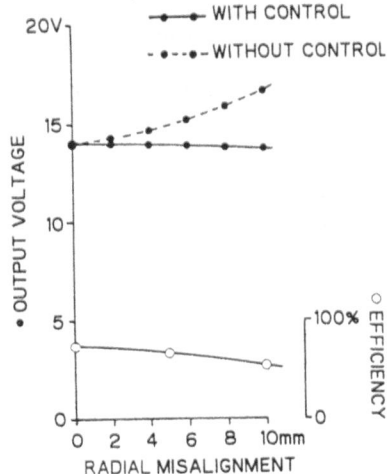

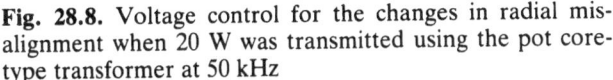

**Fig. 28.8.** Voltage control for the changes in radial misalignment when 20 W was transmitted using the pot core-type transformer at 50 kHz

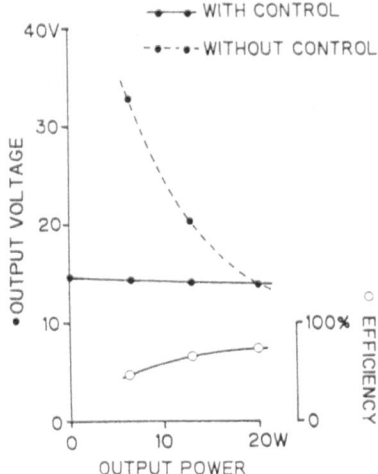

**Fig. 28.9.** Voltage control for changes in the load in the pot core-type transformer

94% in the systems are reasonably high compared with the reported values: The total efficiency was 65%–80% for nominal loads of 12–24 W [6], 53%–67% for 10-W supply [7], and 70%–82% at a 15-W power level [9]; net efficiency of the transformer was 97% at 57 W [1], 90% at 30 W [2], 90% at levels up to 50 W [4], and 95% at 35 W [3].

The optimum number of turns in the coils was determined for a given power requirement, load, frequency, coupling coefficient, and battery voltage. In case of changes in the coupling coefficient during operation, the calculated conditions' become less optimum for minimizing the loss. In this condition, a means for locking the drive frequency to the resonance is effective for reducing the loss [9]. This function is going to be included in the system.

The temperature rise in the tissue when 30 W was transmitted was within 1°C. This temperature rise will not cause harmful effects to the skin. Heat diffusion in the core and heat removal by blood flow probably decreased the temperature rise in the tissue. Similar temperature rises have been reported elsewhere: A maximum tissue temperature of 39.7°C was observed with the transmission of 1 kW of power [5]; temperature rises were less than 1°C at the surface of the implanted coils at a transmission of up to 24 W [6].

With a number of applications, it is important to keep the received power within narrow limits despite coupling variations. Several effective means of achieving this goal were included in the study. To minimize the possibility of lateral motion of the coils, a concave/convex core-type transformer was made. Since the internal device causes a bulge in the skin, the projections on the external portions can engage the internal portion and prevent lateral motion. Although several approaches were developed to prevent lateral motion of the cores, the methods employed involved an additional device such as a shallow cup [2] and annual permanent ferrite magnets [3]. An output voltage control circuit is another effective method for maintaining a constant received power despite coupling variations. The concept of using an implanted, rechargeable cell as a backup battery in case of complete power interruption is attractive and essential for continuous power supply. In this study, a recently developed hermetically sealed lead storage battery was utilized. It has several advantages. The volumetric energy density is as high as 0.066 W h/cm³, while the energy density of the nickel oxide/cadmium cell is 0.056 W h/cm³ [10]. The rate of self-discharge is 0.36%/day at a temperature of 40°C. It is comparable to values of up to 0.3%/day at the body temperature of the nickel oxide/cadmium cell. The sealed lead storage battery can be recharged repeatedly after full discharge. The capacity of 90%–101% can be restored after recharging. The provision of telemetry of the battery voltage would allow continuous battery status assessment to avoid an overcharge.

From the above results, it can be concluded that the developed system is a potential transcutaneous energy transmission system for implanted electric artificial hearts.

**Acknowledgment.** This work was supported in part by a Grant-in-Aid from the Ministry of Public Welfare.

# References

1. Andren CF, Fadall MA, Gott VL, Topaz SR (1968) The skin tunnel transformer: A new system that permits

both high efficiency transfer of power and telemetry of data through the intact skin. IEEE Trans BME BME-15: 278–280

2. Myers GH, Reed GE, Thumin A, Fascher S, Cortes L (1968) A transcutaneous power transformer. Trans Am Soc Artif Int Organs 14: 210–214

3. Sutton GW, Rivera LM, Kirby PT (1981) A miniaturized device for electrical energy transmission through intact skin: concepts and results of initial tests. Artif Organs 5 (Suppl): 437–440

4. Fuller JW (1968) Apparatus for efficient power transfer through a tissue barrier. IEEE Trans BME BME-15: 63–65

5. Schuder JC, Gold JH, Stephenson HE Jr (1971) An inductively coupled RF system for the transmission of 1 KW of power through the skin. IEEE Trans BME BME-18: 265–273

6. Sherman CW, Clay WC, Dasse KA, Daly BDT (1985) A transcutaneous energy transmission system for high-power prosthetics. Proceedings of IEEE 7th Annual Conference of Engineering in Medical Biology Society pp 804–808

7. Koshiji K, Utsunomiya T, Takatani S, Takano H, Nakatani T, Kinoshita M, Noda H, Fukuda S, Akutsu T (1987) Analysis of efficiency and experimental consideration of energy transmission system to drive total implanted artificial hearts. Jpn J Artif Organs 16: 167–170

8. Portner PM, Oyer PE, Jassawalla JS, Chen H, Miller PJ, LaForger DH, Green GF, Shumway NE (1984) A totally implantable ventricular assist device for end-stage heart disease. In: Unger F (ed) Assisted circulation 2, Springer, Berlin, pp 115–141

9. Brugler JS, LaForge DH, Lee J, Beering FK, Jassawalla JS, Portner PM (1986) Transcutaneous power transmission and electronic control of a ventricular assist system. Proceedings of IEEE 8th Annual Conference of Engineering Medical and Biological Society, pp 73–76

10. Holleck GL (1986) Rechargeable electrochemical cells as implanted power sources. In: Owen BB (ed) Batteries for implantable biomedical devices. Plenum, New York pp 275–284

## Discussion

*Yamada* (Shinshu University): What was the flux density between the primary and secondary coils?

*Mitamura* (Hokkaido University): We did not measure the flux density, but we took care to ensure that the density was not over the maximum saturation of the coil.

*Yamada:* I think that the flux density is an important factor and is closely related to the efficiency.

*Moise* (Nimbus Inc.): I was very much interested in your information transmission system. Have any details been published as to the thickness of tissue and the kind of information you can obtain using that photocoupled system?

*Mitamura:* We did not measure this precisely. In our case, the tissue depth is 5 mm; at this depth, infrared light can be transmitted very well. I do not know how much we can transmit this through the skin.

*Moise:* What is the frequency of the light?

*Mitamura:* I do not recall precisely, but I believe it is about 750 nm.

# 29. Linear electromagnetic actuators for implantable artificial heart

Hajime Yamada[1], Masami Nirei[1], Hiroshi Ota[1], Koji Kawakatsu[1], Mitsuji Karita[2], Toshiki Maruyama[2], Makoto Chimura[3], Tsuneo Ogasawara[3], Naotake Nishizawa[4], Toru Takeuchi[4], Yukio Yamamoto[5], and Tetsuzo Akutsu[6]

**Summary.** Three kinds of linear electromagnetic actuator (LEA) have been designed and manufactured for use implantable artificial hearts.

These LEAs were developed with on the principle of the linear motor, and the target was to minimize the occupied space as much as possible. The first actuator (CLOA) was made with a cylindrical linear oscillatory actuator including a permanent magnet. The second actuator (CLPM) and the third actuator (FLPM) were made with a cylindrical and a flat linear pulse motor, respectively.

This paper deals with the configurations, the principle operation, and experimental results of the LEAs developed for implantable artificial hearts.

**Key words:** Artificial heart—Blood pump—Linear electromagnetic actuator—Linear pulse motor—Linear oscillatory actuator

## Cylindrical linear oscillatory actuator

The configuration of a cylindrical linear oscillatory actuator (CLOA-ST87, "CLOA" for short) for implantable use is shown in Fig. 29.1. The CLOA consists mainly of a stator and a rod. The stator has a ring permanent magnet (Nd-Fe-B alloy) and two electromagnets with two coils. The stator is made of low carbon steel (SUM24L), and the rod is composed of two different materials, namely a magnetic (ASK-3500S) and a nonmagnetic material (SUS-304) to obtain the long stroke, Ls, as shown in Fig. 29.1. The rod is supported by the slide bearing set between the stator and the rod.

Fig. 29.2 shows the equivalent electric circuit of the CLOA. The inductances $L_1(x)$ and $L_2(x)$ in the CLOA are excited by an ac $I_1$, $I_2$, and dc $I_{dc}$, alternately. The rod has a reciprocating motion from the exciting current.

The static thrust, $F_s$, of the CLOA is given by [1, 2]:

$$F_s = \frac{1}{2}(2I)^2 \frac{dL(x)}{dx}$$

$$= \frac{1}{2}(2NI)^2 \frac{dP(x)}{dx} \text{ [N]}, \tag{1}$$

where $I = (I_1 + I_{de})/2 = (I_2 + I_{de})/2$ [A], the exciting current; $L(x) = L_1(x) + L_2(x)$ [H], the inductance of the coils; $x$ [m], the displacement of the rod; $N$ the number of turns of the coil; and $P(x) = N^2L(x)$ [H], the permeance of the coils.

Fig. 29.3 shows the static thrust, $F_s$, versus the exciting current, $I$, characteristics of the CLOA. The maximum static thrust of 9 N is obtained under the current of 0.6 A and the magnetomotive force of 1.5 kA. The actuator CLOA has the simplest configuration among LEAs, but it has a comparatively small thrust compared with those of the other actuators mentioned below.

The relation between the kinetic thrust, $F_k$, and driving frequency, $f$, is shown in Fig. 29.4. The rod has resonance at the frequency of around 19 Hz because the magnetic force due to the strong permanent magnet in the CLOA acts like as mechanical spring.

The resonance frequency, $f_r$, of the rod is given as follows [2]:

$$f_r = \frac{1}{2\pi} \frac{\sqrt{2}K}{m} \text{ [Hz]} \tag{2}$$

where $K$ [N/m] is the spring factor and $m$ [kg] the mass of rod. The CLOA for implantable use is shown in Fig. 29.5. The values for the static thrust, mass, and volume are 9 N, 860 g, and 120 ml, respectively, while the input power is 14.4 W.

The mechanical and electromagnetic specifications for the CLOA are given in Table 29.1.

## Cylindrical linear pulse motor

Fig. 29.6 indicates the configuration of a cylindrical linear pulse motor (CLPM-SS85, "CPLM" for short) for implantable use. The CLPM consists mainly of a cylindrical stator and a mover. The stator has a ring permanent magnet and two electromagnets with

[1]Shinshu University, Faculty of Engineering, 500 Wakasato, Nagano, 380 Japan
[2]Shinko Electric Co. Ltd., 100 Takegahana, Ise, 516 Japan
[3]Takahashi Electric Co. Ltd., 2-5-5 Jinmyo-cho, Okaya, 394 Japan
[4]Orion Machinery Co. Ltd., 246 Yukitaka, Suzaka, 382 Japan
[5]Nagano Technical College, 716 Tokuma, Nagano, 380 Japan
[6]National Cardiovascular Center Research Institute, 5-7-1 Fujishiro-dai, Suita, Osaka, 565 Japan

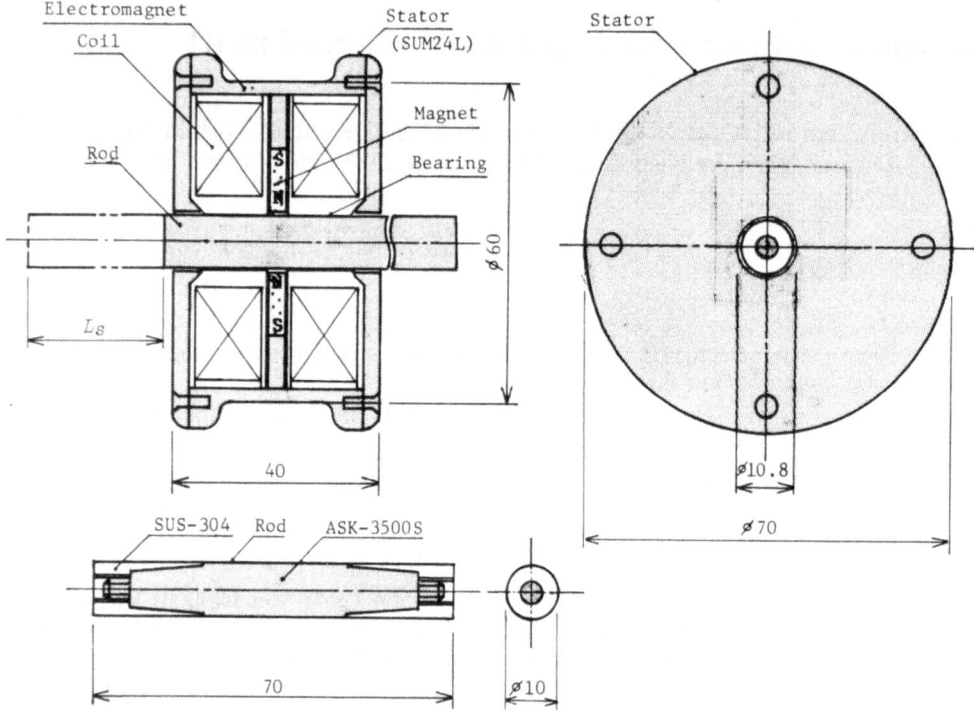

**Fig. 29.1.** Configuration of a cylindrical linear oscillatory actuator (CLOA, units are millimeters)

teeth. The mover has a cylindrical moving rod with many teeth and slots on its surface. The mover is supported by the retainer between the mover and the stator.

In the two-phase excitation, the static thrust, $F_s$, is given as follows [3]:

$$F_s = -\frac{2\sqrt{2}\,\pi NI}{\tau}\Delta\Phi_m \sin\frac{2\pi}{\tau}x \text{ [N]},\qquad(3)$$

where $N$ is the number of turns of the coil, $I$ [A] the exciting current, $NI$ [A] the magnetomotive force per coil, $\tau$ [m] the pitch of teeth, $\Delta\Phi_m$ [Wb] the magnitude of the flux of the permanent magnet, and $x$ [m] the displacement of the mover.

The static thrust, $F_s$, versus the exciting current, $I$, characteristics of the CLPM and FLPM is shown in Fig. 29.7. The static thrust of the CLPM and FLPM are 6.4 N and 48.3 N at the rated current, respectively. The configuration of the FLPM is mentioned below.

Fig. 29.8 shows the CLPM for implantable use. The values of static thrust, mass, and volume are 6.4 N, 175 g, and 27.2 ml, while the input power is 6.2 W.

**Flat linear pulse motor**

Fig. 29.9 shows the configuration of a flat linear pulse motor (FLPM-SS87, "FLPM" for short) for im-

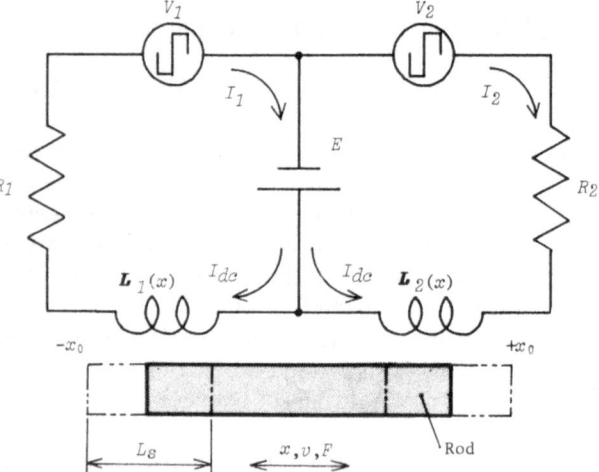

**Fig. 29.2.** Equivalent electric circuit of a cylindrical linear oscillatory actuator (CLOA)

plantable use. The FLPM consists of a flat stator and a mover. The FLPM is double-sided because it has two stators at both sides of the mover [4]. The mover has a moving plate with many teeth and slots on both surfaces; it is made with laminated cobalt steel sheets 0.35 mm thick. The stators are also made with the same material as the mover, because of the maintenance of a high saturation flux density. The static

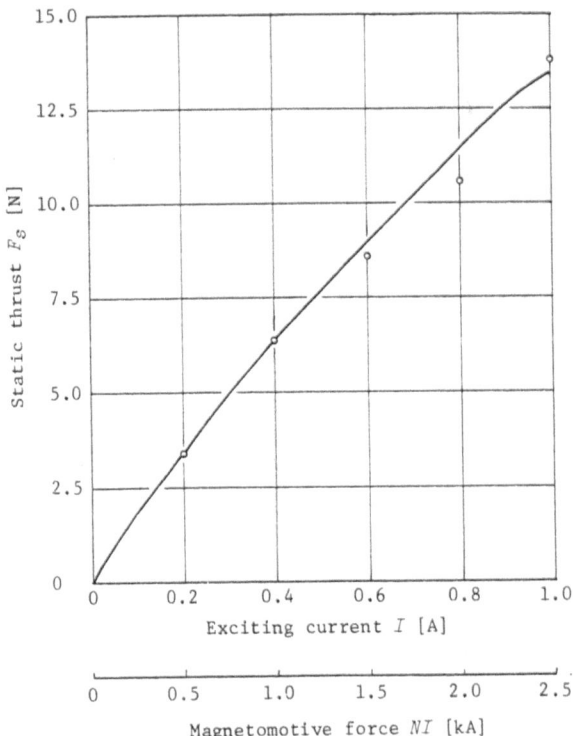

**Fig. 29.3.** Static thrust, $F_s$, exciting current, $I$, characteristics of CLOA

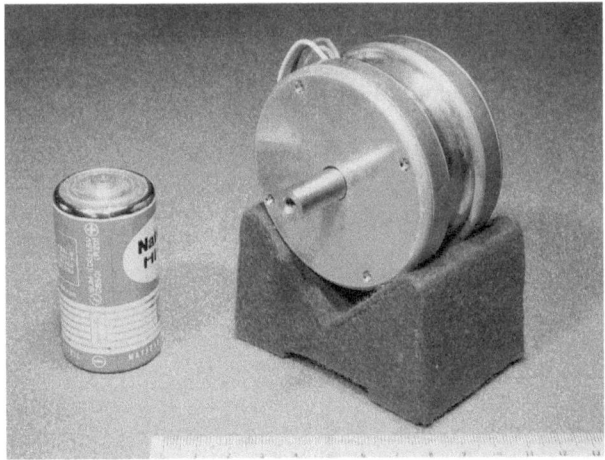

**Fig. 29.5.** Cylindrical linear oscillatory actuator (CLOA-ST87) for implantable use

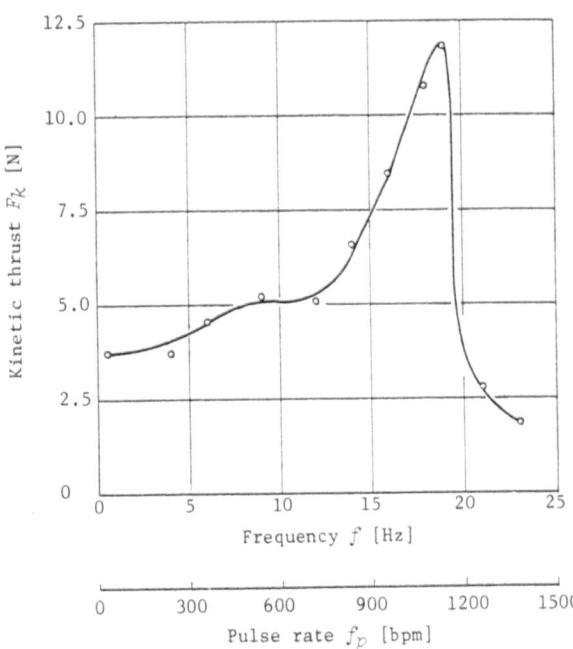

**Fig. 29.4.** Relation between kinetic thrust, $F_k$, and driving frequency, $f$, of a CLOA

**Table 29.1.** Specifications of cylindrical linear oscillatory actuator (CLOA)

| Mechanical specifications | |
|---|---|
| Primary member (stator) | |
| Length (mm) | 40 |
| Diameter (mm) | 60 |
| Volume (ml) | 110 |
| Mass (g) | 820 |
| Materials | SUM24L |
| Secondary member (mover) | |
| Length (mm) | 76 |
| Diameter (mm) | 10 |
| Volume (ml) | 20 |
| Mass (g) | 40 |
| Materials | ASK-3500S and SUS-304 |
| Total mass (g) | 860 |
| Total volume (ml) | 130 |
| Electromagnetic specifications | |
| Number of phases | 2 |
| Number of coils | 2 |
| Number of turns (/coil) | 1250 |
| Diameter of wire (mm) | 0.38 |
| Resistance of coil (ohms) | 19 |
| Exciting current ac (A) | 0.6 |
| Permanent magnet | Nd-Fe-B alloy (Neomax-35) |
| Input power (W) | 14.4 |
| Length of air gap (mm) | 0.35 |
| Stroke of mover (mm) | 26 |
| Driving frequency (Hz) | 0.2–19 |
| Static thrust (N) | 9 (at 0.6A dc) |

thrust characteristics of the FLPM have already been given in Fig. 29.7. The thrust characteristics of the FLPM are superior to those of the CLPM as a result of the use of cobalt steel sheets and rare earth magnets ($Sm_2 Co_{17}$).

Fig. 29.10 shows the FLPM for implantable use. The values of the thrust, mass, and volume are 48.3 N, 320 g, and 56.5 ml, while the input power is

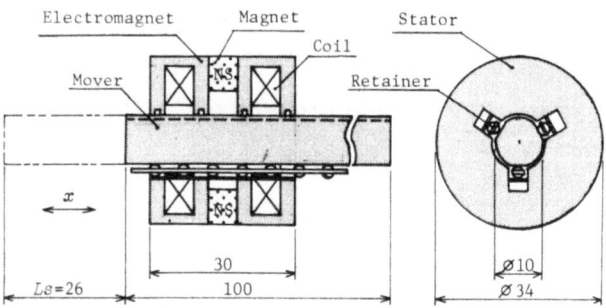

**Fig. 29.6.** Configuration of a cylindrical linear pulse motor (CLPM, units are millimeters)

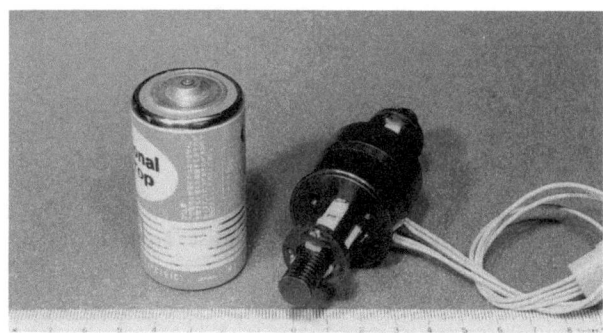

**Fig. 29.8.** Cylindrical linear pulse motor (CLPM-SS85) for implantable use

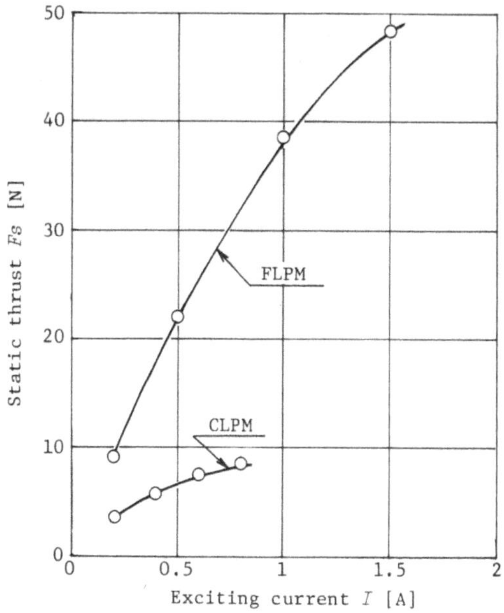

**Fig. 29.7.** Static thrust, $F_s$, exciting current, $I$, characteristics of FLPM and CLPM

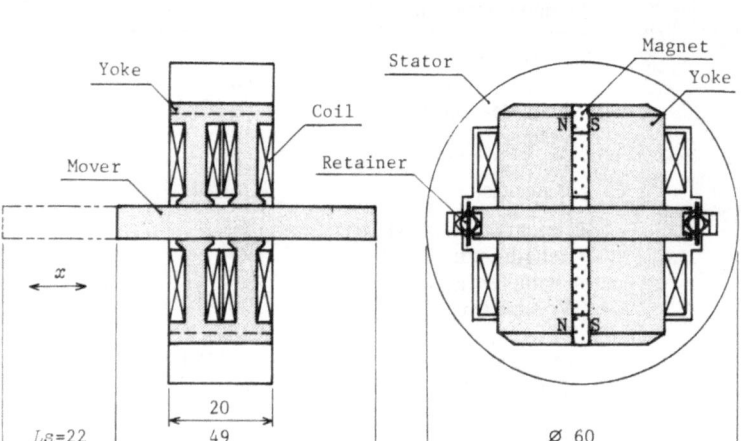

**Fig. 29.9.** Configuration of a flat linear pulse motor (FLPM, units are millimeters)

10.8 W.

The mechanical and electromagnetic specifications of the CLPM and FLPM are given in Table 29.2. The configurations and sizes of these two motors are smaller than those of the linear pulse motor.

Fig. 29.11 shows the relationship between the calculated flow rate, $q$, and the pulse rate, $f_p$, of the actuators CLOA, CLPM, and FLPM. The flow rate, $q$, is calculated by:

$$q = \gamma A L_s f_p \times 10^{-3} \text{ [L/min]}, \qquad (4)$$

where $\gamma$ is the resistance coefficient, $A$ [cm$^2$] the cross section of the pusher plate, $L_s$ [cm] the stroke of the mover, and $f_p$ [bpm] the pulse rate in beats per minute.

Among the three actuators, the actuators CLOA and FLPM have a flow rate of 6–9 l/min in the pulse rate range of 100–150 beats/min. The thrust characteristics of the CLOA and CLPM, however, need more improvement, because of the low thrust.

A comparison of characteristic values (figure of

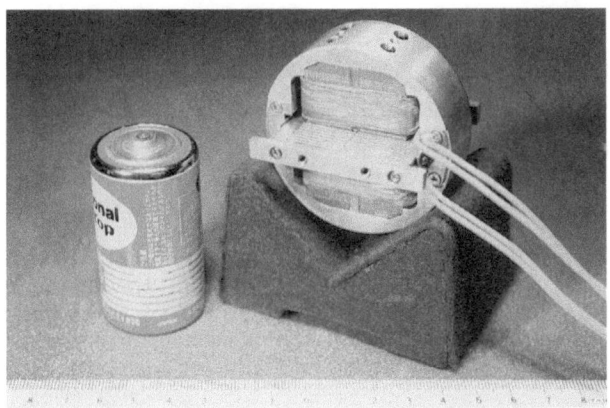

**Fig. 29.10.** Flat linear pulse motor (FLPM-SS87) for implantable use

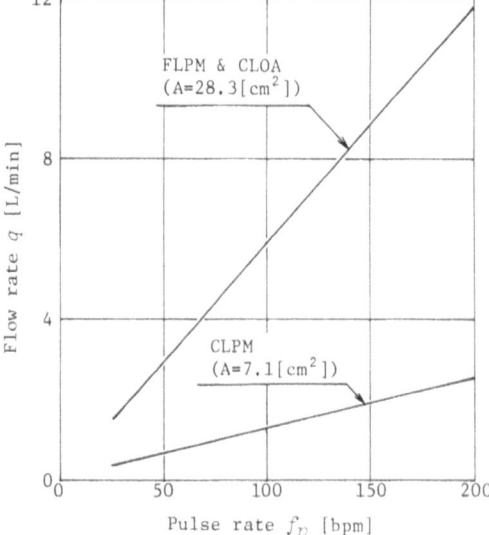

**Fig. 29.11.** Relation between flow rate, $q$, and pulse rate, $f_p$, of three actuators (calculated values)

**Table 29.2.** Specifications of CLPM and FLPM

| Mechanical specifications | CLPM | FLPM |
|---|---|---|
| Primary member (stator) | | |
| Pitch (mm) | 1.6 | 1.6 |
| Number of teeth (/pole) | 2 | 5 |
| Width of tooth (mm) | 0.8 | 0.64 |
| Width of slot (mm) | 0.8 | 0.96 |
| Thickness of lamination (mm) | — | $14.5 \times 2$ |
| Secondary member (mover) | | |
| Pitch (mm) | 1.6 | 1.6 |
| Width of teeth (mm) | 0.8 | 0.64 |
| Width of slot (mm) | 0.8 | 0.96 |
| Thickness of lamination (mm) | — | 34 |
| Total mass (g) | 175 | 320 |
| Total volume (ml) | 27.2 | 56.5 |
| | | |
| Electromagnetic specifications | | |
| Number of phases | 2 | 2 |
| Number of turns (/coil) | 600 | $160 \times 2$ |
| Exciting current (/phase) | 0.4 | 2 |
| Voltage (V) | 7.7 | 2.7 |
| Magnetomotive force (A/phase) | 480 | 320 |
| Resistance of coil (ohms/phase) | 19.3 | 1.36 |
| Permanent magnets | Ferrite | $Sm_2Co_{17}$ |
| Input power (W) | 6.2 | 10.8 |
| Length of air gap (mm) | 0.05 | 0.05 |
| Stroke of the mover (mm) | 26 | 22 |
| Step (mm/pulse) | 0.4 | 0.4 |
| Max. starting pulse rate (pps) | | 1000 |
| Static thrust (N) | 6.4 | 48.3 |

**Table 29.3.** Comparison of characteristic values on four linear actuators

| Item | AHA-H16 | CLOA | CLPM | FLPM |
|---|---|---|---|---|
| Total mass (g) | 1500 | 860 | 175 | 320 |
| Total volume (ml) | 500 | 130 | 27.2 | 56.5 |
| Input power (W) | 16 | 14.4 | 6.2 | 10.8 |
| Static thrust (N) | 86 | 9 | 6.4 | 48.3 |
| Stroke of mover (mm) | 15 | 26 | 26 | 22 |
| Thrust/input ratio (N/W) | 5.4 | 0.6 | 1.03 | 4.47 |
| Thrust/mass ratio (N/g) | 0.07 | 0.001 | 0.037 | 0.15 |
| Thrust/volume ratio (N/ml) | 0.32 | 0.07 | 0.24 | 0.85 |

merits) of the four LEAs are given in Table 29.3. The actuator AHA-H16 listed in Table 29.3 was developed in 1985 [3]. The LEAs do not yet have a pumping action, but a high level of technology has been applied in their development. The data in Table 29.3 signify just the beginning of the development competition of the LEAs.

These four LEAs were exhibited at the Hall of the 2nd International Symposium on Artificial Heart and Assist Device in Tokyo, 1987.

## Discussion

The actuators developed by our group may be likened to the development of Japanese cars in the 1950s. Japanese cars then had many problems, for example, overheating of the engine, poor suspension, and excessive vibration.

It may be possible to solve problems with actuators by applying new ideas, materials, and design [5].

**Acknowledgments.** The authors would like to thank to Mr. A. Nakanishi Sumitomo Special Metals Co. for corporating in the manufacture of special magnets. Part of this research was supported by a Grant-in-Aid from the Ministry of Health and Welfare of Japan.

# References

1. Yamada H (1986) Handbook of linear motor applications, Kogyo-Chosa-Kai, Tokyo, pp 354–379
2. Yamada H, Hamajima T, Ohira Y (1985) Improvement of thrust characteristics of moving iron type linear oscillatory actuator, Trans. IEE Japan, vol 105B, no. 10, p 889
3. Yamada H, Fukunaga S (1986) Artificial heart actuator using linear pulse motor. In: Akutsu T (ed) Artificial heart 1. Springer, Tokyo, pp 77–80
4. Yamada H, Murata K, Nirei M, Fukunaga S, Miwa Z, Yamamoto Y, Wakiwaka H (1987) Developement of an artificial heart actuator using linear pulse motor, Trans. IEE Japan, vol. 107D, no. 6, pp 788–795
5. Yamada H, Yamamoto Y, Miwa Z, Murofushi M, Nirei M, Shu-Jiang Xing, Neng-Qiang Jin, Kawakatsu K (1987) Problems of structure analysis of linear pulse motor magnetic circuit. Technical meeting on magnetics, MAG-87-52, IEE Japan, pp 9–18

## Discussion

*Fukunaga* (Hiroshima University): You showed several kinds of linear motor. Which type is the most promising for the artificial heart?

*Yamada* (Shinshu University): It is difficult to say, but perhaps the linear oscillatory actuator is superior. I do not think that the linear induction motor and linear DC motor are too suitable for the artificial heart.

*Portner* (Novacor Medical Corporation): How much mechanical work is possible with the flat-type motor?

*Yamada:* 50 N multiplied by 20 mm.

*Portner:* Which is about 1 J?

*Yamada:* The linear pulse motor has about 30% efficiency.

*Portner:* So your input power is 4 W and your output power is about 1.25 W?

*Imachi* (University of Tokyo): How about the durability of the flat-type motor?

*Yamada:* It is not yet quite a year since it was first developed so it is difficult to say.

*Imachi:* The force in the flat motor is 40 N. When it is used in the artificial heart acceleration power is required. How much power is generated under conditions of acceleration?

*Yamada:* That type of motor has not yet been specially programed. One of the merits of the linear pulse motor is the great flexibility in the choice of programs.

Part VI

# Total Artificial Heart

# 30. Engineering studies of the Penn State artificial heart

David B. Geselowitz[1]

**Summary.** Development of the Penn State cardiac assist devices and total artificial heart has included intensive engineering studies of fluid flow, control, volume compensation, and transcutaneous transmission of energy and data. Current emphasis is on a brushless dc motor driven device, although many basic techniques were developed previously for our pneumatic devices. An overview of the current status of these several studies is presented.

Fluid flow studies emphasize streak photography to obtain qualitative information concerning flow patterns during the cycle, and pulsed Doppler ultrasound velocimetry and hot film anemometry to obtain quantitative velocity measurements. Newtonian and non-Newtonian blood analogs as well as bovine blood have been studied.

Research continues on a two-phase fluid volume compensation chamber.

Energy will be inductively coupled across the skin using a transcutaneous energy transmission system employing a pair of coils. Separate modulation schemes are required to transmit data to and from the implanted device using the coil pair.

Control studies include development of novel controllers for pusher plate position with consideration of optimization of power consumption. Cardiac output control is based on the approach used for the pneumatic heart. An observer for arterial blood pressure is under development. A mathematical model of the system is used in conjunction with these studies.

**Key words:** Total artificial heart—Electric motor heart—Flow studies—Control—Telemetry—Transcutaneous energy transmission

Pierce has led the Penn State artificial heart program since its inception in 1970. Early efforts were focused on pneumatic pumps, which consist of extremely smooth, seam-free, segmented polyurethane sacs contained within rigid polysulfone cases. Our pneumatic assist device has been undergoing clinical trials for more than a decade [1]. The Penn State total artificial heart (TAH) has been implanted in two patients since 1985 as a bridge to transplant [2].

More recently, our research efforts have turned to an electric motor heart. This paper will review aspects of engineering studies of these systems. Many investigators from our institution including faculty and graduate students have contributed to the work to be described. Rosenberg has been in charge of all aspects of mechanical design. Other contributors will be identified through literature citations.

## General description

The first electric motor-driven artificial heart to be developed by our group consisted of a high torque, low speed brushless dc motor rotating a triple-track drum cam [3]. The TAH configuration utilizes two pusher plate-driven blood pumps attached to a common central housing. The pumps are similar in design to the pneumatic ones and have Bjork-Shiley Delrin disc convexo-convave valves. The pumps are activated reciprocally, one filling while the other ejects blood. This cam-driven system has a nominal 100-cm$^3$ stroke volume and in capable of flow rates in excess of 13 l/min. The cam system has been utilized in ten calves, with the longest calf surviving for 222 days [4] (Fig. 30.1).

Although one calf survived 222 days, concern for durability of the cam follower mechanism and the possibility of achieving reduced size and weight led us to pursue another mechanism to actuate the device, the roller screw [5].

The roller screw mechanism consists of a central screw and a series of external rollers that roll on the screw with complete rolling contact to translate rotary motion into rectilinear motion. The roller screw nut is rotated through six revolutions, stopped, and counter-rotated to complete one cycle. Stroke length is 2.5 cm. The pusher plate is attached directly to the roller screw shaft, and Hall effect sensors are used to determine the relative position of the rotor and stator for commutation (Fig. 30.2).

The motor for the roller screw devices is a three-phase, delta-wound fractional slot brushless dc-type motor with a *vanadium permadore stack* and sama-

---
[1]Bioengineering Program, Pennsylvania State University, University Park, PA 16802, USA

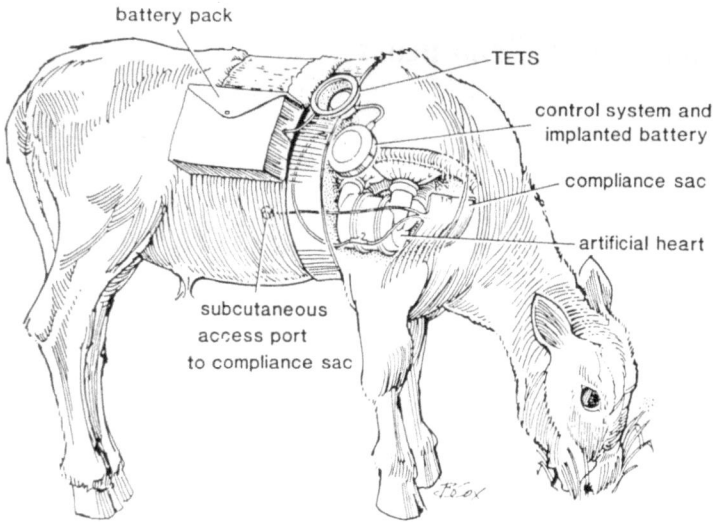

**Fig. 30.1.** Artist's sketch of a calf with an implanted electric motor driven total artificial heart showing various components of the system

rium cobalt magnets. It has low torque and relatively high speed. Initially we used a 36-V motor manufactured by Sierracin Magnedyne. Twelve volts is the highest practical voltage, however, when implanted batteries are required, and we have started testing a 12-V motor. The energy converter utilized with the 100-cm³ stroke volume pump weighs 700 g. Use of neodymium iron magnets may result in some size reduction.

The motor is electronically commutated and controlled by a totally automatic microprocessor-based control system. This automatic control system controls the velocity of the motor throughout the cycle and also varies the beat rate to control overall cardiac output in relation to peripheral vascular resistance. In addition, the outputs of the left and right blood pumps are varied by changing the system stroke time division to balance the outputs of the left and right blood pumps.

In the assist mode, the cardiac output control runs the device in a full-to-empty mode. The motor increases the beat rate until the pump does not fill, then the beat rate is decremented until the pump fills. Thus, the beat rate is automatically adjusted to pump the amount of blood that is returned to the assist device. This control scheme has worked satisfactorily with calves and patients.

The roller screw electric motor-driven TAH has been implanted in five animals thus far, with the longest survival 52 days. It has run continuously on the mock loop for over 50 million cycles (approximately 1 year) with no measurable wear.

Performance of the devices is evaluated in vitro on the Penn State mock circulatory system [6], which provides a reliable analog of the natural circulation. Measurements include efficiency, peak flow rates, adaptability of the control system, and various hemo-

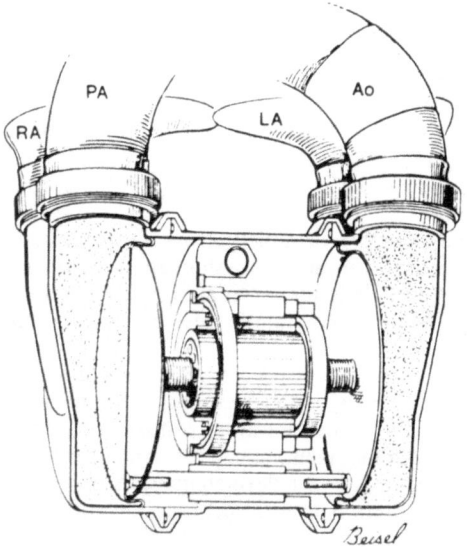

**Fig. 30.2.** Sketch of roller screw total artificial heart. Pusher plates eject blood reciprocally from left and right pumps. *PA* pulmonary artery, *Ao* aorta, *RA* right atrium, *LA* left atrium

dynamic parameters such as pressure drops [7, 8]. Device power consumption is verified to be appropriate for pumping conditions and estimates of left pump stroke volume and arterial pressure are checked for accuracy. A limited number of these systems have been fatigue tested.

## Flow studies

Hemolysis, thrombus formation, and blood sac calcification may be related to the fluid dynamic behavior of blood in artificial blood pumps. Elevated wall shear

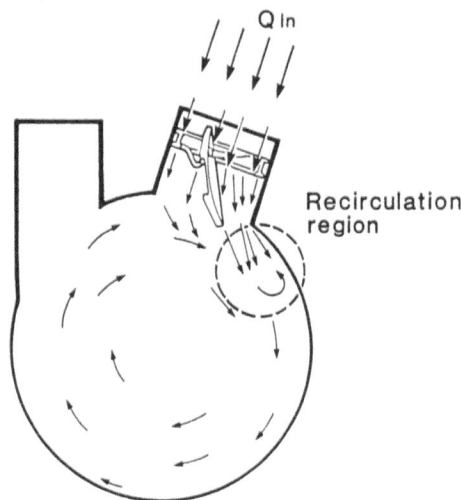

**Fig. 30.3.** Flow pattern in pump chamber during phase of filling. Note small stagnation region. Figure is abstracted from photograph of streak lines reflected from particles suspended in blood analog

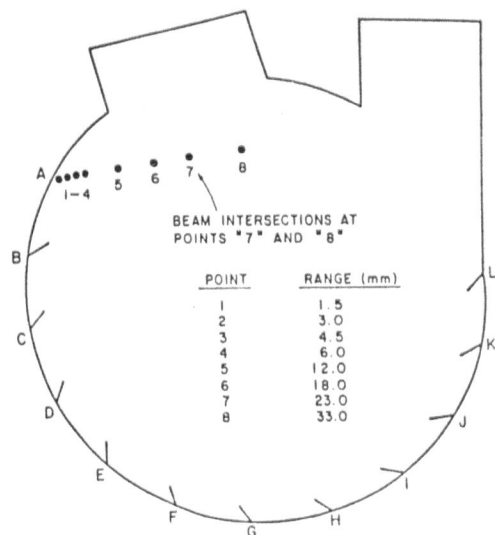

**Fig. 30.4.** Schematic of pump showing positions and orientations of probes for pulsed Doppler ultrasound measurements of fluid velocity. Measurements are made at eight points (ranges) along each beam. These sites are shown for probe A. Ranges are not to scale

stress and turbulent stress (Reynolds stress) can damage blood components, while regions of stasis may lead to prolonged residence time of blood in contact with artificial surfaces and thus may result in thrombus formation [9]. Potentially deleterious fluid dynamic interactions of blood with artificial hearts may be associated with the prosthetic valves, or with the flow patterns inside the pumping chamber itself.

Velocity profiles, wall shear stress, and turbulent stress have been measured in uniform cylindrical tubes distal to artificial heart valves [10–12]. Much less is known about the flow fields inside artificial ventricles. Although particle streak photographs showing the general streamline patterns inside ventricles have been obtained by most research groups, very little quantitative velocity and shear stress information has been reported, and studies to date have, to our knowledge, been conducted only with Newtonian blood analog fluids. The non-Newtonian nature of blood [13] may become important in low shear rate regions such as the spaces behind the heart valve leaflets or regions of flow separation (stasis).

Our laboratory has pioneered in the use of flow visualization techniques for determining flow patterns in the pump chamber and through the valves using qualitative and quantitative techniques. Initial studies, dating from 1970, invloved particle streak photography [14], followed by investigations employing a laser-Doppler anemometer [15]. More recently we have employed pulsed ultrasound-Doppler velocimetry (PUDV). Tarbell now heads these studies.

Fig. 30.3 illustrates the type of information which can be obtained from particle streak photography. The drawing is abstracted from the original photograph and shows the flow pattern at an instant during filling. A small stagnation region is evident near the inlet valve. This effect can be eliminated by redesigning the orientation of the inlet port.

The PUDV studies provide quantitative data on fluid velocities in the pump chamber during a cycle [16, 17]. We used a single probe with a tip-mounted piezoelectric crystal, which was placed successively in a series of holes around the periphery of a specially made flow visualization chamber (Fig. 30.4). The crystal transmitted 10 mHz ultrasound (0.4 $\mu$s pulses) with a pulse repetition frequency of 20 kHz. Velocities were measured at eight range positions (1.4–33.0 mm). Ensemble averaging over 100 cycles was required to determine phasic mean and fluctuating velocity components. The Newtonian test fluid was a water-glycerin mixture having a viscosity of 3.5 cP. The non-Newtonian test fluid was a mixture of polyacrylamide, water, and isopropanol, which displayed shear thinning behavior close to that of both human and bovine blood. Bovine blood was suitably mixed with homologous plasma for study.

Under normal operating conditions, particle streak photography and PUDV measurements confirmed the presence of two counter-rotating vortices in the principle flow plane separated by a stagnation point on the wall distal to the inlet valve over most of the pumping cycle for all three fluids. The location of the stagna-

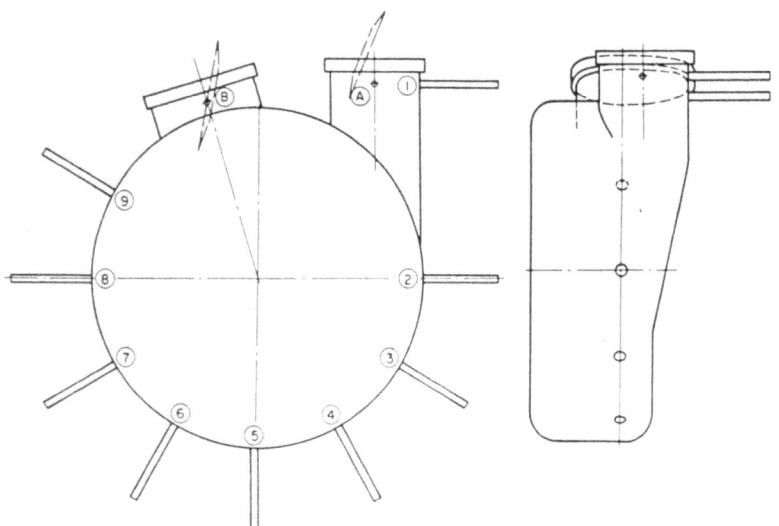

**Fig. 30.5.** Schematic of pumping chamber showing the locations of flush-mounted hot-film probes

tion point varied somewhat with the fluid, and only blood displayed a time interval in which the stagnation point completely disappeared and a single wall washing vortex occupied the entire chamber. These findings emphasize the importance of fluid rheology in pump flows. Because PUDV only measured one component of velocity, it was not possible to measure turbulent stress directly, although order of magnitude estimates based on one componet information were made [16].

PUDV measurements indicated highest rms velocities in the small vortex associated with the inlet valve during diastole. Values in this region for all fluids were typically 10–15 cm/s. The highest rms velocity observed anywhere in the chamber was 23 cm/s. Based on idealized assumptions, this value can be used to estimate a maximum turbulent stress of 212 dynes/cm$^2$.

Wall shear stress estimates based on near wall velocity measurements indicated a maximum value of 25 dynes/cm$^2$ for glycerin/water solutions, with Separan solutions and bovine blood showing values which were about 50% higher. These estimates of wall shear stress and turbulent stress are lower than those measured distal to aortic valve prostheses [10–12] and are well below levels known to damage blood components [9].

One limitation of the PUDV measurements is the relatively large sample volume (order of a cubic millimeter) which is about 1000 times larger than that of a laser Doppler velocimeter. The large sample volume filters the high-frequency components of the turbulence and limits the spatial resolution of velocity measurements. In turn, the limited spatial resolution leads to uncertainty in wall shear stress estimates based on extrapolation of the near wall velocity pro-

file. In addition, since the PUDV measured only a single component of velocity, it was necessary to make idealized assumptions in order to estimate the turbulent stress. A direct measurement of the turbulent stress requires a two-channel instrument capable of simultaneously measuring two components of velocity. The restricted range of the PUDV also limited the region of the chamber which could be interrogated.

To make accurate measurements of wall shear stress, we have employed a flush-mounted hot-film anemometer (FMHFA). Measurement locations are shown in Fig. 30.5 and include several positions near the inlet and outlet valve which were not accessed by PUDV (positions 1, A, and B). The hot-film probe used in our studies was custom made by TSI, Inc. It consists of a flat-ended quartz rod, 1.0 mm in diameter, surrounded by a stainless steel jacket with an outside diameter of 1.5 mm. The sensing element is a platinum film strip, 0.125 mm wide and covered with a 2-$\mu$m quartz coating. The sensing element was flush-mounted to the walls of the test chamber and calibration chamber by means of micrometer-based positioners [18].

Our initial studies used a Newtonian test fluid. Fig. 30.6 shows the ensemble averaged wall shear rate waveform measured at position 1 under operating conditions of 30% and 50% systolic duration at a beat rate of 60 beats/min and a mean flow of 5.8 l/min. The wall shear rate peaks during systole and may be as high as 75 000 s$^{-1}$ for a 30% systolic duration. This shear rate translates into a wall shear stress on the order of 3000 dynes/cm$^2$ for a fluid having a viscosity of blood (4.0 cP). In turn, this value of wall shear stress is the highest one observed anywhere in the chamber and is clearly quite sensitive to operating

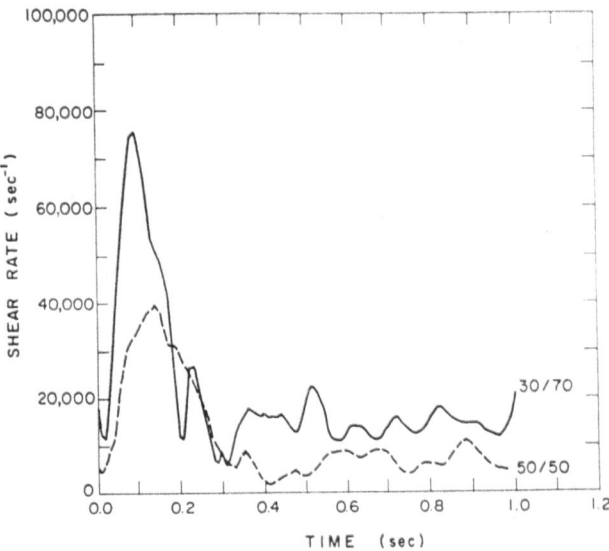

**Fig. 30.6.** Ensemble averaged wall shear rate waveforms obtained with hot-film anemometry at position 1 of Fig. 5 for 30% and 50% systolic duration

conditions as it can be cut in half by increasing the systolic duration. Results at other locations also show a strong sensitivity to operating conditions.

Other interesting results of the FMHFA study were obtained at location 6 (Fig. 30.5), which had been observed to be a region of flow stagnation in our PUDV study. FMHFA measurements in this region showed peak wall shear stress values as high as 480 dynes/cm$^2$, a level seemingly inconsistent with our previous observations of stagnation flow. When the orientation of the probe in the flow field was changed, however, a strong flow perpendicular to the inflow-outflow plane became evident. This perpendicular flow is the source of the observed high wall shear stress value; there is virtually no flow in the inflow-outflow plane. Since PUDV only measured velocities in the inflow-outflow plane, location 6 appeared to be a stagnation region, but no thrombosis had been observed in this area. The FMHFA studies have revealed aspects of the fully three-dimensional nature of the flow field in the artificial ventricle.

We feel that longer term optimization of design and operating conditions will be aided by a computational fluid dynamic model. Ideally, such a model would allow us to compute the velocity, pressure, and stress fields within the ventricle and around the valves for a wide variety of design and operating conditions. The fluid dynamics of the artificial ventricle are extremely complex, involving time-varying three-dimensional fields with complex boundaries and turbulent flow.

## Compliance chamber

The totally implantable, electric motor-drive device is enclosed in a well-sealed casing and cannot be vented to the atmosphere. As a consequence, the space behind the pusher plate, whose volume may vary by 100 ml during the course of a cardiac cycle for a ventricular assist device (VAD), would in the absence of compensation experience a change in pressure which could either impede blood sac filling or increase the work load on the motor [19]. The problem is less severe in the case of the TAH, but exists nonetheless. Tests on the mock circulatory loop have indicated that the VAD could maintain aortic pressure, cardiac output, beat rate, and motor power if the pressure variation over a pumping cycle in the space behind the pusher plate was maintained below 40 mmHg.

Although the sac type compliance chamber has been used successfully in animal experiments [20, 21], the flexible sac materials are susceptible to permeation by noncondensible gases, which can limit the effectiveness of the chamber in long-term applications. The two-phase fluid (TPF) compliance chamber is an alternative which incorporates an impermeable case that may ultimately be more suitable [22–25].

Volume compensation with a two-phase fluid involves placing a fluid which boils (changes phase) at constant temperature and constant pressure in the space behind the pusher plate. Ideally, a substantial change in volume can be achieved at constant pressure as the fluid cycles between liquid and vapor over the pumping cycle. In practice, however, heat must be supplied to the fluid for vaporization and removed for condensation, requiring a temperature differential between the fluid and the heat source/sink. The fluid temperature variation leads to a pressure variation which must be minimized.

A schematic diagram of the TPF compliance chamber under development is shown in Fig. 30.7. The two-phase fluid is isolated from the motor components by a flexible, impermeable diaphragm, e.g., a bellows, and is contained in the space between the bellows and a rigid aluminum external case.

We have tested two FREONs (113 and TMS; E.I. Du Pont) with atmospheric boiling points of 47.7°C and 39.9°C, respectively. FREONs exhibit low heat of vaporization and nonflammability. By mixing two fluids in the appropriate proportions, it is possible to obtain any desired boiling point in the range between the pure component boiling points. About 20 ml FREON is required to produce a minimal pressure swing under typical operating conditions.

In early experiments, metal packing material (e.g., steel wool, metal filings, metal pellets) was placed in the TPF space to act as a heat capacitor. However, too much weight and volume of packing material was

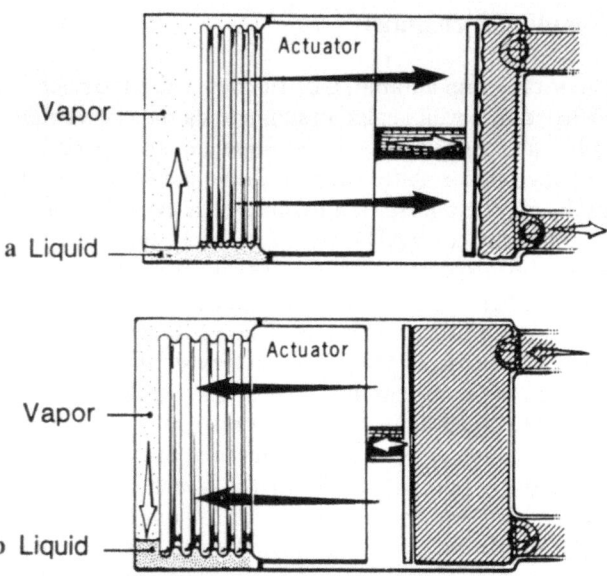

**Fig. 30.7a, b.** Concept of two-phase fluid (TPF) compliance chamber. **a** Pusher plate moves to right, ejecting blood and increasing volume in compartment with TPF, which moves into vapor phase, maintaining pressure behind pusher plate. **b** Process is reversed

required to produce the desired pressure swing. Tarbell and Ojan in our laboratory are currently exploring a technique which involves coating the inside surface of the external aluminum casing with a brazing of fine aluminum particles. The brazed coating greatly enhances the rate of heat transfer between the TPF and the external casing and allows the casing itself to act as an effective heat capacitor.

Tests of the system were carried out by placing the chamber in a heat bath at a controlled temperature and measuring the pressure in the space between the bellows and the pusher plate for various combinations of stroke volume and frequency. Promising results have been obtained with the system incorporating the brazed aluminum coating under the most extreme conditions without additional heat capacitor material.

### Transcutaneous energy transmission system

The transcutaneous energy transmission system (TETS) that was developed by Thermedics, Inc. [26] has been adapted for use with the Penn State electric motor-driven TAH. The Thermedics system uses a transcutaneous double-tuned transformer, thus eliminating the need for percutaneous leads. The transformer consists of a pair of loosely coupled coils separated by approximately 1.5 cm. The external primary coil has an average diameter of 10 cm and contains three turns of Litz wire. The implanted secondary coil consists of 16 turns of Litz wire in the shape of a truncated cone, 7.1 cm in diameter. The slight mound in the skin formed by the implanted coil provides a nearly concentric alignment for the coil pair.

Each coil is part of a 160-kHz series tuned circuit. The TETS primary oscillator converts the 12-V dc input from a battery pack to 160 kHz sinusoidal current in the primary coil. Internally, the TETS output is essentially a constant current source. A nearly constant load voltage is maintained by a voltage regulator, which allows the constant current to flow to the load if the voltage is below nominal ("on" state), but diverts the current through a short circuit if the voltage is above nominal ("off" state). During the "off" state, a corresponding decrease in primary coil current initiates a decrease in the driving voltage of the power oscillator, thereby conserving power. The normal cycle of on-off states depends upon the power required by the load, but typically varies between 10 Hz and 1 kHz.

The original TETS was designed for a maximum output power of 30 W. Although the mean power requirement for the roller screw TAH is typically 10–15 W [27], short duration peak power requirements may be as high as 50 W. A power level of 85 W has been achieved with minor modifications to the external power oscillator [28]. The TETS efficiency is always highest when supplying the maximum design power (i.e., when there is no time spent in the off state). The average efficiency is highest when the peak power levels deviate little from the average. Further studies are necessary to optimize the efficiency of the system.

One topic of current interest is the vulnerability of the TETS to metallic objects placed within a few centimeters of the coil pair. Metal near the coils changes the coil inductances and coupling coefficient, thus upsetting the tuning of the primary and/or secondary circuits. Eddy current and hysteresis losses may also be induced in the metal, reducing efficiency.

### Telemetry

Telemetry is required to transmit data and commands across the skin. Transmission "out" from implanted circuitry provides data on system parameters such as beat rate, velocity profile (i.e., time-course of pusher plate velocity during a stroke), motor power, estimated inlet and outlet pressures, as well as the charge/discharge characteristics of the internal batteries. Transmission "in" permits the control parameters of the internal microprocessor to be modified.

We are exploring the use of the transcutaneous energy transmission system coils and circuitry for telemetry to reduce the number of additional components

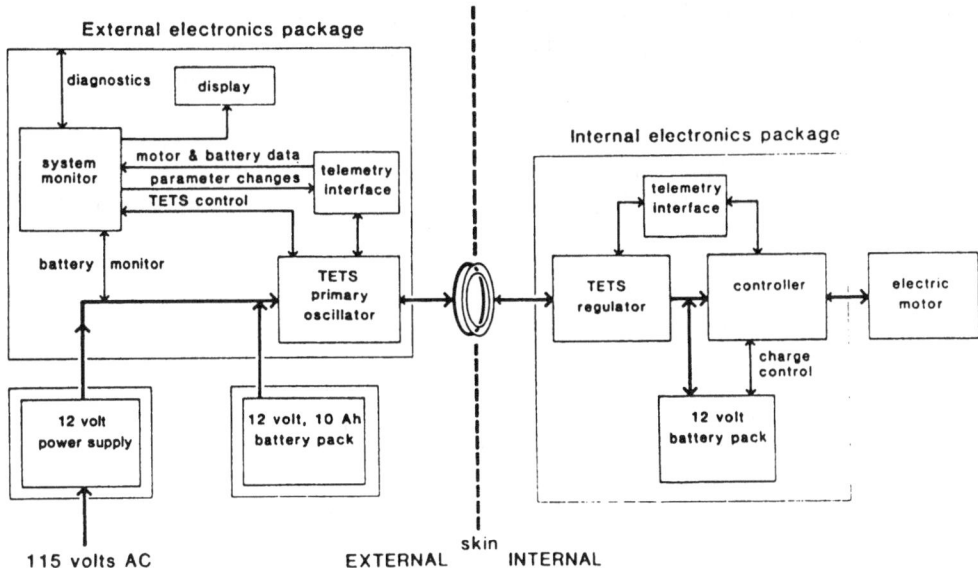

**Fig. 30.8.** Block diagram of electronics including transcutaneous energy transmission, telemetry, and control functions

[29]. Fig. 30.8 shows a block diagram of the electronics system. To transmit input commands, the power oscillator is frequency shift keyed to 161 kHz (mark) or 159 kHz (space) at the beginning of each on state. The normal on-off cycling of the TETS, therefore, serves as a synchronizing signal for each bit change. Since the transmission channel is tuned to 160 kHz, the frequency deviation must be small so as not to interfere with the normal TETS operation.

On the secondary side, demodulation of the carrier is also keyed to the on-off cycling of the TETS. The demodulation signal is sent to a synchronous transmitter/receiver, which interfaces with a control microprocessor. To transmit information from the implanted secondary coil to the primary coil, the impedance of the shorting bridge is modulated during the off state. Since the phase of the current signal in the primary loop is extremely sensitive to the off state impedance in the secondary loop, the change in impedance can be detected, yielding a phase shift keyed data transmission scheme.

Both modulation schemes are synchronized to the on-off cycle of the TETS. One bit of information is transmitted in a single direction during each on-off cycle. Although the resulting transmission rate is relatively slow (approximately 300 BAUD when averaged over one pump cycle), it is sufficient for the intended purposes, and it should be extremely reliable since the information carrier is a strong RF signal. Tests of the telemetry system in unidirectional bit-transmission modes have shown that TETS performance is not measurably affected by inclusion of telemetry functions.

## Simulation and optimal control

We have long used simulation as a tool in our development and engineering studies [6–8, 30, 31]). Simulations are useful in developing controllers for the motor, in developing observers for parameters such as blood pressure, in optimization studies, and in investigating the effects of changes in design parameters.

The current model incorporates the following features:

a) The motor is characterized by a resistance, torque constant, back emf constant, and friction factor
b) The rotary to linear converter is characterized by a mass, moment of inertia, and rotary to linear transformation factor
c) The pump is characterized by volume and pusher plate area
d) The values are characterized by forward and backward resistances, which may be square law, and inertances
e) The circulation is characterized by arterial and venous compliances; a resistance for the pulmonary and systemic circulations, respectively; and an arterial venous shunt resistance

The state variables in our formulation are the pusher plate velocity, pusher plate position, aortic pressure, left atrial pressure, pulmonary pressure, and right atrial pressure. The input is the motor voltage.

During systole, when blood is being ejected from one blood sac, the opposite blood sac is filling. During filling, the sac may or may not be in contact with the pusher plate. The model distinguishes between these modes of operation. If neither pusher plate is in contact with a blood sac, the device and the vascular system are uncoupled.

The systemic and pulmonary circulations in the model are characterized by windkessels. The mock circulatory system used for bench testing is based on a windkessel and is quite accurately modeled. On the other hand, the vascular systems in vivo may be expected to depart somewhat from the windkessel representation.

The brushless dc motor requires electronic communtation utilizing a microprocessor. Magnets are mounted to the rotating portion of the nut and motor rotor assembly. Hall effect switches are mounted stationary relative to the stator portion of the motor. The outputs of these Hall effect sensors provide signals that are used to determine motor position and velocity. The electronic control system controls motor speed throughout the cycle and also changes the beat rate of the device in response to physiological conditions [32, 33]. The motor velocity is controlled in such a manner that inertial forces are minimized throughout the cycle. The motor starts out gradually, accelerates to maximum speed, gradually decelerates and then reverses and begins the second portion of the cycle.

There are, therefore, two controllers required, one for motor velocity during a stroke, the other for cardiac output. Cardiac output is controlled primarily through variation of beat rate. The cardiac output controller must also balance outputs of the left and right hearts. In the case of a pneumatic system, the left and right hearts can be separately controlled to achieve balance. With the electric motor system, as the pair of pusher plates move together in a particular direction, one pump fills while the other ejects blood. Because of this coupling, design of the control scheme becomes more complex. In order to control separately the left and right heart outputs, the duration of the stroke and the wait time at the end of the stroke are varied. We will not discuss further details of this scheme here.

Velocity controllers based on feedback of the error between the actual and desired velocity profile have not proved to be entirely satisfactory, especially at higher beat rates [34, 35]. We use a sample data control system, and sense position. Velocity is determined by a backward difference of sensed position. There is an inherent delay and inaccuracy in the velocity signal, leading to difficulties in the design of the error feedback controller. Therefore, we have been investigating two other approaches to velocity control.

One novel velocity controller developed by Snyder [36] employs a strategy of preprogramming the motor voltage for a cycle and then invoking an adaptive feedforward mechanism that looks at the previous cycle to determine how well the system tracked the desired velocity. Appropriate changes are then made in the control system to insure that the next cycle is tracked more closely. This controller has performed successfully on the bench and in a series of animals.

A second approach involves an output state feedback controller where the values of the states of the system are fed back to achieve a desired velocity profile [37]. Studies with simulation and on the bench have shown that such a controller can be designed using a single state, i.e., pusher plate position.

We are also exploring optimization of the velocity profile to minimize electric power consumption. The mathematical model provies a useful tool for developing the optimization scheme. Since power consumption is dominated by the left heart, our preliminary studies used a simplified model which considered only the left heart. Our approach to optimization has involved the output state controller whose input is a function, instant by instant, of the state variables. An optimal controller would utilize all the state variables. Since these states are not all available, we have developed a suboptimal controller which utilizes only the measured pusher plate position [37].

The controller was designed to drive the pusher plate through its stroke while minimizing the electric energy consumption and forcing the velocity at the turning points to be zero. The latter constraint reduces the contribution of the moving parts to the inertial rocking of the device. Results from the mathematical simulation were implemented and tested on the mock loop.

Preliminary mock loop results indicate that the suboptimal controller saves 11% (0.7 W s) at 60 beats/min and 20% (1.3 W s) at 90 beats/min when compared with the classic triangular velocity controller we have used. Furthermore, the peak power is considerably reduced, a result which can have important consequences for the design of the system.

## Observer

Since we choose to avoid placing pressure transducers in the circulatory system, direct measures of blood pressure are unavailable. Hence, estimates of these pressures are required. In the case of the pneumatic heart, pressures can be derived from measurements of the air pressure waveform [38]. In the case of the electric heart, pressure estimates must utilize quantities we can measure, such as motor voltage and current, and pusher plate position.

One approach we have developed relates the aortic pressure algebraically to the pusher plate linear velocity, armature angular velocity and angular acceleration, and a constant friction torque. The coefficients of this expression are determined empirically. Encouraging preliminary results have been obtained for the average pressure estimated in this fashion [39].

A second approach to the development of an observer for aortic pressure is based on Luenberger's theory [40]. Preliminary results obtained by Tsach with a constant gain observer shown promise in estimating the instantaneous pressure waveform.

Every motor drive which is implanted is bench tested in mock circulation to assure its function and that of the controller. The portion of the control system which is responsible for maintaining left-right output balance is evaluated by plotting the relation of left atrial to right atrial pressure over a range of cardiac outputs and arterial pressures. Within the ability of the electric motor to attain the required speeds, the controller brings the system to the point where the left atrial pressure is at the minimum level required to maintain the cardiac output. The left atrial pressure in such a condition is determined by the mitral valve characteristics, the filling characteristics of the isolated blood sac, and the compliance chamber pressure. The right atrial pressure above which such a condition cannot be maintained is determined by the electromechanical characteristics of the motor, the characteristics of all valves, and the compliance chamber pressure. These interactions of the system parameters provide an interesting challenge for optimization of system design.

## Discussion

In this paper, a number of engineering studies conducted in connection with the development of the Penn State artificial heart have been discussed. They have included flow studies, development of controllers for the dc motor, development of a compliance chamber, transmission of energy and data across the skin, and the development of a mathematical model for the artificial heart and the circulatory system which it drives.

Sufficient progress has been made in all these areas to yield a working heart. On the other hand, there is room for improvement and refinement. Of particular note are efforts to optimize performance, with considerations of power consumption, inertial rocking, interactions with blood, durability of components, etc. From the standpoint of a biomedical engineer, the problems faced are particularly fascinating and challenging.

**Acknowledgment.** This work was supported in part by grants HL-20356 and HL-13426 from the National Heart Lung and Blood Institute.

## References

1. Pierce WS, Parr GVS, Myers JL, Pae WE, Bull AP, Waldhausen JA (1981) Ventricular assist pumping in patients with cardiogenic shock after cardiac operations. N Engl J Med 305 (27): 1606–1610
2. Pennock JL, Pierce WS, Campbell DB, Pae WE, Davis D, Hensley FA, Richenbacher WE, Waldhausen JA (1986) Mechanical support of the circulation followed by cardiac transplantation. J Thorac Cardiovasc Surg 5: 196–202
3. Rosenberg G, Synder A, Weiss W, Landis DL, Geselowitz DB, Pierce WS (1982) A cam-type electric motor-driven left ventricular assist device. Trans ASME J Biomech Eng 104: 214–220
4. Rosenberg G, Snyder AJ, Landis DL, Geselowitz DB, Donachy JH, Pierce WS (1984) An electric motor-driven total artificial heart: Seven months survival in the calf. Trans Am Soc Artif Intern Organs 30: 69–74
5. Rosenberg G, Snyder AJ, Weiss W, Landis DL, Geselowitz DB, Pierce WS (1982) A roller screw drive for implantable blood pumps. Trans ASAIO 28: 123–126
6. Rosenberg G, Phillips WM, Landis DL, Pierce WS (1981) Design and evaluation of the Pennsylvania State University mock circulatory system. ASAIO J 4: 41–49
7. Lewis JB, Hanson KL, Ostroff AH, Sidhwa ED, Geselowitz DB, Rosenberg G, Pierce WS (1984) Simulation studies of the Penn State LVAD: Control. Proceedings 6th Annual Conference IEEE Engineering in Medicine and Biology Society, pp 15–18
8. Fikse TH, Rosenberg G, Snyder AJ, Landis DL, Hanson KL, Kern SE, Geselowitz DB, Pierce WS (1984) Development and verification of LVAD/mock loop system model. Proceedings 6th Annual Conference IEEE Engineering Medicine and Biology Society, pp 33–37
9. Portner PM, Green GF, Ramasamy N (1983) The blood interface at artificial surfaces within a left ventricular assist system. Ann NY Acad Sci 416:471–503
10. Tiederman WG, Steinle MJ, Phillips WM (1986) Two-component laser velocimeter measurements downstream of heart valve prostheses in pulsatile flow. J Biomech Eng 108: 59–64
11. Woo Y-R, Yoganathan AP (1986) *In vitro* pulsatile flow velocity and shear stress measurements in the vicinity of mechanical mitral heart valve prostheses. J Biomech 19: 39–51
12. Tillmann W, Reul H, Herold M, Bruss K-H, van Glise, J (1984) *In vitro* wall shear measurements at aortic valve prostheses. J Biomech 17: 263–279
13. Thurston GB (1979) Rheological parameters for the viscosity, viscoelasticity and thixotropy of blood. Biorheology 16: 149–162
14. Phillips WM, Brighton JA, Pierce WS (1972) Artificial heart evaluation using flow visualization techniques. Trans ASAIO 18: 194–199
15. Phillips WM, Furkay S, Pierce WS (1979) Laser Doppler anemometer studies in unsteady ventricular flows. Trans ASAIO 25: 56–60
16. Tarbell JM, Gunshinan JP, Geselowitz DB, Rosenberg G, Shung KK, Pierce WS (1986) Pulsed ultrasonic Doppler velocity measurements inside a left ventricular assist device. J Biomech Eng 108: 232–238
17. Mann KA, Deutsch S, Tarbell JM, Geselowitz DB, Rosenberg G, Pierce WS (1987) An experimental study

of Newtonian and non-Newtonian flow dynamics in a ventricular assist device. J Biomech Eng 109: 139–147

18. Baldwin JT, Tarbell JM, Deutsch S, Geselowitz DB (1987) Wall shear stress measurements within an artificial heart ventricle. To be presented at Ninth Annual Conf IEEE/EMBS, Boston

19. Lee S, Rosenberg G, Donachy JH, Wisman CB, Pierce WS (1984) The compliance problem: A major obstacle in the development of implantable blood pumps. Artif Organs 8: 82–90

20. Snyder AJ, Rosenberg G, Weiss W, Huang W, Landis DL, Pierce WS (1984) Chronic animal studies with a motor-driven LVAD and an implanted compliance chamber. Trans Am Soc Artif Intern Organs 30: 92–97

21. Sato N, Snow J, Smith W, Kasick J, Kaneko S, Olsen E, Hilleguss D, Harasaki H, Kiraly R, Nose Y (1974) Compliance chamber-system integration studies. Trans Am Soc Artif Intern Organs 30: 545–549

22. van Glise J (1980) Solving the venting problems of pusher plate blood pumps by vaporizing liquids. Proc Eur Soc Artif Organs 11: 51–55

23. McKyton A, Tarbell JM, Geselowitz DB, Pierce WS, Rosenberg G (1982) Volume compensation in a VAD by use of a two-phase fluid. Proceedings 35th Annual Conference Engineering in Medicine and Biology 24: 144

24. McKyton A (1983) The use of a two-phase fluid for volume compensation in a ventricular assist device. M.S. Thesis, The Pennsylvania State University

25. Riggins G (1984) Feasibility of a volume compensator for use with a ventricular assist device. M.S. Thesis, The Pennsylvania State University

26. Sherman C, Daly BDT, Clay W, Dasse K, Handrahan J, Haudenschild C (1984) In vivo evaluation of a transcutaneous energy transmission system. Trans Am Soc Artif Intern Organs 30: 143–147

27. Rosenberg G, Snyder AJ, Weiss WJ, Pierce WS, Geselowitz DB (1987) Power requirements for an electric motor-driven total artificial heart. To be presented at Ninth Annual Conf IEEE/EMBS, Boston

28. Gaumond RP, Geselowitz DB, Gibbons P, Trumble D, Weiss W (1986) Modification of a series-tuned transcutaneous energy transmission system. Proceedings 12th Northeast Bioengineering Conference, pp 3–6

29. Weiss WJ, Gibbons PJ, Gaumond RP, Snyder AJ, Rosenberg G, Pierce WS (1987) A telemetry system for the implanted artificial heart and ventricular assist device. To be presented at Ninth Annual Conf IEEE/EMBS, Boston

30. Geselowitz DB, Miller GE, Phillips WM (1977) Dynamic model of a sac-type pneumatically driven artificial ventricle. Trans ASME (J Biomech Eng) 99 (K): 14–17

31. Kern SE (1986) Control system design for the Penn State electric total artificial heart using computer simulation. M.S. Thesis, The Pennsylvania State University

32. Landis DL, Rosenberg G, Donachy JH, Pierce WS (1980) Automatic control for the artificial heart. IEEE 1980 Frontiers of Engineering in Health Care, pp 305–310

33. Snyder AJ (1986) Introductory lecture on control. In: Bucherl ES (ed) Proceedings of Second World Symposium of the Total Artificial Heart. Vieweg, Braunschweig

34. Greathouse SL, Lewis JB, Ostroff AH, Geselowitz DB, Rosenberg G, Pierce WS (1983) Velocity control of motor-driven ventricular assist device. Proceedings 5th Annual Conference IEEE Engineering in Medicine and Biology Society, pp 433–437

35. Hanson KL, Tsach U, Kern SE, Geselowitz DB, Rosenberg G, Pierce WS (1985) A microprocessor-based feedback control system for the Penn State EVAD. Proceedings 7th Annual Conference IEEE Engineering in Medicine and Biology Society, pp 786–789

36. Snyder AJ (1987) Automatic electric control of an electric motor-driven total artificial heart. PhD Dissertation in Bioengineering, The Pennsylvania State University, University Park

37. Tsach U, Geselowitz DB, Sinha A, Tirinato J, Hsu HK, Rosenberg G, Pierce WS (1987) Minimum power consumption of the electric ventricular assist device through the design of an optimal output controller. ASAIO Trans

38. Rosenberg G, Landis DL, Phillips WM, Stallsmith J, Pierce WS (1978) Determining arterial pressure, left atrial pressure, and cardiac output from the left pneumatic drive line of the total artificial heart. Trans Am Soc Artif Intern Organs 24: 341–344

39. Snyder AJ, Rosenberg G, Landis D (1985) Indirect estimation of circulatory pressures for control of an electric motor-driven total artificial heart. 1985 ASME Winter Annual Meeting, Advances in Bioengineering, pp 87–88

40. Luenberger DG (1971) An introduction to observers. IEEE Transactions on Automatic Control AC-16: 596–602

# Discussion

*Atsumi* (University of Tokyo): The compliance chamber occupies the space in the chest cavity. Therefore, in order to save this space, we made a pump of chamberless design. The blood pump has a moving septal wall that separates the atrium and ventricle. The septal wall has an inflow valve and an outflow valve is also required. Thus, a compliance chamber is not necessary in our blood pump.

*Geselowitz* (Pennsylvania State University): The field is clearly such at the moment that there is still room for many different approaches. What usually happens in technology is that one particular approach emerges as the best, but it is not yet clear with the artificial heart which one that is going to be.

*Nitta* (Tohoku University): What was the direction of the echo beam in the measurement of flow velocity? Flow direction itself has a three-dimensional component.

*Geselowitz:* I tried to show this in my slide. The probes were positioned at different angles. With the pulse Doppler, of course, there is the restriction to the one component of velocity. There are a limited number of points where the beams intersect and the velocity in the plane of the pump can be obtained, though we gain no information about the velocity perpendicular to this. The information is limited, but it did provide us with some interesting data. A number of years ago, we used laser Doppler and we are planning to try this approach again.

*Nitta:* Is the value obtained from the Doppler method accurate, because your flow velocity is low, about 1.10 ml/s?

*Geselowitz:* The low-flow values are of course important near the wall, which is why we used hot-film anemometry.

*Hayashi* (Hokkaido University): With the hot-film anemometry did you detect any turbulences near the wall?

*Geselowitz:* Yes. We do ensemble averaging and obtain an RMS valve which is not the same every cycle. This could be turbulence or it could be just a characteristic of the flow, i.e., a beat-to-beat variation. The RMS values increase as the velocity increases and I think this is due to turbulence.

*Hayashi:* You have been developing two types of electromechanical system—the roller-type and cam-type actuators. Which do you think is better?

*Geselowitz:* We do not have the resources to pursue both of these systems, and about a year ago we had to decide between them. We opted for the roller screw. One of the reasons is that we think we can make a smaller motor with the roller screw. We also believe that as far as wear is concerned the roller screw is preferable. The longest survival though was in fact obtained with the cam.

*Hayashi:* What were the most difficult problems to solve in developing the roller-screw system?

*Geselowitz:* A lot of the technology that I have been discussing could be transferred to the roller screw system. With the cam, there is less than one revolution and there is a one-to-one correspondence between the angle of the rotor and the position of pusher plate. With the roller screw, there are about six revolutions to move the pusher plate from one end to the other. So, care has to be taken to keep track of the fact that each angle of rotation may correspond to six different positions. But in terms of control, the same strategies can be used for both systems. Sometimes, with the cam, there seemed to be some problems with slippage. This does not occur with the roller screw.

# 31. Development of multiparameter automatic control system of total artificial heart for analysis of circulation mechanism

Tsuneo Chinzei[1], Kou Imachi[2], Kiyoshi Maeda[2], Kunihiko Mabuchi[2], Yuusuke Abe[2], Kaoru Imanishi[2], Takumi Yonezawa[2], Iwao Fujimasa[1], and Kazuhiko Atsumi[2]

**Summary.** A fully automatic pneumatically driven total artificial heart (TAH) system was developed with the following objectives: (a) Analysis of the circulatory mechanism under normal and abnormal conditions; (b) clarification of the required performance of the TAH pump under various conditions such as rest and exercise; (c) establishing the data acquisition of biochemical factors, neurological factors, exercise, and their feedback to the TAH system.

This system consists of three decentralized processing and control units with a multimicroprocessor, pneumatic driving unit, data processing unit, and digital servo unit; it achieves a rapid response (each pulse), broad controllable range, flexibility of control algorithm, and multichannel control input.

Using this system, predictive control during treadmill exercise was examined. Predictive blood flow rate curves for the TAH were established based the hemodynamic response of normal goats during and after exercise. The system was able to track well the predictive blood flow rate curves.

**Key words:** Total artificial heart—Automatic control—Simulation—Exercise

The present control method of the artificial heart (AH) is satisfactory for patients confined to bed. However, AH patients cannot enjoy a high quality of life. To develop an AH system which can respond to all circumstances of the patient's daily life, study of the control algorithm of the circulation in the living body is important. For this purpose, an adequate TAH driving system with multiparameter control by computer is necessary. This AH control system makes the following studies possible:

a) Analysis of the circulatory mechanism under normal and abnormal conditions
   1) Simulation of the hemodynamic response of the natural heart in the TAH animal
   2) Analysis of the hemodynamic reaction of the TAH animal under controlled abnormal hemodynamics
b) Clarification of the required performance of the TAH pump under various conditions of the TAH animal such as rest and exercise
c) Establishment of the data acquisition of biochemical factors, neurological factors, and their feedback methods to the TAH system

This paper reports the fully automatic pneumatically driven AH system and its control algorithm, which have been developed in our laboratory.

## Background

The control factors of the natural heart are considered to be the following: intrinsic factors, such as Starling's law and end-systolic pressure-volume relationship; extrinsic factors, such as autonomic nerve and humoral factors. TAH control algorithms which have been reported in many laboratories have mostly been based on an analysis of the intrinsic factors of the natural heart. We have reported that control algorithms based only on Starling's law were inadequate for obtaining long-term survival because of hyper-output syndrome and progressive peripheral circulatory insufficiencies [1]. The reason is that Starling's curve is not a fixed function curve in the living body but is influenced by the contractility and afterload of the natural heart [2]. Moreover, extrinsic factors are dominant in the living body for long-term survival. Thus, it is important to clarify the extrinsic factors and circulatory mechanisms in the living body under various conditions.

With this in mind, we have developed computer-controlled TAH driving systems. In 1965, we reported the first on-line controlled TAH system [3]. In this system, the blood pressure waveform simulated that of the natural heart by computer and the relation between the waveform of each pulse and peripheral circulation was analyzed. In 1977, we reported the computer simulation of hemodynamics on exercise and long-term TAH pumping [4–6]. In this simulation,

[1] Research Center for Advanced Science and Technology, University of Tokyo, 4-6-1 Komaba, Meguro-ku, Tokyo, 153 Japan
[2] Institute of Medical Electronics, Faculty of Medicine, University of Tokyo, 7-3-1 Hongo, Bunkyo-ku, Tokyo, 113 Japan

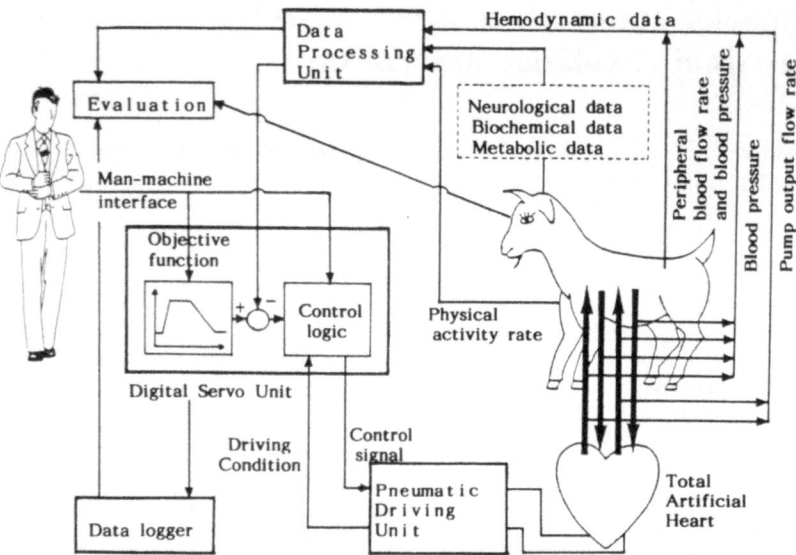

**Fig. 31.1.** Schematic and data flow of
the system

peripheral circulatory distribution and fluid transfer
through the capillary were considered. Since 1980, a
multiparameter automatic control TAH system has
been developed. Using this system, algorithms for
control of the multidriving parameters were studied.
In 1984, the hemodynamic response and multiparameter control of position changes in the TAH animal
were studied.

The advance of technology in microcomputers and
actuators makes real-time control of the TAH with a
compact system possible. Moreover, recent digital
control theory provides the background for multiparameter control algorithms. Following on this, the
new-type pneumatic control system of the TAH was
developed.

### Design concept of TAH control system

The required performance of the TAH control system
was decided to be as follows: (a) rapid response (each
pulse); (b) broad controllable range; (c) flexibility of
control alogrithm; (d) multichannel control input.

To attain these specifications, we employed the following architecture for the TAH control system: (a)
To increase the throughput of the system and software
flexibility, decentralized processing and control units
with multi-microprocessors were used. (b) For rapid
pneumatic pressure response, computer-controlled
electromagnetic valves and air compressors were utilized. (c) The data stream of hemodynamic parameters
was processed to the necessary characteristic values
on each pulse; other parameters such as physical
activity rate were also acquired and reduced to characteristic values. (d) A theoretical model to estimate

the condition of the AH pump and peripheral circulation on each pulse was set up. (e) A network (IEEE-
488) was set up between units; reduced and packed
information was exchanged.

### System description

The scheme and the data flow of the system developed
in this study are shown in Fig. 31.1. Figure 31.2 is a
whole view of the system. The system consists of three
units—pneumatic driving unit (PDU), data processing unit (DPU), and digital servo unit (DSU).

*Pneumatic driving unit*

In the PDU, eight parameters, such as positive and
negative driving pressure, S/D ratio, and pulse rate of
the right and left sides, can be controlled independently and simultaneously within one pulse by sending
a command (five characters/one parameter) from the
DSU. Table 31.1 shows the controllable range of the
driving parameters. To realize rapid response and
accurate setting of the parameters, a digitally controlled electromagnetic valve and air compressor and
local automatically controlled system with five microprocessors were employed. Figure 31.3 shows the outlet air pressure response to the controller command.
In this system, the S/D ratio and pulse rate respond
exactly to the control command at the next pulse.
Positive and negative driving pressures also respond
at the next pulse when the increment or decrement is
within 30 mmHg. The deviation of the positive and
negative driving pressures to the setting value is ±4
mmHg and ±2 mmHg, respectively.

**Fig. 31.2.** Whole view of the system: digital servo unit (*left*), data-processing unit (*middle*), pneumatic driving unit (*right*)

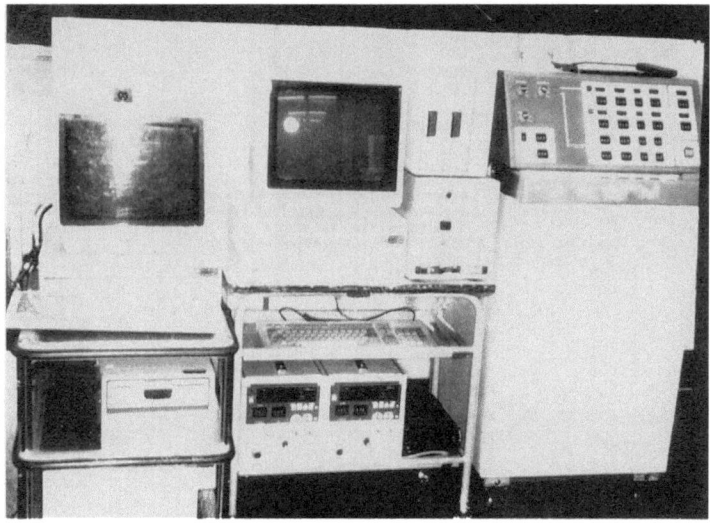

### Data-processing unit

The DPU can calculate mean blood pressures such as aortic pressure, pulmonary artery pressure, and left and right atrial pressure by each pulse. The pump stroke volume can also be measured by the DPU. To obtain rapid system response, it is necessary to process the data pulse-by-pulse. The data-sampling rate of the hemodynamic parameters is 100 Hz with 12 bit accuracy. The DPU can calculate the characteristic parameters as follows on real time: (a) mean pressure and blood flow rates of each pulse; (b) mean systolic and diastolic pressure of each pulse; (c) moving average of pressure and blood flow rate of N pulses.

Figure 31.4 shows a real-time process of the hemodynamic parameters. These parameters are used to estimate the pump movement and hemodynamic change.

The DPU was developed using a high-speed 16-bit microcomputer with the DMA sampler (16-channel analog port and two-channel digital port) and digital processing board. There is much room to sample and process other parameters such as peripheral circulation and physical activity rate.

### Digital servo unit

To construct an AH circulatory model and realize an automatic control system, AH blood pump function must be analyzed theoretically. As the flow-through valve and connector are turbulent and there is limitation in pump volume, the relation between driving parameters and stroke volume is not linear. An electrical circuit model of the AH pump can be expressed in Fig. 31.5a. With the pulsatile pump, the pump output is decided as the minimum between the blood volume

**Table 31.1.** Controllable range of driving parameters

| | |
|---|---|
| Right driving condition | |
| Positive pressure (mmHg) | 0–400 |
| Negative pressure (mmHg) | 0–150 |
| Systolic duration (%) | 10–90 |
| Pulse rate (beats/min) | 20–250 |
| Left driving condition | |
| Positive pressure (mmHg) | 0–400 |
| Negative pressure (mmHg) | 0–150 |
| Systolic duration (%) | 10–90 |
| Pulse rate (beats/min) | 20–250 |

which flows into the sac during the diastolic phase (SVi) and the blood volume which is expelled from the sac during the systolic phase (SVo)[4]. The total head loss on the pump inflow side (hit) and pump outflow side (hot) are given by:

$$h_{it} = K_{it} \times Q_{i2}^2/2g \qquad (1)$$
$$h_{ot} = K_{ot} \times Q_o/2g \qquad (2)$$

where Kit and Kot are the total loss coefficients on the inflow and outflow sides, respectively, and $Q_i$, $Q_o$ are the volume flow rate.

$$SV_i = Q_i/f \times (1 - sd)$$
$$= (2gh_{it}/K_{it})\frac{1}{2}/f \times (1 - sd) \qquad (3)$$

$$SV_o = Q_o/f \times sd$$
$$= (2gh_{ot}/K_{ot})\frac{1}{2}/f \times sd \qquad (4)$$

In pulsatile flow, the inflow volume ($SV_i$) and outflow volume ($SV_o$) per one pulse are given by Eqs. (3) and (4), respectively, where f is the heart rate and $s_d$ the

**Fig 31.3.** Outlet air pressure response to control command

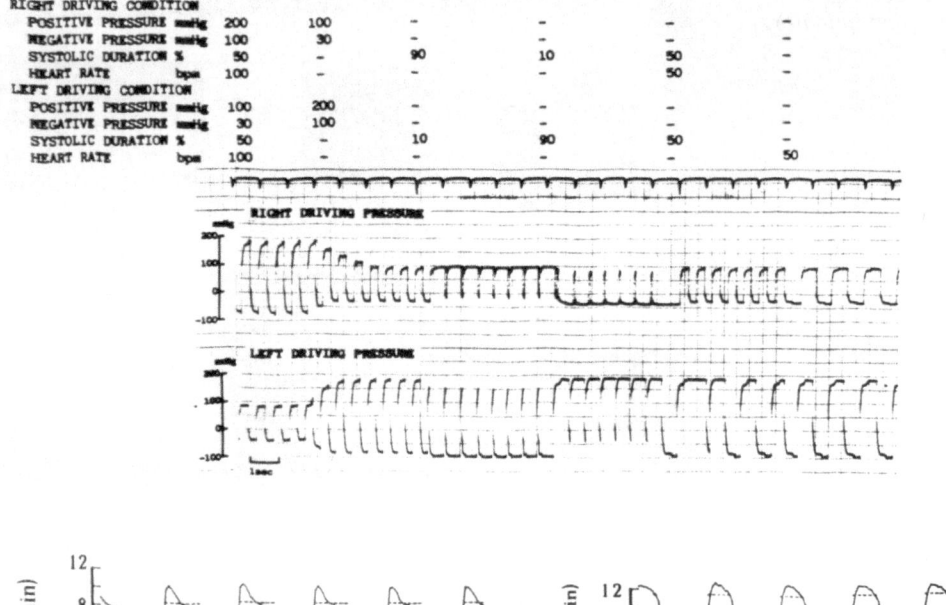

| | | | | | | | |
|---|---|---|---|---|---|---|---|
| **RIGHT DRIVING CONDITION** | | | | | | | |
| POSITIVE PRESSURE | mmHg | 200 | 100 | - | - | - | - |
| NEGATIVE PRESSURE | mmHg | 100 | 30 | - | - | - | - |
| SYSTOLIC DURATION | % | 50 | - | 90 | 10 | 50 | - |
| HEART RATE | bpm | 100 | - | - | - | 50 | - |
| **LEFT DRIVING CONDITION** | | | | | | | |
| POSITIVE PRESSURE | mmHg | 100 | 200 | - | - | - | - |
| NEGATIVE PRESSURE | mmHg | 30 | 100 | - | - | - | - |
| SYSTOLIC DURATION | % | 50 | - | 10 | 90 | 50 | - |
| HEART RATE | bpm | 100 | - | - | - | - | 50 |

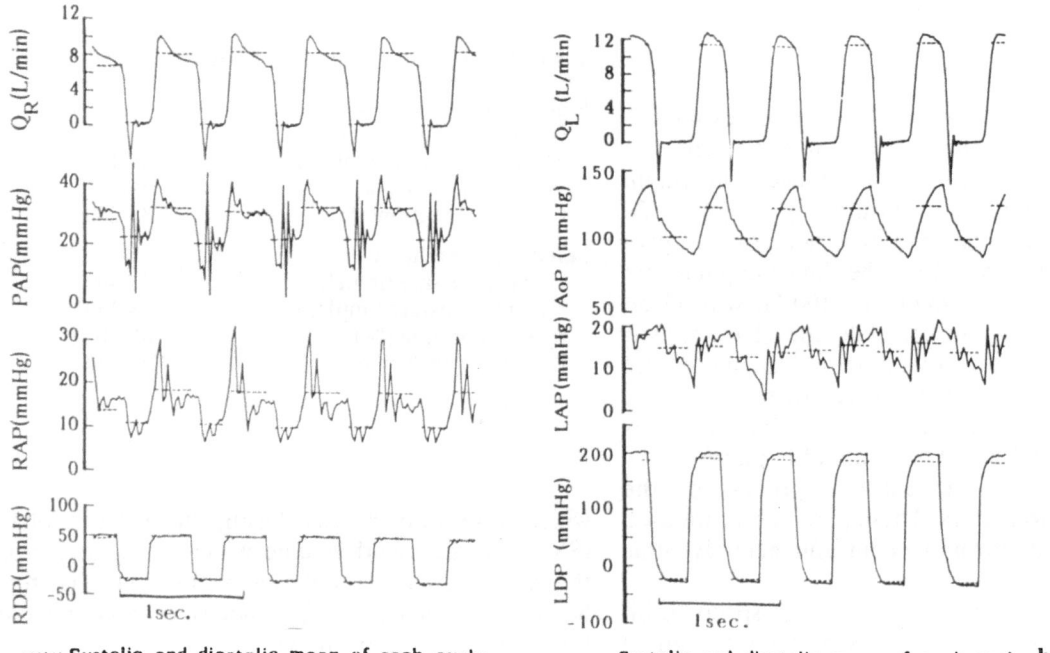

**a**　······ Systolic and diastolic mean of each cycle　　　······ Systolic and diastolic mean of each cycle **b**

**Fig. 31.4. a** Output recording of real-time process of hemodynamic parameters on right side. **b** Output recording of real-time process of hemodynamic parameters on left side

systolic duration. If the sac effective volume is $Vo$, the actual pump stroke volume is given as the minimum value among $VO$, $SV_i$, and $SV_o$. Thus, the stroke volume and the blood flow rate on each pulse are approximated as follows.

$$VD_n = \min (VO, VS_n - 1 + (100 - SD_n)/100 \times$$
$$(60/HR_n) \times \frac{1}{4} h_i \times (PI_n + NDP_n) \P \frac{1}{2}) \quad (5)$$
$$VS_n = \max (O, VD_n - SD_n/100 \times (60/HR_n) \times$$

$$(PDP_n - PO_n) \P \frac{1}{2}) \quad (6)$$
$$SV_n = VD_n - VS_n \quad (7)$$
$$Q_n = SV_n \times HR_n \quad (8)$$

Where $VD$ is the diastolic pump volume (ml), $VS$ the systolic pump volume (ml), $SV$ the stroke volume (ml), $VO$ the effective pump volume (ml), $h_i$ the pump inflow conductance, $h_o$ the pump outflow conductance, $PI$ the pump inflow pressure (diastolic mean; mmHg), *PO* the pump outflow pressure (systolic mean; mmHg), *NDP* the negative driving pressure (mmHg), *PDP* the positive driving pressure (mmHg), *SD* the systolic duration (%), *HR* the pulse rate (beats/min), $Q_n$ the pump output flow rate (ml/min), min $(a, b)$ the minimum value between $a$ and $b$, and max $(a, b)$ the maximum value between $a$ and $b$.

Figure 31.5b shows a comparison between the theoretical value and measured value obtained from the mock circulatory system when the parameter is changed. The figure indicates that the AH blood pump function can be expressed well theoretically.

On this basis, the DSU can execute various control algorithms in real time. The DSU receives hemodynamic data from the DPU and determines the value of control parameters according to loaded control algorithms and sends them to the PDU. The basic control algorithms given below are installed on the DSU.

### Estimation of pump driving condition

Figure 31.5b shows that the relation between cardiac output and systolic duration consists of two slopes and a plateau. The left slope represents the systolic restrict condition, and the right slope the diastolic restrict condition. The plateau indicates that the AH pump works in the full stroke condition. So, the DSU can estimate the pump driving state under given driving parameters and given inflow and outflow conductance and pressure, whether in the systolic, diastolic restrict condition or in full stroke condition, according to Eqs (5)–(7). Moreover, the DSU can determine the parameters and their values which have to be changed to meet a given cardiac output and the necessary pulses to reach the steady state by the iteration method. This routine is the core of the multiparameter control algorithm.

### In vivo automatic calculation of inflow and outflow pump conductance

The DSU can calculate in vivo inflow and outflow pump conductance, changing the driving condition over the cardiac output range of 3–8 l/min automatically. The inflow pump conductance of the left heart is calculated according to the left AH blood flow rate (QL), diastolic mean of left atrial pressure, left negative driving pressure (NDP), left heart rate (HR), and left systolic duration (SD) under various inflow restrict driving conditions. The outflow pump conductance of the left heart is calculated according to QL, systolic mean of aortic pressure, left positive driving pressure (PDP), left HR, and left SD under various outflow restrict driving conditions. The inflow pump conductance of the right heart is calculated according to the right AH blood flow rate (QR), diastolic mean of right atrial pressure, right NDP, right HR, and

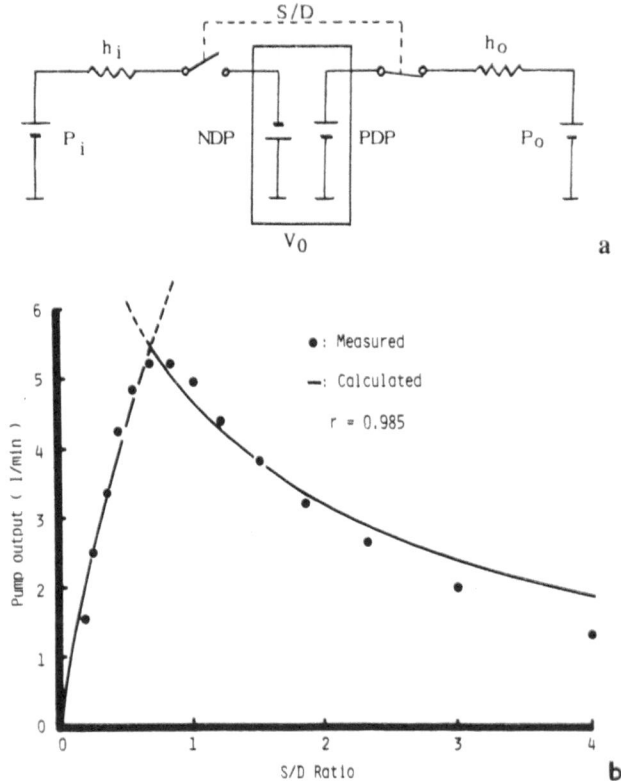

Fig. 31.5. a Schematic model of artificial heart pump. b Comparison between theoretical value and measured value using mock circulation in the cardiac output—S/D ratio relation. Inflow and outflow pressure is 8 cmH$_2$O and 100 mmHg, respectively. Driving pressure is 120–70 mmHg. The heart rate is 91 beats/min. Pump volume is 90 ml

right SD under various inflow restrict driving conditions. The outflow pump conductance of the right heart is calculated according to QR, systolic mean of pulmonary artery pressure, right PDP, right HR, and right SD under various outflow restrict driving conditions.

The blood flow rate of the right and left heart is measured by the electromagnetic flowmeter on the outflow side of the AH pump.

### Tracking control system of AH output blood flow rate

The core of the multiparameter control algorithm mentioned above determines the driving parameters to track a given time function of cardiac output. Since there are many pairs of driving parameters which meet a given cardiac output, the following strategy is employed to select one pair: (a) to change the least number of parameters; (b) each driving parameter has an optimal range according to given cardiac output and the inflow and outflow pressure; (c) the overdrive is used to respond rapidly to the steep cardiac output curve.

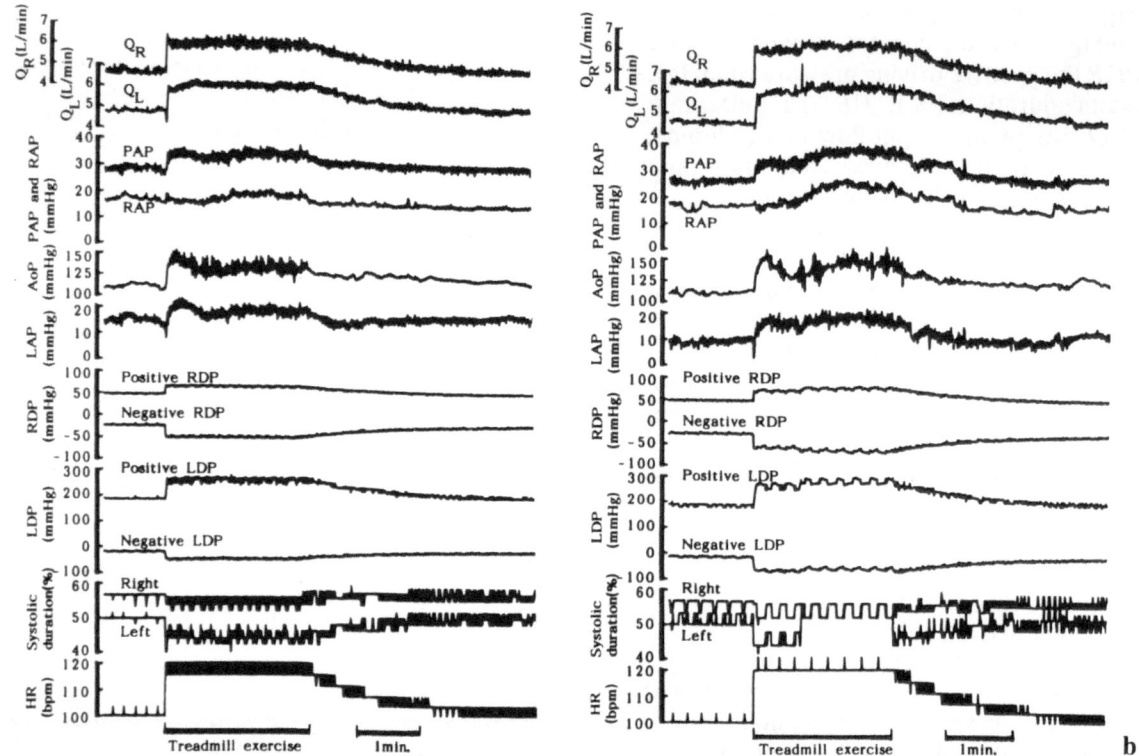

**Fig. 31.6a, b.** Digital recording data of hemodynamic response and control sequence during the treadmill exercise at **a** 1.8 km/h and **b** 3.6 km/h

### Tracking control system of AH inflow or outflow pressure

To control the AH inflow and outflow pressure, a peripheral circulation model between the cardiac output and the inflow and outflow pressure is necessary. We employ an ordinary constant RC network as the model for the peripheral circulation. This model is effective only under resting conditions; it is not effective with position changes, such as a sitting to a standing position or during exercise. It is the major objective with this system to construct a peripheral circulation model which is effective under various circumstances and several studies are in progress.

### Application example

As an application of this system, a study of predictive control in which the AH pump simulates the natural heart response in treadmill exercise has been done with TAH goats (see chapter 32). Digitally recorded and processed data of hemodynamic response and control sequences are shown in Fig. 31.6.

As a first step, in vivo inflow and outflow pump con-

ductance of the right and left AH are measured, changing automatically the pump driving condition. These parameters are supplied to the driving condition optimizing routine in the system. Before this study, predictive curves of blood flow rate during treadmill exercise at various speeds were computed according to measurements of the hemodynamics of natural heart goats during and after exercise. The system tracked well these predictive curves for treadmill exercise, changing eight parameters such as positive and negative driving pressure, systolic duration, and pulse rate of the right and left sides.

Three parameters—treadmill speed, start and end timing of exercise—were input manually in this study. As a next step, feedback control of blood flow rate with physical activity rate in treadmill exercise is planned and experiments are currently under way. The movement sensor detects the start and end timing of exercise and estimates the physical activity rate. According to the relation between physical activity rate and cardiac output of the natural heart, the time function of cardiac output is determined. Various sensing methods for movement are presently being tested.

## References

1. Atsumi K, Sakurai Y, Fujimasa I, Imachi K, Nishisaka T, Mano I, Ohmichi H, Mori J, Iwai N, Kouno A (1975) Hemodynamic analysis on prolonged survival cases (30 days and 20 days) of artificial total heart replacement. Trans Am Soc Artif Int Organs XXI: 545–554
2. Herndon CW, Sagawa K (1969) Combined effects of aortic and right atrial pressures on aortic flow. Am J Physiol 217: 65–72
3. Atsumi K, Sakurai Y, Fujimasa I, Omoto R, Suzuki R, Minami S, Miura H (1965) Artificial control of artificial heart with digital computer. Digest of the 6th International Conference on Medical Engineering and Biological Engineering, Tokyo, pp 333–336
4. Imachi K, Fujimasa I, Miyake H, Takido N, Nakajima M, Iwai N, Kouno A, Ono T and Atsumi K (1980) Computer aided designing system for artificial heart pump. In: Lindberg DAB, Kaihara S (eds) MEDINFO 80 Proceedings of the Third World Conference on Medical Informatics, 29 Sept–4 Oct 1980, Tokyo, North-Holland, pp 1144–1148
5. Fujimasa I, Imachi K, Ohmichi H, Takasugi S, Nishisaka T, Iwai N, Kouno A, Miyake H, Atsumi K (1978) A circulatory dynamic model for artificial heart control. Artif Organs 2 (suppl): 214–216
6. Ohmichi H, Imachi K, Fujimasa I, Nishisaka T, Iwai N, Kouno A, Atsumi K (1978) Hemodynamic and blood gas analysis in a total artificial heart replaced animal during treadmill exercise. Artif Organs 2 (suppl): 230–233

# 32. Predictive control of total artificial heart during exercise

Kiyoshi Maeda, Tsuneo Chinzei, Kou Imachi, Kunihiko Mabuchi, Yuusuke Abe, Kaoru Imanishi, Iwao Fujimasa, and Kazuhiko Atsumi[1]

**Summary.** To establish a total artificial heart (TAH) control method during exercise, we developed a predictive control method in which cardiac output (CO) is controlled predictively based on the objective function curve obtained from natural heart (NH) goats subjected to various grades of exercise. During treadmill exercise, CO of the TAH was controlled to follow the objective function curve by changing the driving parameters, such as positive and negative pressures, S/D ratio, and pulse rate of both artificial heart (AH) pumps under the control algorithm installed in a computer.

The following conclusions were obtained. (a) By using the predictive control method, the time-course of left and right CO in the TAH during exercise was almost the same as in the NH. (2) Blood lactate and blood catecholamine changes during exercise with the predictive control method were lower than with the fixed control method, where the driving parameters did not change during exercise. (3) Blood catecholamine, like blood lactate, was thought to be a suitable parameter for evaluating the CO for the TAH during exercise.

**Key words:** Total artificial heart—Treadmill exercise—Predictive control method—Blood lactate—Blood catecholamine

It has become obvious that the total artificial heart (TAH) recipient can live for a long time under resting conditions, in view of the fact that Mr William Shroeder could survive for 619 days and the TAH goat could survive for 344 days at the University of Tokyo.

As a next step, it is to be hoped that the TAH recipient will be able to return to work and enjoy a high quality of life and engage in such activities as sports. However, the control method of the TAH during exercise has not yet been established. In most papers in the past, it has been asserted that there is no need to change the driving parameters of the artificial heart (AH) during exercise, because TAH animals can adjust to exercise by adapting their peripheral circulatory system. However, it is difficult to achieve a large increase in CO with this intrinsic control method and, in fact, TAH patients and animals cannot tolerate heavy exercise. In general, CO of the natural heart (NH) increase dynamically according to the various grades of exercise. Thus we consider that CO of the TAH should be controlled to increase like the NH during exercise. One of the difficulties in establishing a good TAH control method during exercise is that there is no method of cardiac output (CO) demand in the TAH recipient during exercise. In this study, we propose a new control method for the TAH during exercise, whereby CO is controlled predictively along with the objective function curve obtained from the NH goat according to the grade of exercise.

## Materials and methods

As NH goat (body weight 50 kg) was subjected to various grades of treadmill exercise. An electromagnetic flow probe (EMF) was attached to the ascending aorta and measured the hemodynamic changes. CO changes at each treadmill speed were recorded by microcomputer as a time function; the changes were used for the TAH goat as an objective function in the treadmill exercise. The treadmill speeds were 1.8 and 3.6 km/h. The exercise time was usually 3 min. The treadmill plane was horizontal.

The same treadmill exercise was performed on 8711 TAH goat (body weight 50 kg), the NH of which was resected and replaced by a TAH. Left and right AH pumps are placed on the chest wall. The treadmill exercise was begun after 7 postoperative days (POD) when blood gas showed pH of 7.5, $PCO_2 < 40$ mmHg, and $PO_2 > 100$ mmHg while breathing room air. Treadmill exercise was repeated two to three times/week as long as the TAH animal remained healthy.

The AH control system consisted of a pneumatic AH driver, data-processing module, and control module (Fig. 32.1). The predictive control algorithm was installed to the digital servo-controller in the control module (Fig. 32.2). During the treadmill exercise, CO was controlled to follow the objective function curve by changing the driving parameters such as positive pressure, negative pressure, S/D ratio, and pulse rate

[1] Institute of Medical Electronics, Faculty of Medicine, University of Tokyo, 7-3-1 Hongo, Bunkyo-ku, Tokyo, 113 Japan

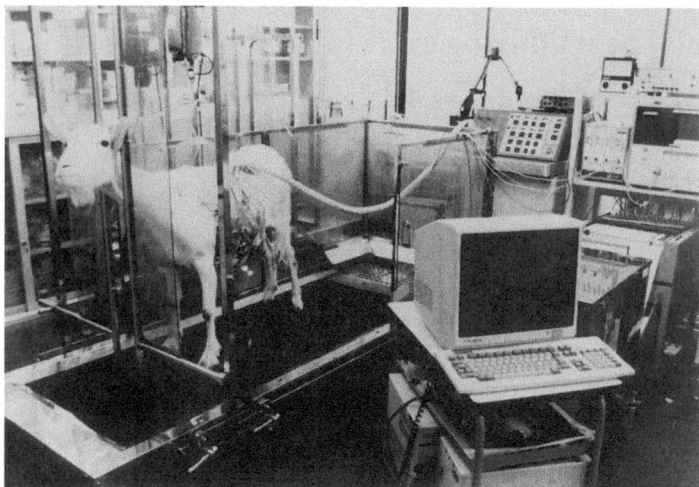

**Fig. 32.1.** 8711 TAH goat on treadmill, pneumatic AH driver, data processing module, and computer

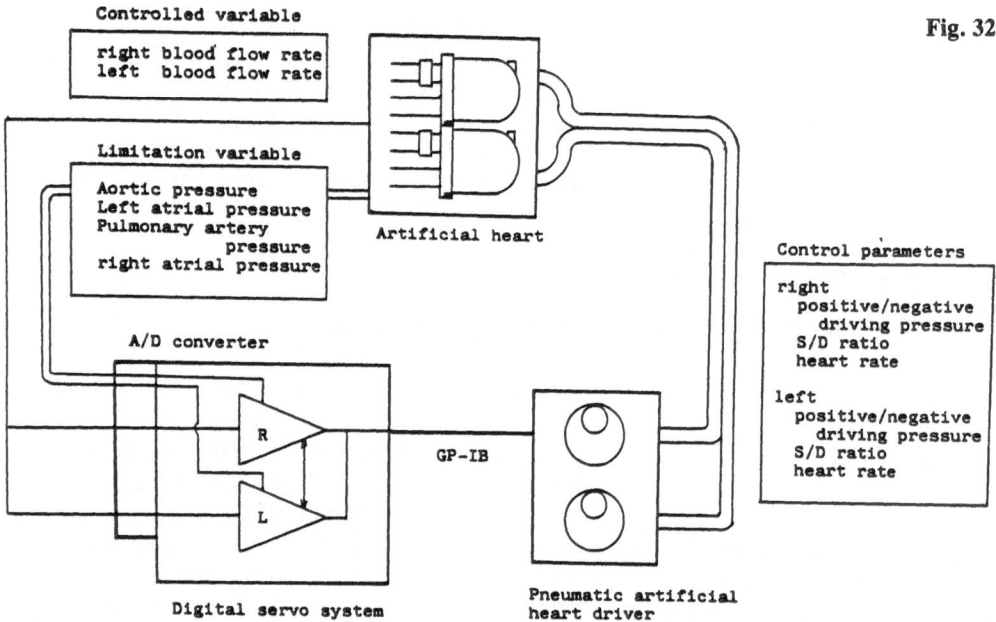

**Fig. 32.2.** System configuration

of both AH pumps under the control algorithm in the control module (Fig. 32.3). The treadmill speed and the start and end timing of exercise were input manually from the computer keyboard.

To evaluate the predictive control method, the following data were measured before, immediately after, and 10 min after exercise: (a) blood lactate as an evaluative measure of metabolism; (b) blood catecholamine as measure of hormonal secretion; (c) blood hemoglobin as a carrier of oxygen to the tissue; and (d) arteriovenous (AV) oxygen difference as an oxygen reception factor in the peripheral tissue. The data were measured three times for each exercise speed.

The predictive control method was compared with the fixed control method, in which the driving para-

meters were not changed during the treadmill exercise. In the fixed control method also, the above data were measured three times for each exercise speed.

## Result

### Hemodynamic changes in NH goat and TAH goat

Figure 32.4 shows the hemodynamic changes in the NH goat and TAH goat with the predictive control method at 1.8 km/h and 3.6 km/h exercise speed. In the NH goat, the most remarkable point was rapid and strong increase in CO during exercise. Even during light exercise, such as a speed of like 1.8 km/h, CO increased by about 1.8 times more than in the

**Fig. 32.3.** 8711 TAH goat during treadmill exercise

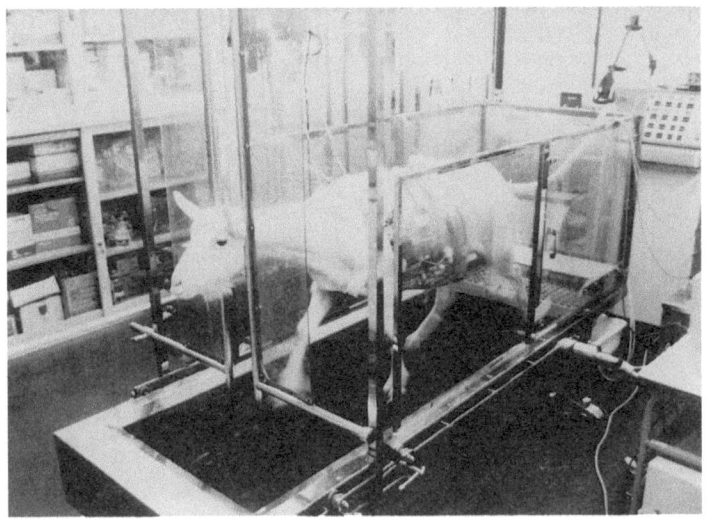

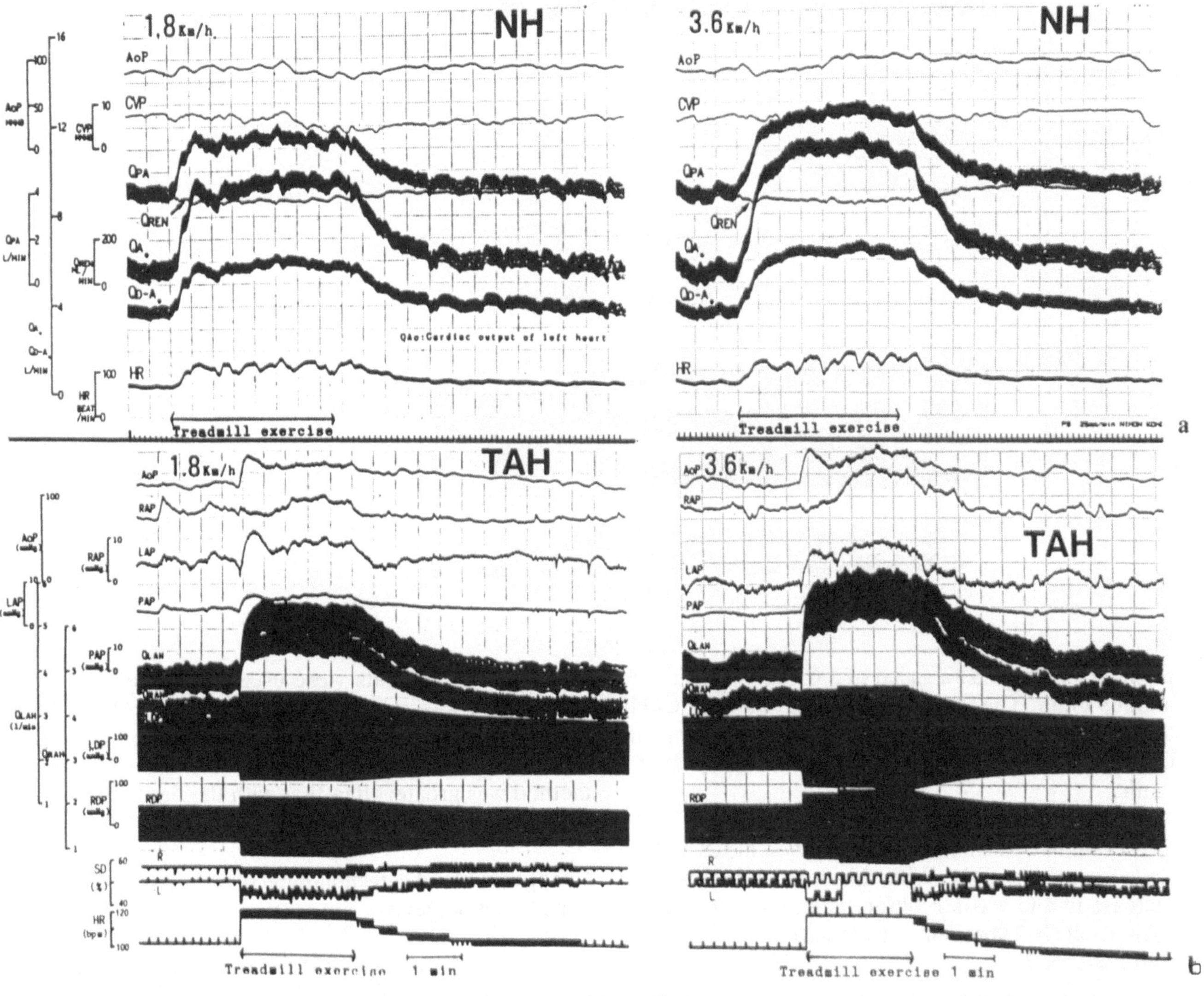

**Fig. 32.4. a** Hemodynamic changes in NH and TAH goat with predictive control method at 1.8 km/h before, during, and after exercise. *AoP* aortic pressure, *LAP* left atrial pressure, *PAP* pulmonary arterial pressure, *RAP* right atrial pressure, *QLAH* cardiac output of left AH, *QRAH* cardiac output of right AH, *LDP* left driving pressure, *RDP* right driving pressure, *SD* systolic duration. **b** Hemodynamic changes in NH goat and TAH goat with predictive control method at 3.6 km/h before, during, and after exercise

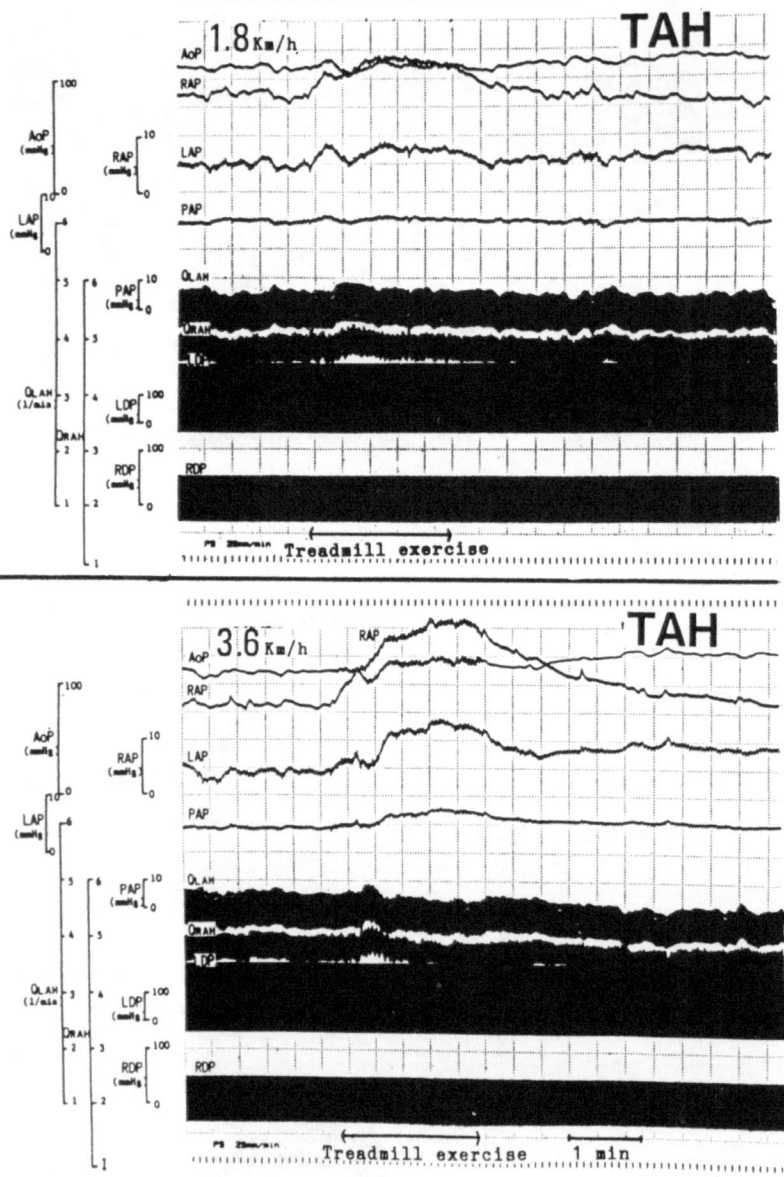

**Fig. 32.5.** Hemodynamic changes in TAH goat with fixed control method at 1.8 and 3.6 km/h before, during, and after exercise. *Abbreviations* as in Fig. 4

resting condition. At a speed of 3.6 km/h CO reached about 9 l/min. The time-course of left and right CO in the TAH was similar to that in the NH. However, the CO of 8711 TAH goat could not be increased over 7 l/min.

Figure 32.5 shows the hemodynamic changes in the TAH goat with the fixed control method at 1.8 and 3.6 km/h exercise speeds. With this control method, the increase in CO was not observed and the increase in right atrial (RA) pressure was remarkable at 3.6 km/h exercise speed.

### Changes in blood lactate level

Figure 32.6 shows blood lactate changes in the NH goat and TAH goat at 1.8 and 3.6 km/h exercise speeds before, immediately after, and 10 min after ex-

ercise. Five NH goats were used. At a speed of 1.8 km/h, there was no significant difference between the predictive and fixed control methods. But at 3.6 km/h, the blood lactate change with the fixed control method was greater than that with the predictive control method.

### Changes in blood catecholamine (adrenaline and noradrenaline) level

Figure 32.7 shows the blood catecholamine (adrenaline and noradrenaline) changes in the NH goat and TAH goat at 1.8 and 3.6 km/h before, immediately after, and 10 min after exercise. At both exercise speeds, the blood catecholamine change with the fixed control method was much greater than with the predictive control method.

**Fig. 32.6.** Blood lactate changes and NH goat and TAH goat at 1.8 and 3.6 km/h before, immediately after, and 10 min after exercise

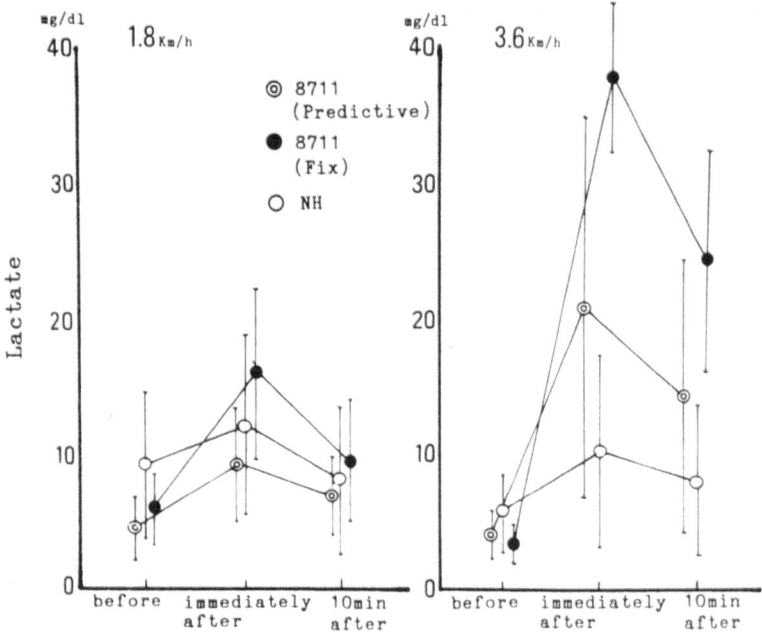

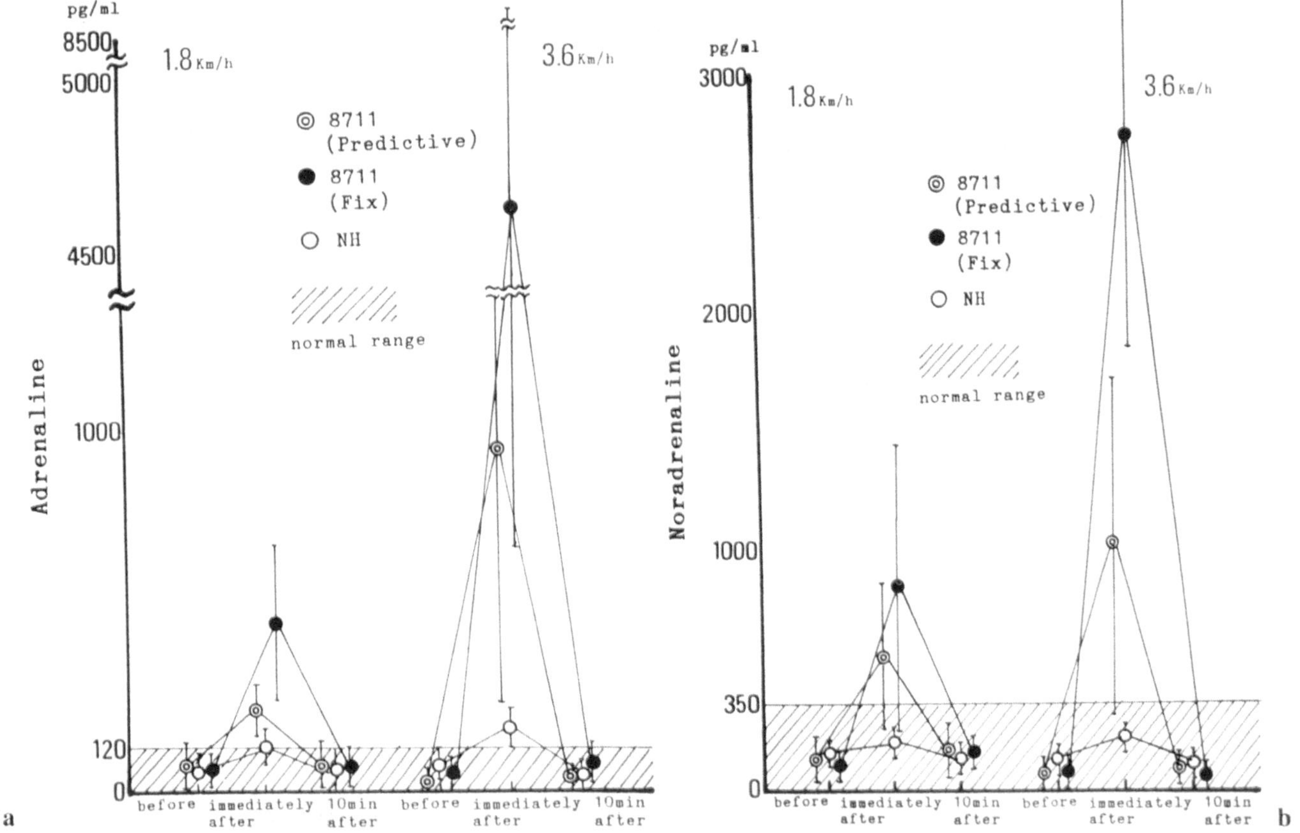

**Fig. 32.7.** **a** Adrenaline changes in NH goat and TAH goat at 1.8 and 3.6 km/h before, immediately after, and 10 min after exercise. **b** Noradrenaline changes in NH goat and TAH goat at 1.8 and 3.6 km/h before, immediately after, and 10 min after exercise

## Changes in blood hemoglobin and AV oxygen difference

Figure 32.8 shows the rate of increase (as compared with the resting condition) of blood hemoglobin and AV oxygen difference in the TAH goat immediately after exercise. Both factors showed a higher rate of increase with the fixed control method and at 3.6 km/h.

## Discussion

There are in the world several control methods of the TAH in the resting condition. Hiller et al. proposed the use of Starling's law as a TAH control method in 1962 [1]. This has been used by many researchers without criticising its propriety due to its simplicity and ease of implementation. Pierce et al. have proposed a control method in which arterial pressure is maintained as a constant value [2]. At the University of Tokyo, CO is restricted within the physiological level (80–100 ml/kg/min) by controlling the right AH pump output [3]

It is doubtful whether these control methods are effective during exercise, because they are designed for the resting condition. However, most past papers have pointed out that the TAH recipient could tolerate exercise to some extent with the same control method as that used for the resting condition. Lunn et al., Stanley et al., and Chiang et al. demonstrated that according to that Starling's law the TAH recipient could tolerated exercise by adapting peripheral vessel resistance without changing the driving parameters

[4–6]. Kito et al. and Mitamura et al. maintained that the TAH recipient increased the AV oxygen difference more than the NH animal and could tolerate exercise by increasing the oxygen intake ratio in the tissues and organs [7, 8]. In the present study, we first analyzed the hemodynamics of the NH in detail. As a result, the CO of the NH increased greatly and rapidly even at 1.8 km/h, just like with a normal walking speed. We considered that CO was the most significant parameter in TAH control and that the essence of TAH control was to achieve adequate CO according to the demand of the peripheral tissues and organs. Thus, it is evident that if CO does not increase significantly only by adaptation in a peripheral circulatory system, the TAH recipient cannot satisfy the oxygen demand sufficiently during exercise and will be subject to great stress.

In the NH, the increase of CO during exercise can be obtained by the following two mechanisms: sympathetic stimulation, with an increase in venous return and heart rate or stroke volume or both, and Starling's law.

In particular, the sympathetic nerve system detects a physiological stress, such as the strain from exercise or excitement, and an abnormal stress, such as a circulatory or respiratory failure, transmits this information to the peripheral organs, and adapts the circulation and metabolism to meet this demand. However, in the present TAH system, there is no feedback loop to transmit this information to the AH control system because there is no sensor which can detect continuously the automatic nerve activity or amount of chemical mediator in the long term. Therefore, we proposed the concept of the predictive control method:

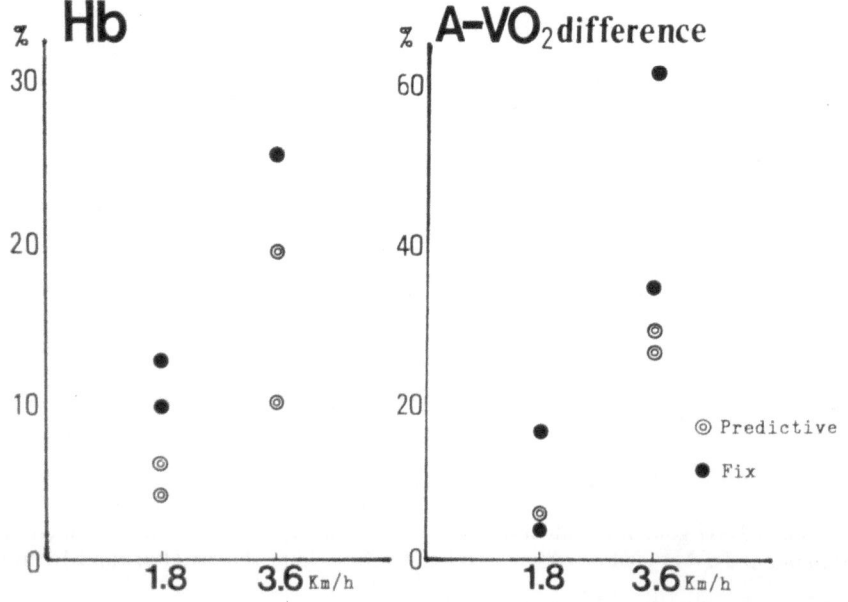

**Fig. 32.8.** Rate of increase (compared with resting condition) of blood hemoglobin and AV oxygen difference in TAH goat immediately after exercise

According to the objective function curve on various grades of exercise, which we predicted from the NH goat, we control the quantity of CO during exercise in the TAH recipient; in order to close the objective function curve, we change the driving parameters such as positive pressure, negative pressure, S/D ratio, and pulse rate of both AH pumps.

In this study, we made an algorithm for the predictive control method and subjected the TAH goat to the treadmill exercise using it. As a result, this new AH control system could simulate the hemodynamic response of the NH in various grades of exercise. On the other hand, when the TAH goat was subjected to the treadmill exercise without the predictive control method (with the fixed control method), no increase in CO was found. If the driving parameters are set at a high value prior to the exercise, CO certainly increases during exercise, reacting to the increase in venous return. But a high driving condition at rest is thought to be undesirable from the viewpoint of durability of the AH pump, pressure stress to the lung, and high output syndrome.

Our position is supported by the following data.

### Blood lactate

Blood lactate is known to increase as a result of anaerobic metabolism and it has been frequently measured in cardiovascular surgery and sports medicine. In 1981, Imachi et al. noted the importance of blood lactate in the evaluation of the metabolic state of the TAH [9]. They measured blood lactate during and after TAH surgical procedures or during treadmill exercise. As a result, they indicated that blood lactate was a suitable parameter for monitoring the prognosis of the TAH animal after a surgical operation and a suitable parameter for the study of TAH control methodologies. In the present study, changes in blood lactate level indicated no significant difference between the predictive control and fixed control methods at 1.8 km/h. But at 3.6 km/h, changes in blood lactate level with the predictive control method had a tendency to be lower than with the fixed control method. This shows that the fixed control method does not satisfy sufficiently oxygen demands in the tissues and organs during exercise because there is no increase in CO.

### Blood catecholamine

The blood catecholamine level dramatically affects the dynamics of the cardiovascular system and, at the same time, plays an important role in protecting the living body from the effects of stress. Measuring its level is thought to be important from the viewpoint of evaluation of the regulation capacity of the sympathetic neuroadrenal medullary system. In the human body, as the level of exercise increases, blood catecholamine levels increase proportional to oxygen consumption [10]. In the present study, and as observed in the NH goat, blood catecholamine levels increased with the increase in the level of exercise, and the changing pattern was similar to that of blood lactates. In the TAH goat, the increase in adrenaline and noradrenaline levels with the predictive control method was lower than with the fixed control method. Inoue and Sato indicated that a patient with heart failure had a low response of positive chronotropic effect and positive inotropic effect for sympathetic nerve stimulation and to maintain normal heart functions, the sympathetic nerves had to be excited more strongly [11]. In severe heart failure, there is a limit for the functions of the heart, even if the sympathetic nerve system is exerted. In this study, the cause of the high level of catecholamine immediately after exercise is thought to be due to the fact that the TAH with the fixed control method cannot supply sufficient CO for the oxygen demand in the tissues and organs, just as in the severe heart failure patient.

This result indicates that in the TAH recipient blood catecholamine shows a normal response to the circulatory dynamics and that it is capable of being used as a parameter for monitoring CO during exercise. Stanley et al. also indicated that the dynamics of blood catecholamine in TAH calves paralleled the changes in oxygen consumption and could be used as a parameter for TAH control [12].

In the present study, the increase in blood lactate and blood catecholamine in the TAH goat with the predictive control method was higher than in the NH goat. The cause of this is thought to be that the maximum CO of 8711 TAH goat was about 7.0 l/min during exercise.

### Blood hemoglobin and AV oxygen difference

Blood hemoglobin and AV oxygen difference increased with the fixed control method. This indicates that the oxygen intake ratio showed a greater increase in the tissues because CO was insufficient in the fixed control method. But even though blood hemoglobin and oxygen difference increased with the fixed control method, there is a limit for the compensation capacity. Moreover, as mild anemia is observed in the TAH recipient [13, 14], the living body with the TAH has to depend more strongly on the increase in CO.

The results of this study can be summarized as follows.

Although the TAH goat with the fixed control method could tolerate the treadmill exercise for speeds of up to 3.6 km/h by adapting the peripheral circulatory system and increasing the blood hemoglobin and AV oxygen difference, the changes in blood lactate and blood catecholamine levels showed that the fixed control method forced an abnormal adaptation and put a big stress on the TAH goat.

At 8711 TAH Goat, the maximum CO was about 7.0 l/min, which was thought to be insufficient for this grade of exercise. However, when the predictive control method was used, the stress to the TAH goat was milder than the stress with the fixed control method.

In this study, the exercise speed, the start and end timing of exercise were input manually. However, the experiment in which these three parameters are automatically detected by acceleration sensor, are undergoing in our laboratory.

## Conclusion

The predictive control method for the TAH recipient during exercise was developed.

By using the predictive control method, the time-course of left and right CO in the TAH during exercise was almost the same as in the NH.

From the viewpoint of changes in blood lactate, blood catecholamine, hemoglobin, and AV oxygen difference, the stress on the tissues and organs with the predictive control method was less than with the fixed control method.

Blood catecholamine is thought to be a suitable parameter for evaluating the adequacy of CO for the TAH during exercise, as demonstrated with blood lactate.

## References

1. Hiller KW, Seidel W, Kolff WJ (1962) A servomechanism to drive an artificial heart inside the chest. Trans Am Soc Artif intern Organs 8: 125
2. Pierce WJ, Landis D, O'bannon W, Donachy JH, White W, Phillips W, Brighton JA (1976) Automatic control of artificial heart. Trans Am Soc Artif Intern Organs 22: 347
3. Imachi K (1981) How to control the total artificial heart. Jpn J Artif Organ 10: 687
4. Lunn JK, Liu WS, Stanley TH, Gentry S, Kolff J, Olsen D (1976) Effects of treadmill exercise on cardiovascular and respiratory dynamics before and after artificial heart implantation. Trans Am Soc Artif Intern Organs 22: 315
5. Stanley TH, Lunn JK, Liu WS, Gentry S (1978) Comparison of cardiovascular responses and left ventricular work during exercise before and after artificial heart implantation. Surgery 83: 542
6. Chiang BY, Olsen DB, Gaykowski R, Dries D, Burns GL, Hamanaka Y, Murray RD, Ilyia E, Dew PA, Hughes SD, Nielsen SD, Kolff WJ (1984) Evaluation of treadmill exercise on total artificial heart recipients. Trans Am Soc Artif Intern Organs 30: 514
7. Kito Y, Honda T, Gibson WH, Nemoto T, Akutsu T (1974) Hemodynamic studies during exercise in calves with total artificial heart. Trans Am Soc Artif Intern Organs 20: 667
8. Mitamura Y, Jacobs G, Kasai S, Morinaga N, Washizu T, Koshino I, Kiraly RJ, Nose Y (1977) Henodynamic studies during exercise on a treadmill in the calf with a total cardiac prosthesis. J Surg Res 23: 75
9. Imachi K, Fujimasa I, Takido N, Nakajima M, Miyamoto A, Tsukagoshi S, Inou N, Motomura K, Kouno A, Ono T, Atsumi K (1982) Blood lactate as an evaluation parameter for artificial heart (AH) control method establishment. Jpn J Artif Organs 11: 305
10. Brooks GA, Fahey TD (1984) Exercise physiology. Wiley, New York, p 176
11. Inoue M, Sato H (1986) The dynamics of sympathetic nerve and blood catecholamine in heart failure. Int Medicine 58: 1317
12. Stanley TH, Liu WJ, Gentry S, Kennard L, Isern-Amaral J, Olsen D, Lunn J (1976) Blood and urine catecholamine concentrations after implantation of artificial heart. J Thorac Cardiovasc Surg 71: 704
13. DeVries WC, Anderson JL, Joyce LD, Anderson FL, Hammond EH, Jarvik RK, Kolff WJ (1984) Clinical use of total artificial heart. New Eng J Medicine 310: 273
14. Imachi K, Fujimasa I, Nakajima M, Mabuchi K, Tsukagoshi S, Motomura K, Miyamoto A, Takido N, Inou N, Kouno A, Ono T, Atsumi K (1984) Overall analysis of the causes of pathophysiological problems in total artificial heart in animals by cardiac receptor hypothesis. Trans Am Soc Artif Intern Organs 30: 591

# Discussion

*Takatani* (National Cardiovascular Center): What kind of algorithm do you use to change the pump output? In Dr. Chinzei's slide, as soon as exercise was initiated, although right and left pump output was increased, left atrial pressure was elevated close to about 20 mmHg. Is there any mechanism to check, for instance, LAP, to adjust relative flow between left and right?

*Maeda* (University of Tokyo): Right flow rate is the main parameter to be controlled. Left atrial pressure is controlled to search for the lowest point. Left outflow resistance was very high, so left atrial pressure was elevated.

*Imachi* (University of Tokyo): On the left, the left atrial pressure is always kept below a certain level; on the right, the cardiac output is controlled along with the predictive control curve. However, we could not decrease the left atrial pressure for the limit of the driving pressure.

*Takatani:* So what is the starting mechanism in your control?

*Imachi:* When the treadmill starts, we manually input the program start.

*Takatani:* So it does not automatically look for some change in the variables? It is especially programmed for the treadmill exercise?

*Imachi:* Only the start point is inputted manually. But once the treadmill exercise has begun, AH is automatically controlled.

# 33. Atrial natriuretic polypeptide in sheep with total artificial heart

Kazunobu Nishimura[1], Hiroyuki Fukumasu[2], Toshihiko Ban[1], Hitoshi Okabayashi[1], Yoshihiko Saito[3], Kazuwa Nakao[3], and Hiroo Imura[3]

**Summary.** The concentrations of atrial natriuretic polypeptide (ANP) in six sheep after implantation of a total artificial heart (TAH) were examined, in order to clarify whether ANP is secreted from the remnant atria, which may receive a little blood supply,. The plasma concentration of ANP in sheep was $45 \pm 11$ pg/ml in the preoperative control period and increased to $151 \pm 32$ pg/ml before cardiopulmonary bypass. The ANP concentration in the coronary sinus was much higher than in the peripheral artery and vein. The ANP concentration was lower after TAH implantation than before operation, especially in the early postoperative period. In a few cases of long survivors, the ANP concentration increased to about half the basal level 1 or 2 weeks after operation. The ANP content in the remnant atrial tissues decreased at autopsy but was still present in sufficient amount to secret ANP.

These results suggest that a small amount of ANP is secreted from the remnant atria in TAH-implanted animals even under the conditions of an adequate level of atrial pressure in the early postoperative period. The secretory function of the remnant atria may recover gradually, because the ANP content in the atrial tissues is still present in sufficient amount to secret ANP at autopsy in spite of marked decreases compared with the control atrial tissues.

**Key words:** Atrial natriuretic polypeptide—Total artificial heart—Coronary sinus—Remnant atrium—Electrolyte-fluid balance

Recently, the clinical indications of the total artificial heart (TAH) have been expanded with its utilization as a bridge bypass to heart transplantation as well as permanent use. Nevertheless, several problems in relation to TAH still remain to be solved prior to general spread of TAH implantation. In addition to improvement of the design and fabrication of the artificial heart and the surgical technique, the pathophysiological implication of TAH-implanted animals must be elucidated [1, 2].

Since de Bold et al. demonstrated that atrial cardiocytes contain a humoral factor capable of stimulating the urinary excretion of salt and water in 1981, the atrium has been recognized as an important endocrine organ for regulating water-electrolyte balance [3]. This cardiac hormone, atrial natriuretic polypeptide (ANP), has been isolated from rat and human atria in various forms with high and low molecular weights [4]. Accumulating evidence indicates that $\alpha$-ANP with 28 amino acids is mainly secreted through the coronary sinus from the heart and circulates in the body [5, 6]. Intravenous administration of synthetic ANP causes rapid diuresis, natriuresis, and vasodilation and inhibits the renin-angiotension-aldosterone system [7]. The secretion of ANP is stimulated by atrial distension, which occurs with increases in atrial pressure [8, 9] and by atrial tachycardia such as paroxysmal supraventricular tachycardia [10-2]. The ANP concentrations in both plasma and the atrial tissues are increased in patients with congestive heart failure, which constitutes a characteristic feature of elevated atrial pressure [7].

After implantation of a TAH, the remnant atria do not received a blood supply via the coronary arteries in our present surgical procedures. Our P-wave studies and histopathological studies of the remnant atria suggested dysfunction over 2 months of TAH implantation [13, 14]. However, the clinical investigation of the ANP concentration in human recipients of the artificial heart demonstrated that the ANP concentration increased after short-term increases in right atrial pressure [15], while it was reported that TAH implantation in calves caused a fall in the ANP level [16]. The discrepancy between the results in human recipients and calves has still not been clarified. Therefore, we examined the changes in the ANP level in sheep during and after TAH implantation in order to elucidate whether ANP is secreted from the remnant atria, which may receive a small supply of blood.

[1]Department of Cardiovascular Surgery, Kyoto University School of Medicine, 54 Shogoin Kawaharacho, Sakyo-ku, Kyoto, 606 Japan
[2]Department of Cardiovascular Surgery, Takeda Hospital, 28–1 Ishidamori-minamimachi, Fushimi-ku, Kyoto, 612 Japan
[3]Second Division, Department of Medicine, Kyoto University School of Medicine, 54 Shogoin Kawahara-cho, Sakyo-ku, Kyoto, 606 Japan

## Materials and methods

### Animal preparation

Six male Suffolk sheep, weighing 45–67 kg, were used in this study. Preoperative feeding was stopped for 3 days before surgery, and water only was given until 24 h before surgery.

### Artificial heart

The artificial heart implanted was the so-called Tomasu heart, which is a modified Utah heart and consists of atrial cuffs, outflow vascular grafts, and ventricles with multisoft layers and a seamless diaphragm [14, 17]. All parts of the Tomasu heart are made of polyurethane only and bonded tightly without wires. Björk-Shiley or Hall-Kaster valves were pushed into the female grooves made in the inflow and outflow polyurethane quick connectors. The outflow grafts were modified to the slip-in connector types, which could be easily connected to both remnant great arteries without suturing [17]. Full stroke volumes were 65 ml on the left and 55 ml on the right ventricle.

### Surgical procedures

After induction of anesthesia with 15–20 mg/kg pentobarbital, the sheep were intubated and maintained on ventilation with optimum doses of GOF. Through a right thoracotomy, the natural heart was exposed and cannulated for preparation of cardiopulmonary bypass (CPB). Under the total CPB, almost all of the ventricular myocardium was excised up to the atrioventricular groove and semilunar cusp rings of both great arteries. Both coronary arteries were divided from the aorta near the ostium. The coronary sinus was closed in two sheep and left open in four. After both cuffs were fixed to the remnant atria with a single running suture of 3–0 prolene, the slip-in connectors were anastomosed to the aorta and the pulmonary artery by ligaturing with an umbilical tape and a large silk thread. Ventricular drive lines were passed out through the right chest wall and connected to the heart driver.

### Driving conditions

The Tomasu heart was optimally driven at 110–130 beats/min with 45%–52% of percent systole. Both driving pressures were adjusted to 160–190 mmHg in the left and 45–65 mmHg in the right ventricle to maintain 90–110 mmHg of mean arterial pressure and less than 15 mmHg of mean left atrial pressure.

### Blood sampling

A preoperative blood sample was obtained from the jugular vein immediately before anesthetic induction. Sampling was then performed from the arterial pressure monitor line at the following times: before CPB, at the end of the operation, on the 1st, 2nd, 4th, 7th, and 14th postoperative days. The ANP concentration in plasma obtained from the coronary sinus was also measured before CPB. Blood samples were transferred to chilled disposable tubes containing aprotinin (1000 kallikrein inactivator units/ml) and EDTA (1 mg/ml) and then immediately centrifuged at 4°C. Aliquots of plasma were stored at −20°C until the time of assay

### Sampling of atrial tissues

Specimens of the auricles in three sheep were obtained at operation, and in two animals they were also obtained at autopsy at almost identical sites. All tissue samples were immediately frozen in liquid nitrogen and stored at −70°C until extraction. The auricles were extracted as previously reported [6]

### Measurement of plasma hormones

The plasma concentrations of aldosterone and antidiuretic hormone (ADH) as well as ANP were measured at the same time as the hormones closely related to the circulation volume. The plasma and auricle concentrations of ANP were measured by a specific radioimmunoassay (RIA) for $\alpha$-ANP, as previously reported [5, 6]. Briefly, this RIA recognizes a carboxy-terminal fragment of ANP and the minimum detectable quantity is 10 pg/ml. The ADH concentration was also measured by RIA with a specific antibody as reported by Yamada et al. [18]. The plasma aldosterone concentration was measured with a commercially available kit (Aldosterone Test Shionogi).

## Results

### Operation results

Table 33.1 summarizes the days of survival and causes of death in six sheep in this series. The days of survival ranged from 4 to 40 days with an average of $15 \pm 13$ days. There were no causes of death as a result of the artificial heart.

**Table 33.1.** Days of survival and causes of death

| Sheep no. | Days of survival | Cause of death |
|---|---|---|
| 1 | 7 | Renal failure |
| 2 | 7 | CNS damage |
| 3 | 4 | LOS |
| 4 | 40 | Late LOS |
| 5 | 15 | GI bleeding |
| 6 | 17 | Pneumonia |

*CNS* central nervous system, *LOS* low output syndrome, *GI* gastrointestinal

### ANP Concentration in plasma and auricles

The ANP concentration was $45 \pm 11$ pg/ml in the preoperative control period and increased to $151 \pm 36$ pg/ml before CPB. The ANP concentration in the coronary sinus was $533 \pm 213$ pg/ml and much higher than in the peripheral artery and vein, resembling observations in human beings (Fig. 33.1). The time-course of the ANP concentration in six sheep from the preoperative period until death showed essentially similar changes. The ANP concentration increased before CPB and decreased to $54 \pm 14$ pg/ml at the end of operation. On the 1st or 2nd postoperative day, it fell to below the minimum detectable value. Subsequently, it generally remained at a low level until death except in one case in which the ANP concentration recovered to 42 pg/ml on the 8th postoperative day (Fig. 33.2). There was no difference between the group with an open and that with a closed coronary sinus. In all cases, the left atrial pressure changed from 6 to 12 mmHg throughout but fell immediately before death. All sheep except one revealed edema in the neck and body throughout the time-course after surgery. One sheep which did not develop edema had a good postoperative course with an adequate circulation volume and showed a relatively higher concentration of ANP than others. The ANP concentration in the atrial tissues was $6.9 \pm 2.4$ μg/g at operation and decreased to less than one-tenth in case 3 on the fourth postoperative day and to about one-third in case 5 on the 15th day (Table 33.2).

### Plasma aldosterone and ADH concentration

Figure 33.3 shows the time-course of the concentration of ANP, aldosterone, and ADH in two sheep. In both cases, the aldosterone and ADH concentrations increased during surgery and decreased 3 days after operation. Although neither aldosterone nor ADH levels showed a correlation with the ANP level, there was a significant positive correlation between aldosterone and ADH levels.

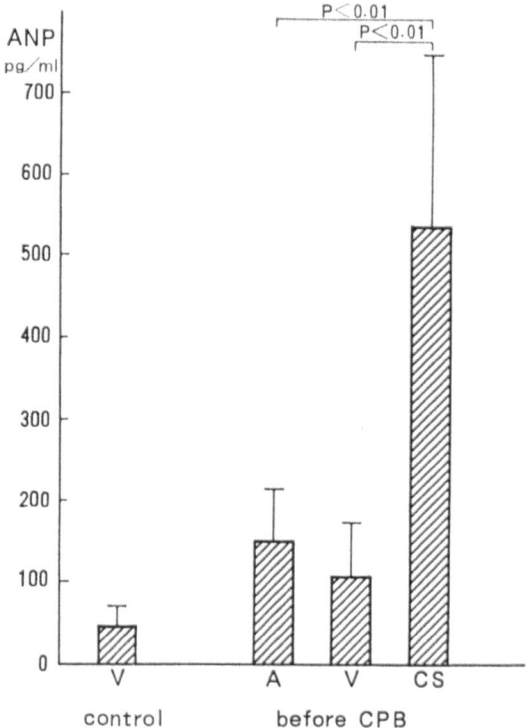

**Fig. 33.1.** Atrial natriuretic polypeptide (ANP) concentrations at various sites. The ANP concentration of plasma obtained from the coronary sinus is three to eight times higher than that of a peripheral artery or vein. *CS* coronary sinus, *A* artery, *V* vein

### Discussion

The present study indicates that a small amount of ANP is secreted from the remnant atria in TAH-implanted sheep in spite of adequate atrial pressure in the early postoperative period. Naturally, such findings may be related to postoperative edema or hypertension although we could not determine this because of the experimental limitations. Westenfelder et al. reported that the plasma concentration of ANP in calves was low after implantation of the Jarvik-7 heart and did not increase with an increase in atrial pressure [16]. On the other hand, a clinical investigation into the changes in ANP concentration in two human recipients of artificial hearts revealed that the ANP concentration increased approximately twofold in response to an elevation of right atrial pressure [15]. Thus, there is a clear contrast in the plasma ANP levels between human recipients of permanent artificial hearts and calves or sheep. These conflicting results may be due to species differences or may be caused by the stage of postoperative studies. The clinical data were obtained over 1 year after implantation in both cases, while the study in calves was

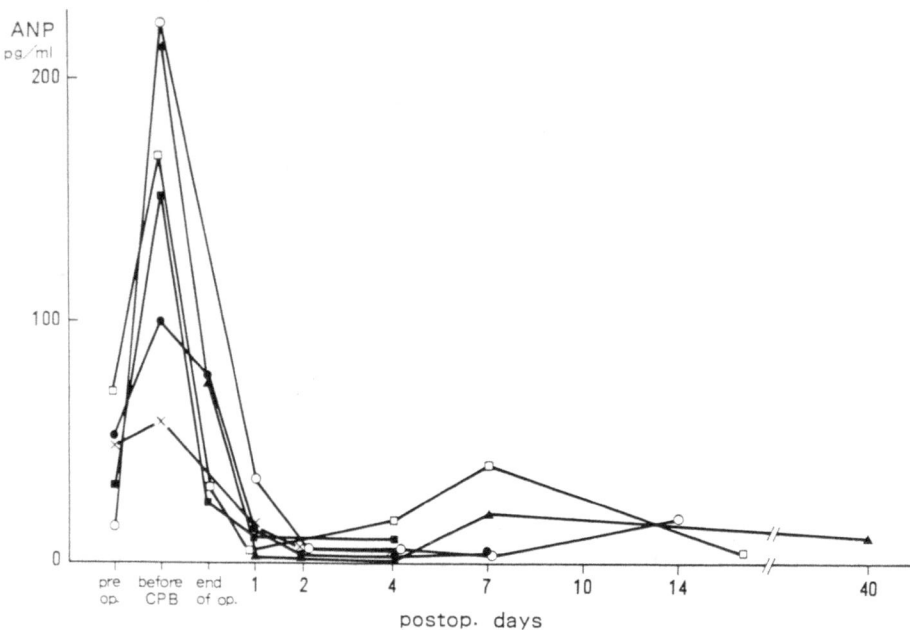

**Fig. 33.2.** Time-courses of ANP changes in six sheep with the total artificial heart

performed 4 weeks and in sheep less than 2 weeks after operation.

The remnant atria do not receive a blood supply via the coronary arteries in our present surgical procedures. Nevertheless, Iwaya et al. have been reported that from histopathological studies remnant atria appear to be viable [13]. They showed that some necrosis was evident in the short-term survival calves, while this was not seen but had been replaced by several degrees of fibrosis in the long-term survivors. Therefore, it was speculated that a blood supply for the remnant atria was maintained by extracardiac vessels, such as the bronchial artery, even if the supply was small. In addition, in terms of atrial electrical activity, the postoperative P-wave was maintained within normal limits during the 1st month after surgery and gradually decreased and often disappeared after 2 months [1, 14]. Therefore, this outcome suggests that the remnant atria are able to maintain electrical viability for at least 1 month, although the role as secretory organ is still undefined.

There are other interesting results concerning the experimental myocarditis mice developed by viral inoculation [19]: The ANP concentration in their atrial tissues decreased 1 week after inoculation and then increased to one and half times the previous level 2 weeks after. This result suggests that the atria injured by myocarditis cause tissue necrosis with little release of ANP. Therefore, it would follow that the ANP concentration is at a considerably low level in TAH-implanted sheep during the early postoperative days,

**Table 33.2.** Atrial natriuretic polypeptide concentrations in the atrial tissues at operation and autopsy

| Case no. | At operation ($\mu$g/g) | At autopsy ($\mu$g/g) |
| --- | --- | --- |
| 3 | 9.4 | 0.8 (4 days) |
| 5 | 4.7 | 1.7 (15 days) |
| 6 | 6.6 | — |

because the evidence of necrosis in the remnant atria was found in the short-term survivors as mentioned already.

In the light of the levels of the ANP concentration in the late phase of human recipients, ANP may be appropriately released into the circulation in association with elevation of atrial pressure. We observed a relatively higher concentration of ANP in one sheep 1 week after surgery. In addition to the results of the plasma ANP concentration, we demonstrated that the remnant atrial tissues still contained a considerable amount of ANP, although the ANP content was decreased compared with the control atrial tissues. The secretory function of the remnant atria may recover gradually as the remaining viable cardiomyocytes develop to be hypertrophic. However, it is as yet doubtful whether ANP is sufficiently secreted from the remnant atria and responds to the hemodynamic changes normally in all long-term survivors; this is because it cannot be determined whether the remnant atria retain the ability to release ANP so as

**Fig. 33.3.** Time-courses of concentrations of
ANP, aldosterone, and ADH in two sheep. *Ald*
aldosterone, *ADH* antidiuretic hormone

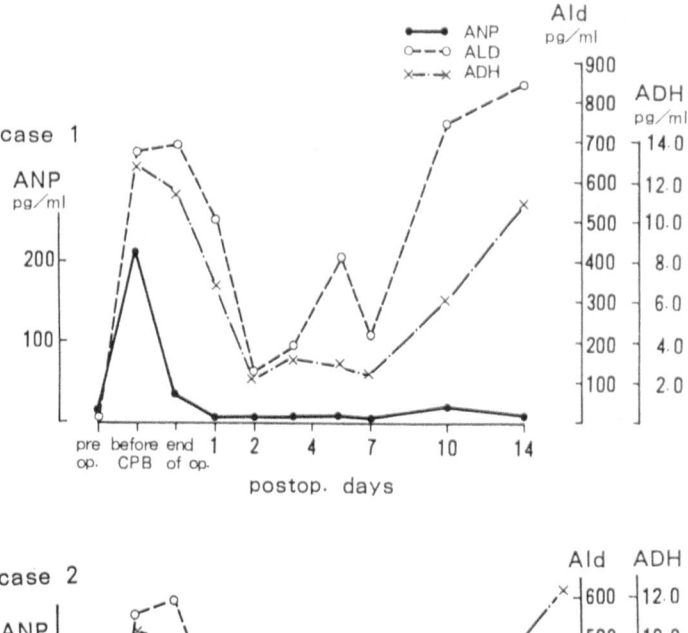

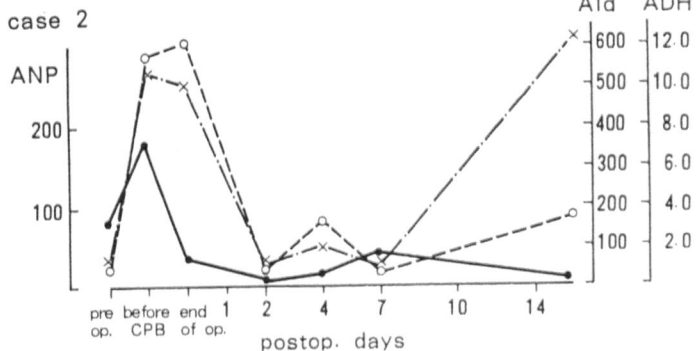

to fit in with various pathophysiological conditions. Further examinations not only into the response of the ANP secretion to various stimulations but also in the ANP content of the remnant atria need to be done in the chronic stage.

We suggest that ANP may be secreted into the right atrium through the small vessels such as thebesian veins by backflow from the coronary sinus under conditions whereby antegrade coronary flow ceases. However, we attained the unexpected result that there was no difference in the ANP concentrations whether the coronary sinus was open or closed. Consequently, it cannot be concluded that it is important for the secretion of ANP to leave the coronary sinus open, since our data are limited in the number of subjects.

ADH was secreted in sheep with TAH in response to the hemodynamic change, as reported by other investigators [20]. There are two main receptors to stimulate the secretion of ADH—osmoreceptors in the hypothalamus and stretch receptors in the atrium. The latter are considered to function here, since ADH increases in the shock state when atrial pressure falls. Thus, it seems that both ADH and aldosterone are

released to regulate electrolyte-fluid homeostasis in TAH-implanted sheep. In addition to these two hormones, ANP must play an important role in the control of body fluid.

In conclusion, we observed the low concentration of ANP in sheep with TAH in the early postoperative period. The surgical disruption of the atrial blood supply may lead to the development of a functional ANP deficiency state. The ANP content in the remnant atrial tissues decreased at autopsy but was still present in sufficient amount to secret ANP. In the long-term survivors, the remaining cardiomyocytes may be able to release ANP, although their ability to secret ANP may be inadequate.

**Acknowledgment.** We acknowledge the assistance of Dr. H. Hirose in the Department of Cardiovascular Surgery and Mr. H. Konishi, Mr. K. Minatoya, Mr. Y. Kawai, and Mr. A. Oyama of Kyoto University School of Medicine in TAH implantation and are grateful to Mr. S. Yuasa of Tomasu Giken for giving us the artificial heart. We thank Miss C. Nakai and Miss I. Yoshida for measurement of hormones. The excellent assistance of Miss Y. Yasui and Miss S. Yuasa in dealing with experimental animals and instrumentation is also gratefully acknowledged.

# References

1. Fukumasu H (1980) Development of total artificial heart. Arch Jpn Chir 49: 225–268
2. Olsen DB, Murray KD (1984) The total artificial heart. Assisted circulation 2. Springer, Berlin, pp 197–228
3. De Bold AJ, Borenstein HB, Veress AT, Sonnenberg H (1981) A rapid and potent natriuretic response to intravenous injection of atrial myocardial extract in rats. Life Sci 28: 89–94
4. Kangawa K, Matsuo H (1984) Purification and complete amino acid sequence of α-human atrial natriuretic polypeptide. Biochem Biophys Res Commun 118: 131–139
5. Sugawara A, Nakao K, Morii N, Sakamoto M, Suda M, Shimokura M, Kiso Y, Kihara M, Yamori Y, Nishimura K, Soneda J, Ban T, Imura H (1985) α-human atrial natriuretic polypeptide is released from the heart and circulates in the body. Biochem Biophys Res Commun 129: 439–446
6. Nakao K, Sugawara A, Morii N, Sakamoto M, Suda M, Soneda J, Ban T, Kihara M, Yamori Y, Shimokura M, Kiso Y, Imura H (1984) Radioimmunoassay for α-human and rat atrial natriuretic polypeptide. Biochem Biophys Res Commun 124: 815–821
7. Saito Y, Nakao K, Nishimura K, Sugawara A, Okumura K, Obata K, Sonoda R, Ban T, Yasue H, Imura H (1987) Clinical application of atrial natricuretic polypeptide to patients with congestive heart failure. Circulation 76: 115–124
8. Ledsome JR, Wilson N, Courneya CA, Rankin AJ (1985) Release of atrial natriuretic peptide by atrial distension. Can J Physiol Pharmacol 63: 739–742
9. Goetz KL, Wang BC, Geer PG, Sundet WG, Needleman P (1986) Effects of atriopeptin infusion versus effects of left atrial stretch in awake dogs. Am J Physiol 250: R221–R226
10. Schiffrin EL , Gutkowska J, Kuchel O, Cantin M, Genest J (1985) Plasma concentration of atrial natriuretic factor in a patient with paroxysmal atrial tachycardia. N Engl J Med 312: 1196
11. Rankin AJ, Courneya CA, Wilson N, Ledsome JR (1986) Tachycardia releases atrial natriuretic peptide in the anesthetized rabbit. Life Sci 38: 1951–1957
12. Nishimura K, Soneda J, Nomoto S, Matsumoto M, Fujiwara Y, Konishi Y, Okamoto Y, Ban T, Sugawara A, Nakao K, Imura H (1986) Atrial natriuretic polypeptide increases during atrial pacing. Jpn Circ J 50: 727 (abstract)
13. Iwaya F, Fukumasu H, Olsen DB, Razzeca KJ, McGill LD, Kolff WJ (1978) Studies of atria of the total artificial heart. Histopathological findings of remnant atria and pannus formation. Jpn J Artif Organs 7: 775–778
14. Fukumasu H (1985) Research on the total artificial heart. Artificial heart 1, Proceedings of the 1st international symposium on artificial heart and assist device, Springer, Tokyo pp 187–192
15. Schwab TR, Edwards BS, DeVries WG, Zimmerman RS, Burnet, Jr JC (1986) Atrial endocrine function in humans with artificial hearts. N Engl J Med 315: 1398–1401
16. Westenfelder C, Baranowski RL, Kablitz C, Olsen DB, Burns G, Jahan S (1986) Atrial natriuretic peptide release in calves with artificial hearts. Kidney Int 29: 389 (abstract)
17. Fukumasu H, Yuasa S, Tatemichi K, Hirose H, Fujita T (1984) Modern technology with the TAH replacement in fully-grown animals. Trans Am Soc Artif Intern Organs 30: 597–602
18. Yamada T, Nakao K, Morii N, Itoh H, Shiono S, Sakamoto M, Sugawara A, Saito Y, Ohno H, Kanai A, Katsuura G, Eigyo M, Matsusita A, Imura H (1986) Central effects of atrial natriuretic polypeptide on angiotensin II-stimulated vasopressin secretion in conscious rats. Eur J Pharmacol 125: 453–456
19. Morii N, Nakao K, Sugawara A, Saito Y, Yamada T, Itoh H, Shiono S, Mukoyama M, Arai H, Matsumori A, Kawai C, Imura H (1987) Atrial natriuretic polypeptide in experimental myocarditis mouse. The 51th annual scientific meeting of Jap Circ Society 294 (in Japanese)
20. Nakajima M, Fujimasa I, Imachi K, Mabuchi K, Chinzei T, Abe Y, Takido N, Atsumi K (1986) Hemodynamic and hormonal study in total artificial heart. Jpn J Artif Organs 15: 686–691

# 34. Plasma atrial natriuretic polypeptide levels during various types of artificial circulation

Yoshiyuki Taenaka, Akihiko Yagura, Hisateru Takano, Takehisa Matsuda, Hiroyuki Noda, Masayuki Kinoshita, Eisuke Tatsumi, Setsuo Takatani, and Tetsuzo Akutsu[1]

**Summary.** Plasma atrial natriuretic polypeptide (ANP) levels were measured in three left ventricular assist device (LVAD) goats with normal hearts, three LVAD goats with fibrillated hearts, and three total artificial heart (TAH) calves. The plasma concentrations of ANP in the LVAD goats with normal hearts were lower than those of the control values, ranging between 6 and 26 pg/ml. The supporting data from similar LVAD experiments suggest that the low levels of plasma ANP of the LVAD animals were due to the low left atrial pressure during LVAD pumping. The ANP levels of the LVAD animals with a fibrillated heart were high, up to 516 pg/ml, because of the high right atrial pressure of 13–21 mmHg. In the TAH calves, the plasma ANP values varied irrespective of the changes in atrial pressure for 2 weeks postoperatively, followed by decreasing to the lower limit of the control value. The plasma ANP levels of one calf did not rise even when the central venous pressure increased suddenly to 18 mmHg due to the failure of the right pump on the 54th postoperative day. In conclusion: (a) the LVAD animals showed a normal response of ANP secretion to the altered atrial pressure; (b) the calves with a TAH did not show a uniform profile of the plasma ANP levels after implantation; (c) the plasma ANP concentration of one TAH calf did not react to the increased right atrial pressure in the chronic phase.

**Key words:** Atrial natriuretic polypeptide—Atrial pressure—Left ventricular assist device—Total artificial heart

Atrial natriuretic polypeptide (ANP) has been investigated in recent years. It is believed that increased atrial pressure, resulting in stretching of the atrial wall, stimulates the secretion of ANP to increase diuresis and cause vasodilation in normal individuals without influencing the nervous system [1, 2]. However, this interesting humoral control of circulation, response of plasma ANP levels to altered atrial pressure, might be affected during artificial circulation such as with the left ventricular assist device (LVAD) and total artificial heart (TAH). The purpose of this study is to investigate the fluctuation of plasma ANP concentration in response to the changes in atrial pressure in animals receiving an LVAD or a TAH.

## Materials and methods

A pneumatic and diaphragm-type LVAD and a pneumatic and pusher-plate type TAH developed at the National Cardiovascular Center were used in this study [3, 4]. Plasma ANP levels were measured in three types of animal model with artificial circulation. They were LVAD animals with a normal heart, single artificial heart (SAH) animals, i.e., LVAD animals with a fibrillated heart, and TAH animals.

### LVAD group

The LVAD was implanted between the left atrium and descending aorta in three goats weighing 28–40 kg with a normal heart. The inflow conduit was inserted into the left atrium through a cuff sutured onto the left atrial appendage and bypass flow was maintained above 2 l/min throughout the experiment.

### SAH group

In three goats weighing 22–31 kg, the LVAD was placed in the same way manner as in the LVAD group. The ventricle was electrically fibrillated following volume loading with fresh frozen plasma 1–2 weeks postoperatively (Fig. 34.1). The LVAD as a SAH yielded 80–120 ml/kg/min of output with a high mean right atrial pressure of 13–21 mmHg. The blood flowed from the right heart to the left atrium with the force of the pressure gradient across the lung [5]. These animals were regarded as LVAD animals with high right atrial pressure.

### TAH group

The TAH was applied to three calves weighing between 97 and 107 kg. The natural ventricles were excised, retaining the atrioventricular ring while the atria were left in place. The aorta and pulmonary artery were separated and their proximal parts from the valve commissure were excised. The coronary sinus was ligated at the orifice to the right atrium.

[1]National Cardiovascular Center Research Institute, 5-7-1 Fujishiro-dai, Suita, Osaka, 565 Japan

Consequently, almost the entire coronary arterial and venous system was removed from the circulation. The variable rate mode, that is, an automatic fill-empty and right-and-left independently pumping mode using Hall-effect position sensors was selected and around 100 ml/kg/min of measured cardiac output was obtained with the TAH.

Blood samples were drawn from the arterial or right atrial sampling line when the animals were standing and stable, and the plasma levels of ANP were measured by means of radioimmunoassay. The samples were taken from three control goats, five control calves, and experimental animals in the LVAD group and TAH group after surgery and in the SAH group after induced ventricular fibrillation. Right atrial or central venous pressure and left atrial pressure were measured continuously in the SAH group and TAH group animals.

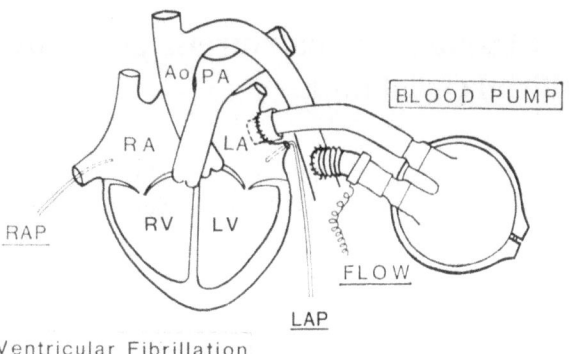

**Fig. 34.1.** Experimental model of single artificial heart. *Ao* aorta, *LA* left atrium, *LV* left ventricle, *PA* pulmonary artery, *RA* right atrium, *RV* right ventricle, *LAP* left atrial pressure monitoring line, *RAP* right atrial pressure monitoring line

## Results

The value of ANP of the control goats was 58.4 ± 14.1 pg/ml and that of the control calves was 39.3 ± 14.9 pg/ml. The ANP concentrations of the LVAD goats with a normal heart were low, ranging between 6 and 26 pg/ml during the experiments, while those of the SAH goats were high, up to 516 pg/ml, for 2–3 weeks after ventricular fibrillation was induced until the termination of the experiments (Fig. 34.2). The right atrial pressure of the SAH goats increased to levels of 13–21 mmHg after ventricular fibrillation. The plasma ANP levels of two TAH calves were within the normal range for 2 weeks after surgery, although the right atrial pressure was high. Conversely, the ANP levels of another calf, whose right atrial pressure was lower than 5 mmHg, were high, with values of 124 pg/ml on the 6th postoperative day (POD) and 116 pg/ml on the 16th POD. In this calf, the plasma ANP values decreased to 23–34 pg/ml, which was lower than the control level, after the 3rd postoperative week. On the 54th POD, even when the central venous pressure rose to 18 mmHg, because of the sudden stop of the right pump due to the rupture of the diaphragm, the plasma ANP level did not increase reactively. The ANP concentration increased to 46 pg/ml just before the termination of the experiment when the animal was critically ill (Fig. 34.3).

## Discussion

The left atrial appendage is damaged at the time of insertion of the inflow cannula in the LVAD recipients when the LVAD is applied between the left atrium and the aorta, and the coronary circulation of the atria is almost totally excluded in the TAH cases. Other than surgical intervention, the artificial pumping may influence the physiological reaction to regulate ANP levels. To investigate the influences of the application of an LVAD or a TAH on ANP secretion, evaluation of the reaction of the plasma ANP levels to the altered atrial pressure in recipients of various kinds of artificial circulation is quite important.

The LVAD goats with a normal heart had low ANP levels compared with the control value throughout the 1-month-experiment. In these animals, neither right nor left atrial pressure was measured. However, the data of the LVAD goats with a normal heart in similar experiments indicated that the mean right atrial pressure ranged between 0 and 4.5 mmHg and the mean left atrial pressure was between −5 and 5 mmHg. These supporting data suggest that the low levels of ANP in the LVAD animals with a normal heart were due to the low left atrial pressure during LVAD pumping. In the SAH goats, the plasma ANP increased to three times the control value on average after induced ventricular fibrillation and remained at high levels. These high levels were caused by the high right atrial pressure in order to maintain adequate cardiac output (Table 34.1). The results obtained from the LVAD and SAH goats proved that the secretion of ANP responding to the changes in right and left atrial pressure was well preserved in animals with an LVAD.

The calves with a TAH did not show uniform tendencies of plasma ANP levels after implantation of the device. The plasma levels of ANP did not correlate with the values of the atrial pressure. Two calves with high right atrial pressure had low ANP levels and another calves with low right atrial pressure had high

**Fig. 34.2.** Profile of the plasma ANP levels in the animals with an LVAD. *ANP* atrial natriuretic polypeptide, *LVAD* left ventricular assist device, *SAH* single artificial heart

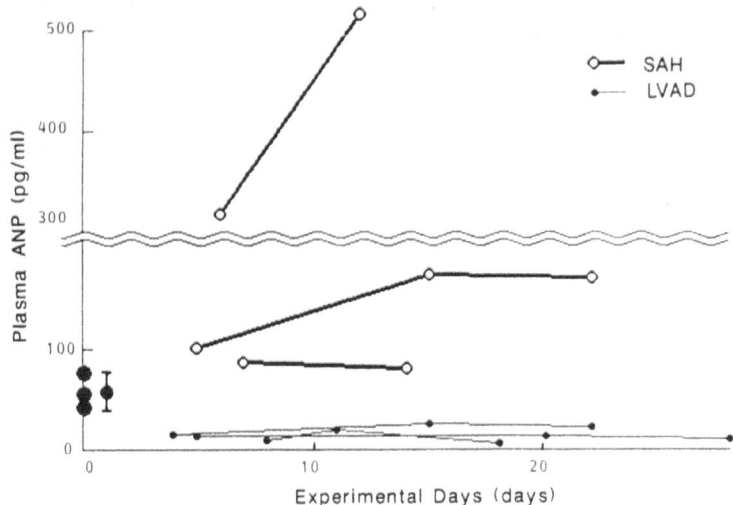

**Fig. 34.3.** Profile of the ANP levels in the animals with a TAH. *ANP* atrial natriuretic polypeptide, *TAH* total artificial heart, *RAP* right atrial pressure, *CVP* central venous pressure

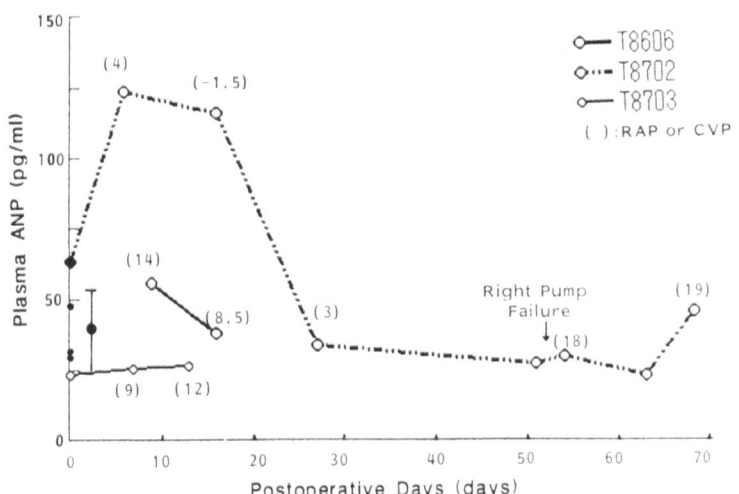

ANP values for 3 postoperative weeks. The ANP levels in the calf decreased to the lower limit of the control value after the 3rd postoperative week and did not respond to the marked increase in right atrial pressure due to the failure of the right pump. A report from the University of Utah described that the intentional decrease in cardiac output from 12 to 4 l/min, resulting in increased right atrial pressure, did not raise the blood levels of ANP in a TAH calf [6]. This result was similar to ours. On the other hand, another study at the Humana hospital in Kentucky with human TAH recipients revealed that the rise in right atrial pressure increased the blood levels of ANP within 5 min [7]. Since the numbers of the subjects in all these experiments are restricted, it is difficult to determine the cause of the differences in the results. One of the reasons may be the differences in the animal species used in the experiments. Another possible reason is the influence of surgical adhesion of the atria. The experimental calf in which we measured the ANP levels was examined within 3 months, while the human subjects were evaluated after 300 days. Tight surgical adhesion of the TAH calves in a relatively early phase after surgery may prevent the atria from stretching to react to the increase in atrial pressure. Further experiments are necessary to clarify the de-

**Table 34.1.** Mean atrial pressure in the experimental animals

|  | RAP (mmHg) | LAP (mmHg) |
|---|---|---|
| LVAD goats | 0–4.5 (2)[a] | −5–5 (0)[a] |
| SAH goats | 13–21 (17) | −2–9 (4.5) |

[a] Data from similar experiments
*LVAD* left ventricular assist device, *SAH* single artificial heart, *RAP* right atrial pressure, *LAP* left atrial pressure

tailed response of the plasma ANP levels in recipients with artificial circulation.

## Conclusion

The goats receiving an LVAD showed normal responses of ANP secretion to the altered atrial pressure. The calves with a TAH did not show a uniform profile of the plasma ANP levels after implantation. The plasma ANP concentration of one TAH calf did not react to the increased right atrial pressure in the chronic phase.

## References

1. Cantin M, Genest J (1985) The heart and the atrial natriuretic factor. Endocrine Reviews 6: 107–127
2. Ledsome JR, Wilson N, Courneya CA, Rankin AJ (1985) Release of atrial natriuretic peptide by atrial distension. Can J Physiol Pharmacol 63: 739–742
3. Takano H, Nakatani T, Taenaka Y, Umezu M (1986) Development of the ventricular assist pump system: Experimental and clinical studies. In: Akutsu T (ed) Springer, Tokyo, pp 141–151
4. Takatani S, Nakatani T, Takano H, Tanaka T, Umezu M, Adachi S, Noda H, Fukuda S, Matsuda T, Iwata H, Nakamura T, Akutsu T (1986) Total artificial heart study in goats and calves with pusher-plate type blood pumpus—Progress and problems. Jap J Artif Organs 15: 654–659
5. Takano H, Nakatani T, Fukuda S, Umezu M, Taenaka Y, Matsuda T, Iwata H, Adachi S, Tanaka T, Noda H, Takatani S, Hayashi K, Nakamura T, Seki J, Akutsu T, Manabe H (1986) Prolonged circulatory maintenance in case of cardiac arrest during LVAD assistance. Progress in Artificial Organs-1985 480–486
6. Olsen DB, Westenfelder C, Burns GL, Kablitz C, Baranowski RL (1986) Neurohormonal responses in total artificial heart recipients. In: Nosé Y, Kjellstrand C, Ivanovich P (eds) ISAO Press, Cleveland, Progress in artificial organs 1985, pp. 112–118
7. Schwab TR, Edwards BS, DeVries WC, Zimmerman RS, Burnett JC (1986) Atrial endocrine function in humans with artificial hearts. N Engl J Medicine 27: 1398–1401

# Discussion

*Taenaka* (National Cardiovascular Center): How high were your right and left atrial pressures? Did you fluctuate the atrial pressure separately to observe the response of the ALP levels?

*Nishimura* (Kyoto University): I did not do these measurements. You closed the coronary sinus. We carried out experiments in sheep in which the coronary sinus was open in four animals and closed in two. What would be your comments on this?

*Taenaka:* How can you implant the total artificial heart without closing the coronary sinus? It will be difficult and cause bleeding.

*Nishimura:* There is a clear discrepancy between the clinical data and the results in calves or sheep with our total artificial heart. What do you think the cause of discrepancy is?

*Taenaka:* The number of our experiments and those performed in the USA is very limited. Perhaps a species difference may play a role here. I have carried out experiments with the implantation of the total artificial heart in sheep, and sometimes in them it is very difficult to control the circulatory volume after surgery. They are not so reactive to the administration of diuretics such as Lasix or furosemide.

Another factor may be that in Utah the sampling for the experiments was carried out in the 1st or 2nd postoperative month. The surgical adhesion may have affected the results of this experiment. In Kentucky, they use patients 300 days after operation. Perhaps, the adhesion is not tight around the atrium. In our case, even if the right atrial pressure increases, stretching of the atria might be prevented by the adhesion.

*Nishimura:* The discrepancy between the results in clinical cases and those in our laboratory may be partly due to a difference in species. However, I believe it is mainly due to the stage of research. They carried out their clinical research 1 year after operation whereas in our cases it was within 1 month. In the acute stage, the atria shows some degree of necrosis; in the chronic stage, this is replaced by fibrosis. The remnant viable cardiomyocytes become hypertrophic and secrete ANP.

*Fukumasu* (Takeda Hospital): A point that was not answered concerned closing the coronary sinus and how it is possible to carry out surgery. At first, I used to close the coronary sinus, but now I leave it open.

*Imachi:* Why did you measure the ANP? Did you have any pathological evidence from AH animal or clinical AH patients?

*Taenaka:* Mainly just because of interest. In left ventricular assist patients, renal failure after surgery sometimes occurs. So I thought that poor secretion of ANP may have been responsible for this renal dysfunction. In TAH cases, the animals sometimes show a refractory response to diuretics after surgery.

*Nishimura:* I think the remnant atria may have a little blood supply, which depends on various extracardiac collateral arteries. So I speculated there would be very little secreted ANP.

*Imachi:* In our laboratory, we measured ANP to clarify two causes of pathophysiological phenomena such as high CVP and hypertension in TAH animals. Dr. Mabuchi will present our results concerning ANP.

*Mabuchi:* (University of Tokyo): Our plasma levels of ANP were similar to those of Dr. Taenaka. There was no correlation between the ANP level and plasma-renin activity. I suspect that the hypertension that appears in TH animals is not due to ANP.

*Fukumasu:* How many cases does your study include?

*Mabuchi:* Only three.

*Fukumasu:* So you cannot really arrive at a definite conclusion until you have studied more. If there is no coronary flow to the atrium, this will bring about a lot of changes there. This kind of study should be continued until we obtain more data.

*Geselowitz* (Pennsylvania State University): I would just like to make the comment that with the artificial heart we have a very powerful tool in physiology in that we are able to separate the cardiac and vascular elements aspects of the cardiovascular system.

# 35. Design criteria of implantable blood pump in the goat's chest cavity

Kou Imachi, Kunihiko Mabuchi, Tsuneo Chinzei, Yuusuke Abe, Kiyoshi Maeda, Kaoru Imanishi, Masahiro Asano, Akimasa Kouno, Toshiya Ono, Iwao Fujimasa, and Kazuhiko Atsumi[1]

**Summary.** It is desirable to use the adult goat as an experimental animal for the TAH with an implantable pneumatic driven blood pump since the calf has the problem of growth during the study period. Adult animals are also much more similar to adult human patients in physiological terms than immature animals such as the calf. However, it has not yet been possible to design a blood pump that fits well into the narrow space of the goat chest cavity. To solve this problem, a new design of the blood pump fitted to the goat chest cavity was investigated in this study. A bullet-shaped blood pump, which has two sack-type ventricles, was designed and fabricated together with a low-profile atrial cuff. The pump fitted well into goats weighing 47–67 kg and easily produced normal pump output. The results show the promise of future success in obtaining long survival with goats using this blood pump.

**Key words:** Artificial heart—Blood pump—Design of blood pump—Fabrication method—Goat

In experiments concerning the total artificial heart (TAH), it is preferable to use an adult animal for the following reasons: (a) an immature animal, such as the calf, grows quickly during the experiments [1]; (b) an adult animal is more similar to an adult human physiologically than an infant animal. So, many laboratories have made great efforts to attain long-term survival in goats with implantable pneumatically driven TAH over the past 10 years. However, none of these laboratories have succeeded in achieving survival in the goat of more than 12 days except for one case of 184-day survival at Purkyne University [2]. It is supposed that the cause of these failures lies in the blood pump not fitting well into the goat's chest cavity, which is a very narrow space; the goat consistently survived with a TAH when the blood pumps were placed on the chest wall [3].

The objective of the present study is to establish the design criteria for an implantable pneumatically driven blood pump for a 50- to 60-kg

## Design and fabrication of blood pump

### Measurement of goat's chest cavity dimension

The shape and size of the heart and chest cavity of 50- to 60-kg goats were measured by left thoracotomy. As shown in Fig. 35.1, the shape of the natural heart and chest cavity of the goat has the following features: (a) the apex is very sharp; (b) the diameter of the heart at the atrioventricular ring is about 80 mm and the distance between the atrioventricular ring and the apex is 85–100 mm; (c) the angle between the sternum and diaphragm is acute; (d) the thickness of the chest cavity is about 120–130 mm. Following these measurements, it became obvious that the sac-type blood pumps developed in our laboratory and other conventional diaphragm pumps, such as the Jarvik type, are difficult to implant into the chest cavity of the goat.

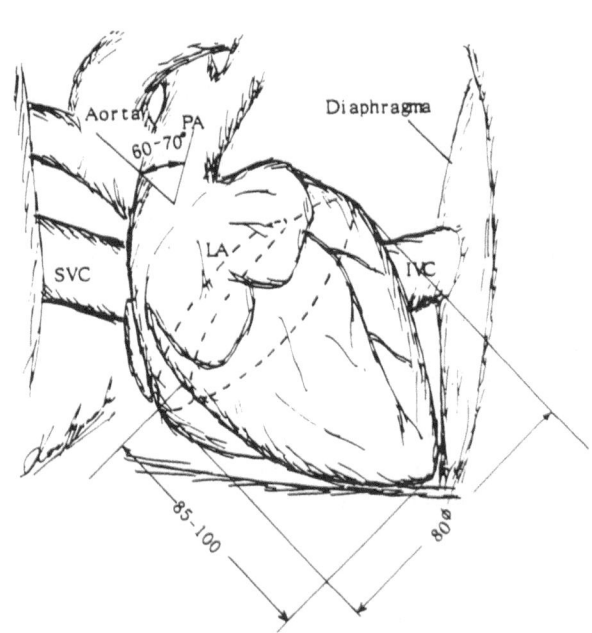

**Fig. 35.1.** Dimensions of goat's natural heart

[1]Institute of Medical Electronics, Faculty of Medicine, University of Tokyo, 7-3-1 Hongo, Bunkyo-ku, Tokyo 113 Japan

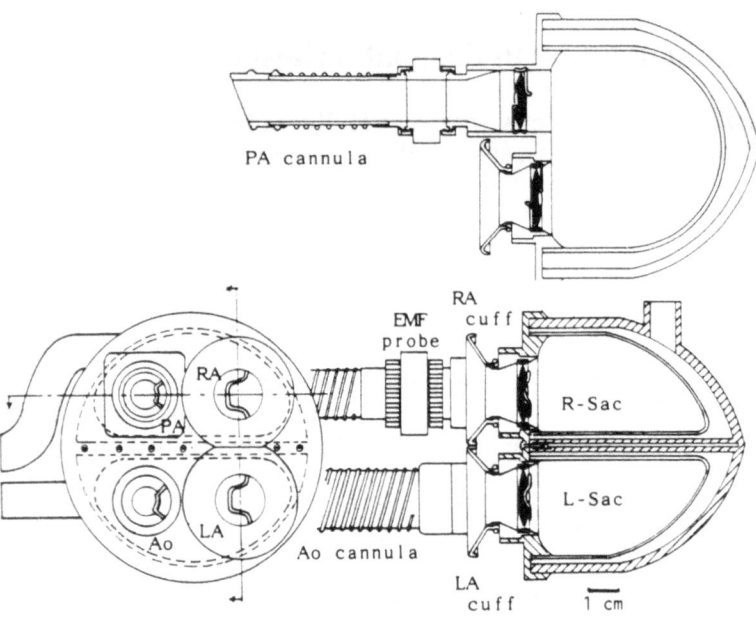

**Fig. 35.2.** Schematic figure of a new blood pump

### Basic design of blood pump

The specifications of the blood pump were decided as follows:

a) The blood pump to have a similar outer shape to the natural heart
b) The outer diameter and length of the blood pump to be less than 90 and 80 mm, respectively
c) The sack-type blood pump to be designed from the viewpoint of durability and calcification, because the sac-type blood pump has few stress concentration points
d) The maximum pump output to be 5 l/min at 100 beats/min
e) Björk-Shiley valves with an 18-mm orifice diameter, used in our laboratory, to be used as inflow and outflow valves
f) The distance between atrial cuff and the blood pump to be as short as possible

With these specifications, a blood pump was designed as shown in Fig. 35.2. To diminish the pump total volume and to fit well into the chest cavity, a bullet-shaped outer case with 80-mm diameter and 75-mm length was designed, in which a partition divided the lumen into left and right air chambers. Two sack-type ventricles with a volume of 60 ml were installed into each air chamber. To shorten the distance between the atrial cuff and the pump, each inflow valve was mounted in a screw-type connector, and the atrial cuff was also connected with the connector.

### Fabrication of blood pump

The blood pump (sacks, housing, and outer case) is made of polyvinylchloride (PVC) paste by the dipping or casting method or by a combination of both [4]. The whole blood-contacting surface was coated with Cardiothane to achieve blood compatibility. The cannulae connecting to the aorta and pulmonary artery (PA) were made by combining an EPTFE ring graft with PVC [5]. The atrial cuff was made of a Gore-Tex sheet by cutting and sewing, and fixed to the screw-type connector made of stainless steel. The inner surface of the cannulae and atrial cuff was also coated with Cardiothane. Figure 35.3 shows the blood pump, atrial cuffs, and cannulae.

### Measurement system

The pump output was measured and controlled by a specially designed small electromagnetic flow probe, which was inserted between the PA cannula and blood pump. The aortic blood pressure and right and left atrial pressure were measured by the pressure transducers through a side tube of the cannula and each atrial cuff. The displacement of the sack was detected by a Hall sensor fixed between the sack and outer case.

### Evaluation of blood pump

#### In vitro performance

The pump performance was tested in a mock circulatory system. Figure 35.4 shows the relationship of pump output to systolic duration at 10 cmH$_2$O of inflow head, 100 mmHg of outflow load, and 100 beats/min. The pump output increased according to the increase in positive air pressure, and the max-

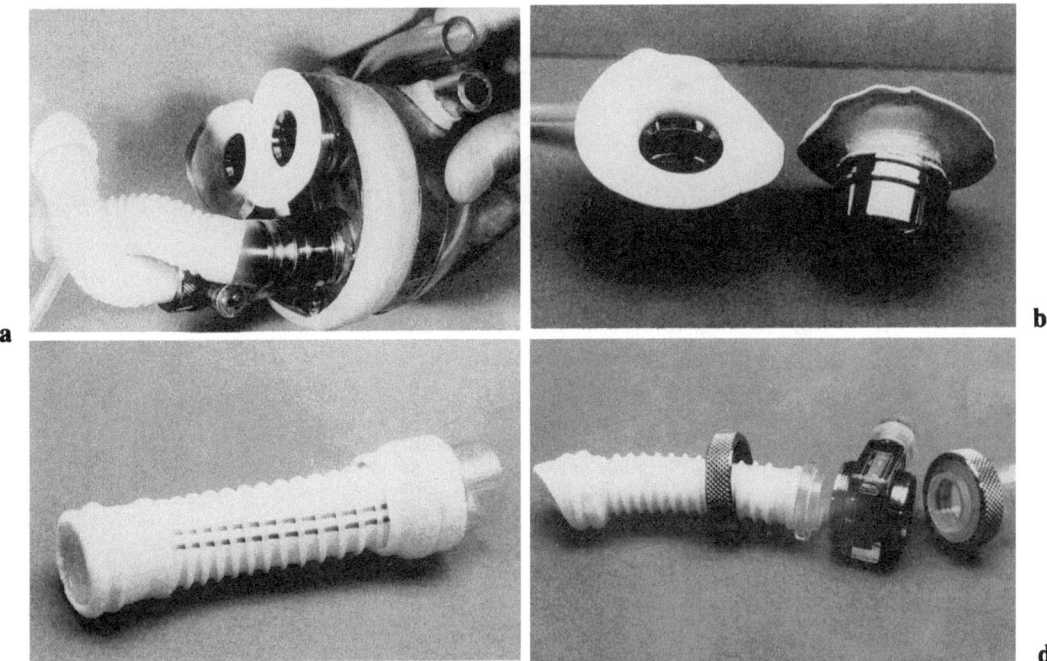

**Fig. 35.3.** **a** New blood pump, **b** atrial cuff, **c** aorta cannula, and **d** pulmonary artery cannulae with electromagnetic flow probe

imum output was 5.1 l/min. Figure 35.5 shows the relationship between pump output and pulse rate at 50% of systolic duration. The pump output increased in proportion to the increase in pulse rate when the positive and negative driving air pressures were set at a high value. The maximum pump output was 9.3 l/min at 200 beats/min. These results reveal that the pump has sufficient performance for a 60-kg goat, including when the animal undergoes light exercise.

**In vivo evaluation of blood pump**

Goats with a body weight of 47–67 kg were used in this study. The animals were anesthetized with halothane and the chest was opened by a left fifth rib resection. For the extracorporeal circulation (ECC), the specially designed inflow cannulae with air cuffs were inserted into the superior (SVC) and inferior venae cavae (IVC) through the right atrium, and an outflow cannula was inserted into the left carotid artery. These cannulae were connected to the ECC circuit. After ECC was started, the natural heart was resected. The aorta and PA cannulae were inserted into the ascending aorta and main PA, respectively, and were ligated by strings. The left and right atrial cuffs were sutured together to the atrial septum and then sutured to the left and right atria, respectively. The right and left atrial connectors were inserted into the inflow ports of the blood pump. After the right side pump was filled with blood by deflating the air

cuff of the IVC cannula, the PA cannula with electromagnetic flow probe was connected to the outflow port of the right side pump. After the left pump was filled with blood from the bronchial artery, the aorta cannula was connected, and both pumps were started. To close the chest completely and to prevent infection, a specially designed artificial chest wall, through which air tubes and cables of the flow probe and Hall sensor were guided to the body surface, was used. During the experiment, right pump output was maintained between 80 and 100 ml/kg/min, and the left pump was controlled so as not to elevate the left atrial pressure.

Following experimental trials, the blood pump fitted well in the goat's chest cavity, as shown in Fig. 35.6. No bleeding and no air sucking were observed after surgical operation in spite of the absence of protamine. Except for a few cases, the tracheal tube was removed within 1 or 2 h of surgery and the goat could stand up within few hours. No anticoagulant was used after the operation. The postoperative recovery course was almost the same with the other types of TAH goat in which the blood pumps were placed outside the body. The blood pump could be controlled well. Figure 35.7 shows the hemodynamic data of the TAH goat. Thus far, three goats have survived for 2 weeks (Fig. 35.8). The main cause of death was infections by eumycetes, which have invaded our laboratory over the past 2 year. No thrombus was formed in the blood pump and cannulae except for the

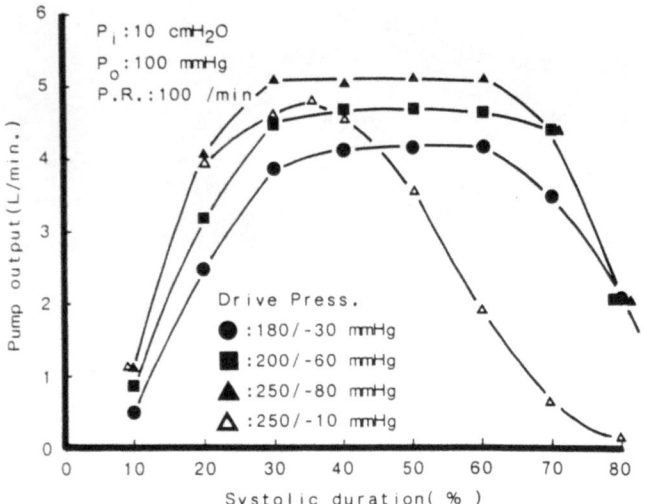

**Fig. 35.4.** Relation between pump output and systolic duration

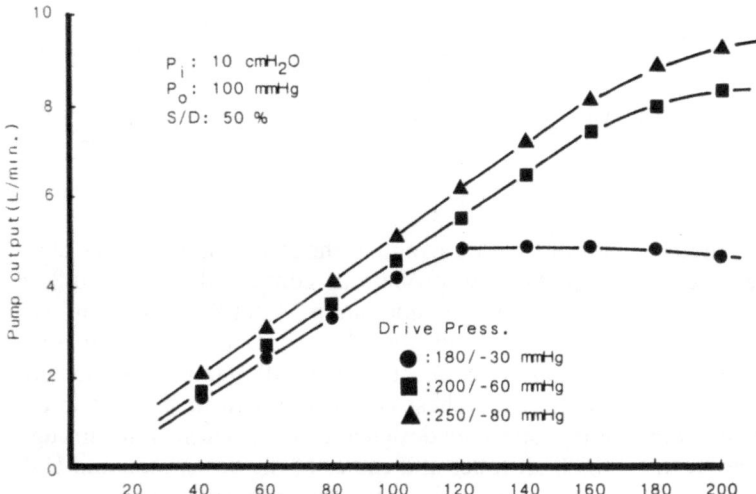

**Fig. 35.5.** Relation between pump output and pulse rate

infectious cases in which a heavy infectious thrombus was formed inside the aorta, PA cannula, and atrial cuff.

## Discussion

In TAH animal experiments, the calf has been used worldwide in many laboratories. However, with the longer survival of the TAH calf, the following problem has become apparent: The calf grows fast in the course of the TAH experiment and a low cardiac output state is induced, which makes it difficult to maintain the animal in a physiological condition. Thus, many laboratories have been trying to change from the calf to the adult goat over the past 10 years. At the Free University of Berlin, attempts were made to use a goat around 1979 but without success. The University of Utah also failed to achieve survival with the goat with the TH, and they successfully changed from the

goat to the sheep. The Hershey Medical Center has also attempted using the goat with the TAH. However, they reported that their TAH goat acted violently after the surgical operation and did not recover completely. The longest survival period was 12 days [6]. At Purkyne University, Vasku has been experimenting with the goat. However, he could only achieve survival for a few days except in one case that survived for 184 days [2]. In Japan, the National Cardiovascular Center and Kobe Central City Hospital have used the goat but with no greater survival than 7 days. They cited the following as causes of failure: (a) the goat has a very narrow chest cavity, which makes it difficult to fit the blood pump and obtain sufficient cardiac output; (b) the erythrocytes of the goat have very weak mechanical properties compared with other animals such as the calf and sheep; (c) the goat is week in TAH surgery, especially for ECC, and its management after the operation is very difficult.

In our laboratory, on the other hand, the goat has

**Fig. 35.6.** Pump was fitted well into chest cavity of goat

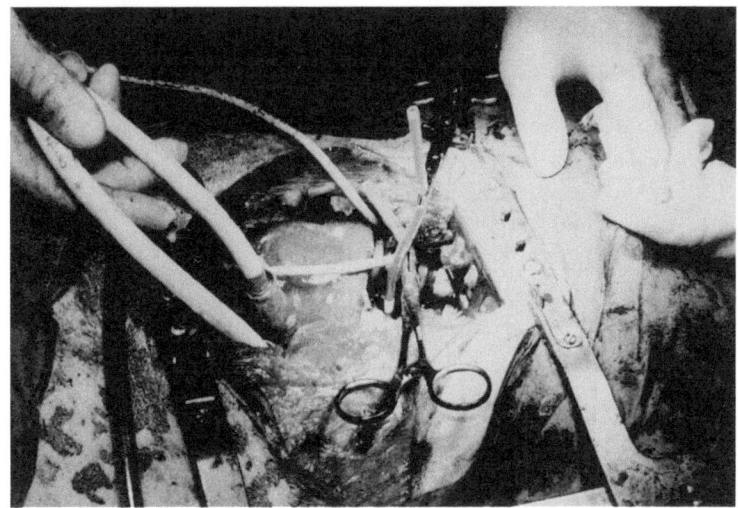

**Fig. 35.7.** The new blood pump implanted in a goat

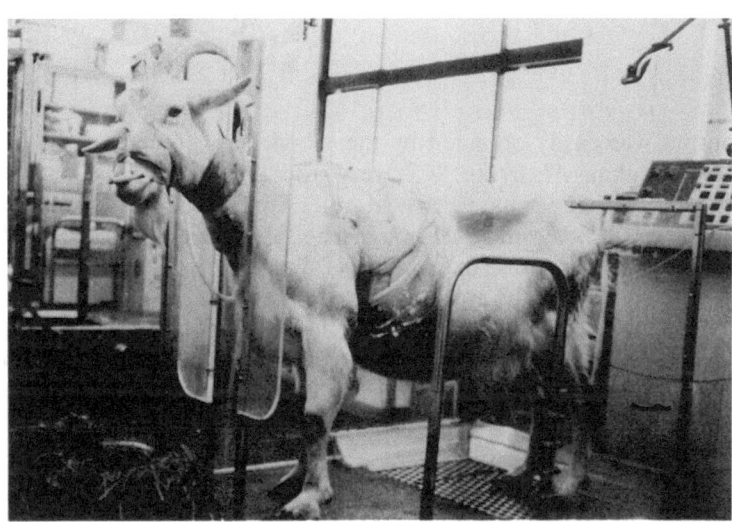

been used as an experimental animal for many types of TAH since 1972 [7]. In 1979, the TAH was used in conjunction with the fibrillated natural heart and the goat survived for 174 days. In 1980, the TAH was used with the natural heart still beating only from perfusion of the animal's own coronary circulation; here, the goat survived for 288 days. In the TAH in which the natural heart was resected, one goat survived for 344 days in 1984, which was the longest survival in the world at the time [8].

Although the blood pumps were placed on the chest wall in these experiments, the results have proved that the goat could withstand TAH surgery and ECC, and the erythrocytes of goat were not so weak for TAH pumping. Following these results, we conclude that fitting of the blood pump was the main problem in long-term survival of the goat where the pump was implamtable and pneumatically driven. From the results of fitting trails of various types of blood pump, it became obvious that the conventional types of blood pump, such as the sack-type pump which we have used externally and the Jarvik pump, were difficult to fit into the goat's chest cavity because of: (a) the chest cavity is very thin; (b) the angle between the sternum and diaphragm is acute and the pump requires a sharpe configuration. In the present study, we designed a bullet-shaped blood pump, which has a sharp configuration at the pump end, and succeeded in diminishing total volume of the pump. Another important problem was how to shorten the distance between the atrial cuff and blood pump: If the distance is too great, both atria will be pressed in the cranial direction and the blood return from the vein and lung will be disturbed. To solve this problem, a very low-profile atrial cuff and screw-type connector were designed, which facilitated blood return from the vein and lung. The blood pump developed in this study has shown a very good fit into the goat chest cavity, and normal cardiac

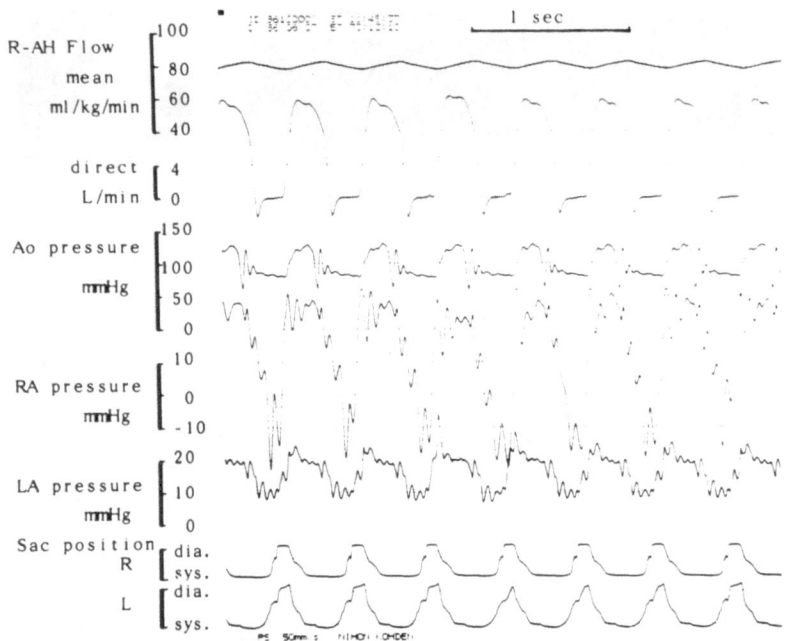

**Fig. 35.8.** In vivo flow and pressure wave form with the new blood pump

output was easily obtained by the blood pump for a goat weighing 47–67 kg. Recovery from surgery was more or less the same as that in other types of TAH goats in our experience. Although, the TAH goats did not survive for more than 2 weeks due to infection problems, the results are promising for future success in obtaining long survival with the blood pump.

## Conclusion

Criteria for designing an artificial heart blood pump fitted to the goat chest cavity were proposed.

It became obvious that the pump configuration for a goat was highly restricted at points such as the blood pump diameter, shape of the pump end, and the distance between the atrial cuff and blood pump.

To satisfy the criteria, a bullet-shaped blood pump and low-profile atrial cuff were designed and fabricated.

The pump fitted well into the narrow chest cavity of the goat and normal pump output was obtained for animals weighing 47–67 kg.

Recovery of the TAH goat from surgery was almost the same as with other types of TAH in our laboratory with long survival.

The results are promising for the future success in obtaining long survival with the goat under this blood pump.

## References

1. Hastings WL, Aaron JL, Deneris J, Kessler TR, Pons AB, Razzecca KJ, Olsen DB, Kolff WJ (1981) A re-trospective study of nine calves surviving five months on the pneumatic total artificial heart. Trans Am Soc Artif Intern Organs 27: 71–76
2. Vasku J (1987) Recent actual problems on the total artificial heart research in Czechoslovakia. Artif Organs 11: 298
3. Fujimasa I, Imachi K, Nakajima M, Mabuchi K, Tsukagoshi S, Kouno A, Ono T, Takido N, Motomura K, Chinzei T, Abe Y, Atsumi K (1986) Pathophysiological study of a total artificial heart in a goat that survived for 344 days. In: Nose Y, Ivanivich P, Kjellstrand C (eds) Progress in artificial organs—1985. ISAO Press, Cleveland, pp 345–353
4. Imachi K, Fjuiimasa I, Miyake H, Takido N, Nakajima M, Motomura K, Kouno A, Ono T, Atsumi K (1981) Evaluation of antithrombogenicity, durability and biocompatibility of an artificial heart system for more than 100 days. Artif Organs 5: 423–429
5. Imachi K, Nakajima M, Fujimasa I, Miyake H, Takido N, Motomura K, Tsukagoshi S, Kouno A, Ono T, Atsumi K (1981) A new composite materials for smooth-surface vascular prosthesis. Artif Organs 5: 484–487
6. Gaines WE, Pierce WS, Prophet GA, Holtzman KL (1985) The goat: an animal model for implantable blood pumps. Asaio J 8: 135–138
7. Atsumi K, Fujimasa I, Imachi K, Nakajima M, Tsukagoshi S, Mabuchi K, Motomura K, Kouno A, Ono T, Miyamoto A, Takido N, Inou N (1985) Long-term heart substitution with an artificial heart in goats. Asaio J 8: 155–165
8. Fujimasa I, Imachi K, Nakajima M, Mabuchi K, Tsukagosi S, Kouno S, Ono T, Takido N, Motomura K, Chinzei T, Abe Y, Atsumi K (1986) Pathophysiological study of a total artificial heart in a goat that survived for 344 days. In: Nose Y, Ivanivich P, Kjellstrand C (eds) Progress in artificial organs. ISAO Press, Cleveland, pp 345–353

# Discussion

*Takatani* (National Cardiovascular Center): You said that you use the Hall device to track the movement of the diaphragm. Your device is of the sac type. Can you linearly detect the position of the sac movement?

*Imachi* (University of Tokyo): No. As in the sac type pump, both sides of the sack walls are moved, we cannot calculation the stroke volume from the output of the Hall sensor. But we can determine the conditions of sac movement.

*Portner* (Novacor Medical Corporation): You seem to have done a good job in designing a heart that addresses the concern raised by, I believe, Prof. Copeland, which is the elimination of the dead space by having smooth contours around both ventricle. However, do you not think that you should be designing an artificial heart suitable for the human anatomy and then trying to adapt that to the experimental animal shape rather than developing a device that is specifically intended for a particular animal model?

*Imachi:* I have never tried to fit the pump for humans, but I suppose that it would fit by only minor changes such as the angle of the inflow and outflow tracts.

# 36. New valve-containing systems for the total artificial heart

Hiroyuki Fukumasu[1], Sadao Yuasa[2], Fumio Iwaya[3], and Kiyoshi Tatemichi[4]

**Summary.** Two common sites of thrombus formation are observed in the use of the total artificial heart (TAH) in the valve-containing portion of the quick-connect system: the connector junction of the vascular graft and atrial cuff to the TAH, and the valve-mounting junction. To reduce thrombus formation, an improved method has been devised, whereby commercially available valves are seated and sealed into the convex groove formed in the high-durometer polyurethane, which is a part of the male quick-connect system; a layer of the antithrombogenic segmented polyurethane is then coated over the inner surface, including the metal ring of valves.

The new connector and valve-mounting systems have been evaluated in the calf, goat, and sheep implants of the Tomasu TAH. All connections were evaluated by noting the presence or absence of macroscopic thrombus formation at the junctions. Animal testing to date has included evaluation of 294 quick-connector junctions (83% incidence of thrombus) and 68 new valve-mounting portions (6% incidence of thrombus). A previous evaluation of thrombus formation of around 204 valve mounts fabricated with the old Utah type of convex notch-mounting techniques and 226 valve mounts with our previous preliminary techniques revealed, respectively, 87% and 64.2% incidence of thrombus formation. These results have demonstrated promising results of the newly developed valve-mount systems toward eliminating thrombus formation in the current TAH design.

**Key words:** Total artificial heart—Thrombus formation—Valve-mounting junction—Quick-connect system—Polyurethane

For the past couple of decades, thrombus formation in the total artificial heart (TAH) has been one of the major problems to be solved to achieve successful clinical application [1, 2]. With the introduction of a smooth surface on the blood-contacting layer of segmented polyurethane, it has been possible to reduce dramatically thrombus formation in the TAH down to an acceptable level [3]. Advanced design and fabrication techniques of a seamless diaphragm-housing (DH) junction have eliminated macroscopic thrombus formation almost completely inside the ventricular blood pump [4]. However, recent experimental [5] and clinical use [6] of the TAH reveals two major sites of thrombus formation in the valve-containing portion of the quick-connect system: the connector junction of the vascular graft and the atrial cuff to the TAH, and the valve-mounting junction.

To reduce thrombus formation at those junctions, many investigators through the world have developed new types of valve-containing connector systems, such as high-precision, screw-type connector systems (Fig. 36.1) made of stainless steel [7] or a high-durometer polyurethane (Isoplast 301) [8]. The incidence of macroscopic thrombus formation, however, around the junction has remained in the range of 36% [9] to 86% [8] without the use of special fabrication techniques [10]. More recent clinical reports have revealed that the incidence of cerebrovascular thromboembolic

[1]Department of Cardiovascular Surgery, Takeda Hospital, 28-1, Ishidamoriminamicho, Fushimi-ku, Kyoto, 601-13 Japan
[2]Tomasu Giken, 722 Yashiroshinmichi, Himeji, 670 Japan
[3]First Department of Surgery, Fukushima Medical School, 1 Hikarigaoka, Fukushima, 960-01 Japan, and
[4]Department of Cardiovascular Surgery, Kobe Central Municipal Hospital, 4-6 Minatoshimanakamachi, Chuo-ku, Kobe, 650 Japan

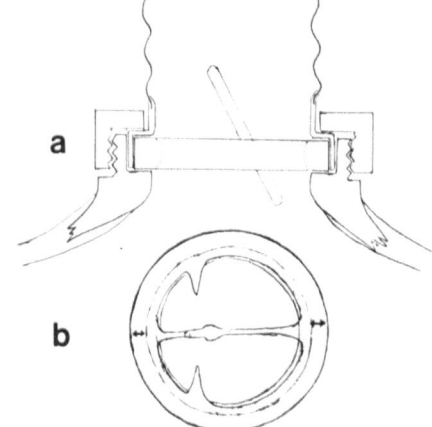

**Fig. 36.1a, b.** The screw type of valve containing the connector with a specially designed Medtronic Hall™ valve. To reduce thrombus formation around **a** the screw-type valve-containing connector, **b** the specially designed valve was produced by Medtronic Co. Ltd. (Mineapolis, USA)

events in humans is high compared with results in animals surviving extended periods. This discrepancy may be due, in part, to the difficulty in achieving precise neurological evaluation of animals but also may be due to differences in the vascular anatomy, including the presence of an intracranial vascular plexus acting as a filter in animals, and differences in the distribution of cardiac output [10]. Therefore, a small amount of macroscopic thrombus formation around the junctions causes severe injuries in humans and remains one of the major problems to be solved prior to the future successful use of long-term TAH implantation.

## Historical valve-containing systems

The oldest and simplest artificial valves [11] applied to the TAH were hinge types of unileaflet valves mainly because of reasons of economy; they had limited long-term survival with the TAH because of the huge amount of thrombus formation, especially around the valve. It was not before the commercially available valves started to be successfully implanted in patients that attempts were made at placing the hingeless types of mechanical valve directly in the inflow and outflow ducts, connected to a ventricular blood pump. However, the connecting portion of the metal ring of the valves in the inlet and outlet ducts had not been satisfactorily treated, and so the untreated narrow blood-static slit spaces remained as one of the major sources of thrombus formation in the TAH under development, even at the early stages of the postoperative course. Thus, many workers have made efforts to eliminate all of the blood-static, narrow spaces by coating the junctions with an additional polyurethane or silastic layer.

The previous old type of the Jarvik 7 heart consisted of the polycarbonate male duct of the "quick-connector" system [9], which held a metal ring of the mechanical disc (Björk-Shiley) valve placed on a convex notch build in the middle part of the polycarbonate duct. Several slits were made on the polycarbonate quick connector in order to allow placing a Björk-Shiley valve on the convex notch; they were coated with a polyurethane membrane to avoid leaking blood and eliminate thrombus formation around the valve. However, the dimethylformamid (DMF) solution, which was a solvent for the segmented polyurethane, induced fragility of the polycarbonate. The result of this was that the split spaces remaining between the valve ring and the convex polycarbonate notch could not be completely covered with the segmented polyurethane, becoming one of the main sources of thrombus formation after extended periods of TAH implantation.

## Selection of valves for TAH

Several types of mechanical disc valve (Fig. 36.2) and experimental prosthetic membrane leaflet valve have been considered as candidates for clinical use of the TAH, by considering the valvular functions, including the loss of energy across the valve, long-term durability, and tendency toward thrombus formation, not only on the valves but also around the valves. In general, if the valves are fixed directly and simply as mentioned before in the semirigid or rigid inflow and outflow ducts, they easily suffer greater damage than the valves implanted in the natural heart because of

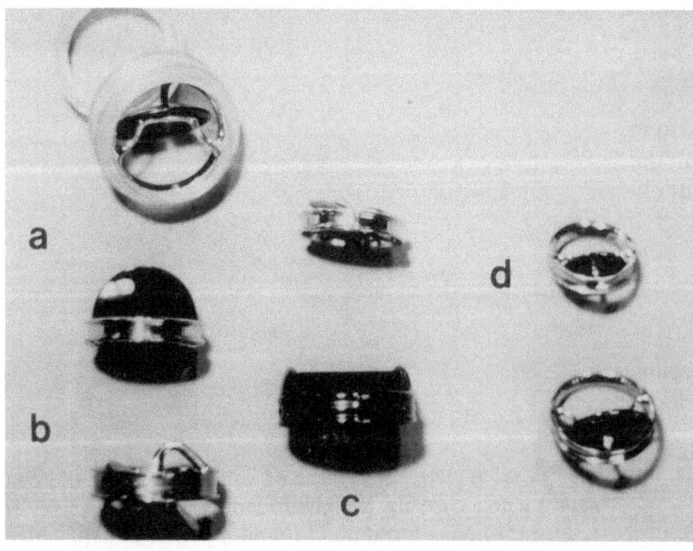

**Fig. 36.2a–d.** Several types of mechanical valve applied to the artificial heart. **a** Björk-Shiley valve; **b** Medtronic Hall™ valve; **c** St. Jude Medical valve; **d** Brazilian modified Björk-Shiley type valve. Each valve has a different outer shape of the valvular ring without the sawing ring

the lack of cushioning effects of the perivalvular soft tissues or the sewing cloth materials to avoid high stress from the higher dp/dt-raising driving pressure (3000–4500 mmHg/s) of the TAH compared with that (ca. 2500 mmHg/s) of the natural heart [12].

There is a little difference in the loss of energy measured across the various valves, and the mechanical valves reveal generally higher loss of flow energy than the soft membranous leaflet valves. However, the high loss of energy across the valve is a small problem in the artificial heart because there is no fatigue of the myocardium but full control of the driving power supplied to the artificial blood pump. Therefore, the most important critical factors in selecting the best valves are considered to be durability and the low tendency of thrombus formation both on and around the valves.

To reduce the incidence of thrombus formation around the valves and the valve-containing ducts, many workers have attempted to change the design of the valve-containing systems and have performed various comparison studies concerning the fabricating process and carried out animal experiments. For example, the Utah group has successfully developed an improved, high-precision, screw-type connector system, which contains a commercially available mechanical disc valve or a specially designed Medtronic Hall™ valve, and have evaluated it in calf and sheep implants of the U-100 TAH. Some other investigators have unsuccessfully developed several types of membranous three-leaflet valve constructed in the soft outflow or inlet, Valsalva-sinus like shaped duct and have evaluated the incidence of thrombus formation in short- and long-term animal experiments.

We have also made efforts to develop a good valve-containing system by investigating the best commercially available mechanical valves, including the St. Judie Medical (SJM) bileaflet disc valve, the Björk-Shiley valves, the Brazilian modified Björk-Shiley valve, the Medtronic Hall valve, and our own ball valves with the specially designed streamlined valve-containing duct. The SJM bileaflet valve was seen to have the least loss of energy across the valve, especially when placed in a rigid, straight inlet or outlet duct of the TAH; however, a definite disadvantage was evident with the outer surface of the valvular pyrolate carbon ring, which could only be fixed into a specially designed valve-containing system. Our own ball valve was excellent in terms of energy loss across the valve [13], although it definitely takes up the largest space around the TAH. Thus, the Björk-Shiley valve, the Brazilian modified Björk-Shiley valve, and the commercially available Medtronic Hall valve were selected for our comparative studies with the Tomasu TAH heart and some clinical Tomasu ventricular assist device (VAD) hearts.

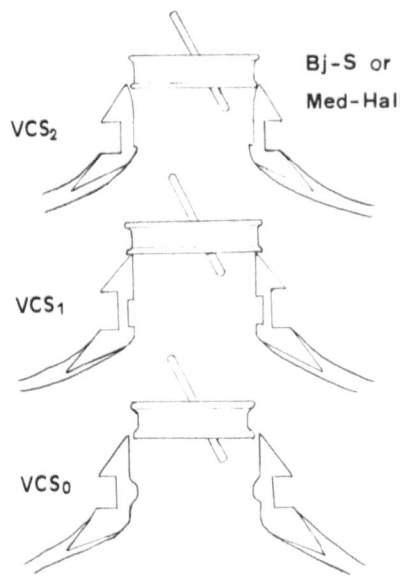

**Fig. 36.3.** Valve-containing systems (VCS) used in the Tomasu heart. $VCS_0$ is the oldest VCS; it has a convex notch in the middle of the polyurethane male quick-connect system (QCS). The outer diameter of the valve ring must be less than the inner diameter of the QCS. $VCS_1$ was our original VCS with a concave groove, in which a valve was placed. $VCS_2$ is the improved VCS; it shows the best fit with the various commercially available mechanical valves

## Design of our new valve-containing system

The newly designed valve-containing system (VCS) of the Tomasu heart are made of durometer polyurethane (Niporan 4327) and fabricated in two types ($VCS_1$ and $VCS_2$) with a concave groove in the middle of the male quick-connector system, as shown in Fig. 36.3. A special tool was developed and applied to place the various valves without a sawing ring into the groove (Fig. 36.4). The polyurethane is heated to approximately 70°C so that a selected valve with a slightly large diameter, which cannot be inserted without breaking the polyurethane container, can be gently pushed into the groove (Fig. 36.5); it then cools down to room temperature so that the dilated softened polyurethane duct shrinks to the previous diameter and clings tightly to the metal ring of the inserted valve. Additionally, a layer of segmented polyurethane is coated to reduce the remaining slit spaces between the groove and metal ring.

The original concave groove we made in the polyurethane duct was approximately 0.5–0.8 mm deep; the improve groove was 0.0–0.1 mm deep on one side and 0.4–0.5 mm deep on the other. A selected valve is inserted through the shallower side and pressed toward the deep edge of the improved groove, as shown in Fig. 36.6. The best fit of the valve

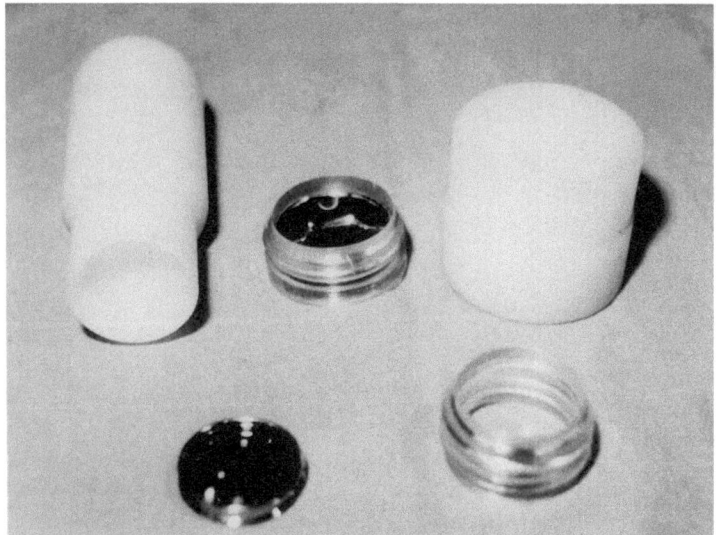

**Fig. 36.4.** A special tool for inserting a valve into the high-durometer VCS₂. See Fig. 5

**Fig. 36.4.** A special tool for inserting a valve into the high-durometer VCS$_2$. See Fig. 5

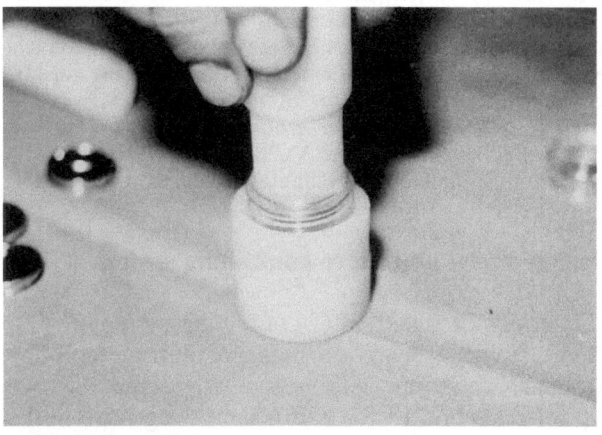

**Fig. 36.5.** A special tool for inserting a valve into the high-durometer VCS$_2$

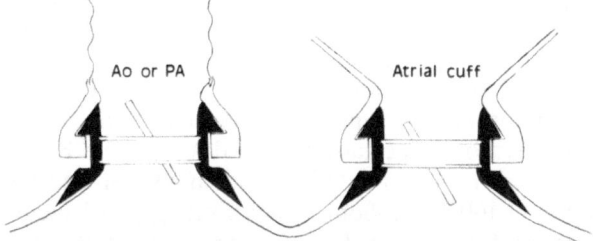

**Fig. 36.6.** Quick-connector systems used for the Tomasu TAH. The valve-containing systems with the Medtronic Hall™ valves are connected to both the outflow vascular graft and inflow atrial cuff with the male and female push-in quick-connect systems

in the groove was obtained with the commercially available Medtronic Hall™ valve, which has two short small edges of the outer concave metal ring produced by machine from a piece of metal with a perfectly circular outer shape; the Björk-Shiley valve and the Brazilian modified Björk-Shiley valve have individually shaped metal rings.

## Materials and methods

The Thomasu TAH with the original concave grooves containing four Björk-Shiley valves in the rigid polyurethane connectors was implanted in 20 calves, 24 sheep, and 12 goats; the longest survivals were 226 days in sheep, 67 days in calf, and 8 days in goat experiments [14]. The Tomasu TAH with the im-

proved concave groove in the hard polyurethane ducts containing two regular Björk-Shiley valves and two of the commercially available Medtronic Hall™ valves was recently implanted in 14 calves, 12 sheep, and eight goats, whereby the longest survivals were respectively 37, 41, and 4 days. Six stainless steel, screw-type valve-containing systems with a Björk-Shiley type of Delrin disc valve placed in the Pierce-Donachy VAD heart were applied in three patients at our institutes as a left ventricular assist device (LVAD) in one case and as right ventricular assist device (RVAD) in two patients for up to 4 days [15]. Four semirigid polyurethane outlet or inlet tubes, containing the Brazilian modified Björk-Shiley valve placed in the original concave groove (Fig. 36.7) and tied tightly from the outside of the segmented polyurethane tube by Tigan nylon tape, were applied as a LVAD in two

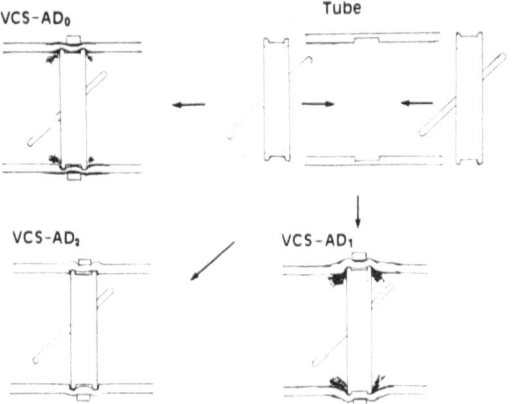

**Fig. 36.7.** The valve-containing systems, made of semi-rigid segmented polyurethane in the Tomasu ventricular assist device. The VCS-AD has a concave groove, which is 0.3 mm deep; the length varies with the size of the valve ring. When a large-diameter Brazilian modified Björk-Shiley type valve was placed in the VSC-AD$_1$, a relatively high degree of thrombus formation occurred at the supra- and subvalvular junctions. If the optimum size of the Björk-Shiley valve is used in the VCS-AD$_0$, the thrombus formed around the valve is minimal. Junctions like the VCS-AD$_2$ can be used with a Medtronic Hall™ valve

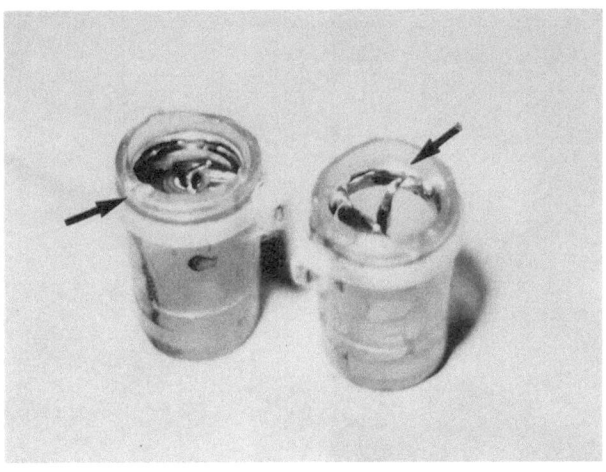

**Fig. 36.8.** Thrombus formation (*arrows*) in the VCS-AD$_0$ with a Björk-Shiley valve. This system had been implanted successfully in a patient for 12 days with a left ventricular assisting device. There was, however, no evidence of thrombo-embolism

patients for up to 14 days. Of these, one who was assisted for 7 days could be discharged from hospital [16]. Twelve semirigid segmented polyurethane ducts with the Björk-Shiley valves placed in the original concave groove with Tigan tape on the outside were implanted in six patients as five LVADs and as an RVAD for up to 12 days. Four of the six patients could be weaned from the assist devices and two of them could be successfully discharged from hospital.

In the long-term survivors in animal experiments with the Tomasu heart, 3–5 mg warfarin was given orally every day after the 4th or 5th postoperative day as anticoagulant, while no anticoagulant was used in the seven patients with the LVAD or RVAD. However, adequate doses of heparin were given in the remaining three patients with the Tomasu LVAD to keep the active clotting time (ACT) at around 200 s [15].

At the time of animal autopsy or surgical removal of the assist devices, all connections were washed gently of fresh blood only with ca. 500–1000 ml of normal saline solution. They were evaluated by noting the evidence of the presence or absence of macroscopic thrombus formation at the valve-containing junctions and comparing this with evidence of thrombus formation at the junctions of the male and female quick connectors or at the diaphragm and housing junctions.

## Results

When the commercially available Björk-Shiley valve was placed in the stainless steel screw-type valve-containing system of the Pierce-Donachy VDA heart, several slit types of blood stationary spaces were found at both sides of the valve and acted as major sources of thrombus formation at the junctions. However, in the valve-containing systems with a modified Björk-Shiley Derlin disc valve placed in the Pierce-Donachy VAD [16], the thrombus formation was found to be minimal because there are almost no splitting spaces between the specially fabricated metal ring of the modified Derlin, Björk-Shiley type valve and the stainless steel valve-containing system. On the other hand, the commercially available Björk-Shiley valvular junction in the semirigid polyurethane ducts of the Tomasu VAD heart revealed a little thrombus formation in all cases (Fig. 36.8), but which was smaller than that found at the junctions containing the Brazilian modified Björk-Shiley valve. The latter has a thicker metal ring, leading to thrombus formation more at the blood-static areas separated from the turbulent bloodstream behind the valve, as shown the Fig. 36.9.

One of the Björk-Shiley valves placed in the original concave groove of the Tomasu TAH slipped out of the groove and killed the calf, which had been in

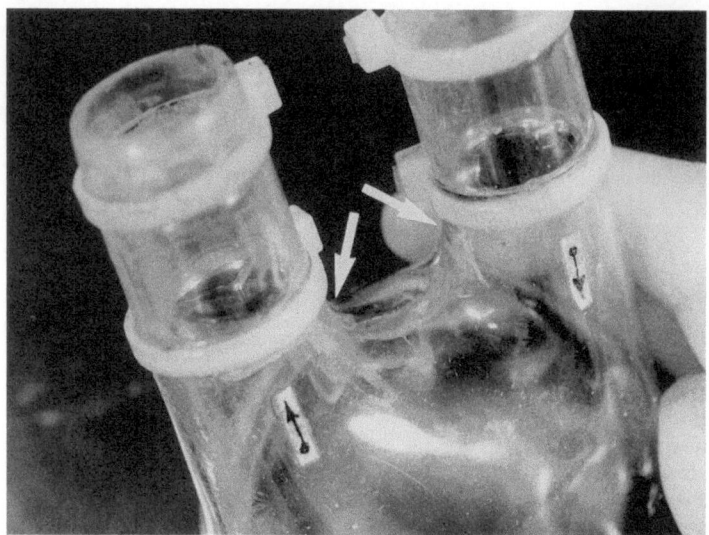

**Fig. 36.9.** Thrombus formation (*arrows*) in the VCS-AD₁ (see Fig. 7). A large amount of thrombus was found at the junctions in the Tomasu LVAD implanted in a patient for 14 days without giving any anticoagulants; there was no evidence of thrombus formation at any other parts of the LVAD. The patient could not be weaned from the LVAD assist

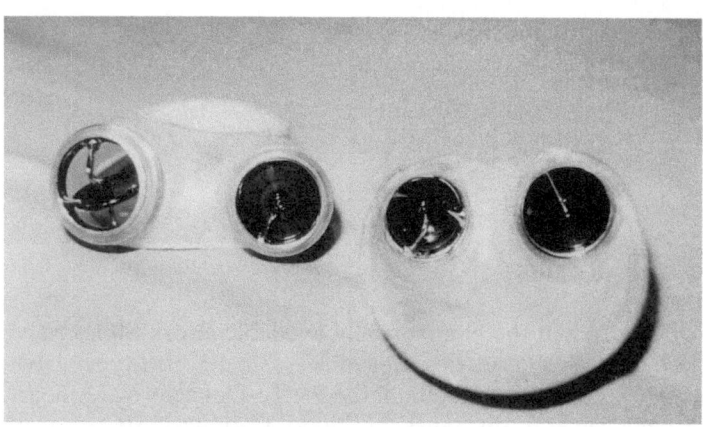

**Fig. 36.10.** No thrombus formation at the valve junctions in the Tomasu TAH. The improved valve-containing systems with a Björk-Shiley valve and three Medtronic Hall™ valves were constructed into the Tomasu TAH and implanted into a sheep for 41 days. The main causes of death of this sheep was not due to thrombus formation or any other mechanical failure of the Tomasu heart but to the excess dehydration created by giving too much diuretic in order to reduce ascites

a very healthy condition for more than a month. Another two Björk-Shiley valves placed in the original concave groove of the Tomasu TAH failed due to sticking of a disc leaflet in the transformed metal ring; the cause of this was overshrinkage of the durometer polyurethane valve containers. Also, there was much evidence of small pieces of old thrombus formed around 145 Björk-Shiley valves (64.2%, of total 226 valves) placed in the original groove. The Björk-Shiley valves placed in the improved concave groove (Fig. 36.10) revealed a 23.5% incidence of thrombus formation (8 of 34 cases), whereas the commercially available Medtronic Hall™ valve (Fig. 36.10) showed minimum thrombus formation in only 1 of 34 cases (3%). Thus far, there have been no valvular troubles with any of the Björk-Shiley and Medtronic Hall™ valves placed in the improved concave groove in the Tomasu TAH.

## Discussion

Recently, the Utah group has reported current evaluation studies of thrombus formation in the newly developed valve-containing portion of the quick-connect systems used experimentally and clinically in the Jarvik and U-100 TAH hearts [8, 10]. In animal testing to date, a 36% incidence of thrombus formation has been observed around the quick connectors. Evaluation of supra- and subvalvular thrombus formation of 12 valve mounts fabricated without special techniques revealed an 83% incidence of thrombus formation, while 44 valves specially mounted in the new Isoplast rings exhibited only a 7% incidence.

From the studies investigated by the Utah group, our original concave valve-containing system holding the Björk-Shiley valve has shown very similar incidence of thrombus formation to that induced on the screw-type valve-containing system fabricated without special techniques. Our improved concave valve-containing system with the Medtronic Hall™ valve has exhibited a similar incidence of thrombus formation to that around the valves specially mounted in the new screw-type (Isoplast 301) rings; of the latter, an outer flat shape of the valvular metal ring has been specially designed for the Utah TAHs.

We have also tried to mount the newly designed Medtronic Hall valve with the flat outer shape of the valvular ring into the improved concave groove of our Tomasu TAH. However, the flat metal ring did not fit sufficiently into the concave groove because of the large contacting area of the metal ring on the softened and dilated polyurethane, which transforms the inner surface of the male quick connector, resulting in the necessity of additional special techniques to eliminate the splitting spaces under the valve ring.

## Conclusion

Our improved newly developed valve-containing system with a Medtronic Hall™ valve revealed almost no incidence of macroscopic thrombus formation in the Tomasu TAH as well as in the new screw type of valve-containing system developed by the Utah group. In the latter, the specially designed Medtronic Hall valve can be seated and sealed prior to incorporation into the Jarvik 7 or U-100 TAH. Thus, the preliminary results of our improved valve-containing system with a concave groove in the high-durometer polyurethane quick connectors are promising in terms of eliminating thrombus formation around the valves in current TAH designs.

However, our quick-connect systems of the vascular graft and the atrial cuff to the TAH are still under development and evaluation in calf, sheep, and goat implants of the Tomasu TAH. If the female quick connector could be fabricated to a perfect size and fit completely on the male connector, though, a great reduction in thrombus formation in the junctions between the male and female quick connect systems could be obtained.

## References

1. Lawson J, Hershgold E, et al. (1975) A comparison of polyurethane and silastic artificial heart in the long sur-

vival experiments in calves. Abst Am Soc Artif Intern Org 4: 36
2. Lawson J, Olsen D, et al. (1976) A three month survival of calf with an artificial heart. J Lab Clinic Med 87: 848–858
3. Murakami T, Ozawa K, Harasaki H, Jacobs G, Kiraly R, Nose Y (1979) Transient and permanent problems associated with the total artificial heart implantation. Trans Am Soc Artif Intern Org 25: 239–247
4. Kessler TR, Pons AB, Jarvik RK, Lawson JH, Razzeca KJ, Kolff WJ (1978) Elimination of predilection sites for thrombus formation in the total artificial heart—before and after. Trans Am Soc Artif Intern Org 24: 532–535
5. Imachi K, Fujimasa I, et al. (1978) How to protect the thrombus formation in artificial heart. Proc ISAO (Artif Org) 2: 141–143
6. Joyce LD, Devries WC, Hastings WL, Olsen DB, Jarvik RK, Kolff WJ (1983) Response of the human body to the first permanent implant of the Jarvik-7 total artificial heart. Trans Am Soc Artif Intern Org 29: 81–85
7. Pierce WS, Rosenberg G, Donachy JH, Weiss WJ, Wisman CB, Richenbacher WE, Snyder AJ, Landis DL, Geselowitz DB (1984) Successful coupling of a compliance chamber to implanted motor-driven assist pumps. Prog Artif Org—1983 1: 226–230
8. Burns GL, Olsen DB (1987) The calf as a model for thromboembolic events with the artificial heart. Abst Am Soc Artif Intern Org 16: 4
9. Fukumasu H (1980) Development of total artificial heart. Arch Jpn Chir 49: 225–268
10. Holfert JH, Riebman JB, Dew PA, Paulis RD, Olsen DB (1987) Early preliminary results of a new total artificial heart connector system. Abst Am Soc Artif Intern Org 16: 4
11. Akutsu T, Kolff WJ (1958) Permanent substitutes for valves and hearts. Trans Am Soc Artif Intern Org 4: 230–236
12. Fukumasu H, Jinno K, Kim K, Yamaguchi K, Daito N (1981) Experimental and retrospective clinical evaluation of various artificial valves. Jpn J Artif Org 10: 975–979
13. Kijima T, Akamatsu T, Shiroyama T, Takaki K, Fukumasu H (1984) The development of ducted ball valve. Jpn J Artif Org 13: 275–278
14. Fukumasu H, Iwaya F, Yuasa S, Tatemichi K, Okamoto Y, Ban T (1985) Recent progress in total artificial heart (TAH). RBM (Revue Europeenne de Technologie Biomedicale) 7: 39–42
15. Fukumasu H, Yamazato A, Ban T, Soneda J, Fujiwara Y, Nishimura F, Iwaya F, Hoshino S, Yuasa S (1987) Initial application of ventricular assist devices (VAD). Arch Jpn Chir 56: 3–16
16. Ban T, Fukumasu H, Soneda J, Iwaya F, Hoshino S, Yuasa S (1987) Clinical application of left ventricular assist devices. J Cardiac Surg 21: 21–30

## Discussion

*Imachi* (University of Tokyo): Does the polyurethane ring completely adhere to the metal ring? Doesn't it come loose with long-term use?

*Fukumasu* (Takeda Hospital): It is obvious that it is impossible for molecules of the segmented polyurethane to adhere to the metal ring, but clearly the metal ring of the valve melts into the softer polyurethane quick connecter and is tightly held, after the connector has cooled down to room temperature (body temperature)

*Copeland* (Arizona Health Science Center): I think it's very important that you have developed a new valve mounting. This is, I believe, an area of major problems. I would like to ask a question about the so-called quick connectors. It has been our experience that they are anything but quick; they are difficult and clumsy and often result in the tearing of atrial tissue, which can destroy everything that the surgeon has done to try and achieve hemostasis. Are there any efforts underway to redesign quick connectors and make them easier to use?

*Fukumasu:* The Utah group have, I believe, recently developed a new quick connector, which is of the screw type, not a valve-containing system. The screw is on top of a connector on the atrial cusp or vascular graft. This idea sounds good. They say that special treatment is required to avoid thrombus formation around this junction, not around the valve-containing system.

# 37. Implantable motor-driven artificial heart

Shintaro Fukunaga, Yoshiharu Hamanaka, Hiroshi Ishihara, Taijiro Sueda, and Yuichiro Matsuura[1]

**Summary.** An implantable artificial heart was made using a flat-type brushless dc motor, a cylindrical cam, and Harmonic Drive as a reduction gear. A specially designed cylindrical cam makes the one-directional slow revolution into the reciprocating motion, then two sacs inside the driver are pushed alternately by the pusher plates located at both ends of the cam. The percentage systole of the driver is fixed at 50%. The two sacs, blood chambers, are 87 ml (left) and 81 ml (right) in volume and are made of polyurethane rubber. Björk-Shiley monostrut valves are placed at the inflow and outflow of the sacs.

The artificial heart worked at the driving rate of 39–125 beats/min with a flow rate of 2.9–7.3 l/min, consuming 15–43 W of electric power. The temperature at the surface of the driver increased by 3.9°C, while that of the saline in the mock circulatory system rose by 0.4°C. This artificial heart was implanted in a 120-kg calf, and various problems were clarified.

**Key words:** Brushless dc motor—Cylindrical cam—Harmonic Drive—Implantable driver—Total artificial heart

Toward a totally implantable cardiac prosthesis, various designs have been proposed [1–3]. One of them uses a modified Stirling cycle machine to actuate a blood pump [4], while another utilizes an electrohydraulic energy converter [5]. Most studies have dealt with a variety of artificial hearts composed of electric motors and pusher-plate blood pumps.

Artificial hearts with high-speed electric motors and ball screws [6–8] do not require reduction gears, but the motors have to rotate forward and backward alternately according to the systolic and diastolic period of the artificial hearts, resulting in energy loss owing to acceleration and retardation of the motors. On the other hand, a low-speed high-torque motor and cylindrical cam are introduced to the energy converter [2, 9–11]. This driver does not need reversal of the revolution of the motor, but low-speed motors generally have low energy density.

Two types of motor-driven artificial hearts were studied at Pennsylvania state University—a drum cam system and a roller-screw system—and 7 months survival in the calf was reported with the drum cam-drive artificial heart [12, 13].

Yamada and Fukunaga reported that linear motors were promising candidates for artificial heart actuators [14], but that there was still room for improvement to increase their thrust for totally implantable use.

We have developed a motor-driven artificial heart composed of a flat-type brushless dc motor, Harmonic Drive as a reduction gear, a specially designed cylindrical cam, and polyurethane sacs as blood chambers. The purpose of this paper is to present the structure and function of this artificial heart and the results in an animal experiment.

## Materials and methods

The structure of the motor-driven artificial heart is shown in Fig. 37.1. The high-speed one-way rotation of the motor is transmitted to the cylindrical cam by the reduction gear. The cylindrical cam then reciprocates to push the two sacs, blood chambers, alternately by the pusher plates located at both ends of the cam.

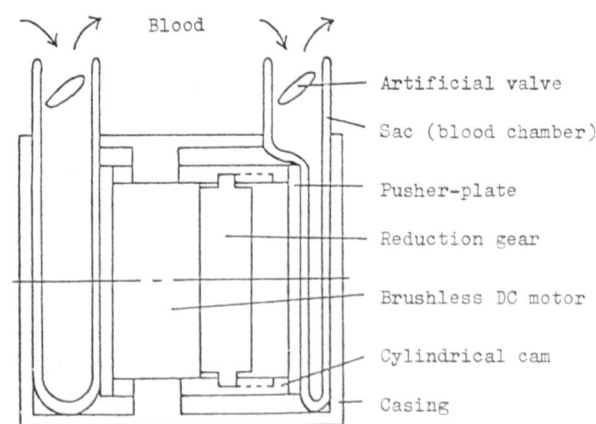

**Fig. 37.1.** Structure of motor-driven artificial heart

[1] First Department of Surgery, Hiroshima University School of Medicine, Research Institute for Artificial Heart, Hiroshima University, 1-2-3 Kasumi, Minami-Ku, Hiroshima, 734 Japan

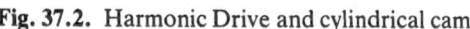
**Fig. 37.2.** Harmonic Drive and cylindrical cam

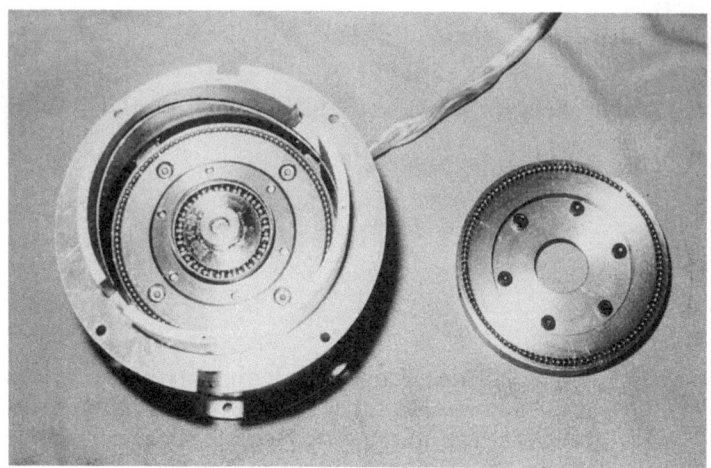

**Fig. 37.3.** External view of motor-driven artificial heart

The actuator used is a flat-type brushless dc motor, 69 mm in diameter and 38 mm in length. The rated speed, torque, and output power of the motor are 5500 rpm, 480 g-cm, and 27 W, respectively. The flat-type Harmonic Drive component is used as a reduction gear. It provides a high-gear ratio of 88 with an output torque of 0.8 kg-m through coaxial input and output shafts. It is 50 mm in diameter and 15 mm long.

A specially designed cylindrical cam has an endless groove for the cam followers, which makes one-directional slow revolution into reciprocation without reversing the revolution of the motor. The groove of the cylindrical cam and Harmonic Drive are shown in Fig. 37.2. As the cam moves from one side to the other, the two sacs inside the casing are pushed alternately by the pusher plates located at both ends of the cam. Then, the phase of pushing the two sacs, one for the left ventricle, the other for the right, is reversed and the percentage systole of the driver is fixed at 50%.

The two sacs are 87 ml (left) and 81 ml (right)

and are made of polyurethane rubber. Bjök-Shiley monostrut valves of 29 mm and 25 mm are placed at the inflow and outflow of the sacs. The external view of the artificial heart and its controller is presented in Fig. 37.3. The main body of the driver is made of aluminum alloy and carbon steel. Its maximum diameter, length and weight are 110 mm, 108 mm and about 2 kg, respectively

An in vitro total artificial heart test was performed using a Donovan-type mock circulatory system. A schematic diagram of the mock test is presented in Fig. 36.4. Aortic pressure (AoP), pulmonary arterial pressure (PAP), central venous pressure (CVP), left atrial pressure (LAP), and cardiac output (CO) at the aorta were recorded. The electric power consumed by the motor and the temperature of the saline inside the mock circulatory system and at the surface of the driver were also measured. The artificial heart with its controller, mock circulatory system, pressure transducers, and an electromagnetic blood flow meter probe are shown in Fig. 37.5

Experiments were then carried out using a 120-kg

**Fig. 37.4.** Schematic diagram of mock test

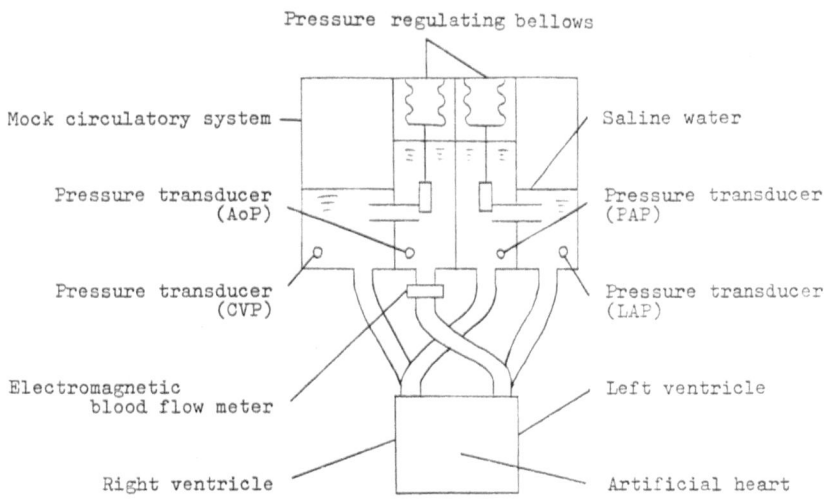

Pressure regulating bellows

Mock circulatory system

Pressure transducer (AoP)

Pressure transducer (CVP)

Electromagnetic blood flow meter

Right ventricle

Saline water

Pressure transducer (PAP)

Pressure transducer (LAP)

Left ventricle

Artificial heart

**Fig. 37.5.** Mock circulatory system with artificial heart

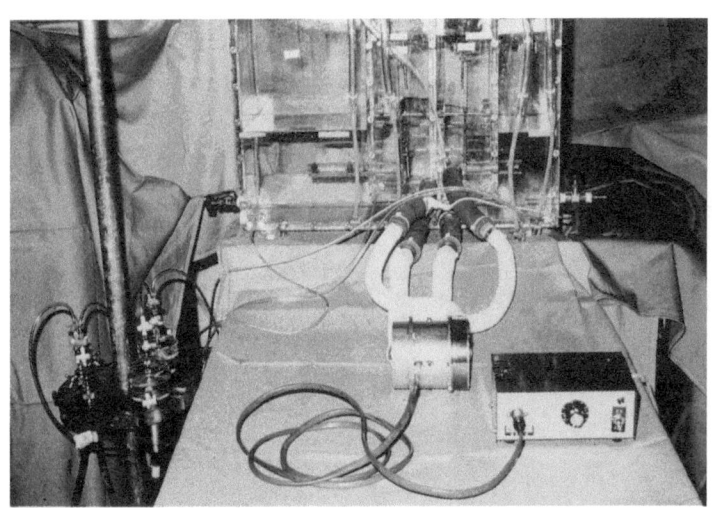

calf, as shown in Figs. 37.6 and 37.7. Blood was bypassed from the left atrium to the descending aorta, and from the right atrium to the pulmonary artery by the artificial heart. Impra-flex grafts of 30 mm were used as withdrawal cannulae and those of 25 mm as return cannulae. Flow rate was measured at the pulmonary artery (COPA) and at the withdrawal cannula of the left sac of the artificial heart (COAH). Electrocardiogram (ECG), AoP, CVP were also recorded simultaneously

## Results

The recordings of AoP, PAP, CVP, LAP, and CO in the mock test are shown in Fig. 37.8. Results of the mock test are also summarized in Table 37.1. The artificial heart worked at the driving rate of 39–125 beats/min, with CO in the range of 2.9–7.3 l/min. The phase of AoP to PAP is inverted because of the mechanism

of this artificial heart. Power consumed by the motor was 15–43 W according to the driving rate. The temperature at the surface of the driver increased by 3.9°C, while that of the saline (about 12 l) in the mock circulatory system rose by 0.4°C after about 2 h of driving in the ambient temperature of 25°C.

Hemodynamic recordings during the experiment with the animal under anesthesia are shown in Fig. 37.9. When the artificial heart was not working, the ECG showed the calf's own heart rate to be about 100 beats/min. The value of COPA showed the cardiac output of the calf's own heart to be about 6 l/min while the value of COAH indicated that there was no blood flow in the artificial heart. When the calf's heart and the artificial heart worked simultaneously, the AoP curve showed an irregular pattern. The cardiac output of the artificial heart, however, was almost negligible at that time because of the strong function of the calf's own heart and poor filling of the artificial heart. When the calf's own heart was under fibrilla-

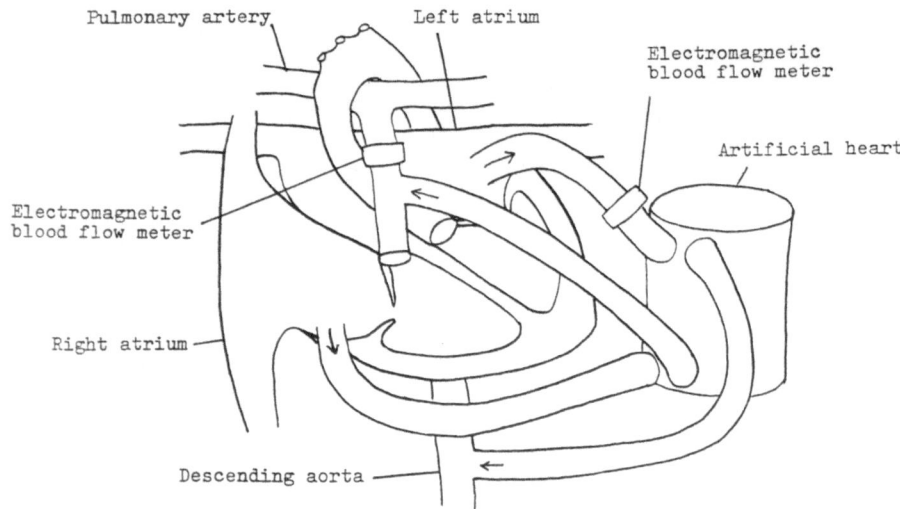

Pulmonary artery

Left atrium

Electromagnetic
blood flow meter

Artificial heart

Electromagnetic
blood flow meter

Right atrium

Descending aorta

**Fig. 37.6.** Biventricular bypass using motor-driven artificial heart

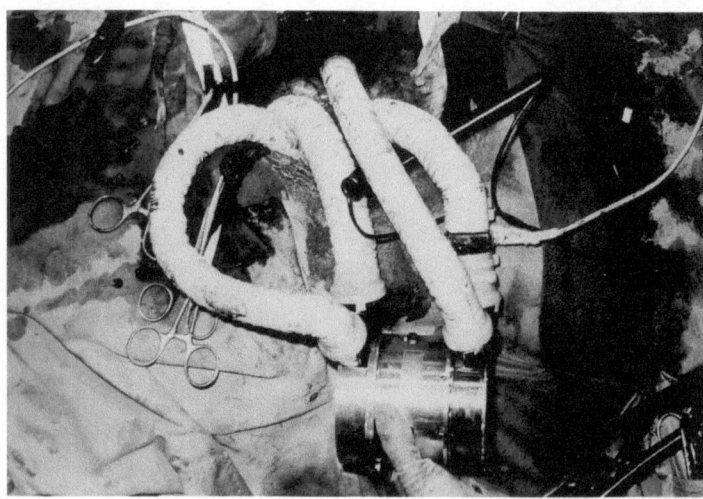

**Fig. 37.7.** Animal experiment

tion, the value of COPA decreased to about 3 l/min at the driving rate of 103 beats/min, which was equal to the value of COAH. The calf recovered from anesthesia without any sign of brain damage after about 30 min of circulation with the artificial heart alone, but at this point the calf was killed to terminate the experiment because there was little prospect of long-term survival.

## Discussion

An artificial heart, using a flat-type brushless dc motor, Harmonic Drive as a reduction gear, a specially designed cylindrical cam, and polyurethane rubber sacs, was made for totally implantable use. Its performance was tested in a mock circulatory system and

in an animal experiment.

The artificial heart was able to adjust its driving rate in the range 39–125 beats/min in a mock circulatory system. Cardiac output from the artificial heart varied from 2.9 to 7.3 l/min according to the driving rate. The stroke volume of 58–77 ml was observed in the mock test, thus the efficiency of the left sac was 67%–89% of the designed value of 87 ml, and that of the right sac was 72%–95% of the designed value of 81 ml. The flow rate of the left sac was the same as that of the right in spite of the different volumes of the two sacs. The filling of the sacs completely depends on the left and right atrial pressures; the present device has no active filling function, and so the flow rate between the left and right sacs is automatically balanced. As seen in Fig. 37.8, percentage systole of the artificial heart is fixed at 50%, and the phase of Aop to PAP is

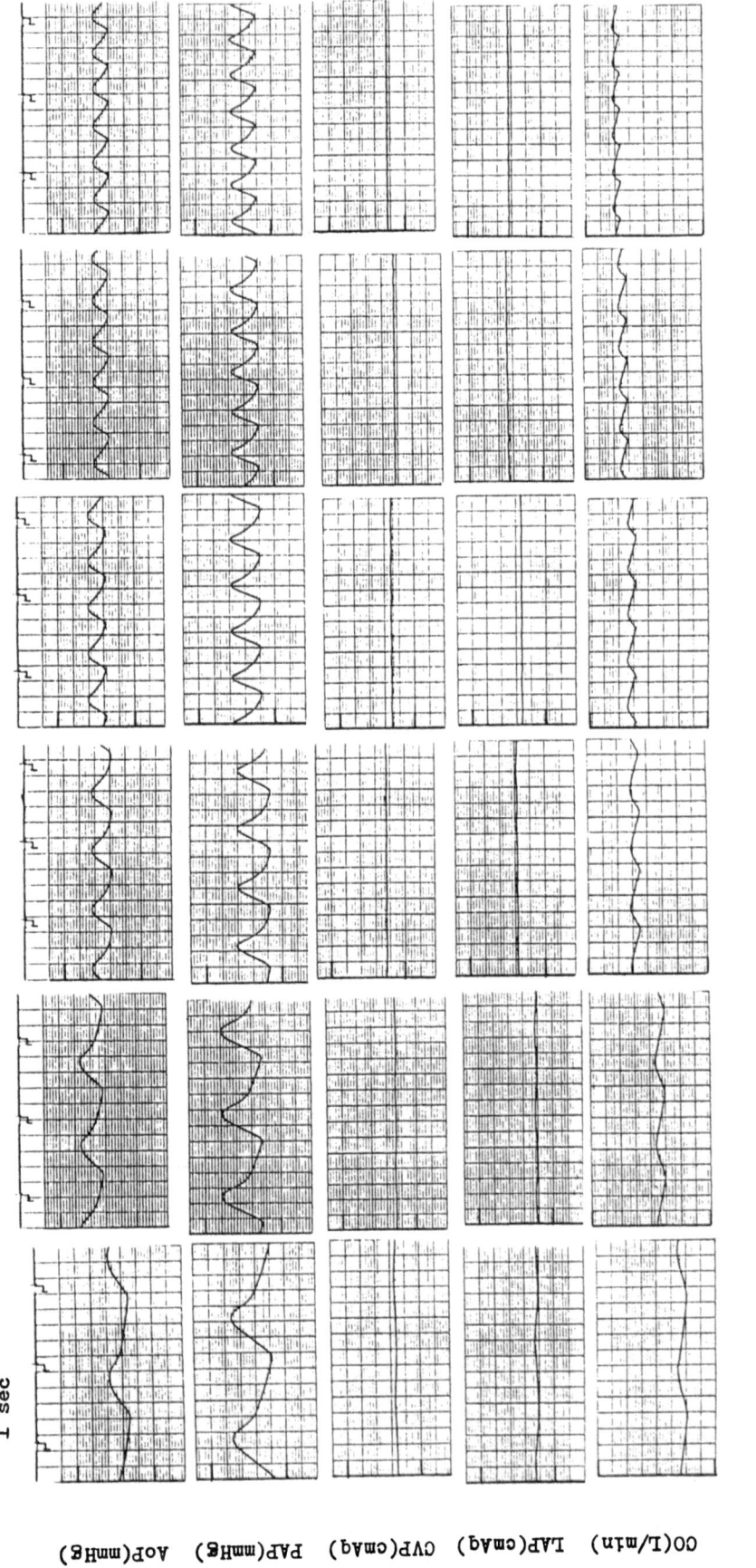

**Fig. 37.8.** Data of mock test

**Table 37.1.** Results of mock test

| Driving rate (beats/min) | 39 | 56 | 80 | 100 | 113 | 125 |
|---|---|---|---|---|---|---|
| AoP (mmHg) | | | | | | |
|    Mean | 84 | 98 | 98 | 96 | 98 | 104 |
|    Max/min | 112/64 | 144/88 | 128/80 | 120/74 | 120/80 | 120/84 |
| PAP (mmHg) | | | | | | |
|    Mean | 40 | 48 | 34 | 34 | 36 | 36 |
|    Max/min | 72/18 | 80/26 | 60/16 | 56/18 | 56/21 | 54/22 |
| Mean CVP (cmAq) | 17 | 16 | 13 | 15 | 12 | 12 |
| Mean LAP (cmAq) | 12 | 11 | 18 | 16 | 24 | 22 |
| Cardiac output (l/min) | 2.9 | 4.3 | 6.1 | 6.5 | 6.8 | 7.3 |
| Stroke volume (ml) | 74 | 77 | 76 | 65 | 60 | 58 |
| Power consumption (W) | 15 | 20 | 25 | 30 | 35 | 43 |

*AoP* aortic pressure, *PAP* pulmonary arterial pressure, *CVP* central venous pressure, *LAP* left atrial pressure

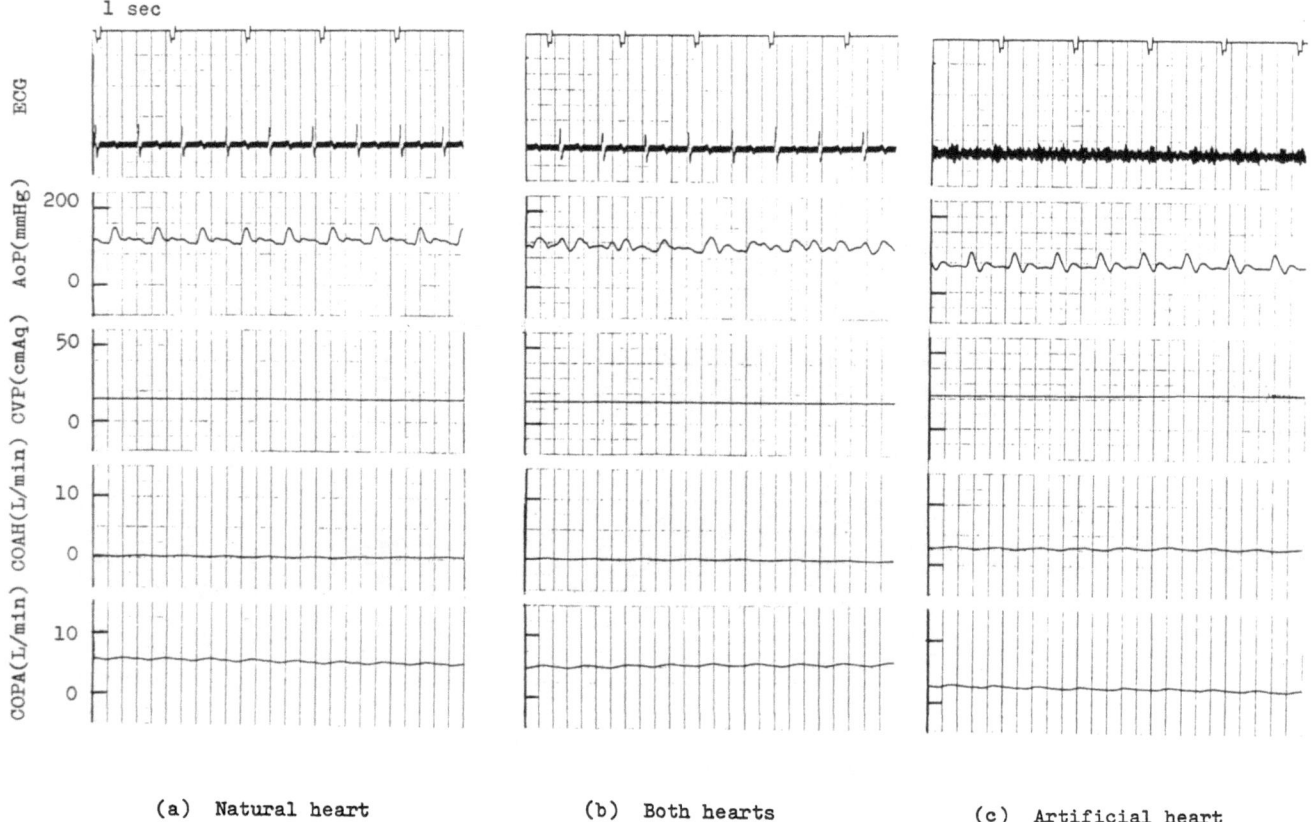

    (a)   Natural heart            (b)   Both hearts           (c)   Artificial heart

**Fig. 37.9.** Hemodynamic recordings of animal experiment

inverted. Cardiac output and the waveforms of blood pressure, however, seemed to be satisfactory in the mock test.

Cardiac output of the artificial heart in the experiment using a 120-kg calf was rather less than expected. The main reasons for this were considered to be as follows: (a) severe bending and obstruction occurring at the withdrawal cannulae; (b) lack of an active filling function in the artificial heart; and (c) a relatively short diastolic period as a result of fixed percentage systole at the value of 50%. Improvement of the artificial heart by equipping it with an active filling function without imbalancing the cardiac output between the left and right ventricles remains as a major problem for future studies.

**Acknowledgement.** Part of this work was supported by a Grant-in-Aid for Scientific Research from the Ministry of Education, Science and Culture of Japan.

## References

1. Pierce WS (1983) Protable artificial heart systems. Trans Am Soc Artif Intern Organs 29: 754–759
2. Takatani S (1986) Toward a completely implantable total artificial heart system. In: Akutsu T (ed) Artificial heart 1. Springer, Tokyo, pp 51–57
3. Harasaki H, Sugita Y, Fujimoto L, Sato N, Smith W, Navarro R, Kiraly R, Miose J, White M, Nose Y (1987) Implantable left ventricular assist system. Jpn J Artif Organs 16: 183–189
4. White MA (1986) Implantable energy source for artificial hearts. In: Akutsu T (ed) Artificial heart 1. Springer, Tokyo, pp 33–48
5. Moise J, Butler K, Payne J, Wampler R, Smith W, Fujimoto L, Golding L, Kiraly R, Harasaki H, Nose Y (1985) Experimental evaluation of complete electrically powered ventricular assist system. Trans Am Soc Artif Intern Organs 31: 202–205
6. Hayashi K, Seki J, Nakamura T, Fukumasu H (1986) Portable drive unit for artificial heart: Toward a totally implantable system. In: Akutsu T (ed) Artificial heart 1. Springer, Tokyo, pp 97–102
7. Jufer M (1986) Brushless dc motor for an electrical artificial heart. Proceedings of International Conference on Electric Machines, 8–10 Sept., Munich, Part 3, pp 1172–1174
8. Steiner HL, Hanitsch R (1986) Electromechanic driving unit for an artificial heart. Proceedings of International Conference on Electric Machines, 8–10 Sept., Munich, part 3, pp 1179–1182
9. Takatani S, Takano H, Nakatani T, Kinoshita M, Noda H, Fukuda S, Tsuchimoto K, Akutsu T, Konishi T, Koshiji K, Utsunomiya T (1987) Development of a permanent use motor driven total artificial heart system. Jpn J Artif Organs 16: 179–182
10. Gernes DB, Bernhard WF, Clay WC, Sherman CW, Burke D (1983) Development of an implantable, integrated, electrically powered ventricular assist system. Trans Am Soc Artif Intern Organs 29: 546–550
11. Takatani S, Tanaka T, Nakatani T, Noda H, Fukuda S, Adachi S, Takano H, Akutsu T (1985) Simultaneously ejecting left-or-right triggered total artificial heart actuated by a single electromechanical system. Trans Am Soc Artif Intern Organs 31: 367–371
12. Rosenberg G, Pierce WS, Landis DL, Snyder AJ, Richenbacher WE, Weiss W, Felder G (1984) Progress in the development of the Pennsylvania State University motor-driven artificial heart. In: Unger F (ed) Assisted circulation 2. Springer, Berlin, pp 270–285
13. Rosenberg G, Snyder AJ, Landis DL, Geselowitz DB, Donachy JH, Pierce WS (1984) An electric motor-driven total artificial heart: seven months survival in the calf. Trans Am Soc Artif Intern Organs 30: 69–74
14. Yamada H, Fukunaga S (1986) Artificial heart actuator using linear pulse motor. In: Akutsu T (ed) Artificial heart 1. Springer, Tokyo, pp 77–80

# Discussion

*Nakamura* (National Cardiovascular Center): How do you control the input power for the various arterial pressures?

*Fukunaga* (Hiroshima University): The motor power is controlled by the external controller.

*Nakamura:* What is the algorithm to control the power?

*Fukunaga:* We have no algorithm as yet. We just use the rotation speed. At this stage, the heart rate is controlled manually.

*Imachi* (University of Tokyo): What company made this motor?

*Fukunaga:* Aichi Denki Co.

*Imachi:* Is it easy to produce this motor according to the special specifications?

*Fukunaga:* It is a mass-production model, a conventional motor.

# 38. Left-right simultaneously ejecting motor-driven total artificial heart system

Setsuo Takatani[1], Hisateru Takano[1], Yoshiyuki Taenaka[1], Masayuki Kinoshita[1], Hiroyuki Noda[1], Mitsuo Umezu[1], Tetsuzo Akutsu[1], K. Koshiji[2], Eimei Shuu[2], and Toshio Utsunomiya[2]

**Summary.** As a completely implantable total artificial heart (TAH) system, a motor-driven TAH system powered by a transcutaneous transformer system has been designed and built. The TAH system consists of a high-torque and low-speed dc brushless motor sandwiched between a pair of pusher-plate type ventricles. The unique aspects of this system include: (a) the left and right ventricles eject simultaneously like the natural heart; and (b) ejection of the ventricles is controlled by the filling of either ventricle, thus pump output can vary in response to changes in either left or right atrial pressure.

The system is cylindrical with a diameter of about 90 mm and a height of 80 mm, and the overall weight, including the two ventricles and connectors, is approximately 900 g. The pump output of 6–7 l/min is possible against the afterload of 100 mmHg. The system efficiency is about 10%–15%. It was confirmed in acute studies that the motor-driven TAH as powered by a transcutaneous transformer system is a possible way of attaining a completely implantable TAH system. Currently, the durability test is underway and in vivo implantation will ensue when the anatomical fitting study is completed.

**Key words:** Total artificial heart—Transcutaneous energy transmission

In the last decade, research into the artificial heart has made remarkable progress and human survival for over 1 year with the natural heart replaced by an artificial one has become a reality [1]. However, in terms of the patient's quality of life and from the scientific point of view, limitations of the currently available artificial heart systems have become apparent. They include: (a) tethering of the patients to the bedside control drive systems: (b) risk of infection through the drive lines that penetrate the chest wall; (c) thromboembolic complications that can lead to stroke; and (d) inadequacy of pump output control to meet patient's changing cardiac demand. Continued efforts have been made to try and solve these problems and to obtain a completely implantable system which is durable, reliable, and thromboresistive [2–4].

Since 1983, we have been engaged in the development of a completely implantable total artificial heart (TAH) system. We selected the pusher plate-type blood pump for TAH application because of its excellent controllability and mating capability with implantable energy coverters such as electrical motors or thermal engines. Initially, a pneumatic TAH was designed and built to establish the technical problems associated with replacement of the natural heart and maintenance of the entire circulation with the TAH [5]. To date, we have been successful in obtaining survivors for a duration of 68 and 81 days with the pneumatic pusher plate-type TAH system. One of the problems that has been observed in the pneumatic model is finding the most suitable left-right control method for the completely implantable TAH system. In terms of hardware, anatomy, control, and physiological factors, left-right independent, simultaneous, and alternate ejection modes were studied in the TAH animal, leading to selection of the left-right simultaneous ejection mode for the completely implantable TAH system. An electromechanical system utilizing a dc brushless motor was designed and fabricated [6]. Concerning the energy supply for the electric motor, in order to isolate the implanted system from the external device, the concept of transcutaneous energy transmission utilizing a transformer system was incorporated into the system [7]. This paper describes the progress to date in the development of a completely implantable most-driven TAH system powered by a transcutaneous energy transmission device.

## Transcutaneous energy transmission device

The concept of transcutaneous energy transmission was proposed by Schuder et al. [8]. In this concept, the energy is first converted into high-frequency energy and transmitted through air or a dielectric material using a coupled coil system. Thus, transmission efficiency and energy loss become the main problem, particularly in a biological environment, in designing an efficient transformer system.

[1]National Cardiovascular Center Research Institute, 5-7-1 Fujishiro-dai, Suita, Osaka, 565 Japan
[2]Science University of Tokyo Department of Electronics, 2641 Yamazaki, Noda, Chiba, 278 Japan

## Transformer model analysis

In Fig. 38.1, an equivalent circuit for a transformer system is shown. Based on this model, transmission efficiency is expressed [7] as:

$$\eta = \frac{\omega_0^2 k_m^2 N_1^2 N_2^2 R_L}{(k_{r2}N_2 + R_L)^2 k_{r1} N_1 + \omega_0^2 k_m^2 N_1^2 N_2^2 (K_{r2}N_2 + R_L)}$$

where $N_1$, $N_2$ are the number of turns of the primary and secondary coils, $k_{r1}$, $k_{r2}$ are the resistance per unit turn of the primary and secondary coils, respectively, and $k_m$ is the mutual inductance per unit turn between the primary and secondary coils. This equation indicates that when $N_1$, $R_L$ (load resistance), $\omega_0$ (angular frequency), and dimensions of the coils are determined, $N_2$ value can be determined to yield the maximum efficiency. Figure 38.1b shows the efficiency versus the $N_2$ value for two types of coil whose dimensions are defined in Fig. 38.2. Maximum efficiency of about 70%–80% can be obtained for the two types of coil at $N_2$ values of about 10–15.

## In vivo study

To study transmission efficiency and the effects on the biological tissue, the type 1 type 2 coils specified in Fig. 38.2 were fabricated using insulated copper wire. The secondary coil was placed in the subcutaneous tissue of a goat and the primary coil was paced externally, directly above the secondary coil. The skin thickness was approximately 5 mm. The output from the secondary coil was connected to the resistive load that was located outside the body. To evaluate the effects on the biological tissue, tissue temperature was monitored at five different locations, as indicated in Fig. 38.2. Figure 38.2b,c shows the temperature changes with time for type 1 and type 2 coils when 10 W power was transmitted. For type 1, the temperature rise on the skin surface and in the tissue between the two coils was significant. This was mainly due to heat dissipation in the primary coil that was directly transmitted to the surrounding tissue. In the type 2 coil, temperature increases measured at the same locations were lower, and the temperature rise of the primary coil was also less. These differences stemmed from the fact that the impedance matching between the power source and primary coil was not appropriate in the type 1 coil, and thus a high power loss occurred in the primary coil. The transmission efficiency of the type 1 and 2 coils was 66% and 86%, respectively, and these values agree fairly well with the theoretical values. In the type 1 coil, approximately 27% of the entire power was dissipated as heat in the primary coil, while in type 2 it was only 6%. The power loss in the secondary coil of both types was 6.7%–8.5%. This result indicates that appropriate design of the primary

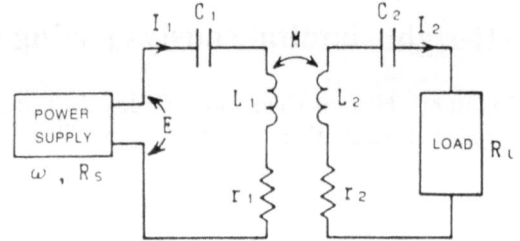

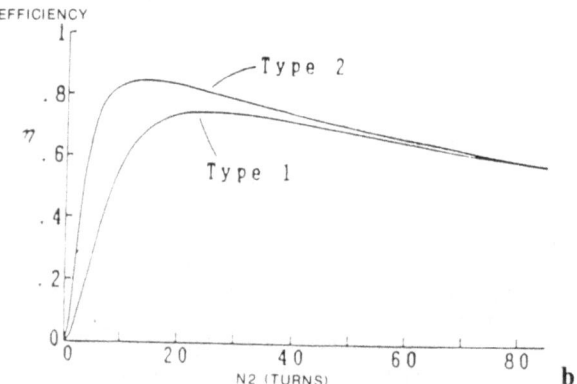

**Fig. 38.1.** **a** An equivalent circuit model for a transformer system and **b** efficiency vs. number of turns for the secondary coil

coil is a key factor in optimization of the transmission efficiency and power loss in the transformer system. The type 2 coil was later used in the benchtop study to power the mother-driven artificial heart.

## Motor-driven TAH system

### Left-right simultaneous ejection mechanism

To achieve left-right simultaneous ejection utilizing a single electric motor, a mechanical system to convert the rotational motion of the motor to a left-right simultaneous rectilinear motion is necessary. Though a roller screw or ball screw has been utilized to drive blood pumps, its application is limited for a reversing alternate operation. The only possibility is a modification of a cam which has been used for reversing left-right alternate ejection. To obtain left-right simultaneous ejection using a cam, a coaxial double-cam mechanism having a double-cam track was proposed and designed [6, 9]. Though the original design incorporation different tracks for the left and right cam follower, there was a problem at the crossover point of

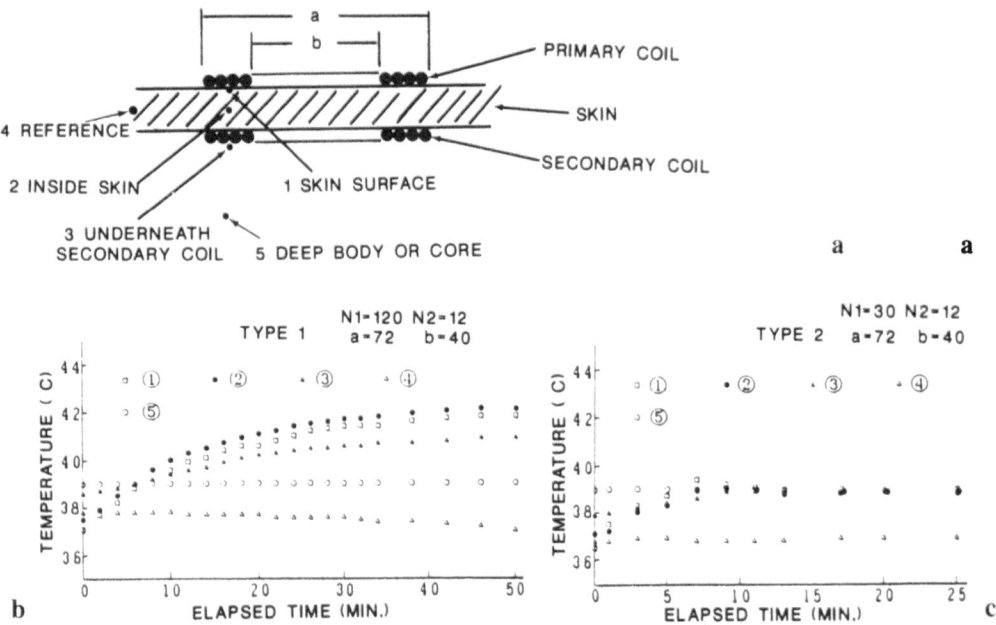

**Fig. 38.2. a** Location of temperature measurement inside the subcutaneous tissue during energy transmission study in the goat; **b** temperature vs. elapsed time for type 1; and **c** type 2 coil

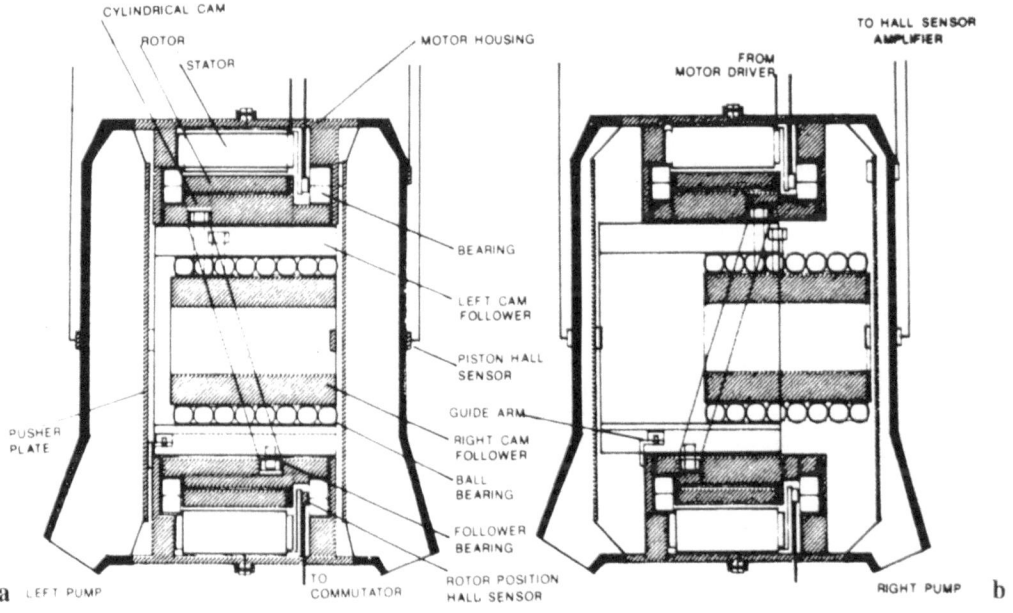

**Fig. 38.3a, b.** Simultaneous ejection mechanism showing **a** the end-diastolic and **b** end-systolic phase

the two tracks. Hence, in the later design, a single-track system was employed to eliminate the problem of crossover between the two tracks [10]. Figure 38.3 is a schematic diagram of the cylindrical cam-double cam-follower mechanism to achieve left-right simultaneous ejection. The follower mechanism is a coaxial two-layer piston where the outer and inner piston move in opposite directions to attain simultaneous rectilinear motion. The cylindrical cam has a single-track cut at its inner surface, where the follower bearing of the follower pistons slides as the motor-cam assembly rotates. Since the cam followers are prevented from rotational motion by the slide bearing attached to the motor housing and since the follower bearings of the followers are separated by 180° from one another, the follower pistons move in opposite directions to activate the ejection of the pusher plate located on either side of the motor housing.

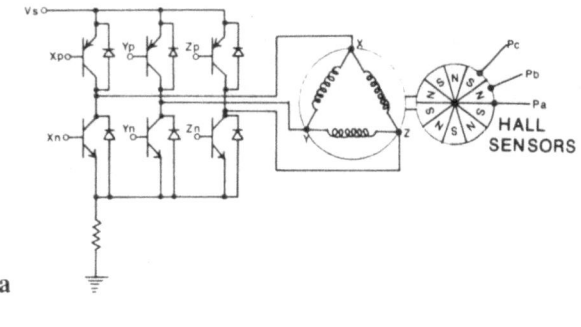

a

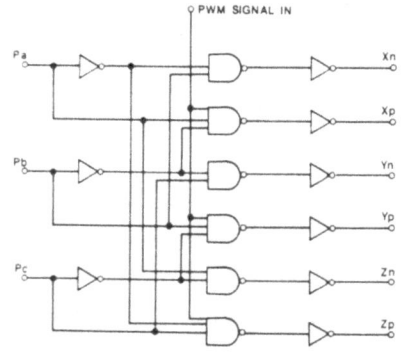

b

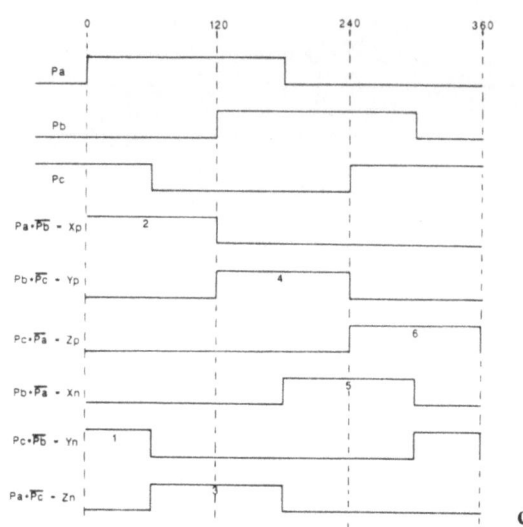

c

**Fig. 38.4a–c.** Circuit diagrams of **a** the rotor commutator and motor driver, **b** pulse distributor, and **c** timer

**Fig. 38.5.** Block diagram of a motor-driven TAH control system

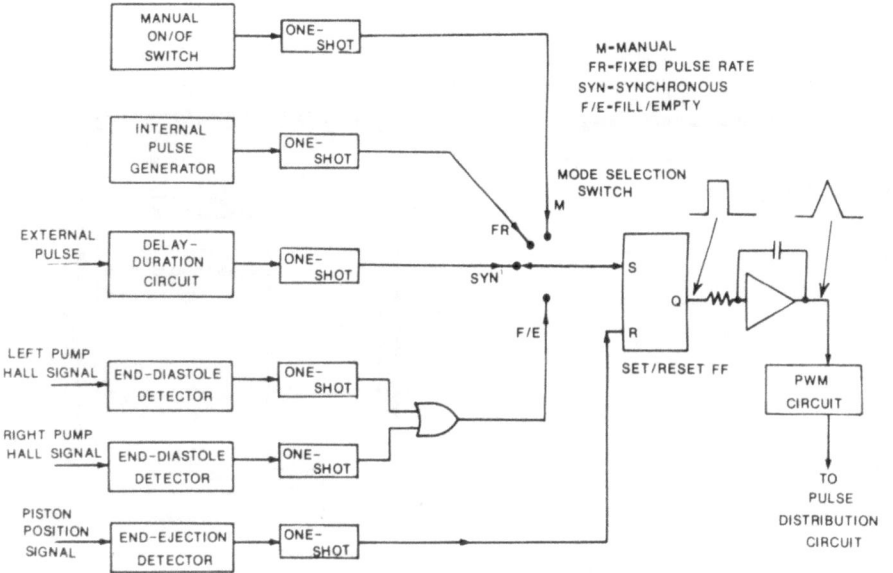

### Control-drive mechanism

The unique feature of this system is utilization of two sets of sensor system to control rotation of the motor: one is a set of three Hall sensors attached to the end of the motor stator to detect rotor position, and the other is a set of three Hall sensors to detect the position of the follower piston and position of the pusher plate of the left and right blood pumps.

**Motor commutation circuit**. To detect the position of the rotor and to commutate the rotor rotation, three Hall sensors are attached to the edge of the stator. Since the motor is a ten-pole and three-phase winding machine, three Hall devices are placed 24° apart to generate commutation signals. The driver circuit consists of a set of three NPN-PNP transistors whose midpoints are connected to the widings of the motor. The commutation circuit and its timing diagram are shown in Fig. 38.4.

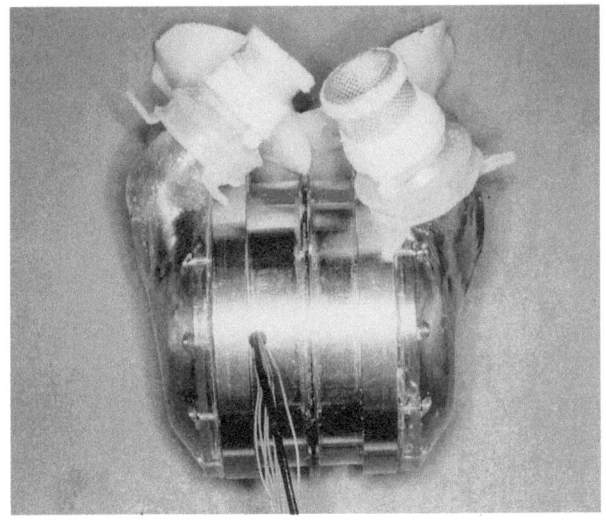

**Fig. 38.6.** Prototype motor-driven TAH system

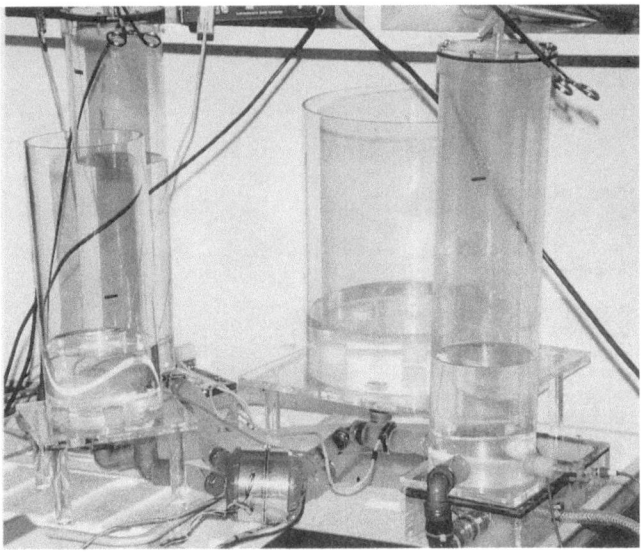

**Fig. 38.7.** Bench-top mock circuit, including the prototype motor-driven TAH system

**Fig. 38.8.** Hydrodynamic performance of a motor-driven TAH. Response of the system as the left pump afterload was increased from 20 to 110 mmHg

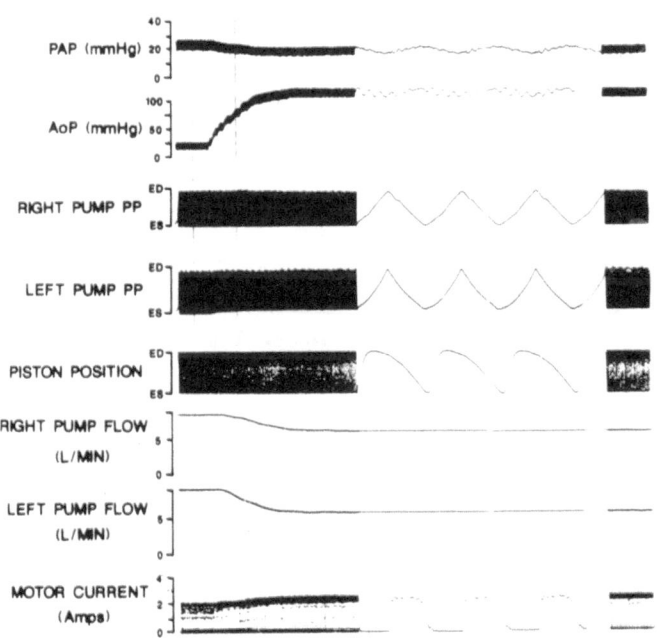

**Control-drive system.** Figure 38.5 is a block diagram of the control-drive system. The drive modes are: (a) manual; (b) fixed pulse rate; (c) variable pulse rate; and (d) synchronous. In each mode, the Hall-effect position signal of the cam-follower piston is used to terminate the ejection process. In the variable rate mode, filling of either ventricle is detected from the Hall-effect position signal to trigger ejection of both ventricles.

**Prototype TAH**

Figure 38.6 shows the prototype motor-driven TAH. The system is cylindrical with a diameter of 90 mm and height of 80 mm. The overall weight, including both ventricles, is about 900 g. The stroke volume of the ventricle is about 60 cm³.

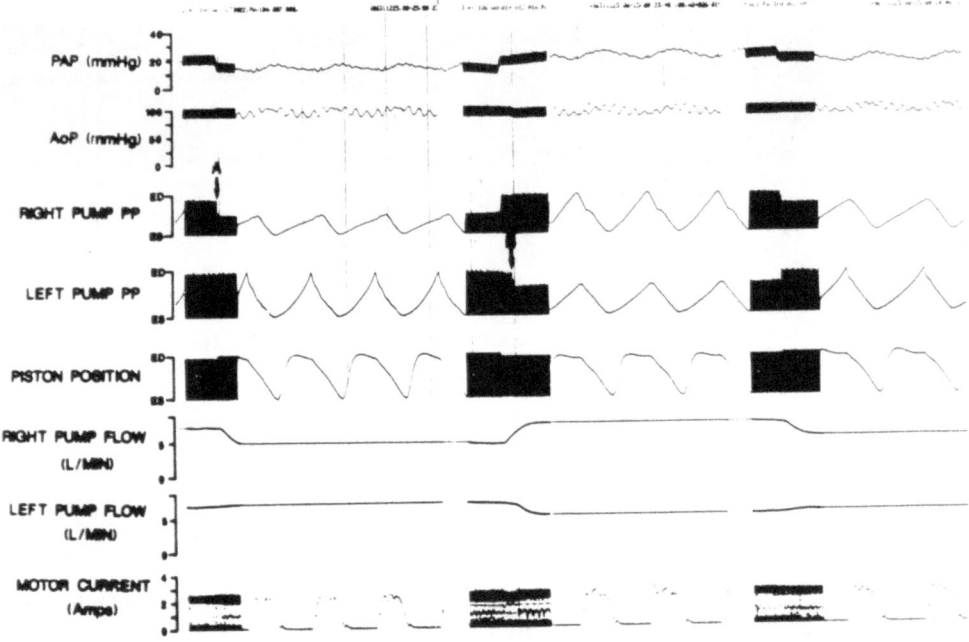

**Fig. 38.9.** Hydrodynamic performance of a motor-driven TAH. Response of the left-or-right triggered fill/empty system as the right and left pump filling rate was varied

$$P_r = 1/T \int_0^T P_{ap}(t) \times Q_r(t)\, dt$$

$$P_l = 1/T \int_0^T A_{op}(t) \times Q_l(t)\, dt$$

$$P_i = 1/T \int_0^T V(t) \times I(t)\, dt$$

$$\eta = (P_r + P_l)/P_i$$

## In vitro and in vivo evaluation

### In vitro bench-top test

Prior to study in vivo, the performance of the prototype system was tested in vitro using a mock circulatory system. The mock circuit consisted of a simulated systemic and pulmonary circuit. Figure 38.7 shows the mock circulatory system with a prototype motor-driven TAH. Compliance and resistance were simulated using an air chamber and back-pressure regulator, respectively.

Figure 38.8 depicts the performance of the system when the left afterload was increased 20 to 110 mmHg with the right afterload fixed at a mean of 20–55 mmHg. The drive mode was in the left-or-right triggered fill/empty mode. With an increase in the left afterload, the ejection time increased and thus the overall pump rate decreased, resulting in a net reduction of pump output. Figure 38.9 shows the performance of the system operated in the left-or-right triggered fill/empty mode when the left or right pump filling rate was varied. The system respond quickly to changes in the filling rate and the pump control alternated between the two ventricles. In Fig. 38.10, the electric power input and fluid power output of the sys-

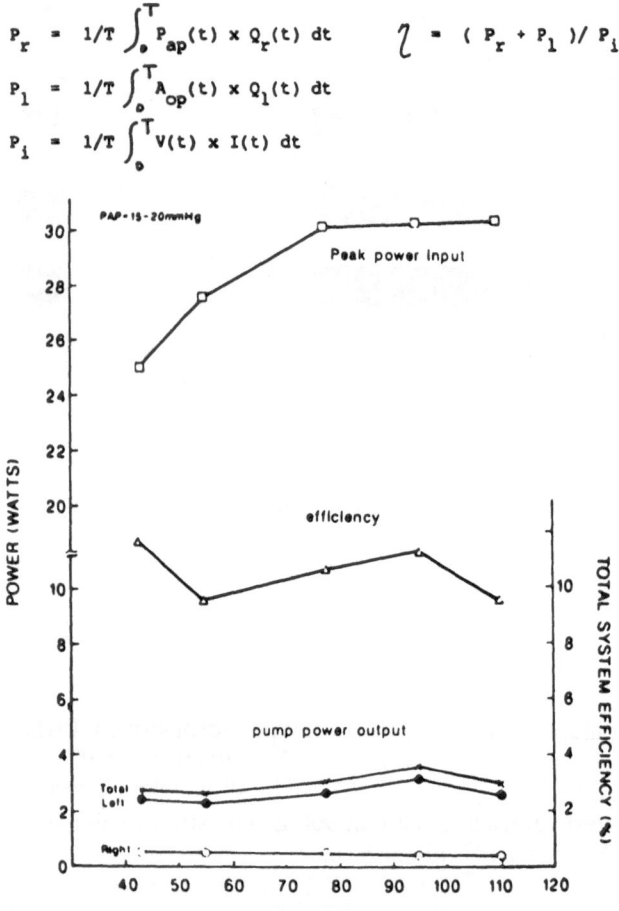

**Fig. 38.10.** Electric input power, fluid power output, and system efficiency of the motor-driven TAH system

**Fig. 38.11.** Hemodynamic trace during acute biventricular experiment with a prototype motor-driven TAH in the goat

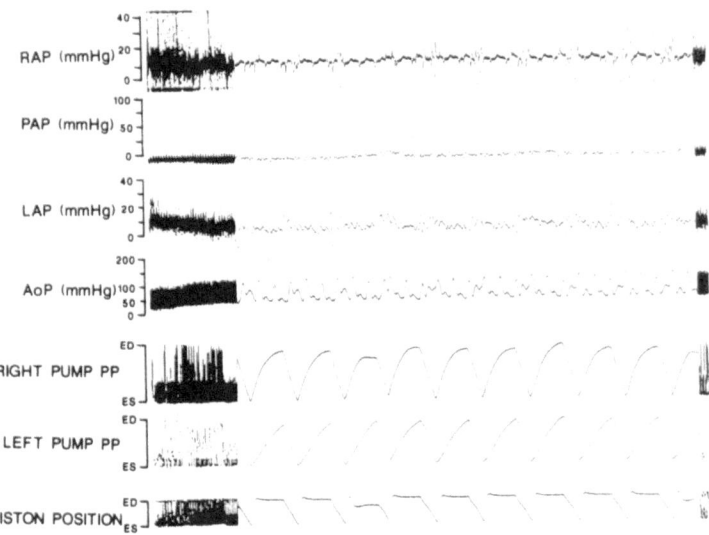

tem are illustrated together with the system efficiency as the left afterload was varied from 40 to 110 mmHg. The input power to the system ranged from 24 to 30 W, with the system efficiency being between 10% and 15%.

## Acute biventricular bypass experiment

Prior to in vivo study, the prototype system was used to bypass the fibrillating ventricles of the goat in acute experiments. The motor power was supplied using a transcutaneous transformer described earlier. Figure 38.11 shows the hemodynamic trace during the biventricular bypass using the prototype system. It was confirmed that the motor-driven TAH powered by a transcutaneous transformer can adequately maintain circulation of the animal.

**Acknowledgment.** This research was partially supported by grants-in-Aid from the Japanese Ministry of Education under #61870058 and from the Japanese Ministry of Health and welfare.

## References

1. Pierce WS (1987) The artificial heart—1986: Partial fulfillment of a promise. Trans Am Soc Artif Intern Organs 32(1): 5–10
2. Rosenberg G et al. (1984) An electric motor-driven total artificial heart: Seven months survival in the calf. Trans Am Soc Artif Intern Organs 30: 69–74
3. Moise JC et al. (1978) Development of compact thermal and electrical energy converters for left heart assist systems. Trans Am Soc Artif Intern Organs 29: 77–83
4. Kim SW, Okano T (1986) Prevention of platelet adhesion and agregation at blood-polymer interfaces. In: Akutsu T (ed) Artificial heart 1. Springer, Tokyo, pp 3–7
5. Takatani S et al. (1984) Development of high performance inplantable type total artificial heart system. Life Support System 249
6. Takatani S et al. (1985) Simultaneously ejecting left-or-right triggered total artificial heart actuated by a single electromechanical system. Trans Am Soc Artif Intern Organs 31: 367–371
7. Koshiji K et al. (1987) Analysis of efficiency and experimental consideration of energy transmisssion system to drive total implanted artificial heart. Jpn Artif Organs 16(1): 167–170
8. Schuder JC et al. (1971) An inductively coupled RF system for the transmission of 1 KW of power through the skin. IEEE Trans Biomed Eng BME-18: 265
9. Takatani S (1986) Toward a completely implantable total artificial heart system. In: Akutsu T (ed) Artificial heart 1. Springer, Tokyo, pp 51, 58
10. S. Takatani et al. (1987) Toward a completely implantable TAH: Left-right simultaneously ejecting motor driven TAH system. Trans Am Soc Artif Intern Organs

## Discussion

*Imachi* (University of Tokyo): How do you maintain the balance between left and right flow?

*Takatani* (National Cardiovascular Center): This is taken care of by the animal's system. The system learns whichever fills first. If the left flow or the left atrial pressure increase, the filling becomes much faster on the left side. So we try to increase the flow on the right side, and then, in return, the right atrial pressure may increase and take over control. It is not like the alternate system. When it is run simultaneously you do not have to worry about left and right flow difference.

*Imachi:* In that case is the pump filled with only the atrial pressure?

*Takatani:* In addition there is a recoil force from the diaphragm to assist the filling.

*Imachi:* Can you quantify the thickness of the diaphragm of the right and left with the same sensitivity for the atrial pressure? If the sensitivity is different then control perhaps becomes quite difficult.

*Takatani:* It is quite difficult to control precisely the thickness of the diaphragm. It is possible with a small difference and the resulting difference in sensitivity does not present a major difficulty in controlling the left and right flow difference.

# Keywords Index

# Scientific Exhibition

1. Total Artificial Heart at NCVC
   (Research Institute, National Cardiovascular Center)

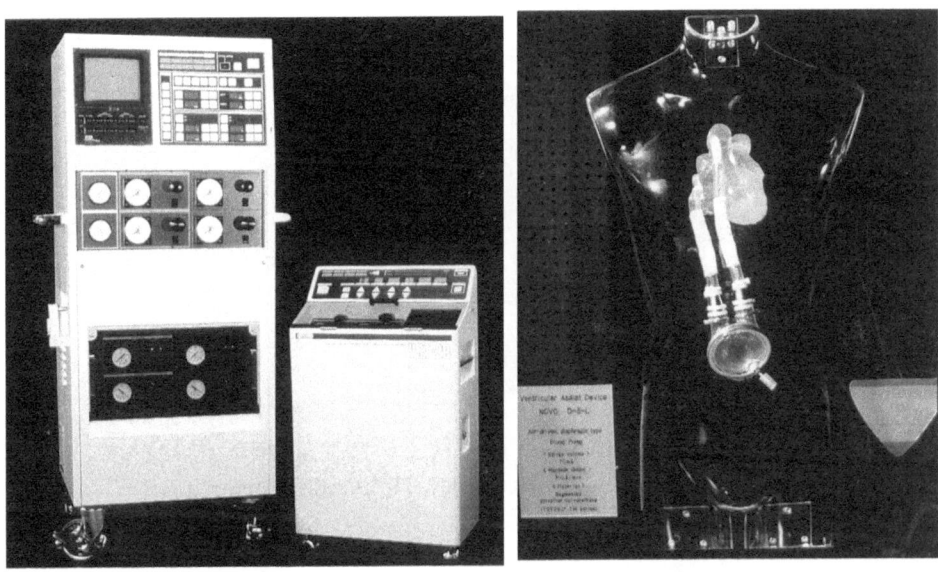

2. Motor-Driven Artificial Heart
   (1st Department of Surgery and Research Institute for Artificial Heart, Hiroshima University)

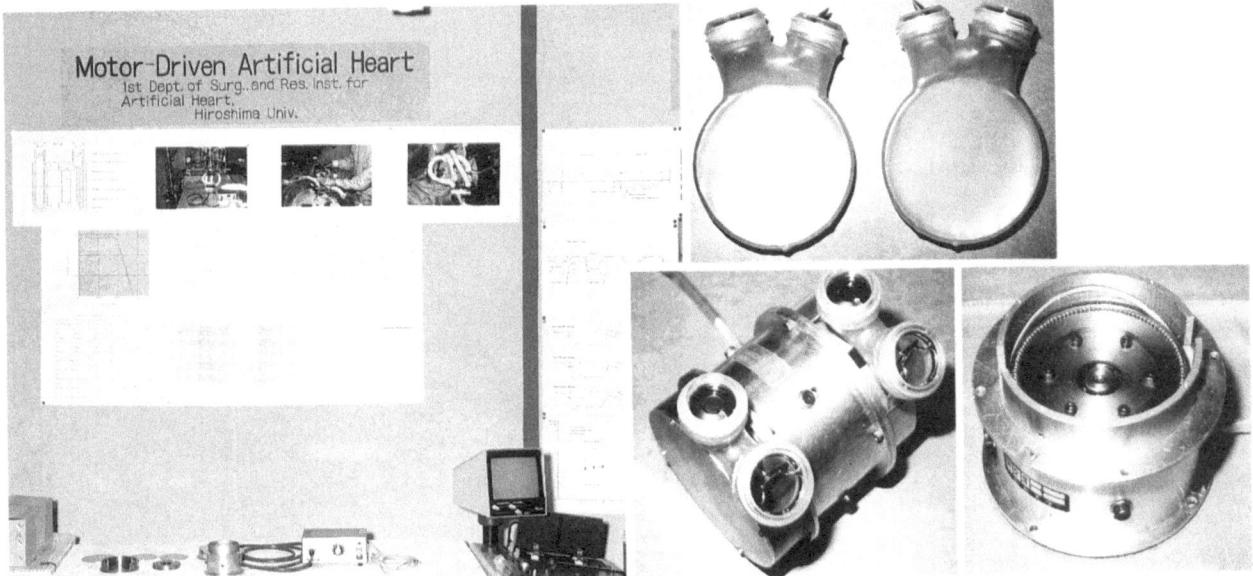

3. Artificial Heart at University of Tokyo
   (Institute of Medical Electronics, University of Tokyo)

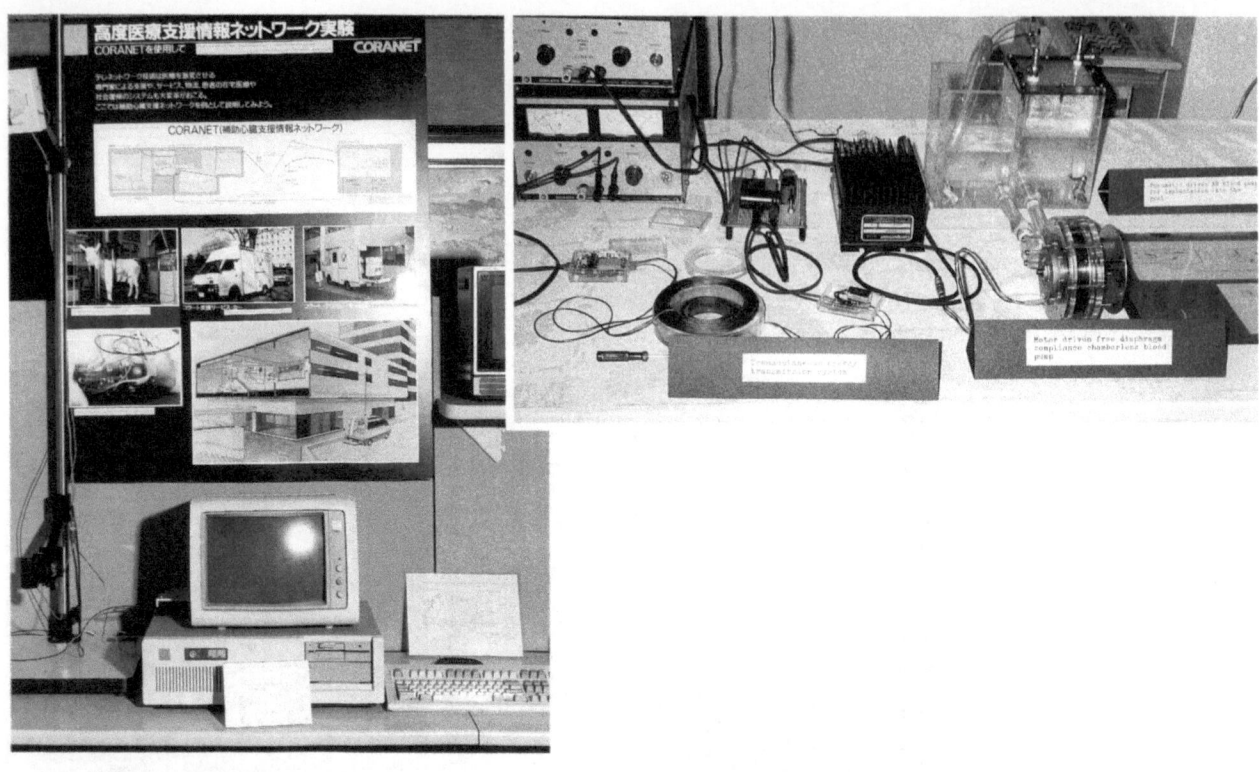

4. Ballscrew-Driven Artificial Heart
   (Research Institute of Applied Electronics, Hokkaido University)

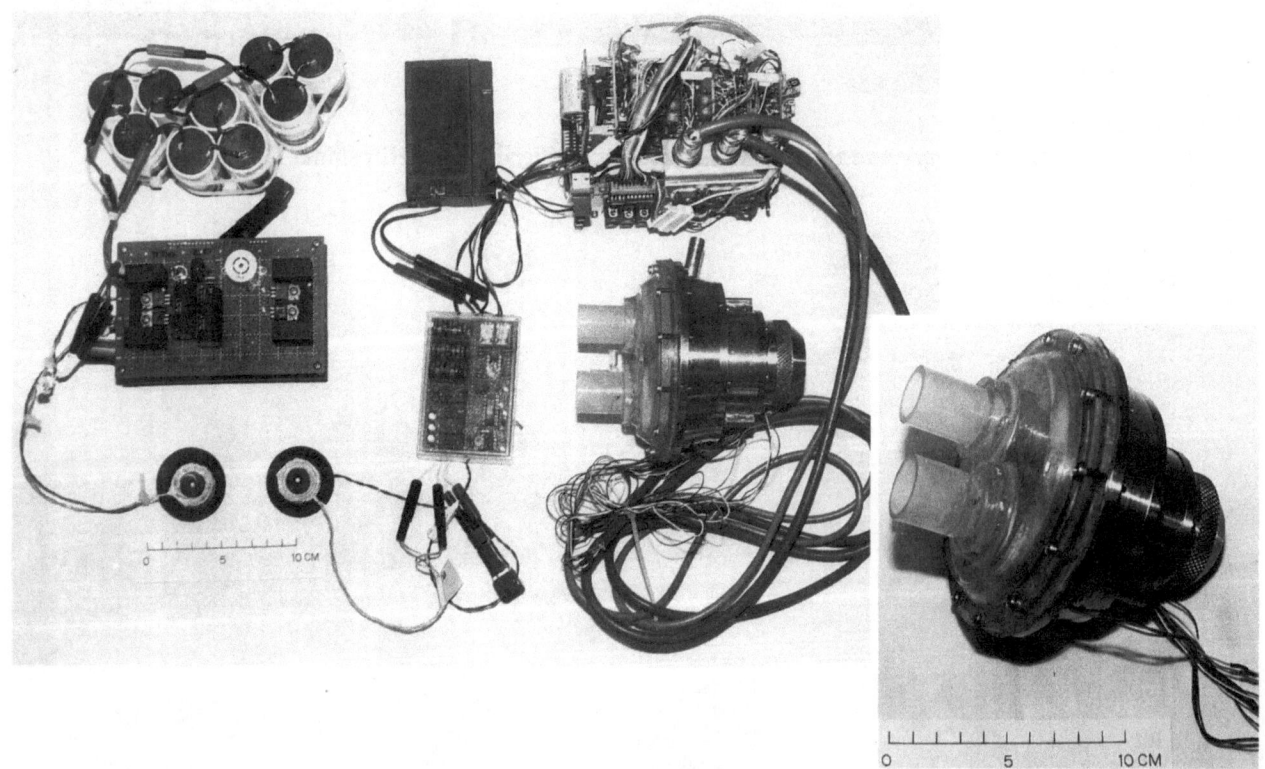

### 5. Air-Driven Sac-Type VAD
(Department of Thoracic Surgery, Tohoku University)

### 6. Double-Chambered Alternate Pumping System
(Shizuoka-Saiseikai General Hospital)

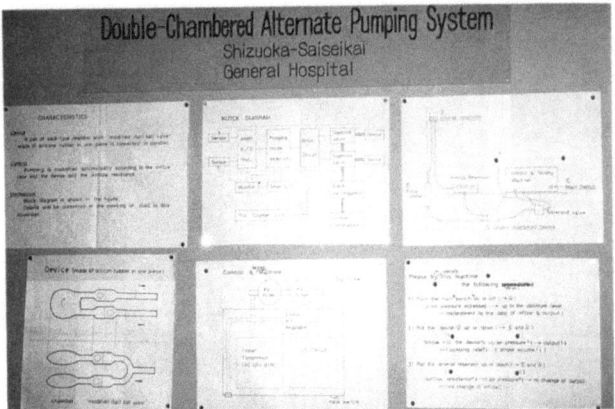

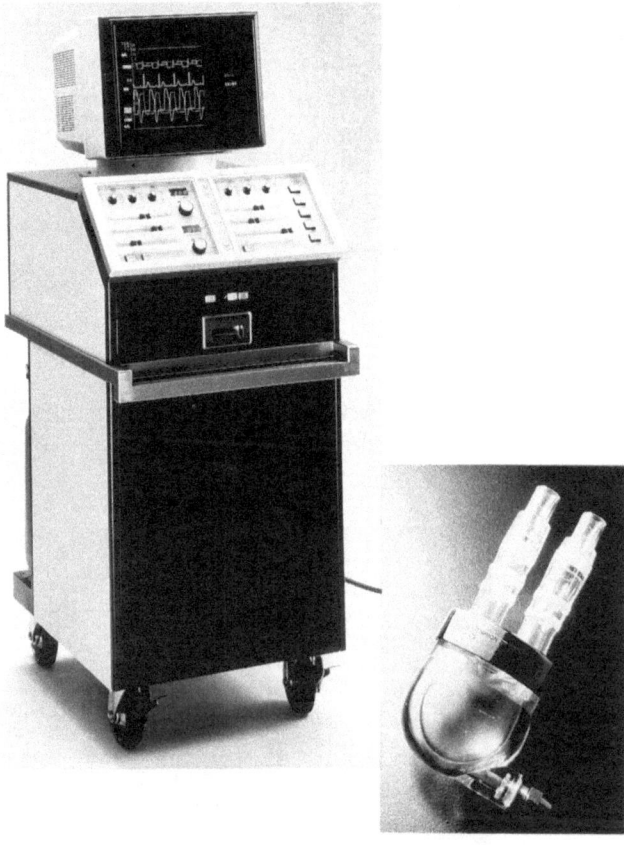

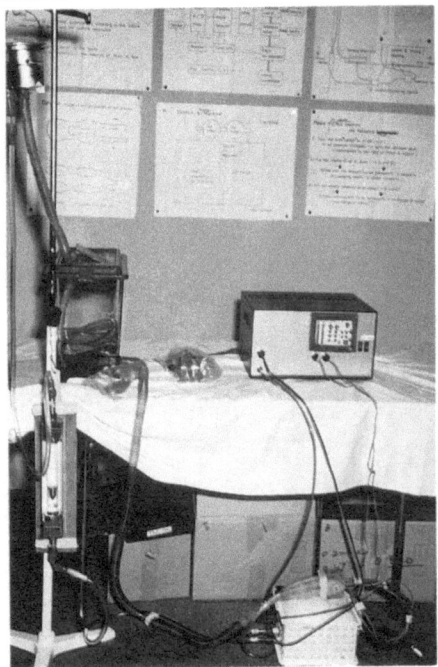

### 7. Portable Artificial Heart Driver
(Institute of Biomedical Engineering, Tokyo Women's Medical College)

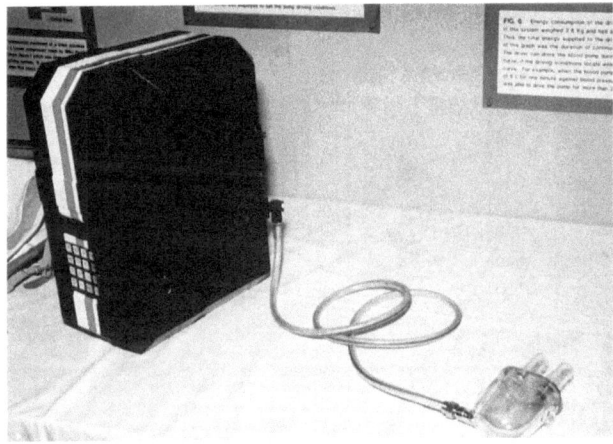

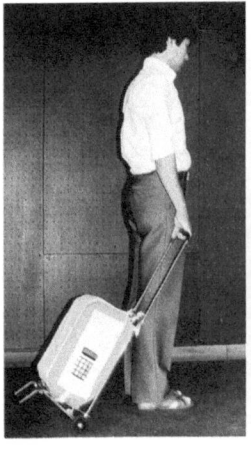

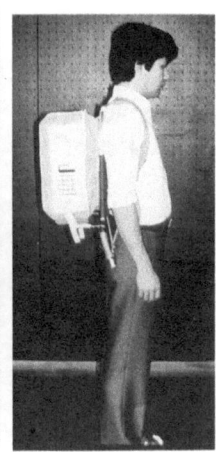

## 8. Linear Electromagnetic Actuators for Artificial Heart
   (Faculty of Engineering, Shinshu University)

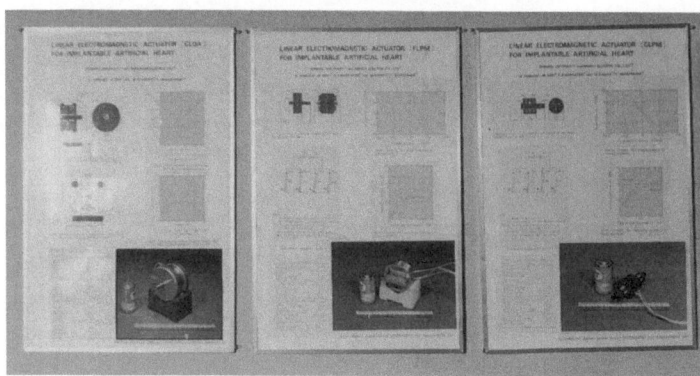

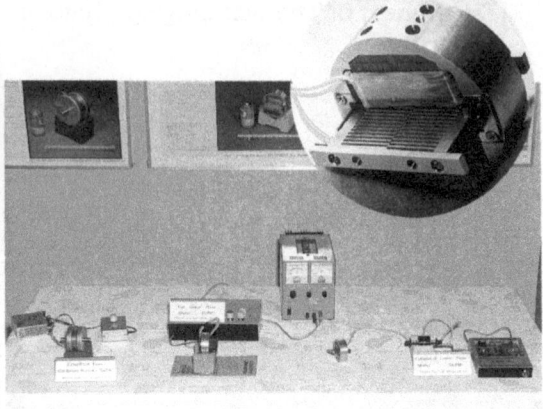

## 9. Tomasu Heart
   (Tomasu Giken; Takeda Hospital;
   Kyoto University)

## 10. JARVIK-7 Total Artificial Heart and Ventricular
   Assist Device (Symbion Inc.)

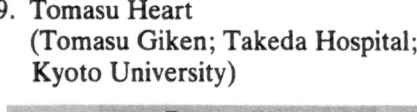

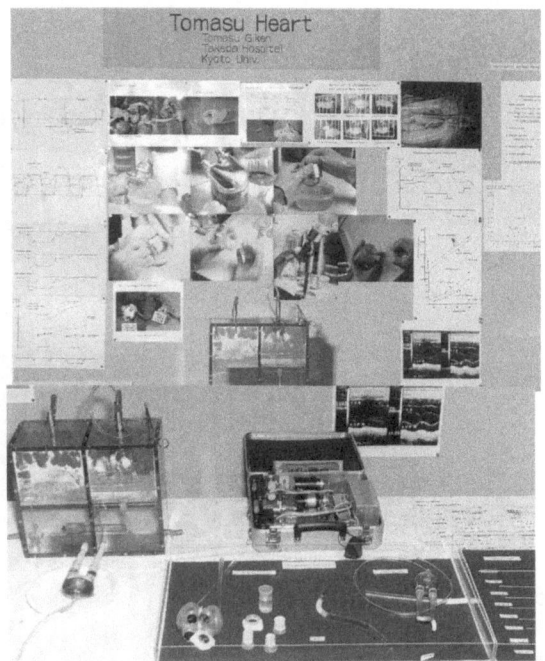

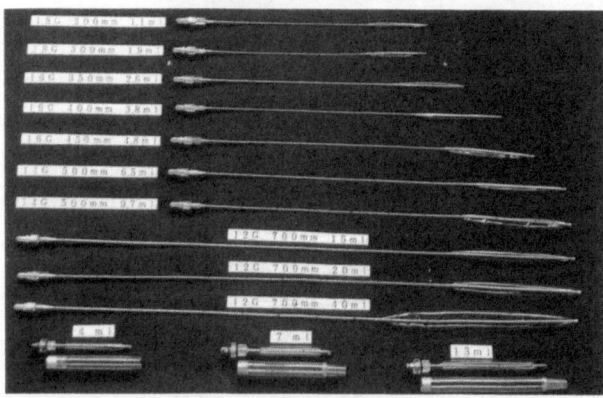

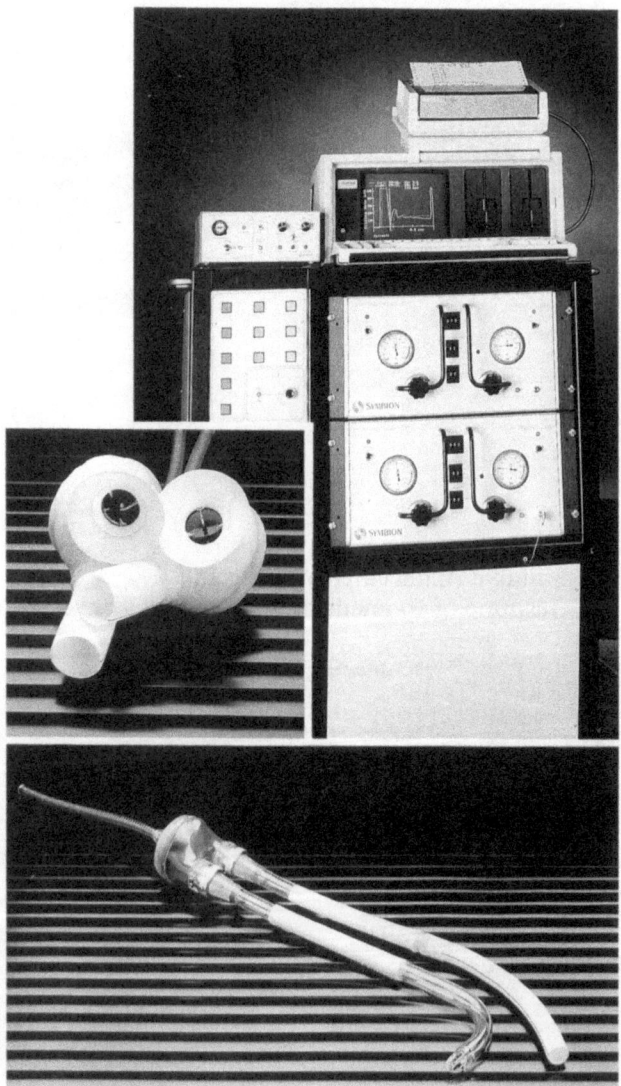

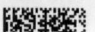